James B. Stiehl

Werner H. Konermann

Rolf G. Haaker

Anthony M. DiGioia III

Navigation and MIS in Orthopedic Surgery

James B. Stiehl

Werner H. Konermann

Rolf G. Haaker

Anthony M. DiGioia III

Navigation and MIS in Orthopedic Surgery

With 515 Figures and 56 Tables

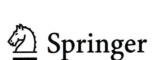

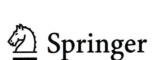 Springer

Stiehl, James B., Associate Professor, M.D.
Columbia St Mary's Hospital,
575 W River Woods Parkway, Milwaukee,
Wisconsin 53211, USA

Konermann, Werner H., Professor, M.D.
Orthopaedic Hospital,
Am Mühlenberg 3,
37235 Hessisch-Lichtenau, Germany

Haaker, Rolf G., Associate Professor, M.D.
Orthopedic Clinic, St. Vincenz-Hospital,
Danziger Str. 17, D-33034 Brakel, Germany

**DiGioia, Anthony M. III, Clinical Associate Professor
of Orthopaedic Surgery, M.D.**
University of Pittsburgh School of Medicine and
Renaissance Orthopaedics, P.C. 300 Halket Street
Pittsburgh, PA 15213, USA

ISBN 978-3-540-36690-4   Springer Medizin Verlag Heidelberg

Cataloging-in-Publication Data applied for
A catalog record for this book is available from the Library of Congress.

Bibliographic information published by Die Deutsche Nationalbibliothek
Die Deutsche Nationalbibliothek lists this publication in the Deutsche Nationalbibliografie;
detailed bibliographic data is available in the Internet at http://dnb.d-nb.de.

Springer Medizin Verlag
springer.com
© Springer Medizin Verlag Heidelberg 2007
Printed in Germany

SPIN 11678861
Cover Design: deblik Berlin, Germany
Typesetting: TypoStudio Tobias Schaedla, Heidelberg, Germany
Printer: Stürtz GmbH, Würzburg, Germany

Printed on acid free paper   18/5135/ud – 5 4 3 2 1 0

Foreword

The reader is enthusiastically encouraged to tackle this second edition text in two ways. The first is simply to scan chapters with their introductions, summaries and conclusion points. Second, is to delve into those sections of seeming greater interest depending upon one's specialty and role.

The expansion and quality of this material speak to the success of the first edition by these editors and many similar authors. In addition, the continued and enlarged interest in computer assisted Orthopedic surgery indicates the relevance and enduring importance of this advance in our field of musculoskeletal surgery.

I suggest that no other discipline in surgery is so appropriately suited to computer assistance including robotic performance. Orthopedics has always seemed unique to this author in that it focuses more than any other medical field on gross physical, mechanical structure. We deal nearly exclusively in physical repair of broken elements, rearrangement of deformed ones, and resurfacing or refurbishing those that are diseased in a way that has altered their mechanical integrity, shapes, and other structural aspects.

Certainly there are biochemical, physiologic, cell biologic, and immunologic even infectious and neoplastic issues involved to major degrees in the injuries, treatments and basic pathology of all that we treat. Our methods attempt to take advantage of these aspects of the biology and structure involved. Nonetheless, what we actually do in the operating room, what we spend so many years learning to do safely, correctly and accurately is to rebuild and repair the physical structures which are the musculoskeletal system. It is my belief that this rather gross structural character of Orthopedic surgery is what makes so ready-made for computer assistance, even robotic preparation and interaction.

The anatomic and physiologic nature of the human body makes physical intervention much more variable and complex than tasks done on inanimate objects in factories. These factors also present more difficulty than addressing many problems and studies in physical and biological science. It was only natural that computer assistance in general and the employment of robots in particular factory processes were first seen in those applications. However, the need for precision is as great and in many ways greater when we commence treatment of the deranged or diseased human structure.

Clearly there is resistance to the introduction of these hi-tech changes into our field. We first fear their cost, second their complexity as it relates to the uninitiated user, and also the sense of losing control of our surgical processes. Nonetheless, the need is there – the need to maximize the accuracy, consistency, and safety of our surgical procedures.

It is this writer's prediction that our future, within the next 10 to 15 years will see an evolution in computer applications and mechanical, plus robotic methods that will revolutionize the way our surgeries are performed. It will be routine practice that our procedures are done thru incisions that are only as large as necessary to either introduce or remove the material which is involved in an operation. And, this surgery will be done with maximal computer assistance in the form of navigation and other aspects. Furthermore, retraction, tissue cutting and reformation, as well as implant placement, will be done by robots. Like it or not today, the importance of accuracy and consistency, together with technologic changes and software development will allow and drive this revolution. That said, it is time for all of us to understand the bases of these techniques and appreciate the applications and success of the methods developed so far.

Kenneth A. Krackow, MD

In memoriam Thomas Günther from Springer,
who unexpectedly died during this book project.

He will be greatly missed.

Short Biography of the Editors

Stiehl, James B., Associate Professor, M.D.
Orthopaedic Hospital of Wisconsin
575 West Riverwood Parkway, Suite 204
Milwaukee 53212, USA
Born in 1949, Adult Reconstructive Orthopaedic Surgeon. Residency at the University of Texas Health Science Center in San Antonio Texas under Drs. Charles Rockwood and David Green, and Fellowships at the Princess Margaret Rose Hospital, Edinburgh and Swiss AO Fellowship, Zurich. He is in private practice at Columbia St Mary's Hospital in Milwaukee, Wisconsin, USA. His main interests are in total joint arthroplasty and adult reconstructive surgery and he has a longstanding interest in biomechanical research in orthopaedics.

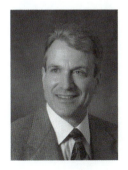

Konermann, Werner H., Professor, M.D.
Hospital of Orthopaedics and Traumatology
Am Mühlenberg 3, D-37235 Hessisch-Lichtenau, Germany
Born in 1959, Specialist Orthopaedic Surgeon and Rheumatologist. Residencies in three German Universities at Tübingen, Münster and Mannheim. His thesis was done in biomechanics of the lumbar spine. He is now a Consultant Orthopaedic Surgeon for orthopaedics and traumatology in Hessisch Lichtenau, Germany. His main interests are in total joint arthroplasty, adult reconstructive surgery and computer assisted surgery.

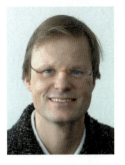

Haaker, Rolf G., Associate Professor, M.D.
Hospital for Orthopaedics and Rheumatology
St. Vincenz-Hospital, Danziger Str. 17, 33034 Brakel, Germany
Born in 1959, Specialist Orthopaedic Surgeon and Rheumatologist. Residencies at the Sportsmedical Division, Military Hospital in Warendorf and Koblenz followed by a recidency at the University in Bochum, Germany. His thesis was done in biomechanics of the multilevel lumbar spinal fusion. He is now a Chief Consultant Orthopaedic Surgeon in Bad Driburg-Brakel, Germany. He has a main interests in revision surgery of hip and knee arthroplasty, spine surgery and computer assisted surgery.

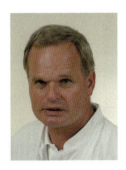

DiGioia, Anthony M. III, MD
Magee-Womens Hospital of the University of Pittsburgh Medical Center and Renaissance Orthopaedics, P.C.
Adult Reconstructive Orthopaedic Surgeon and Clinical Researcher. Undergraduate and Masters degrees in engineering from Carnegie Mellon University. Medical degree from Harvard University School. Residency in Orthopaedic Surgery at the University of Pittsburg Medical Center. Fellowship in Adult Reconstructive Surgery at the University of Pittsburgh Medical Center. He is in private practice at Magee-Womens Hospital in Pittsburgh, PA. He was a founder of the Innovation Center at the UPMC Health System in Pittsburgh. His main interest is in applied research and development of new technologies for training simulations, process re-engineering and programs in Patient Focused Care.

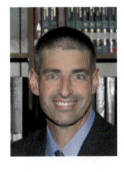

Stiehl, James B., Associate Professor, M.D.
Orthopaedic Hospital of Wisconsin
575 West Riverwoods Parkway Suite 206
Milwaukee, USA

Born in 1948, full-time attending orthopaedic surgeon. Residency at the University of Iowa, Iowa, he also trained in Salt Lake City under Dr. Charles Rockwood and David Green, and fellowship at the Brooke Medical for bone hospital, Bethesda and Shriner for fellowship. Currently. He is in private practice in Columbia St. Mary's Hospital in Milwaukee, Wisconsin, USA. His main interests are in total joint arthroplasty and adult reconstructive surgery, and he has a long-standing interest in biomechanical research in orthopaedics.

Kremer-mann, Werner H., Professor, M.D.
Department of Orthopaedics and Traumatology
Am Mühlenberg 1, D-34212 Hessen/Kassel, Germany

Born in 1962, Director of Orthopaedic Surgery and Rheumatological Rehabilitation at the University of Tübingen, Stuttgart. He trained in surgery at the Director of the University hospital. He is now a Chief Orthopaedic Surgeon for orthopaedics and traumatology in Hessen/Tübingen, Germany. His main interests are in total joint arthroplasty, adult reconstructive surgery and computer-assisted surgery.

Haaker, Rolf G., Associate Professor, M.D.
Hospital for Orthopaedics and Rheumatology
St. Vincenz Hospital, Danziger str. 17, 33611 Brakel, Germany

Born in 1956, consultant orthopaedist for bone and Rheumatological Rehabilitation at the orthopaedic hospital. He trained in surgery. December 1 in 1997 as Assistant Medical Director at the University hospital. He was a consultant in the orthopaedic hospital at the same university hospital, and he is now a Chief Consultant orthopaedic Surgeon in St. Bad Driburg/Brakel, Germany. His main interests are in surgery and surgery of hip and knee arthroplasty, adult surgery and computer-assisted surgery.

Gioia, Anthony M. di, M.D.
Magee-Womens Hospital of the University of Pittsburgh, Medical Center and Renaissance Orthopaedics, USA

Anthony DiGioia is an Orthopaedic Surgeon and Clinical Researcher. Undergraduate and graduate degrees in engineering from Carnegie Mellon University, medical degree from Harvard University School. Residency in Orthopaedic Surgery at the University of Pittsburgh Medical Center. Fellowship in Adult Reconstructive Surgery at the University of Pittsburgh Medical Center. He is in private practice at Magee-Womens Hospital in Pittsburgh, PA. He was a founder of the innovation Center at the UPMC Health System in Pittsburgh. His main interest is in applied research and development of new technologies for tracking, simulation processes, engineering and programs in Patient-Focused Care.

Preface

Computer assisted Orthopedic surgery has made significant advances since our first textbook was completed in 2003, not only in refinement of existing methods but in newer ideas such as early robotic applications and validation concepts. The basic platforms from which we work have been long established fixtures in the computer and technology world. One might conclude that the medical profession has been late to get into this game. Machines aren't necessarily better than humans when it comes to artistic creations, but they can certainly have become more reproducible and precise. Any surgeon who dismisses this concept faces the likely hood of becoming a surgical anachronism. Surgical navigation is an enabling technology that has limited side effects and promises to advance the art of Orthopedic surgery in ways not imagined. This contrasts with Minimally Invasive Surgery which is a new and different surgical technique done through less intrusive methods that enhance postoperative recovery and minimize tissue damage. Many surgeons have learned that MIS techniques can be difficult and may add significant complications to previously straight forward operations. This textbook importantly discusses the marriage of surgical navigation with minimally invasive surgery as we believe »virtual reality« in surgery makes MIS a safer venture.

The other important point we would like to make about these technologies, is that they are fickle mistresses and takes no hostages. Scientific advancement celebrates only the innovators and practioners of today and tomorrow, not of yesterday. There are no 'giants' in this field comparable to the days of Mueller, Charnley and Insall who literally held court throughout their lifetimes following the hegemony of their primary innovations. In contrast, going to the 'computer store' to buy your first new personal computer will quickly put you on equal footing with the guy who has been doing it for ten years. This simple collaborative fact makes computer assisted surgery extremely attractive to the future generation of »millenial« Orthopedic surgeons, who thrive on teamwork and system consensus. This is how they have been raised. The editors celebrate our friendship with all the world-wide group of contributors to this current volume and offer our gratitude for their participation in this exciting field.

October 2006
The Editors
James B. Stiehl, Werner H. Konermann, Rolf G. Haaker (Senior Editors), Anthony M. DiGioia III

Sections

Contents

Editors

Stiehl, James B.,
Associate Professor, M.D.
Columbia St Mary's Hospital,
575 W River Woods Parkway,
Milwaukee, Wisconsin 53211, USA

Konermann, Werner H.,
Professor, M.D.
Orthopaedic Hospital,
Am Mühlenberg 3,
37235 Hessisch-Lichtenau, Germany

Haaker, Rolf G.,
Associate Professor, M.D.
Orthopedic Clinic, St. Vincenz-Hospital,
Danziger Str. 17, D-33034 Brakel,
Germany

DiGioia, Anthony M., III
Clinical Associate Professor
of Orthopaedic Surgery, M.D.
University of Pittsburgh School
of Medicine and Renaissance
Orthopaedics, P.C. 300 Halket Street
Pittsburgh, PA 15213, USA

List of Contributors

Alan, R.K.
Institute for Advanced
Orthopaedic Study,
The Orthopaedic Center
of New Jersey, USA

Arand, M.
Department of Orthaepedic
Trauma Surgery, Hand- and
Reconstructive Surgery,
University of Ulm, Steinhövelstraße 9,
89075 Ulm, Germany

Argenson, J.-N.
The Aix-Marseille University,
Department of Orthopaedic Surgery,
Hopital Sainte-Marguerite,
Service de Chirurgie Orthopédique,
270 Boulevard Sainte-Marguerite,
13009, Marseille, France

Aubaniac, J.-M.
The Aix-Marseille University,
Department of Orthopaedic Surgery,
Hopital Sainte-Marguerite,
Service de Chirurgie Orthopédique,
270 Boulevard Sainte-Marguerite,
13009, Marseille, France

Babisch, J.
Department of Orthopedic Surgery,
University of Jena, Waldkrankenhaus
»Rudolf Elle«, Eisenberg,
Klosterlausnitzer Straße 81,
07607 Eisenberg, Germany

Bach, J.M.
Colorado School of Mines,
1610 Illinois St., Golden, CO 80401, USA

Balicki, M.A.
New York University-Hospital for Joint
Diseases Orthopaedic Program,
New York City, USA

Bäthis, H.
Department of Trauma and
Orthopaedic Surgery, University of
Witten-Herdecke, Cologne-Merheim
Medical Center (CMMC),
51109 Cologne, Germany

Benazzo, F.
Clinica Ortopedica e Traumatologica
dell'Università di Pavia – Fondazione
IRCCS Policlinico San Matteo,
P.le Golgi 2, 27100 Pavia, Italy

Benecke, P.
Chirurgische Abteilung,
Kreiskrankenhaus Ratzeburg, Germany

Berend, K.R.
Associate, Joint Implant Surgeons, Inc.,
New Albany, OH USA, Clinical Assistant
Professor, Department of Orthopaedics,
The Ohio State University, Columbus,
OH USA, Vice Chairman of the Board,
New Albany Surgical Hospital,
New Albany, OH USA

Berger, R.
Assistant Professor of Orthopaedics,
Department of Orthopedic Surgery,
Rush-Presbyterian-St. Luke's Medical
Center, 1725 W. Harrison St.,
Suite 1063, Chicago, Illinois 60612, USA

Bolognesi, M.P.
Assistant Professor, Duke University
Medical Center, Division of Orthopaedic
Surgery, Hospital South, Orange Zone,
Room 5315, Durham,
North Carolina 27710, USA

Bonutti, P.M.
Bonutti Clinic
1303 West Evergreen Ave.
Effingham, IL 62401, USA

Bouillon, B.
Department of Trauma and
Orthopaedic Surgery, University of
Witten/Herdecke, Cologne-Merheim
Medical Center (CMMC),
Ostmerheimer Straße 200,
51109 Cologne, Germany

Brandenberg J.E.
OrthoZentrum St. Anna,
St. Annastrasse 32, 6006 Luzern,
Switzerland

Briard, J.L.
Clinique du cèdre – Bois Guillaume,
76235 Rouen-Cedex, France

Buckup, K.
Orthopädische Klinik des Klinikum
Dortmund gGmbh, Beurhausstr. 40,
44137 Dortmund, Germany

Busch, C.L.
Anatomisches Institut der
Medizinischen Universität zu Lübeck,
Germany

Cazzamali, S.
Clinica Ortopedica e Traumatologica
dell'Università di Pavia – Fondazione
IRCCS·Policlinico San Matteo,
P.le Golgi 2, 27100 Pavia, Italy

Chelule, K.L.
Research Fellow, Academic Unit of
Musculoskeletal and Rehabilitation
Medicine, University of Leeds, Leeds,
United Kingdom

Cheung, K.-W.
Department of Orthopaedics and
Traumatology, Prince of Wales Hospital,
Shatin, Hong Kong

Chiu, K.-H.
Department of Orthopaedics and
Traumatology, Prince of Wales Hospital,
Shatin, Hong Kong

Chiu, K.-Y.
Department of Orthopaedics and
Traumatology, Queen Mary Hospital,
Pokfulam, Hong Kong

Christ, R.M.
Orthopaedic Hospital Auguste-Viktoria,
Am Kokturkanal 2,
32545 Bad Oeynhausen, Germany

Citak, M.
Trauma Department, Hannover Medical
School, Carl-Neuberg-Str. 1,
30625 Hannover, Germany

Cobb, J.
Professor of Orthopaedics,
Imperial College, Charing Cross Hospital,
London W4, United Kingdom

Conditt, M.A.
Institute of Orthopedic Research
and Education, The Methodist Hospital,
and Baylor College of Medicine,
Houston, Texas, USA

Cook, J.L.
Florida Joint Replacement and Sports
Medicine Center
5243 Hanff Lane
New Port Richey, FL 34652

De Simoni C.
OrthoZentrum St. Anna,
St. Annastrasse 32, 6006 Luzern,
Switzerland

Decking, R.
Orthopädische Abteilung des Rehabilitationskrankenhauses Ulm, Orthopädische
Klinik mit Querschnittgelähmtenzentrum
der Universität Ulm, Oberer Eselsberg 45,
89081 Ulm, Germany

DiGioia, Anthony M., III
Clinical Associate Professor
of Orthopaedic Surgery, M.D.
University of Pittsburgh School
of Medicine and Renaissance
Orthopaedics, P.C. 300 Halket Street
Pittsburgh, PA 15213, USA

Dong, X.
MEM Research Center for Orthopaedic
Surgery, Institute for Surgical
Technology and Biomechanics,
University of Bern, Bern, Switzerland

Dorr, L.D.
The Arthritis Institute,
501 E. Hardy Street, Suite 300,
Inglewood, CA 90301, USA

Duncan, C.P.
Professor and Head
Department of Orthopaedics
UBC and Vancouver Acute
910 West 10th Avenue, Room 3114
Vancouver BC V5Z 4E3, Canada

Ecker, T.M.
Department of Orthopaedic
Surgery, Inselspital, University of Bern,
Bern, Switzerland,
and Center for Computer Assisted and
Reconstructive Surgery, New England
Baptist Hospital, Tufts University,
Harvard Medical School, Boston, MA,
USA

Eckman, K.
The Robotics Institute, Carnegie Mellon
University, Pittsburgh, Pennsylvania, USA

Eichhorn, H.-J.
Orthopaedic Praxis Cooperation,
Hebbelstraße 14a, 94315 Straubing,
Germany

Fadel, M.
Professor of Orthopaedics, El-Minia
University Hospital, El-Minia, Egypt

Flecher, X.
The Aix-Marseille University,
Department of Orthopaedic Surgery,
Hopital Sainte-Marguerite,
Service de Chirurgie Orthopédique,
270 Boulevard Sainte-Marguerite,
13009, Marseille, France

Forman, R.A.
New York University-Hospital for
Joint Diseases Orthopaedic Program,
New York City, USA

Fritsch, E.
Orthopaedic University Hospital,
Homburg, Kirrberger Straße,
66421 Homburg/Saar, Germany

Fuiko, R.
Gersthof Orthopaedic Hospital, Vienna,
Austria

Garbuz, D.S.
Division of Lower Limb Reconstruction
and Oncology, University of British
Columbia Department of Orthopaedics,
910 West 10th Avenue, Vancouver, BC,
Canada V5Z 4E3

Gebhard, F.
Assistant Medical Director,
Department of Orthaepedic Trauma
Surgery, Hand- and Reconstructive
Surgery, University of Ulm,
Steinhövelstraße 9, 89075 Ulm,
Germany

Geerling, J.
Trauma Department,
Hannover Medical School,
Carl-Neuberg-Str. 1, 30625 Hannover,
Germany

Gleichmann, A.
Orthopedic Clinic, St. Vincenz-Hospital,
Danziger Str. 17, D-33034 Brakel,
Germany

Gösling, A.
Trauma Department,
Hannover Medical School,
Carl-Neuberg-Str. 1,
30625 Hannover, Germany

Gösling, T.
Trauma Department,
Hannover Medical School,
Carl-Neuberg-Str. 1,
30625 Hannover, Germany

Granchi, C.
Praxim Inc, 4, av de l'Obliou
38700 La Tronche, France

Grifka, J.
Department of Orthopaedic Surgery,
University of Regensburg,
93042 Regensburg, Germany

Grote, S.
Department of Trauma and
Orthopaedic Surgery, University of
Witten/Herdecke, Cologne-Merheim
Medical Center (CMMC),
Ostmerheimer Straße 200,
51109 Cologne, Germany

Grundei, H.
Fa. Eska Implants, Lübeck, Germany

Grützner, P.A.
Ärztlicher Direktor, Klinik für Unfall-
und Wiederherstellungschirurgie,
Klinikum Stuttgart, Katharinenhospital,
Kriegsbergstraße 60,
70714 Stuttgart, Germany

Haaker, R.G.
Orthopedic Clinic, St. Vincenz-Hospital,
Danziger Str. 17, D-33034 Brakel,
Germany

Hackbart, M.
Orthopaedic Hospital Auguste-Viktoria,
Am Kokturkanal 2,
32545 Bad Oeynhausen, Germany

Hafez, M.A.
Adjunct Clinical Scientist, The Institute
for Computer Assisted Orthopaedic
Surgery, Western Pennsylvania Hospital,
Pittsburgh, PA, USA

Hagena, F.-W.
Orthopaedic Hospital Auguste-Viktoria,
Am Kokturkanal 2,
32545 Bad Oeynhausen, Germany

Halder, A.M.
Hellmuth-Ulrici-Kliniken Sommerfeld,
Klinik für Endoprothetik,
Fachklinik für operative Orthopädie,
Waldhausstraße 1, 16766 Kremmen/
OT Sommerfeld, Germany

Hartzband, M.A.
Director, Total Joint Replacement
Service, Hackensack University Medical
Center, Hackensack, NJ, USA

Hassenpflug, J.
Department for Orthopaedic Surgery,
University of Schleswig-Holstein,
Campus Kiel, Michaelisstraße 1,
24105 Kiel, Germany

Hebecker, A.
Siemens AG, Medical Solutions,
Hartmannstr. 48, 91052 Erlangen,
Germany

Heck, D.A.
Baylor Health Care System, Dallas,
Texas, USA

Hernández, V.H.
3661 South Miami Ave. Ste 610
Miami, FL. 33133, USA

Hess, Th.
Chefarzt der Abteilung für
Orthopädie und Gelenkchirurgie
Dreifaltigkeitshospital,
59555 Lippstadt, Germany

Hoeher, J.
Department of Trauma and
Orthopaedic Surgery, University of
Witten/Herdecke, Cologne-Merheim
Medical Center (CMMC),
Ostmerheimer Straße 200,
51109 Cologne, Germany

Hommen, J.P.
Orthopaedic Institute at Mercy,
3659 S. Miami Ave Ste 4008,
Miami, FL 33133, USA

Hosny, G.
Professor of Orthopaedics,
Faculty of Medicine, Benha University,
Benha, Egypt

Hüfner, T.
Trauma Department,
Hannover Medical School,
Carl-Neuberg-Str. 1,
30625 Hannover, Germany

Ismaily, S.K.
Institute of Orthopedic Research
and Education, The Methodist Hospital,
and Baylor College of Medicine,
Houston, Texas, USA

Jaramaz, B.
Institute for Computer Assisted
Orthopaedic Surgery, The Western
Pennsylvania Hospital and Robotics
Institute, Carnegie Mellon University,
Pittsburgh, Pennsylvania, USA

Jenny, J.Y.
Centre de Traumatologie et
d'Orthopédie, 10 avenue Baumann,
67400 Illkirch-Graffenstaden, France

Joskowicz, L.
School of Engineering and Computer
Science, The Hebrew University of
Jerusalem, Jerusalem 91904, Israel

Josten, M.I.C.
Universitätsklinikum Leipzig,
Zentrum für Chirurgie, Klinik für
Unfall-, Wiederherstellungs- und
plastische Chirurgie,
Liebigstr. 20a, 04103 Leipzig, Germany

Julliard, R.
Surgeon emeritus
Impasse du petit Vial
38320 Herbeys, France

Kahler, D.M.
Associate Professor, University of
Virginia, Department of Orthopaedic
Surgery, Charlottesville, VA 22908, USA

Kalteis, T.
Department of Orthopaedic Surgery,
University of Regensburg, 93042
Regensburg, Germany

Keil, C.
Berufsgenossenschaftliche Unfallklinik
Ludwigshafen, Klinik für Unfall- und
Wiederherstellungschirurgie an der
Universität Heidelberg

Kendoff, D.
Unfallchirurgische Klinik
Medizinische Hochschule
30625 Hannover, Germany

Kettrukat, M.
Orthopaedic Hospital Auguste-Viktoria,
Am Kokturkanal 2,
32545 Bad Oeynhausen, Germany

Kiefer, H.
Department of Orthopaedic and
Trauma Surgery, Lukas Hospital,
Hindenburgstraße 56,
32257 Bünde, Germany

Kistner, S.
Orthopaedic Hospital,
Am Mühlenberg 3,
37235 Hessisch-Lichtenau, Germany

Klein, G.R.
Hackensack University Medical Center,
Hackensack, NJ, USA, and New York
University-Hospital for Joint Diseases
Orthopaedic Program, New York City,
USA

Köhler, S.
Hellmuth-Ulrici-Kliniken Sommerfeld,
Klinik für Endoprothetik,
Fachklinik für operative Orthopädie,
Waldhausstraße 1, 16766 Kremmen/
OT Sommerfeld, Germany

Komistek, R.D.
Professor of Biomedical Engineering,
University of Tennessee; Center
Director, Center for Musculoskeletal
Research

Konermann, W.H.
Orthopaedic Hospital,
Am Mühlenberg 3,
37235 Hessisch-Lichtenau, Germany

Kowal, J.
MEM Research Center for Orthopaedic
Surgery, Institute for Surgical
Technology and Biomechanics,
University of Bern, Bern, Switzerland

Krackow, K.A.
Dept. of Orthopaedic Surgery, The
State University of New York at Buffalo,
Orthopaedic Surgery B 2, Buffalo
General Hospital, 100 High Street, B-2,
Buffalo, New York 14203–1126, USA

Krettek, C.
Medizinische Hochschule Hannover,
Zentrum Chirurgie, Unfallchirurgische
Klinik, Carl-Neuberg-Str. 1,
30625 Hannover, Germany

List of Contributors

Kubiak-Langer, M.
MEM Research Center for
Orthopaedic Surgery,
Institute for Surgical Technology
and Biomechanics, University of Bern,
Bern, Switzerland

Langlotz, F.
M.E. Müller Research Center for
Orthopaedic Surgery,
Institute for Surgical Technology
and Biomechanics, University Bern,
Bern, Switzerland

Laskin, R.S.
Chief of the Arthroplasty Division,
Professor of Orthopaedic Surgery,
Hospital for Special Surgery,
Weill Medical College of
Cornell University

Lavallée, S.
PRAXIM, Grenoble, France

Lavernia, C.
Orthopaedic Institute at Mercy,
3659 S. Miami Ave Ste 4008,
Miami, FL 33133, USA

Layher, F.
Department of Orthopedic Surgery,
University of Jena, Waldkrankenhaus
»Rudolf Elle«, Eisenberg,
Klosterlausnitzer Straße 81,
07607 Eisenberg, Germany

Lazovic, D.
Clinic for Orthopedics,
Pius-Hospital,
Georgstraße 12,
26121 Oldenburg, Germany

Lefevre, C.
Centre Hospitalier et Universitaire
de Brest, Hôpital de la Cavale Blanche,
Brest, France, and Laboratoire de
Traitement de l'Information Médicale,
INSERM, U650, Brest, France

Liebergall, M.
Department of Orthopaedic Surgery,
Hadassah-Hebrew University Medical
School, Jerusalem, Hadassah Medical
Center, POB 12000, Jerusalem 91120,
Israel

Linke, C.L.
Orthopädische Klinik des Klinikum
Dortmund gGmbh, Beurhausstr. 40,
44137 Dortmund, Germany

Lionberger, D.R.
Baylor College of Medicine,
6550 Fannin St, #2625, Houston,
Texas 77030, USA

Lombardi, A.V. Jr.
Clinical Assistant Professor,
Department of Orthopaedics and
Department of Biomedical Engineering,
The Ohio State University, Columbus,
OH USA

Lucente, L.
Clinica Quisisana, Via Gian Giacomo
Porro n. 5, OO197 Roma, Italy

Lüring, C.
Gesundheitsökonom, Orthopädische
Klinik, Universität Regensburg,
Asklepios Klinikum Bad Abbach,
Kaiser-Karl-V.-Allee 3,
93077 Bad Abbach, Germany

MacDonald, M.
Northwestern Center for Orthopedics,
676 North St. Clair, Ste. 450, Chicago,
Illinois, USA

Machacek, F.
Gersthof Orthopaedic Hospital, Vienna,
Austria

Malik, A.
The Arthritis Institute, 501 E. Hardy
Street, Suite 300, Inglewood,
CA 90301, USA

Mathis, K.B.
Institute of Orthopedic Research
and Education, The Methodist Hospital,
and Baylor College of Medicine,
Houston, Texas, USA

Mattes, Th.
Orthopädische Abteilung des
Rehabilitationskrankenhauses Ulm,
Orthopädische Klinik mit
Querschnittgelähmtenzentrum
der Universität Ulm,
Oberer Eselsberg 45, 89081 Ulm,
Germany

Mont, M.A.
Reubin Institute of Advanced
Orthopaedics
2401 W. Belvedere Ave.
Baltimore, MD 21215

Mosconi, M.
Clinica Ortopedica e Traumatologica
dell'Università di Pavia – Fondazione
IRCCS Policlinico San Matteo,
P.le Golgi 2, 27100 Pavia, Italy

Mosheiff, R.
Department of Orthopaedic Surgery,
Hadassah-Hebrew University Medical
School, Jerusalem, Hadassah Medical
Center, POB 12000, Jerusalem 91120,
Israel

Murphy, S.B.
Center for Computer Assisted and
Reconstructive Surgery, New England
Baptist Hospital, Tufts University,
Harvard Medical School, Boston, MA,
USA

Neumann, W.
Orthopädische Klinik der Otto-
von-Guericke Universität Magdeburg,
Leipzigerstr. 44, 39120 Magdeburg,
Germany

Noble, P.C.
Institute of Orthopedic Research and
Education, The Methodist Hospital, and
Baylor College of Medicine, Houston,
Texas, USA

Nolte, L.P.
M.E. Müller Research Center for
Orthopaedic Surgery. Institute for
Surgical Technology and Biomechanics,
University Bern, Bern, Switzerland

Othman, A.
Department of Orthopaedic and
Trauma Surgery, Lukas Hospital,
Hindenburgstraße 56, 32257 Bünde,
Germany

Ottersbach, A.
Orthopaedic Department, Brig,
Switzerland

Paffrath, Th.
Department of Trauma and
Orthopaedic Surgery, University of
Witten/Herdecke, Cologne-Merheim
Medical Center (CMMC),
Ostmerheimer Straße 200,
51109 Cologne, Germany

Pagnano, M.W.
Associate Professor of Orthopedic
Surgery, Mayo Clinic College of
Medicine, Mayo Clinic, 200 First Street
SW, Rochester, MN 55905, USA

Pap, G.
Orthopädische Klinik der Otto-
von-Guericke Universität Magdeburg,
Leipzigerstr. 44, 39120 Magdeburg,
Germany

Parratte, S.
The Aix-Marseille University, Depart-
ment of Orthopaedic Surgery, Hopital
Sainte-Marguerite, Service de Chirurgie
Orthopédique, 270 Boulevard Sainte-
Marguerite, 13009, Marseille, France

Pearle, A.
Assistant Attending Orthopedic
Surgeon, Hospital for Special Surgery
Assistant Attending Orthopedic
Surgeon, New York Presbyterian
Hospital
Clinical Director, Hospital for
Special Surgery Computer Assisted
Surgery Center
Hospital for Special Surgery
535 East 70th Street
New York, NY 10021, USA

Perlick, L.
Department of Orthopaedic Surgery,
University of Regensburg,
93042 Regensburg, Germany

Perrin, N.
Laboratoire de Traitement de
l'Information Médicale, INSERM,
U650, Brest, France, and PRAXIM,
Grenoble, France

Piovani, L.
Clinica Ortopedica e Traumatologica
dell'Università di Pavia – Fondazione
IRCCS Policlinico San Matteo,
P.le Golgi 2, 27100 Pavia, Italy

Plaskos, C.
PRAXIM, Grenoble, France

Plate, J.F.
Reubin Institute of Advanced
Orthopaedics
2401 W. Belvedere Ave.
Baltimore, MD 21215

Plaweski, S.
Orthopedic department
University of Joseph Fourier
CHU Grenoble
BP 217
38043 Grenoble, France

Pohlemann, T.
Medizinische Hochschule Hannover,
Zentrum Chirurgie, Unfallchirurgische
Klinik, Carl-Neuberg-Str. 1,
30625 Hannover, Germany

Prymka, M.
Department for Orthopaedic Surgery,
University of Schleswig-Holstein,
Campus Kiel, Michaelisstraße 1,
24105 Kiel, Germany

Puls, M.
MEM Research Center for Orthopaedic
Surgery, Institute for Surgical
Technology and Biomechanics,
University of Bern, Bern, Switzerland

Recum J. von
Berufsgenossenschaftliche Unfallklinik
Ludwigshafen, Klinik für Unfall- und
Wiederherstellungschirurgie an der
Universität Heidelberg

Reichel, H.
Orthopädische Abteilung des
Rehabilitationskrankenhauses Ulm,
Orthopädische Klinik mit Querschnitt-
gelähmtenzentrum der Universität
Ulm, Oberer Eselsberg 45, 89081 Ulm,
Germany

Richter, M.
Department for Trauma, Orthopaedic
and Foot Surgery, Coburg Clinical
Center, Ketschendorfer Str. 33, 96450
Coburg, Germany

Ritschl, P.
Gersthof Orthopaedic Hospital, Vienna,
Austria

Sagbo, S.
MEM Research Center for Orthopaedic
Surgery, Institute for Surgical
Technology and Biomechanics,
University of Bern, Bern, Switzerland

Sander, K.
Department of Orthopedic Surgery,
University of Jena, Waldkrankenhaus
»Rudolf Elle«, Eisenberg,
Klosterlausnitzer Straße 81,
07607 Eisenberg, Germany

Saragaglia, D.
Service de chirurgie Orthopédique
et de Traumatologie du Sport, CHU
de Grenoble, Hôpital Sud, 38130,
Echirolles, France

Saur, M.A.
Orthopaedic Hospital,
Am Mühlenberg 3,
37235 Hessisch-Lichtenau, Germany

Schemitsch, E.H.
Orthopaedic Department,
St Michael Hospital, University of
Toronto, Canada

Schemitsch, E.H.
Professor, Division of Orthopaedics,
Department of Surgery, University of
Toronto, St. Michael's Hospital, Suite
800, 55 Queen Street East, Toronto,
Ontario M5C 1R6, Canada

Scuderi, G.R.
Insall Scott Kelly Institute
210 East 64th St. 4th Floor
New York, NY 10021

Seedhom, B.B.
Reader, Academic Unit of
Musculoskeletal and Rehabilitation
Medicine, University of Leeds, Leeds,
United Kingdom

Senkal, M.
Department for General Surgery
and Orthopaedic Surgery,
Ruhr University Bochum, Germany

Seyler, T.M.
Reubin Institute of Advanced
Orthopaedics
2401 W. Belvedere Ave.
Baltimore, MD 21215

Shafizadeh, S.
Department of Trauma and
Orthopaedic Surgery, University of
Witten/Herdecke, Cologne-Merheim
Medical Center (CMMC),
Ostmerheimer Straße 200,
51109 Cologne, Germany

Sherman, K.P.
Consultant Orthopaedic Surgeon,
Castle Hill Hospital, Cottingham,
Hull, UK

Siebenrock, K.A.
Department of Orthopaedic Surgery,
Inselspital, University of Bern, Bern,
Switzerland

Stiehl, J.B.
Columbia St Mary's Hospital, 575 W
River Woods Parkway, Milwaukee,
Wisconsin 53211, USA

Stindel, E.
Centre Hospitalier et Universitaire de
Brest, Hôpital de la Cavale Blanche,
Brest, France, and Laboratoire de
Traitement de l'Information Médicale,
INSERM, U650, Brest, France

Stroppa, S.
Clinica Ortopedica e Traumatologica
dell'Università di Pavia – Fondazione
IRCCS Policlinico San Matteo,
P.le Golgi 2, 27100 Pavia, Italy

Stulberg, S.D.
Professor of Clinical Orthopaedic
Surgery, Northwestern University
Feinberg School of Medicine, Director,
Joint Reconstruction and Implant
Service, Northwestern Memorial
Hospital, 633 Clark Street, Evanston,
IL 60208, USA

Suhm, N.
Department of Surgery, University
Hospital Basel, Basel, Switzerland

Sussman-Fort, J.
Department of Biomedical Engineering,
Columbia University, New York City, USA

Tannast, M.
Department of Orthopaedic Surgery,
Inselspital, University of Bern, Bern,
Switzerland, and Center for Computer
Assisted and Reconstructive Surgery,
New England Baptist Hospital, Tufts
University, Harvard Medical School,
Boston, MA, USA

Thomas, W.
Clinica Quisisana, Via Gian Giacomo
Porro n. 5, 00197 Roma, Italy

Thompson, M.T.
Institute of Orthopedic Research and
Education, The Methodist Hospital, and
Baylor College of Medicine, Houston,
Texas, USA

Tiling, Th.
Department of Trauma and
Orthopaedic Surgery, University of
Witten/Herdecke, Cologne-Merheim
Medical Center (CMMC),
Ostmerheimer Straße 200,
51109 Cologne, Germany

Tingart, M.
Department of Orthopaedic Surgery,
University of Regensburg,
93042 Regensburg, Germany

Tria, A.J. Jr.
Institute for Advanced Orthopaedic
Study, The Orthopaedic Center
of New Jersey, 1527 State Highway 27,
Suite 1300, Somerset,
New Jersey 08873, USA

Troccaz J.
TIMC Laboratory, Grenoble University,
France

Trottenberg, G.
Orthopedic Clinic, St. Vincenz-Hospital,
Danziger Str. 17, 33034 Brakel, Germany

Vail, T.P.
Professor of Orthopaedic Surgery,
Director of Adult Reconstructive
Surgery, Duke University Medical
Center, Durham, North Carolina, USA

Victor, J.
Department of Orthopaedics
AZ St-Lucas, Brugge, Belgium

Walker, P.S.
Director, Laboratory for Minimally-
Invasive Surgery, Department of
Orthopaedics, NYU Hospital for Joint
Diseases, New York City, USA

Wan, Z.
The Arthritis Institute, 501 E. Hardy
Street, Suite 300,Inglewood, CA 90301,
USA

Wasielewski, R.C.
Adjunct Professor of Biomedical
Engineering, University of Tennessee

Wei, C.-S.
Cooper Union for the Advancement of
Science and Arts, New York City, USA

Weidner, A.
Spine Center
Lengericher Landstr. 19b
49078 Osnabrück, Germany

Weil, Y.
Department of Orthopaedic Surgery,
Hadassah-Hebrew University Medical
School, Jerusalem, Hadassah Medical
Center, POB 12000, Jerusalem 91120,
Israel

Wendl, K.
Berufsgenossenschaftliche Unfallklinik
Ludwigshafen, Klinik für Unfall- und
Wiederherstellungschirurgie an der
Universität Heidelberg

Wentzensen, A.
Berufsgenossenschaftliche Unfallklinik
Ludwigshafen, Klinik für Unfall- und
Wiederherstellungschirurgie an der
Universität Heidelberg

Willburger, R.
Department for General Surgery and
Orthopaedic Surgery, Ruhr University
Bochum, Germany

Wixson, R.L.
Professor of Clinical Orthopaedic
Surgery, Feinberg School of Medicine,
Northwestern University, Chicago,
Illinois, USA

Yau, W.-P.
Department of Orthopaedics and
Traumatology, Queen Mary Hospital,
Pokfulam, Hong Kong

Yildirim, G.
Laboratory for Minimally-Invasive
Surgery, Department of Orthopaedics,
NYU Hospital for Joint Diseases,
New York City, USA

Zech, S.
Trauma Department,
Hannover Medical School,
Carl-Neuberg-Str. 1,
30625 Hannover, Germany

Zhang, X.
MEM Research Center for Orthopaedic
Surgery, Institute for Surgical
Technology and Biomechanics,
University of Bern, Bern, Switzerland

Zheng, G.
MEM Research Center for Orthopaedic
Surgery, Institute for Surgical
Technology and Biomechanics,
University of Bern, Bern, Switzerland

I

Basics of Computer-Assisted Orthopaedic Surgery

J. Kowal, F. Langlotz, L.-P. Nolte

Introduction

Computer-assisted orthopaedic surgery (CAOS) aims at improving the perception that a surgeon has of the surgical field and the operative manipulation that he/she carries out. Conventional surgical handwork requires competences such as dexterity or fine motor skills, which are complemented by visual and tactile feedback. Current CAOS systems offer enhanced visualization by displaying a virtual model of the operated anatomy together with relevant information about the position of a surgical instrument or implant on a computer monitor thus improving the surgeon's visual feedback by complementing the direct visual impression of the operation site. They present greater details, three-dimensional views or sights of internal structures, which are invisible to the naked eye. The anticipated effect on surgical performance is manifold: the increased visual perception of the operator leads to an increased precision with which surgical tasks can be carried out. Bony manipulation such as drilling, chiseling, or sawing can be performed more accurately and implants can be placed more exactly. This reduces the risk of harming the patient intra-operatively by damaging sensitive structures. As a result, numerous studies have reported smaller variations of the outcome of patients who underwent navigated surgery when compared to the corresponding conventional approaches. It can be expected that recent trends in CAOS research and development will result in navigation systems that also complement the surgeon's tactile sensation by providing haptic feedback when appropriate.

This chapter will present the basic elements that are common to all navigation systems and will describe optional features that have been implemented in the products of some manufacturers or the prototypes of some researchers.

Building Blocks of a CAOS System

The core of each CAOS system presents virtual representations of the operated anatomy and the performed surgical action and ensures, by linking this virtual model to the operated patient, that the replayed scene matches with what is performed at the surgical situs [9]. The following subsections will explain the building blocks that make such systems reality and will present a review of available technologies.

Appropriate Patient Anatomy Representation

Operating with the support of a surgical navigation system requires an image of the treated anatomy to be used as virtual object. A large variety of image modalities can potentially be employed for this purpose, but not all of them are ideal for use in CAOS.

Using established methods of medical imaging is surely most obvious and, consequently, the CAOS systems of the first generation used preoperative computed tomography (CT) scans to represent the bone structures that were involved in the respective surgery. CTs are an almost ideal preoperative image modality for the needs of CAOS: they present the outer shape and inner structures of bony anatomy with high resolution and good contrast and without any geometrical distortions. Magnetic Resonance Imaging (MRI) in contrast suffers from poor hard tissue representation and sometimes considerable geometric distortions. Although special acquisition protocols have been suggested to overcome these difficulties at least partially, MRIs are not widely used in orthopaedic navigation nowadays. The same is true for preoperative, conventional X-rays. Their geometrical imprecision and the fact that they capture only a two-dimensional (2D) projection of a three-dimensional (3D) scene have made developers refrain from building navigation systems based on X-rays.

In any case when a preoperative image serves as a virtual object, a so-called registration or matching procedure is required to align the operated anatomy with its »canned« preoperative image, assuming that the represented topology of the bone has not changed between image acquisition and surgical intervention. Numerous registration approaches have been described [10]. Each of them requires certain features to be interactively or semi-automatically identified in both, the patient's anatomy and the image. Based on the inherent knowledge of correspondence between these feature sets, the spatial relation between virtual object and operated anatomy is extrapolated. While feature extraction from the image dataset is performed either »manually« using the computer mouse or with the help of image processing algorithms, intra-operative digitization of the corresponding features is done by the surgeon using a digitizing stylus, laser scanners, ultrasound probes, fluoroscopic imaging or similar devices. Since the perfect alignment of image and reality is crucial for the accuracy of the subsequently available navigation feedback, this usually interactive step requires careful execution and, as an element of safety, subsequent verification of the achieved result.

Alternatively, intra-operative imaging using 2D or 3D fluoroscopy can be applied [5]. Using such intra-operative images as a replacement of preoperative CT scans allows for intra-surgical image update when the operated morphology does not any more correspond to what is frozen in the preoperative image, e.g., in cases of fracture reduction or repositioning osteotomies. Moreover, using an intra-operative means of image acquisition permits the imaging device to be integrated into the coordinate space of the navigation system. Provided a pre-calibration

of the device, the link between image space and surgical space can be determined automatically effectively making the aforementioned interactive registration procedure obsolete.

As another alternative that goes entirely without »classical« radiological images, so-called »image-free« systems construct virtual models of the operated anatomy exclusively based on interactively acquired position data. Such data is either recorded by digitization methods as described above for the registration of preoperative images or is derived from the kinematic analysis of joint motion [18], which lets the CAOS system determine, e.g., the rotation center or axis of a joint. Resulting models are rather abstract since they are constructed from very sparse data only [16]. To improve the realism with which the surgical field is represented on the screen, statistical shape atlases can be combined with the recorded data. The technological background of this method is described in greater detail in Chapter 76 (»Advanced Technologies in Navigation«) of this book.

Passive Navigation Systems

Passive navigation systems utilizing a device called *tracker* to determine the spatial 3D positions and orientations of objects in real time. Different physical modalities have been investigated and used to remotely sense the spatial location of objects.

Nowadays optical tracking is by far the most commonly used tracking modality. It utilizes infrared light that is either actively emitted or passively reflected from the tracked objects. The basic principles of navigation are outlined in the following using an optical tracking system but they apply for other physical modalities as well.

To track objects such as surgical instruments or the patient anatomy light emitting or reflecting markers are rigidly attached to the tracked objects. A system consisting of an object to be tracked and markers rigidly attached to it is called »rigid body«. The optical trackers also known as cameras detect the reflected or emitted light signals and reconstruct the corresponding markers' 3D positions in the camera's coordinate system.

From mathematics it is known that the positions of three non-collinear marker positions are required to uniquely define the 3D position and orientation of an object in space. Therefore, the markers are usually grouped in rigid constellations of three or more forming their own local coordinate system. By increasing the number of markers together with an optimized spatial arrangement the »visibility« of a tracked object can be improved. Additionally, it has been shown that increasing the number of markers on a rigid body up to six improves the navigation accuracy significantly. With increasing number of markers the accuracy gradually converges against a maximum.

By means of calibration or registration the real object geometry will be defined in the local rigid body coordinate system. Knowing the individual marker positions of a rigid body and the orientation of the real object within the local rigid body coordinate system the absolute position and orientation of the real object in the camera coordinate system can be computed. If more than one object is tracked simultaneously by the camera the relative positions of all tracked objects can be determined as well.

For tracked patient anatomies similar mechanisms are used: By the help of mechanical supports (e.g. Dynamic Reference Bases [14]) a marker constellation will be rigidly attached to the anatomy during the surgical intervention. As long as the marker arrangement stays rigid in relation to the anatomy, the rigid body concept is not violated and the relative position between patient anatomies and/or surgical tools can be computed. ◻ Figure 1.1 illustrates this tracking concept by showing the individual transformations between the camera coordinate system (C-cos), the tool coordinate system (T-cos) and a DRB attached to a patient anatomy forming a rigid body and defining a local coordinate system (A-cos).

Tracking based on video images and symbolic patterns attached as markers to the tracked objects has been proposed as an alternative [3, 4], but proved less accurate than infrared light based tracking system.

Ultrasound-based tracking systems are established in the area of biomechanical motion analysis [7] but due to this technology's limited accuracy and rather complex marker handling and calibration it did not prove to be competitive for surgical navigation.

Both tracking modalities – optical as well as ultrasound – have a common major drawback: For proper functioning both require a direct line of sight between the tracker and the tracked objects, which might be problematic with respect to the setup in the operating room.

Electromagnetic fields as tracking modality do not have this restriction. Such a system consists of a field generator (emitter coil) and receiver coils attached to the surgical tools or the patient anatomy similar to the marker concept for optical tracking. By measuring magnetic field interferences the system can detect the spatial positions of the receiver coils within the generated field of the emitter coil. The electromagnetic field propagates unimpeded through bones or soft tissue, which is of advantage because this implies that a direct line of sight is not mandatory for the system to work, but on the other hand such an electromagnetic field might be strongly distorted by ferromagnetic materials within the field such as surgical tools. Newer systems are able to cope with these distortions to some extend. However, this ferromagnetic sensitivity restricts the application of magnetic navigation systems to fields where less metal is involved, e.g., catheter navigation for cardiac surgeries.

Nowadays, navigation systems are only able to visualize the spatial relationship between tracked objects. More recent developments [1] try to incorporate other physical modalities such as acting forces or moments of surgical tools into the navigation system. This will provide a more complete picture of the surgical procedure. From a technical point of view the incorporation of additional input such as video streams or analog signals (e.g., forces) demand for special synchronization mechanisms to be

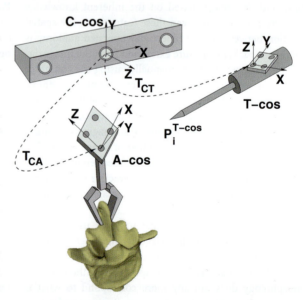

◻ **Fig. 1.1.** Optical navigation system overview: Relationships between the camera coordinate system (C-cos), a tool coordinate system (T-cos), and an anatomy coordinate system (A-cos). After the dynamic reference base is attached the DRB and the patient anatomy are a considered to be a single rigid body

implemented. Such synchronization mechanisms guarantee that all used modalities, e.g., forces, video streams, and tracker information are handled in the right temporal order.

Active or Robotic Navigation Systems

For this group of navigation systems the robot itself plays the role of a navigator. The robotic actuator system in conjunction with the position sensors attached to the individual joints of the robotic arm is used to precisely position mounted surgical tools to perform specific tasks as part of the therapeutic treatment. Knowing the geometric relation of the robotic system a treatment plan can be established within the patient anatomy representation. Before executing the treatment plan a registration between the patient anatomy representation and the real anatomy has to be established. This registration has to stay valid during the whole execution phase.

After the registration step, the robotic system performs a planned surgical task autonomously without additional support by the surgeon.

Robotic systems for a number of clinical applications such as total joint replacement [11, 15] have been developed but their clinical benefit is discussed controversially [6, 12, 13]. Compared to the considerable investment they require, the field of application that individual robotic systems can cover is rather limited. The fact that the first robotic systems were basically slightly adapted industrial robots turned out to be another disadvantage because they required a rather big surgical approach in order to realize a rigid attachment between the patient anatomy and the robot itself. Those systems have not been especially designed for application in the surgical environment with all its specialties and constrains in terms minimal invasiveness or sterilizability. Moreover, surgeons are reluctant to fully embrace this new technology due to the inherent autonomous workflow of a robotic navigation system.

However, more recent developments try to better respect the constraints and requirements of the surgical field. For example, a semi-active robotic system called ACROBOT has been proposed by Jakopec et al. [8]. This system is still based on an industrial robot; however, it differs in the purpose that it serves intra-operatively. Instead of actively milling the femur shaft, the system allows the surgeon to move the reamer freely in order to resect bone as long as this motion stays within a preoperatively defined safety volume. When the milling action is about to leave this volume causing more tissue than planned to be resected, the robot would actively intercept to block the unwanted movements. This approach enables the surgeon to carry out the actual resection process manually while being assured that the planned cuts are realized precisely.

As an example of a robotic system that has been especially designed for the use in a surgical environment the MiniAture Robot for Surgical procedures (MARS) by Shoham et al. [17] should be mentioned. The device is a 5×5×7cm^3, 200 g, six degree of freedom parallel manipulator. The device will be directly attached on the bony anatomy and supports spinal pedicle screw placement or drill guidance for distal locking screws during intramedullary nailing.

Nevertheless, the importance of active robotic navigation systems is currently rather low compared to passive surgical navigation. This might change in the future if robotic systems are better adapted to the surgical environment and if there is clear evidence that robotic navigation has significant advantages compared to passive surgical navigation.

Visualization for CAOS Systems

After the introduction of patient anatomy representations with their implicit or explicit registrations and real-time tracking methods for objects together with the rigid body concept nearly all building blocks necessary for a computer-assisted surgery system have been explained. In a last step, the individual parts are put together with visualization techniques to form a complete CAOS system. This section introduces common visualization concepts used in CAOS systems.

In general the visualization type is driven by the clinical application. The classical visualization in CAOS systems is based on arbitrarily cut slices through volumetric data sets such as CT data. During a surgical planning step the slices' positions and orientations can be changed by user interaction in order to plan, for example, implant positions or trajectories for fixation screws. During a subsequent navigation step the slice positions within the slice stack are continuously updated, for example, by the tip of a tracked surgical tool using the real-time position updates from the tracking system. The surgical tools or additional information from a previous planning step like screw positions are then displayed as overlays on top of

1

the rendered slices. ◘ Figures 1.2 and 1.3 show typical CT data-based planning and navigation applications.

Other navigation solutions are based on surface models. These surface models can be created during an additional segmentation and model creation step based on a volumetric data set or using statistical models refined by digitized patient specific anatomy information. The accuracy of such generated surface models is a critical issue especially if treatment decisions are made based on visualized surgical scenes. Therefore, reliable automatic segmentation procedures, especially for pathologic degenerated anatomies, are still challenging research topics. Manual segmentation is not a real option for daily clinical use. The applicability of surface models generated from statistical models is limited to surgical areas where neither pathologic changes of the bones are very prominent nor the existence of fractures must be represented by the created models. Usually, these models are used to improve the overview in a surgical scene, for example, in image free navigation systems for total knee arthroplasty.

Volume-rendering techniques based on volumetric datasets have just started to emerge in CAOS systems, but existing hardware limitations prevent this technique from being used in an extensive manner, although this technique together with automatically computed transfer functions for the rendering process offers very interesting and helpful alternative visualizations. Up to now CAOS systems utilize volume rendering techniques just to provide an anatomy overview based on down-sampled volumetric data sets. The lower right view in ◘ Figure 1.2

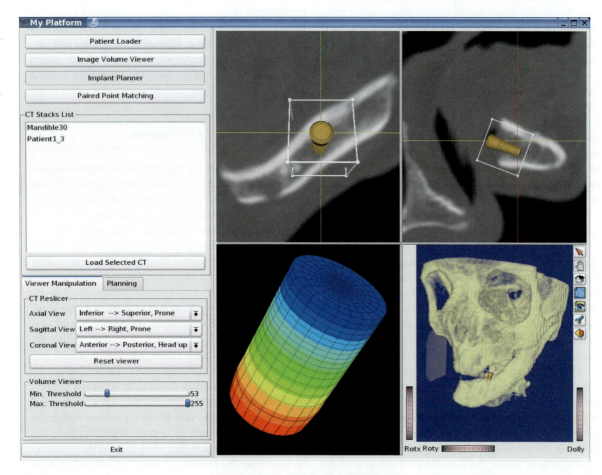

◘ **Fig. 1.2.** Typical CT data-based planning application showing an implant positioned as overlay on top of arbitrary slices across a CT data set. The lower right view show the CT slice stack in a down sampled volume rendered version as well with the planed implant

demonstrates a view of a volume rendered skull used in a planning application.

If the anatomy representations are 2D data sets such as fluoroscopic images originated from navigated intra-operative X-ray devices the visualization has to respect and simulate the correct underlying projection model of the imaging device in order keep the spatial relation between the image itself and the overlaid surgical tools correct.

Intra-operatively, CAOS systems normally use conventional computer monitors to visualize the surgical scene. This approach has two disadvantages: First, due to the spatial distance between the surgical situs and the computer monitor the surgeon is enforced to continuously change his/her viewing direction. The second disadvantage is the monitor itself, which finally displays just a 2D projection of the computed 3D scene. The depth perception of such a displayed scene is almost lost despite using shading effects and other visualization techniques.

To overcome the first problem, solutions have been proposed using semi-transparent mirrors as a projection plane for the computed scene. These devices are mounted directly in the line of sight between the surgeon's eyes and the surgical situs [2].

Real 3D perception can be simulated by the use of recently introduced 3D monitors or glasses with stereoscopic displays also known as *look-through displays*.

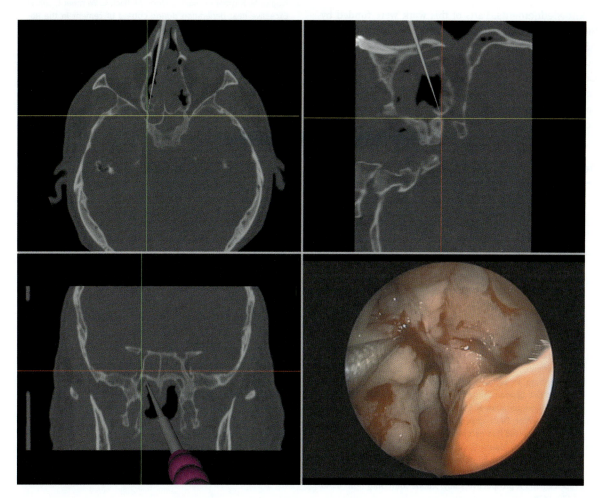

◘ **Fig. 1.3.** Typical CT data-based navigation application with a surgical tool as overlay whereas the re-slice positions of the CT data set are defined by updated tip position of the surgical tool. Additionally the lower right view shows simultaneously injected video stream coming from an endoscope

However, surgical navigation systems using such glasses, or half transparent projection mirrors, or microscopy-based navigation system, where the simulated scene is injected directly into the view channel of the surgeon will have to cope with one problem in order to gain further acceptance in the community: The stronger the injected or overlaid simulated surgical scene is the less visible the real surgical situs will become and vice versa. The major challenge will be to find either innovative solutions allowing for the coexistence of the unimpeded view to the surgical scene and the injected computed scene or the right balance in overlaying both scenes without loosing valuable information.

Acknowledgements. Parts of this work were funded by the M.E. Müller Foundation, Bern Switzerland, the AO/ASIF Foundation, Davos Switzerland, and the Swiss National Science Foundation through the National Center of Competence in Research CO-ME, Zürich Switzerland. All Screenshots show in this article are originating from the open source application framework for medical applications MARVIN (https://choroidea.unibe.ch/marvin).

References

1. Ambrosetti S, Burger J, Piotrowski W et al. (2003) Smart surgical instrument for spinal interventions. Computer Assisted Orthopaedic Surgery – Proceedings of 6th Annual Meeting of CAOS-International 2006
2. Blackwell M, Nikou C, DiGioia AM, Kanade T (1998) An image overlay system for medical data visualization. In: Wells WM (ed) Medical image computing and computer-assisted intervention – MICCAI'98. Springer, Berlin Heidelberg New York Tokyo, pp 232–240
3. Colchester A, Zhao J, Holton-Tainter K, Henri C, Maitland N, Roberts P, Harris C, Evans R (1996) Development and preliminary evaluation of VISLAN, a surgical planning and guidance system using intra-operative video imaging. Med Image Anal 1(1): 7390
4. de Siebenthal J, Langlotz F (2003) Video tracking for intra-operative guidance – A complementary solution to tracking in CAOS interventions. In: Langlotz F, Davies BL, Bauer A (eds) Computer Assisted Orthopaedic Surgery – Proceedings of 3rd Annual Meeting of CAOS-International. Steinkopff, Darmstadt, pp 86–87
5. Foley KT, Simon DA, Rampersaud YR (2001) Virtual fluoroscopy: computer-assisted fluoroscopic navigation. Spine 26: 347–351
6. Honl M, Dierk O, Gauck C, Carrero V, Lampe F, Dries S, Quante M, Schwieger K, Hille E, Morlock MM (2003) Comparison of robotic-assisted and manual implantation of a primary total hip replacement. A prospective study. J Bone Joint Surg (Am) 85A8: 1470–1478
7. Huitema RB, Hof AL, Postema K (2002) Ultrasonic motion analysis system--measurement of temporal and spatial gait parameters. J Biomech 356: 837–842
8. Jakopec M, Harris SJ, Rodriguez y Baena F, Gomes P, Cobb J, Davies BL (2001) The first clinical application of a „hands-on" robotic knee surgery system. Comput Aided Surg 66: 329–339
9. Langlotz F, Nolte LP (2004) Technical approaches to computer-assisted orthopedic surgery. Eur J Trauma 30: 1–11
10. Maintz JB, Viergever MA (1998) A survey of medical image registration. Med Image Anal 2(1): 1–36
11. Mittelstadt B, Kazanzides P, Zuhars J, Williamson B, Cain P, Smith F, Bargar WL (1996) The evolution of a surgical robot from prototype to human clinical use. In: Taylor RH, Lavallée S, Burdea GC, Mösges R (eds) Computer integrated surgery. MIT Press, Cambridge, pp 397–407
12. Nogler M, Maurer H, Wimmer C, Gegenhuber C, Bach C, Krismer M (2001) Knee pain caused by a fiducial marker in the medial femoral condyle: a clinical and anatomic study of 20 CAOSes. Acta Orthop Scand 72: 477–480
13. Nogler M, Krismer M, Haid C, Ogon M, Bach C, Wimmer C (2001) Excessive heat generation during cutting of cement in the Robodoc hip-revision procedure. Acta Orthop Scand 72: 595–599
14. Nolte LP, Visarius H, Arm E, Langlotz F, Schwarzenbach O, Zamorano L (1995) Computer-aided fixation of spinal implants. J Imag Guide Surg 1: 88–93
15. Paul A (1999) Operationsroboter in der Endoprothetik: Wie CAOSPAR Hand an die Hüfte legt. MMW Fortschr Med 141(33): 18
16. Sati M, Stäubli HU, Bourquin Y, Kunz M, Käsermann S, Nolte LP (2000) Clinical integration of computer-assisted technology for arthroscopic anterior cruciate ligament reconstruction. Oper Tech Orthop 10(1): 40–49
17. Shoham M, Burman M, Zehavi E, Joskowicz L, Batkilin E, Kunicher Y (2003) Bone-mounted miniature robot for surgical procedures: concept and clinical applications. IEEE T Robotic Autom 19: 893–901
18. Stulberg SD, Picard FD, Saragaglia D (2000) Computer-assisted total knee replacement arthroplasty. Oper Tech Orthop 10(1): 25–39

CT-Based Navigation Systems

B. Jaramaz, A.M. DiGioia III

Introduction

Medical imaging modalities in diagnostic and clinical use today offer a wide range of possibilities for design and implementation of computer assisted surgical systems. Among those modalities, Computed Tomography (CT) scan has a prominent role, since it provides three dimensional (3D) images of relatively high accuracy. It is especially well suited for orthopaedics, since the bone separates from the rest of the tissue by its intensity, which makes the bone segmentation a relatively simple task.

CT scanners are large machines, typically housed in the hospital's radiology departments or at separate imaging facilities. Attempts to integrate CT scanners in the operating room, or to develop navigation systems integrated with CT scanners did not have much success so far, especially in orthopaedics. However, because bones don't change shape between the time of the scan and the time of the surgery, it was possible to design procedures in which the imaging, planning and image guided intervention could be done at different times, as three separate consecutive events. Most of the early surgical navigation procedures and all of the robotic procedures in orthopaedics have been designed this way – sometimes referred to as »canned reality« procedures.

This overview identifies the most important technical components of CT-based CAS systems, using the example of the HipNav system, developed by our team. HipNav (CASurgica, Inc.) is the surgical navigation system developed initially to address the problem of cup alignment in total hip replacement [3]. It has introduced several new concepts in the computer-assisted surgery, most notably the concept of patient-specific pre-operative simulation for joint replacement procedures. Proper alignment of implant components is one of the most important factors that contribute to the joint stability; Misalignment of components reduces the safe range of motion and can lead to dislocation of the joint, or repeated impingement of components that can result in excessive wear and generation of wear debris. Especially sensitive is the alignment of the cup part, since the orientation of the cup is not restricted by the shape of the bone cavity. Currently used mechanical tools for positioning of the cup aligns the cup with respect to global body landmarks, often resulting in inadequate cup alignment. HipNav relies on the CT-scan image for planning, and both the cup and the femoral stem of the desired type and size are selected from the 3D model database and placed in the respective bones.

Image Segmentation, Pre-operative Planning and Simulation

With CT technology, three-dimensional image is created by a reconstruction of the transverse planar images acquired in a systematic and sequential order from a source-receiver assembly that rotates in a circular pattern. Because of its relatively high accuracy and the bone imaging characteristics CT scans are very suitable for surgical navigation, especially in orthopaedics. The bones can be easily distinguished from any other tissue, and can be easily segmented out. The

2

bones are also the least deformable parts of the body, and therefore the most stable references for navigation, making it possible for different phases of surgical planning and execution to be performed well after the patient imaging.

Pre-operative planning is typically done in three orthogonal cross-sectional views made through the CT

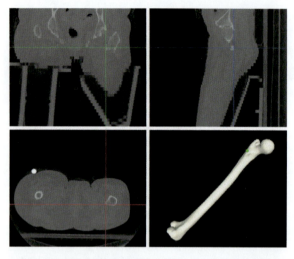

◘ **Fig. 2.1.** Cross sections through a CT scan and a surface model of the femur derived from the scan. The same point is identified with the cross hairs in the CT cross sections and with a small sphere in the surface model

scan volume. The target bone can also be visualized as a three-dimensional object and rendered in the perspective view from an arbitrary viewpoint, which can be useful in some planning and navigation tasks (◘ Fig. 2.1). In order to create this kind of renderings, the organs and tissues of interest need to be segmented out from the rest of the image, and their boundaries have to be determined. Surface models are then built, which describe the surface of the bone of interest as a contiguous set of triangles fully encompassing the bone's volume.

Early applications of image-guided surgery where the goal is to accurately and precisely reach the target and to choose the access trajectory so that the damage to the collateral tissue is minimized (such as tumor removal, fracture stabilization and biopsy tasks) were fairly simple from the planning point (◘ Fig. 2.2).

In contrast, HipNav has introduced more complex planner enhanced with a simulator, providing analytical capability that can aid the surgeon in making the critical pre-operative planning decisions. As a 3D imaging modality, CT scan provides a basis for complex three dimensional planning, which can greatly enhance surgeons capability to visualize the surgical task, examine the potential solution and explore the alternatives. HipNav planner incorporates a range of motion (ROM) simulator that can aid the surgeon in the optimal selection and orientation of implant components (◘ Fig. 2.3).

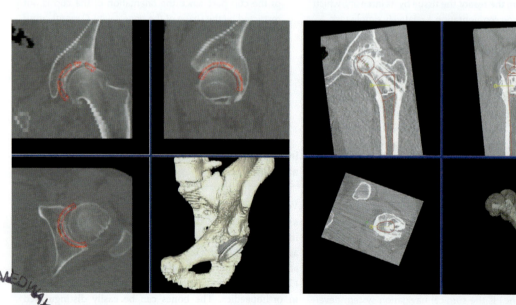

◘ **Fig. 2.2.** Surgical planning with HipNav: Planning of the cup implant; planning of the femoral implant (© CASurgica, Inc.)

Planning is performed with respect to the anatomic coordinate systems derived from the anatomic landmarks. In the pelvis, the anterior pelvic plane is defined with the most anterior points – anterior iliac spines and the mid-pubis symphysis point. In the femur, the reference system is defined with the center of the femoral head and the plane defined by the lesser trochanter and the posterior condyles [4]. After the landmarks are automatically detected in the planner, the alignment of implant components can be uniquely defined. The surgeon selects the implant components from the database and places them in a desired position and orientation, using both cross-sectional CT views and 3D surface models. In the final stage, the virtual replacement joint is assembled and tested for the range of motion simulation. The range of motion analysis is performed for any desired leg motion path, to test the impingement limits of that motion. Both prosthetic and bone impingent limits are detected. The effects of the change of any relevant parameter (orientation, size, position, pelvic flexion) on ROM and on component offset and leg length can be examined in real time, helping surgeon in optimizing the plan. The implants orientation can be modified, or alternative components can be selected, so that the safe range of motion is maximized, and the leg length change is properly considered. Once the surgical plan is developed, it becomes a blueprint for surgical intervention. Its surgical execution is typically dependent on several technical steps, in particular on tracking, registration, and navigation.

Intraoperative Steps

Tracking

The key component of surgical navigation is the ability to determine accurately and precisely at every step where the target bones and surgical tools are in space and how their position corresponds to the pre-operative image that was used for planning. This is typically achieved by using tracking systems and by rigidly attaching tracking markers to bones of interest and to the surgical tools, and by tracking those markers using localizing devices (◘ Fig. 2.4).

The most commonly used tracking systems are the optical and electromagnetic ones. The optical localizers consist of two (Polaris, NDI, Ontario, Canada) or three (OptoTrak, NDI, Ontario) CCD cameras placed in the rigid enclosure that detect the position of either infrared light emitting diode markers (active) or reflective spherical markers (passive) in space. Typically four to six markers are placed on one rigid object, called dynamic reference body (DRB), allowing calculation of the 6 degree of freedom position of that object in space. If a DRB is then attached rigidly to another object such as medical instrument or bone, one can inherently track the position of those objects in space, as well. The orientation of tools relative to the bone of interest can then be calculated and compared to

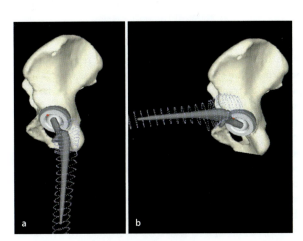

◘ **Fig. 2.3a,b.** Surgical planning with HipNav: Range of motion test **a)** Neutral position **b)** Internal rotation in flexion. Red dot indicates the impingement point. (Copyright CASurgica, Inc.)

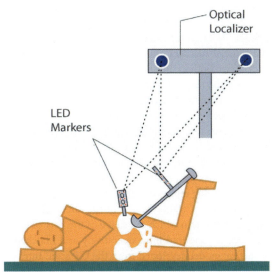

◘ **Fig. 2.4.** Tracking with an optical system: Optical localizer tracks the positions of markers attached to a bone and a surgical tool

Optical
Localizer

LED
Markers

the planned one. While the accuracy of optical tracking systems is currently the highest of all tracking systems, they require a line of sight to be maintained throughout the surgery, which sometimes represents a difficulty in the organization and ergonomics of the operating room. An alternative tracking modality is electromagnetic (EM) tracking. In EM tracking the emitting coil emits an electromagnetic field that induces the electricity current in the receiving coil. The position of the receiving coil is detected by measuring the induced current and solving the EM field equation for spatial variables. This method does not require the line of sight between the localizer and its target and can therefore enable better OR ergonomics. While it approaches the accuracy of the lower-end optical trackers, it is susceptible to the presence of ferromagnetic objects and other disturbances in the EM field.

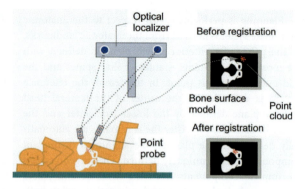

Fig. 2.5. Shape based registration. Bone surface coordinates are measured using a point probe. The resulting point cloud is matched with the surface model

Registration

In order to implement the surgical plan, the position of the patient's bone in the operating room has to be correlated with the position of the same bode in the plan image. This involves finding the geometric transformation that would map the patient's intra-operative position to coincide with the position in the plan space. The calculation of this position is called registration. The simplest registration is the fiducial registration. It involves the insertion of fiducials (implanted physical markers) into the bone before a 3D image (CT scan) is obtained, and keeping them inserted throughout the surgical procedure.

The fiducial markers are designed to be clearly and easily identified both in the image space and in the tracker space during the surgery. Three such markers placed in predetermined anatomical areas are sufficient for registration. Although this type of registration is conceptually and computationally simple, it requires that additional screws are placed in bone for their attachment, typically several days before surgery, causing inconvenience and increasing the risk of infection, and whenever possible this method is being replaced with alternative methods.

Shape based registration is one of the alternatives to fiducial registration, in which the shape of the part of the bone surface is measured intra-operatively and matched to the surface model developed from the CT scan. Intra-operative shape measurement of the bone surface can be done by a tracked point probe, an ultrasound probe or a laser range scanner. If the point probe is used, coordinates of a discrete set of points (point cloud) on the bone surface are acquired. Registration is achieved by minimizing the distance between the perturbed point cloud and the surface model of the bone (**Fig. 2.5).

Ultrasound registration is based on measuring the bone surface profiles with an ultrasonic probe and it is a promising alternative [1], especially for less and minimally invasive applications, where the bone surface exposure is not sufficient to acquire a widely distributed cloud of points. Some CAS applications use intra-operative imaging for navigation, and with the tracking markers are inserted before the image is acquired, can avoid the need for the explicit registration.

Navigation

Once the tracking is established and the registration is performed, the surgeon can learn at any time what is the position of tracked surgical tools relative to the target bones, and how does it compare to the planned one. The computer interfaces then enable the surgeon to interactively reposition the tools in order to match the planned positions and trajectories and in effect assist them in navigating the patient's anatomy. Typical interfaces show the tools' current position in the cross sections through the patient's image, or as a three-dimensional view from the chosen point of view. Simple interfaces similar to those used by airplane pilots guide the surgeon to desired tool alignment.

In HipNav surgery, one tracking marker is attached to the iliac wing of the pelvis through a small incision and the other markers are attached to the cup placement tool and the pointing probe, respectively. Shape based registration is performed by collecting coordinates of 46 points through the incision and percutaneously at the iliac spine using the pointing probe and by matching those points to the surface model of the pelvis. Once the registration is completed (typically 1–2 min), the pelvis can be tracked in real-time. The current orientation of the cup alignment tool is compared against the planned one and displayed as a simple cross hair interface, that allows the surgeon to interactively align the tool in accordance with the pre-operatively planned alignment. ■ Figure 2.6d shows the navigation interface for cup tool alignment in HipNav. Two circles with crosses represent the opposite ends of the tool axis. The cup guide is aligned in the pre-operatively planned position when the circles' centers coincide.

Intra-operative Feedback

It is important to provide the surgeons with the feedback on their actions. In orthopaedic procedures, this providing updated images ranges from showing relative positions of tools and bones, bone images modified for the cuts that are made. This also means that the relevant updates, such as updated range of motion or the measurements of stress in bone, can be provided. Some of this information is simply geometry updates and some require more elaborate and complex measurements.

The amount of information available to surgeons in the OR can already be overwhelming and is going to increase even more with increased sophistication and complexity of computer assisted procedures. One of the goals of application developers is to make this information

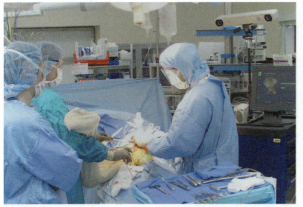
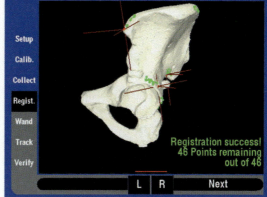
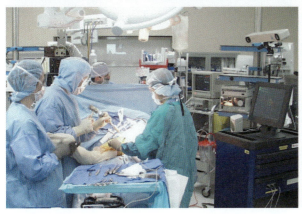
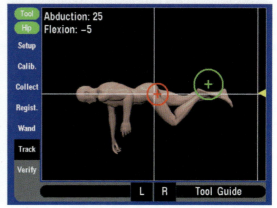

■ **Fig. 2.6a–d.** Characteristic steps of HipNav surgery: Collection of registration points (optical localizer is in the top right), point cloud and a surface model of the pelvis after registration; the surgeon is inserting the acetabular cup implant; navigation interface during cup insertion (© CASurgica, Inc.)

easier to comprehend. This is achieved by prioritizing and simplifying the information, by using visual means wherever possible, making it intuitive and logical and by not diverting the surgeons attention from the main task. With the increased emphasis on minimally invasive procedures, it is important to find the ways to replace direct vision with surrogates that enable confident navigation. Supplemental information can be brought into surgeon's field of view by using »hybrid reality« devices that can combine display information with the real view of the operating field. Head-mounted display can provide surgeon with vital statistics, relevant patient pre-operative information and images while they look at the operating field. The remaining problems with these devices are the additional weight that is carried on surgeon's head throughout the surgery and the need to focus at two different planes at the same time, which can cause headache. Devices such as Image Overlay [2] can eliminate both concerns by independently supporting the display system and placing the virtual image in the same plane with the real image.

Discussion

CT-based navigation procedures can improve the ways surgery is planned and performed by increasing the accuracy and reducing the invasiveness of those procedures. They hold the promise to improve the patient outcomes and permanently change the way many surgical procedures are done today.

Because of the cost of CT scan, additional effort for image segmentation and intra-operative registration, image-free (Aesculap AG, Tuttlingen, Germany) and fluoroscopic (Medivision, Oberdorf, Switzerland) procedures have been developed as alternative surgical navigation approaches. Recently, fluoroscopy has been used to create intra-operative 3D images similar to CT scans (Siremobil – Siemens Medical, Germany). This method combines the advantages of three-dimensional CT scan with the reduced cost of imaging and eliminated need for registration, since the images are acquired after the bone tracking is initiated.

However, new developments that eliminate the need of manual processing of the CT data, improvement in the imaging speed, and the overall trend in medical imaging to make CT scanners widely available and less expensive, combined with the superb performance, ability to provide the best guidance interface, amount of information and its

performance in minimally invasive procedures will ensure that CT-based procedures will have a place it deserves in the CAS family in the future.

References

1. Amin DV, Kanade T, DiGioia AM III, Jaramaz B, Nikou C, LaBarca RS (2001) Ultrasound based registration of the pelvic bone surface for surgical navigation. 1st Annual Meeting, International Society for Computer Assisted Orthopaedic Surgery (CAOS-International), Davos, Switzerland
2. Blackwell M, Morgan F, DiGioia A (1998) Augmented reality and its future in orthopaedics. Clin Orthop Rel Res 345: 111–122
3. DiGioia AM III, Jaramaz B, Nikou C, LaBarca RS, Moody JE, Colgan B (2000) Surgical navigation for total hip replacement with the use of HipNav. Oper Tech Orthop 10:3–8
4. Nikou C, Jaramaz B, DiGioia AM III, Levison TJ (2000) Description of anatomic coordinate systems and rationale for use in an image-guided total hip replacement system. In: Delp, DiGioia, Jaramaz (eds) Medical image computing and computer assisted intervention – MICAI 2000. Springer, Berlin Heidelberg New York Tokyo, pp 1188–1194

C-Arm-Based Navigation

A. Hebecker

Concepts of Image-Based Surgical Navigation

The common feature of CT- and C-arm-based surgical navigation is the coupling of the medical image and the surgical action: The surgeon sees the instrument displayed as a virtual instrument in the medical image in real time. This is achieved by using surgical instruments equipped with infrared (IR) LEDs (active markers) or with reflecting spheres (passive markers), enabling the instrument to be »seen« by a camera.

The terms *CT-* or *C-arm-based navigation* indicate the origin of the medical images and until recently have been used as synonyms for navigation on *3D image data with manual registration* or on *2D projection images without*

manual registration. However, in order to simplify differentiation between the concepts of image-based navigation after the introduction of the isocentric 3D C-arm SIREMOBIL Iso-C^{3D} and its successor ARCADIS Orbic 3D (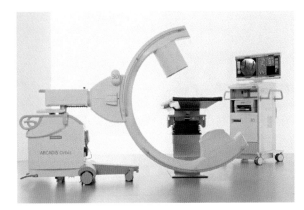 Fig. 3.1) it is more helpful to refer only to *navigation with manual registration* as opposed to *navigation without manual registration* or *direct navigation*, and then to differentiate between 2D and 3D navigation in that context (□ Table 3.1).

These two concepts of image-based surgical navigation can be described as follows:

Navigation with Manual Registration. Navigation on 3D image data sets, for example on CT data acquired pre-operatively or on 3D data acquired intra-operatively by the ARCADIS Orbic 3D C-arm. The individual steps in the workflow are as follows:

Step 1: (*Image transfer*): The medical images are loaded onto the navigation computer via a network or from portable data media.

□ Fig. 3.1. ARCADIS Orbic 3D: an isocentric mobile C-arm for intra-operative two- and three-dimensional imaging

□ Table 3.1. Overview of the concepts of image-based surgical navigation

	With manual registration	Without manual registration
2D navigation	–	ARCADIS Orbic 3D, conventional C-arms
3D navigation	ARCADIS Orbic 3D, CT	ARCADIS Orbic 3D

Step 2: (*Tracking*): The surgical instruments are fitted with active or passive markers and are tracked by a camera.

Step 3: (*Referencing*): An active or passive reference marker is attached to the patient in the OR. This is to allow automatic detection of and compensation for relative movements of the patient and the camera.

Step 4: (*Registration*): Correlation between the patient and the image is established by defining certain prominent points in the image and assigning them to corresponding points on the patient using a tracked device referred to as the pointer. There are two different methods: one is paired-point matching, involving a small number of correlation points, and the other is surface matching, which is more exact and involves a greater number of points. In paired-point matching the correlation points on the patient can either be unique anatomical points or markers applied either pre-operatively or intra-operatively, known as fiducial markers.

Step 5: (*Navigation*): The surgical instrument is displayed as a virtual instrument (as an animated object) in the medical images in real time.

Navigation Without Manual Registration/Direct Navigation.

Navigation on one or more C-arm 2D projection images acquired intra-operatively or on intra-operatively acquired 3D image data sets from the ARCADIS Orbic 3D C-arm. This simplifies the workflow compared to navigation with manual registration, and the surgical intervention can be carried out as a less invasive procedure:

Step 1: (*Tracking*): The surgical instruments are fitted with active or passive markers and are tracked by a camera.

Step 2: (*Referencing*): A reference marker is attached to the patient in the OR. This is to allow automatic detection of and compensation for relative movements of the patient and the camera.

Step 3: (*Image acquisition and transfer*): Images are taken using the C-arm and loaded into the navigation computer. For this purpose the C-arm is equipped with active or passive markers and is tracked by the camera during image acquisition. This means that there is no need for manual registration.

Step 4: (*Navigation*): The surgical instrument is displayed as a virtual instrument (as an animated object) in the medical images in real time.

Direct Navigation in Two-Dimensional Projection Images

A common feature of both techniques of direct navigation, i.e. 2D and 3D navigation, is that the navigation system's camera tracks not only the surgical instrument but also the C-arm representing the imaging system.

In direct 2D-navigation a device with the following functions is attached to the image intensifier of the C-arm (◘ Fig. 3.2):

- Making the C-arm visible to the navigation system: The attachment is fitted with either active or passive markers. This enables the navigation system's camera to detect the position of the C-arm from which an X-ray image is being taken. Through the use of calibration, the location and the relative position of the projection image are therefore known.

- Compensating for image distortion in the image intensifier: The electron optics and the earth's magnetic field causes images to be distorted in 2D projections. The magnitude of these distortions is determined using a metal marker plate in front of the input window of the image intensifier. Compensation is performed by software.

- Online or offline calibration of the mechanical twisting of the C-arm: Calibration is necessary because the C-arm is subject to mechanical twisting in different

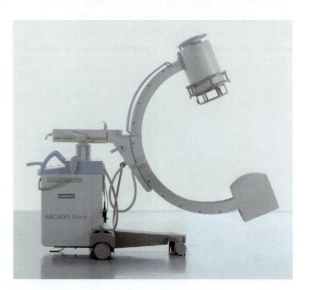

◘ **Fig. 3.2.** Conventional C-arm with navigation attachment for direct 2D navigation ways depending on its position. This intrinsic movement of the C-arm is measured with the help of a two-plate attachment to the image intensifier either intra-operatively during image acquisition (online calibration) or once only during installation of the navigation system on the C-arm (offline calibration) and is taken into account in the software. With the given reproducibility of the twisting, the advantage of offline calibration is that the distance between the patient and the image intensifier is hardly reduced during surgery. In this case, only the metal marker plate that compensates for the image distortion in the image intensifier is used intra-operatively.

Direct 2D navigation can be carried out with both isocentric and non-isocentric C-arms.

Direct Navigation in Three-Dimensional Image Data

Direct 3D navigation is based on intra-operative 3D imaging with an isocentric mobile C-arm and on automatic correlation between the region of interest (ROI) in the patient and the corresponding 3D image data set by the navigation system.

3D Imaging with an Isocentric Mobile C-Arm

ARCADIS Orbic 3D makes 3D imaging possible as a result of its isocentric design and 190° orbital motion supported by its hidden cable routing. In contrast with non-isocentric C-arms, the central beam always crosses the center of rotation of the C-arm, irrespective of the orbital angle (◘ Fig. 3.3). This means that the ROI always remains in the cone angle, regardless of the current projection angle, allowing a 3D image data set to be generated around the isocenter.

During 3D operation of the C-arm a defined number of 2D projection images are acquired at fixed angular intervals during a continuous motorized orbital rotation through 190°. Simultaneously a high-resolution 3D data cube with an edge length of approximately 12 cm and an isotropic spatial resolution of around 0.5 mm is reconstructed on the basis of these projection images. As soon as the rotation is completed, the reconstructed 3D data cube can be used to produce any required multiplanar

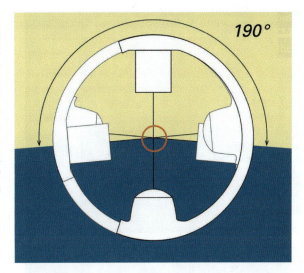

◘ **Fig. 3.3.** The isocentric mobile C-arm ARCADIS Orbic 3D is automatically rotated through 190° for intra-operative 3D image acquisition. The central beam always crosses the isocenter of the C-arm during the orbital movement

reconstructions (MPR) in real time at the monitor trolley (◘ Fig. 3.4).

The field of application for ARCADIS Orbic 3D has so far been limited to high-contrast objects such as bones and joints because of the lack of soft tissue differentiation, as with CT.

Automatic Registration

During installation of the navigation system, the correlation between the 3D reconstruction volume and a special reference point on the C-arm is determined in an offline calibration procedure. The reference point can be located by the navigation system's camera because there is a fixed correlation between this point and the active or passive markers on a marker ring attached to the C-arm.

During 3D image acquisition the navigation system's camera detects the position of the reference point with the aid of the marker ring. Because of the measurements taken during offline calibration, the navigation system's computer immediately knows the position and orientation of the 3D data cube in the OR. The position of the surgical instrument – which is tracked by the same camera during the surgical procedure – can therefore be

3

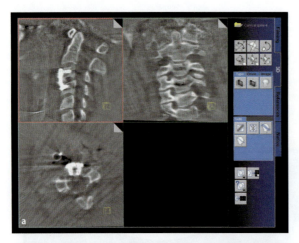

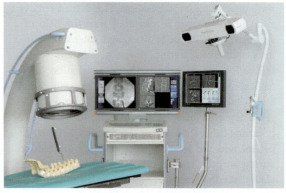

Fig. 3.5. Direct 3D navigation with ARCADIS Orbic 3D: The C-arm is fitted with a marker ring, so that its position can be detected during 3D image acquisition by the navigation system's camera. The position of the surgical instrument is detected during surgery by the same camera. On the navigation monitor the instrument is displayed in real-time as a virtual object in 3 MPRs of the reconstructed 3D image data set

displayed in real-time as a virtual object in the 3D image data set without manual registration (Fig. 3.5).

The solution for this automatic registration described here follows the approach of an open interface, which means that fundamentally it can be implemented by all manufacturers of navigation systems. Under simulated clinical conditions, i.e. if movements of the C-arm and the camera system are allowed, an overall accuracy of less than 2 mm is achieved for the surgical intervention [16].

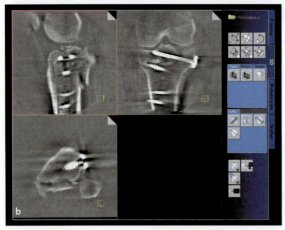

Advantages of Direct Navigation

The biggest advantage of direct 2D and 3D navigation is that the surgical instrument can be displayed in the intra-operatively acquired image data immediately, i.e. without the time-consuming and error-prone manual registration procedure. The underlying principle can be expressed as »shoot and navigate«. In addition, the large surgical incisions necessary for manual registration can be avoided, which means that direct navigation supports minimally invasive surgery to a considerable extent. And as the C-arm is used in the OR, the image acquisition for the navigation procedure can be repeated as often as required, e.g. after repositioning of bone fragments.

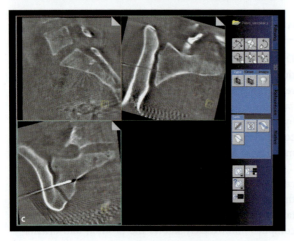

Fig. 3.4a–c. Examples of the presentation of the 3D image data set, acquired with ARCADIS Orbic 3D, in three MPRs: Screw osteosynthesis of a cervical spine (**a**), a tibia (**b**) and a pelvis (**c**)

For the sake of completeness it is worth mentioning some other advantages of navigation based on the use of the C-arm in the OR:

- Increased accuracy of the surgical intervention. 2D navigation achieves this by displaying the surgical instruments in several projection images at the same time (for example A-P and lateral), while 3D navigation does so by providing up-to-date 3D information during the operation with less registration errors that might otherwise occur. Any required sectional image can be freely selected from within the 3D data cube for the purposes of navigation. In addition it is possible to display other views, such as axial images along the spine which cannot be generated using projection techniques.
- Removal of the C-arm after image acquisition. This allows better use of the available space and reduces the risk of the spread of infection during the surgical procedure.
- Continuous display of the surgical instrument in the stored image. Additional X-ray radiation from the C-arm can therefore be avoided.
- Considerable reduction in radiation exposure compared to the conventional technique. The most pronounced decrease in the emission of ionizing radiation can be achieved with direct 3D navigation [8].

Indications for Direct Navigation

So far, compared to the conventional method, the use of navigation systems based on pre-operatively produced CT image data has already resulted in a considerable reduction in the number of positioning errors occurring when inserting pedicle screws to stabilize fractures of the spine [14]. However, situations can arise where the position of the bones relative to each other during the surgical intervention is no longer the same as the position shown in the pre-operative CT, for example as a result of repositioning of the patient on the operating table or because of the surgical procedure [6, 9]. Another important factor causing irregularities is the manual registration procedure. These problems can be avoided by using direct 2D navigation [15] or direct 3D navigation [10].

The indications for which the direct navigation technique is predestined arise from its advantages. In general, direct navigation is always helpful in positioning guide wires, screws and implants accurately and quickly in a minimally invasive intervention. This is achieved by displaying images in different projections simultaneously (e.g. A-P and lateral), or by generating 3D image data sets

during the surgical procedure. Although the distinction proposed below will doubtlessly not apply in all case, it is possible to distinguish between typical indications for direct 2D navigation on the one hand and 3D navigation on the other. This distinction follows the principle of choosing the easiest way to acquire the required information. Typical indications for direct 2D navigation:

- Long bones: Insertion of intramedullary nails including distal locking [18, 19].
- Corrective osteotomy of long bones.
- Hip endoprosthetics, especially acetabulum and shaft navigation.
- Insertion of screws in the femoral neck [2].

Typical indications for direct 3D navigation:

- Fractures which include the joint region: upper and lower limbs (elbow, distal radius, scaphoid bone, knee, distal tibia, calcaneus, talus, etc.), and acetabulum [10].
- Spine: positioning of pedicle screws in the lumbar and thoracic spine, cervical spine fixation, e.g. from C1 to C2 [1, 10, 12].
- Pelvis: fractures, insertion of screws in the iliosacral region, osteotomies [10].

However, especially when checking the position of dislocated fragments and of implants (for example bone plates and screws for osteosynthesis) and also during reconstruction of joint surfaces, simply using ARCADIS Orbic 3D for intra-operative 3D imaging alone, i.e. without navigation, provides a considerable information gain and consequently results in higher quality and greater safety in the OR [4, 5, 11, 13, 17, 20, 21]. One crucial factor for the OR workflow is the possibility of using ARCADIS Orbic 3D both in conventional 2D mode and in 3D mode without reducing access to the patient, which would require additional logistical efforts. When performing a repositioning of bone fragments of this nature without navigation, the workflow can be outlined as follows [3]:

1. 2D mode: repositioning of bone fragments and preliminary fixation with Kirschner's wire.
2. 3D mode (»preliminary scan«): checking of position in the 3D reconstruction.
3. 2D mode: definitive osteosynthesis.
4. 3D mode (»definitive scan«): final 3D reconstruction. This avoids the need for a post-operative CT and avoids a follow-up operation in the event of fragments or implants being incorrectly positioned.

As mentioned earlier, the use of intra-operative direct 3D navigation enables navigation to be carried out in a current 3D image data set, for example in order to proceed with an a.m. osteosynthesis procedure accurately and quickly after repositioning of the bone fragments is completed. It is even feasible that the use of image segmentation will in future support the navigated repositioning of bone fragments as well.

Conclusion and Outlook

The use of direct 3D navigation with ARCADIS Orbic 3D allows surgeons to move a vital step closer to their real aim, which is to perform minimally invasive interventions accurately and speedily with online visualization of their instruments in always updated 3D image data of the patient.

In contrast with CT-based navigation – which relies on 3D image data obtained pre-operatively – ARCADIS Orbic 3D enables the 3D data cube to be updated repeatedly during the operation, without manual registration and hence with the minimum of invasive interventions. While it is true that CT and MRI units have recently found their way into operating theaters, with the result that updated intra-operative images are also available for navigation from these devices, the effort and expenditure is typically much higher.

Until recently, working without manual registration has only been possible when using C-arm-based 2D navigation on projection images – with the associated effect that the images have a relatively low information content.

In future the use of image fusion during the surgical intervention will lead to new application opportunities. New technologies, such as the use of flat-panel detectors, may widen the scope of use of mobile C-arms, especially with respect to the differentiation of soft tissue which will then be possible. A virtual intra-operative »view inside the bones and joints« [7] is finally entering the realm of the feasible.

References

1. Arand M, Hartwig E, Hebold D, Kinzl L, Gebhard F (2001) Präzisionsanalyse navigationsgestützt implantierter thorakaler und lumbaler Pedikelschrauben. Unfallchirurg 104: 1076–1081
2. Arand M, Schempf M, Kinzl L, Fleiter T, Pless D, Gebhard F (2001) Präzision standardisierter Iso-C-Arm-basierter navigierter Bohrungen am proximalen Femur. Unfallchirurg 104: 1150–1156
3. Euler E, Heining S, Fischer T, Pfeiffer KJ, Mutschler W (2002) Initial clinical experiences with the SIREMOBIL Iso-C3D. electromedica 70: 64–67
4. Euler E, Wirth S, Pfeifer KJ, Mutschler W, Hebecker A (2000) 3D-Imaging with an Isocentric Mobile C-Arm. electromedica 68: 122–126
5. Euler E, Wirth S, Linsenmaier U, Mutschler W, Pfeifer KJ, Hebecker A (2001) Vergleichende Untersuchung zur Qualität C-Bogen-basierter 3D-Bildgebung am Talus. Unfallchirurg 104: 839–846
6. Gebhard F, Kinzl L, Arand M (2000) Grenzen der CT-basierten Computernavigation in der Wirbelsäulenchirurgie. Unfallchirurg 103: 696–701
7. Gebhard F, Arand M, Fleiter T et al. (2001) Computer assistierte Chirurgie, Entwicklung und Perspektiven 2001. Orthopäde 30: 666–671
8. Gebhard F, Kraus M, Schneider E, Arand M, Kinzl L, Hebecker A, Bätz L (2003) Strahlendosis im OP – ein Vergleich computerassistierter Verfahren. Unfallchirurg 106: 492–497
9. Grützner PA, Vock B, Köhler T, Wentzensen A (2002) Rechnergestütztes Arbeiten an der Wirbelsäule. OP Journal 17: 185–190
10. Grützner PA, Wälti H, Vock B, Hebecker A, Nolte LP, Wentzensen A (2004) Navigation using fluoro-CT technology. Eur J Trauma 30: 161–70
11. Heiland M, Schmelzle R, Hebecker A, Schulze D (2004) Intraoperative 3D imaging of the facial skeleton using the SIREMOBIL Iso-C3D. Dentomaxillofacial Radiology 33: 130–132
12. Kandziora F, Stöckle U, König B, Khodadadyan-Klostermann C, Mittlmeier Th, Haas NP (2001) C-Bogen-Navigation zur transoralen atlantoaxialen Schraubenplatzierung. Chirurg 72: 593–599
13. Kotsianos D, Rock C, Euler E, Wirth S, Linsenmaier U, Brandl R, Mutschler W, Pfeifer KJ (2001) 3D-Bildgebung an einem mobilen chirurgischen Bildverstärker (Iso-C-3D): Erste Bildbeispiele zur Fracturdiagnostik an peripheren Gelenken im Vergleich mit Spiral-CT und konventioneller Radiologie. Unfallchirurg 104: 834–838
14. Laine T, Lund T, Ylikoski M, Lohikoski J, Schlenzka D (2000) Accuracy of pedicle screw insertion with and without computer assistance: A randomised controlled clinical study in 100 consecutive patients. Eur Spine J 9: 235–240
15. Nolte LP, Slomczykowski MA, Berlemann U, Strauss MJ, Hofstetter R, Schlenzka D, Laine T, Lund T (2000) A new approach to computer-aided spine surgery: fluoroscopy-based surgical navigation. EuroSpine J 9: 78–88
16. Ritter D, Mitschke M, Graumann R (2002) Markerless navigation with the intra-operative imaging modality SIREMOBIL Iso-C3D. electromedica 70: 47–52
17. Rock C, Linsenmaier U, Brandl R, Kotsianos D, Wirth S, Kaltschmidt R, Euler E, Mutschler W, Pfeifer KJ (2001) Vorstellung eines neuen mobilen C-Bogen-/CT-Kombinationsgerätes (Iso-C-3D): Erste Ergebnisse der 3D-Schnittbildgebung. Unfallchirurg 104: 827–833
18. Suhm N (2001) Intraoperative accuracy evaluation of virtual fluoroscopy – a method for application in computer-assisted distal locking. Comp Aid Surg 6: 221–224
19. Suhm N, Jacob AL, Nolte LP, Regazzoni P, Messmer P (2000) Surgical navigation based on fluoroscopy – clinical application for computer-assisted distal locking of intramedullary implants. Comp Aid Surg 5: 391–400
20. Wich M, Spranger N, Ekkernkamp A (2004) Intraoperative Bildgebung mit dem Iso-C3D. Chirurg 75: 982–987
21. Rübberdt A, Feil R, Stengel D, Spranger N, Mutze S, Wich M, Ekkernkamp A (2006) Die klinische Wertigkeit des Iso-C3D bei der Osteosynthese des Fersenbeins. Unfallchirurg 109: 112–118

CT-Free-Based Total Knee Arthroplasty Navigation with a Minimally Invasive Surgical Technique

S.D. Stulberg

Introduction

Computer-assisted surgery (CAS) is beginning to emerge as one of the most important technologies in orthopaedic surgery. Many of the initial applications of this technology have focused on adult reconstructive surgery of the knee. The value of CAS in TKA has been established in many studies. Minimally invasive surgical (MIS) techniques for performing TKA are also receiving extensive and intensive attention. The goals of this chapter are to 1) present the rationale for the use of image-free CAS in knee surgery; 2) describe the hardware and software components of image-free CAS systems; 3) explain the rationale for combining CAS with MIS techniques and, 4) illustrate a typical CAS-MIS surgical technique; 5) summarize the early results with this technique.

Rationale for the Use of Computer-Assisted Surgery in Knee Reconstruction

A successful surgical reconstruction of the knee requires proper patient selection, appropriate peri-operative management, correct implant selection and accurate surgical technique. The consequences of performing a knee reconstruction inaccurately have been well documented for total knee arthroplasties, uni-condylar arthroplasties, anterior cruciate ligament reconstructions and high tibial osteotomies [1, 2, 3, 6, 9, 15, 16, 20, 21, 25, 27, 29–31, 33, 34, 41, 54–56, 69, 70, 75, 76, 82–85, 91, 94, 106, 107, 109, 111, 112].

Although mechanical instrumentation has significantly increased the accuracy and reliability with which knee reconstructions are performed [28], errors in implant and limb alignment continue to occur, even when the procedures are performed by experienced surgeons. The accuracy with which these procedures are performed using manual instrumentation is dependent upon the knowledge and experience of the surgeon and the frequency with which the surgeon performs the procedures.

Computer-assisted surgical techniques have been developed to address the inherent limitations of mechanical instrumentation [11, 12, 17–19, 22–24, 37, 41–47, 51, 52, 57, 58, 61, 62, 67, 68, 74, 77, 79–81, 86, 89, 90, 97, 103–105, 108]. The goals of integrating CAS with knee reconstruction techniques are to increase the accuracy of these procedures and reduce the proportion of alignment outliers that occur when these procedures are performed [7, 10, 12, 35, 36, 38–40, 48, 49, 53, 63–66, 71–73, 78, 87, 88, 90, 92, 93, 95, 97, 99, 102, 113, 114].

Errors in the alignment of bone resection can occur at numerous points during the performance of a knee reconstruction (50, 101). The placement of the cutting blocks or ligament alignment jigs may be inaccurate. The attachment of these tools to bone may produce an error in their placement. The actual performance of the cut or drilling of the hole may be inaccurate (e.g. the saw blade may deflect). The final insertion of the implant may be inaccurate. Mechanical instrumentation does not provide a method for checking the accuracy of each of these steps of a knee reconstructive procedure. Integrating CAS with knee reconstruction allows the surgeon with a means of placing cutting blocks accurately and measuring the accuracy with which each step of the procedure is performed. During the performance of an MIS-TKA, visualization of each step of the procedure is difficult. Therefore, the ability to measure each step of the TKA procedure using CAS may be particularly important for MIS TKA (50, 98, 101, 110).

The goal of knee reconstructive procedures is to align limbs and implants correctly. They also seek to restore appropriate kinematic relationships and ligamentous stability to the knee (8, 48, 96). Mechanical instrumentation can not measure the precision with which knee kinematics and ligament stability is restored. CAS techniques make it possible to determine the pre-surgical kinematic relationships and ligamentous stability of the knee and help guide the surgeon restore the desired kinematic relationships and ligamentous balance.

Hardware and Software Requirements for Surgical Navigation

A detailed description of the hardware and software needed to perform computer-assisted reconstructive knee surgery is beyond the scope of this chapter. However, it is important that knee surgeons understand the basic components of a computer-assisted orthopaedic system so that they can use the system correctly, safely and efficiently and so that they can make intelligent choices regarding the appropriateness of various systems for their surgical needs.

The hardware devices common to CAS systems are: 1) imaging devices; 2) computers and the peripherals and interfaces to allow them to function in the operating room; and 3) localizers and trackers (◘ Fig. 4.1).

The imaging devices that are currently available for use with computer-assisted orthopaedic surgery systems include computed tomography (CT), magnetic resonance imaging, (MRI), and fluoroscopy (4, 5, 22, 60, 67, 71–73, 79, 81). These devices are used to acquire anatomical information upon which a pre-surgical or intra-operative surgical plan is made. This plan becomes the basis for placing cutting tools intra-operatively and for establishing the alignment and stability of the knee. Although potentially extremely useful for knee reconstruction surgery, especially for robotic or customized surgery, imaging devices as currently employed with CAS knee systems have been perceived by surgeons as requiring additional and cumbersome steps to well-established knee procedures without providing significant benefits. Consequently, **image-free**

computer-assisted systems have emerged as the most desired form of CAS for knee reconstruction. As a result, the role of imaging when **image-free** CAS systems are used remains largely identical to its role when CAS is not used. Imaging is used pre-operatively to develop a plan (e.g. applying a goniometer on a long-standing anterior-posterior X-ray to determine desired frontal alignment) and is used post-operatively to assess the results of the procedure.

The computers used in CAS are obviously the core of these systems. They integrate information from medical images, implant data, intra-operative tracking and surgical plans to guide the surgeon in the performance of a knee procedure. The speed of computing, memory, storage capacity and communication ability with peripherals have reached a level where even mid-range, less expensive personal computers can satisfy the needs of image-free CAS knee applications. All current CAS knee applications use a range of platforms based usually on either UNIX or Windows operating systems. It is likely that applications will soon be written on the open Linux operating system. The computers are currently mounted on transportable carts (or operating room booms) that include the computer, monitor, key board, mouse, power transformer and isolation unit and tracker controller unit with ports to plug in the tracker and tracking markers. Communication between the surgeon and computer is necessary for the continuous monitoring of the procedure. This communication can be achieved with single or double foot pedals, keypads, touch screens, pointer integrated controls or voice-activated controls (◘ Fig. 4.1a).

A CAS knee-navigation system can be thought of as an aiming device that enables real-time visualization of surgical action with an image of the operated structures. In order for this navigation to occur, it is necessary that the position and orientation of an instrument be visualized with respect to the anatomical structures to which it is attached. Although this objective could be met by attaching tools to a rigid, multi-linked arm attached to a pedestal, such a device would be unsuitable for knee surgery, where the limb must be freely moved. Therefore, contactless systems are used to communicate between the extremity and the computer system. Information can be transmitted using infra-red light, electro-magnetic fields or ultrasound. Each method has its advantages and drawbacks. All of these methods allow several objects (e.g. 2 bones) to be viewed simultaneously.

Optical localization using infra-red light is currently the most widely used method of communication between

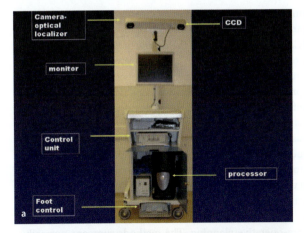

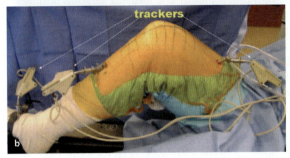

◻ **Fig. 4.1.** A typical image-free computer assisted hardware system consisting of an optical tracker with charged coupled devices (the »cameras«), a computer monitor, control unit and processor, and a foot control system for communication between surgeon and the system. Active trackers (also called rigid bodies or fiducials) attached to bicortical screws rigidly fixed to the femur and tibia

the operated extremity and computer. Two types of optical tracking are used, active or passive. Systems utilizing active tracking use markers (also called trackers or rigid bodies) that have light emitting diodes (LED) which send out light pulses to a camera (optical localizer). Three or (for redundancy) more of these LEDs are attached to screws or wires which are rigidly attached to the femur and tibia. The camera system to which the light is sent consists of 2 planar or 3 linear charge couples devices (CCD) that are rigidly mounted onto a solid housing (The Polaris system, Northern Digital, is a commonly used camera system). Passive systems use reflecting spheres that are placed on tracking markers that are attached to screws or pins rigidly implanted in the femur and tibia. Infra-red flashes sent by LED arrays on the camera housing illuminate the spheres. The 2 planar or 3 linear charged couple devices (CCDs) observe the reflections and interpolate the spatial location of each light source. It is important for surgeons and their staffs to realize that the arrays on the tracking markers, whether active or passive, are specific to each CAS system. One company's trackers can not be used on another companies CAS system, even though the trackers may appear to be similar (◻ Fig. 4.1).

The advantages of optical localizing systems are that they are reliable, flexible, and highly accurate and have good operating room compatibility. A disadvantage of these systems is that it is necessary to provide free line of sight between the LED/spheres and the CCD arrays on the camera (optical localizer). Active trackers may require cables in order to power and synchronize the LED's. These cables may be cumbersome. Active trackers can be driven by batteries which eliminate the need for cables. These require recharging, making their use for sequential procedures more difficult. Passive trackers do not require cords. However, automatic tool identification is more difficult for passive systems, because all spheres in view reflect the light flashes equally. A unique identification of each tracker is possible with the sequentially pulsed LED's of the active trackers. The reflecting spheres must constantly be kept clean to obtain accurate signal transmission. Moreover, the spheres are disposable and, therefore, a source of additional per-case expense.

Magnetic fields can be used to measure the position and orientation of objects in space. A generator coil is used to erect a homogeneous magnetic field. Specially designed »coils« can be implanted into the femur and tibia or attached to tools. These »coils« measure the changes in magnetic field characteristics during the performance of the procedure. The computer can integrate these changes with the implant data and surgical plans to guide the surgeon in the performance of a knee procedure. There are a number of potential advantages of these systems. The equipment (»coils«) attached to the bones and tools can be small. The accuracy of many systems is very good. The need for a camera and its associated »line of sight« requirement are eliminated. However, the presence of ferro-magnetic items such as implants, instruments and operating room equipment made of steel can disturb precise measurements dramatically and in *unpredictable* ways. Moreover, the »coils« are disposable and, therefore, a source of additional per-case expense.

The function of software in CAS systems is to integrate medical images and mathematical algorithms with surgi-

4

cal tools and surgical techniques [19, 22, 24]. A relatively small number of software components underlie most CAS image-free systems. These components include: registration, navigation, procedure guidance and safety.

Image- free CAS knee systems use as their pre-operative plan concepts of limb and implant alignment that are currently used with manual instrumentation (e.g. restoration of the mechanical axis). In order to accomplish this plan, anatomic and kinematic information about a patient must be transmitted to the software on the computer and geometrically transformed using registration algorithms. Because bones are rigid and assumed unlikely to deform during the procedure, the algorithms used are termed *rigid*. These algorithms also require that the trackers attached to bones do not move during the procedure. Fiducial-based registration is a type of rigid registration. Therefore, the objects to which the LED's are attached may be referred to as fiducials, trackers or rigid bodies. Fiducial registration requires that at least three sets of markers be implanted into each bone or attached to each tool to determine the object's position and orientation. Therefore, each tracker must have at least 3 LED's or reflecting spheres. Some CAS knee systems currently use shaped-based registration as an alternative to fiducial based registration. These systems measure the shape of the bone surface intra-operatively and match the acquired shape to a surface model created from medical images and stored in the computer. The registration process for image-free knee navigation systems requires that information be acquired using kinematic techniques (e.g. circumducting the leg to determine the center of the femoral head) and/or surface registration techniques (e.g. touching bone landmarks with a probe).

Once the software takes anatomic and kinematic input from the extremity and geometrically transforms it, the surgeon is presented with a user interface that depicts in sequence the steps of the knee procedure. One of the most important objectives of software development in CAS knee surgery is to depict procedure sequences that are familiar to surgeons and with which they have become comfortable using manual instrumentation.

Example of an Image-Free, Minimally Invasive CAS Surgical Technique for TKA

Computer-assisted surgical technologies require that surgeons incorporate new tools into surgical routines with which they are experienced and comfortable. In fact, the most successful application of CAS occurs when surgeons are very familiar with all aspects of the procedure in which CAS is used. Although the details of the CAS application for one knee procedure (e.g. TKA) vary from those of another knee procedure (e.g. ACL reconstruction), the basic principles and intra-operative steps are very similar for all of them. Because the TKA image-free CAS application is currently the most rapidly developing and most widely used, a brief description of a typical CAS-MIS-TKA will be described [32, 103, 104]. It is important for surgeons to understand that the goal of CAS is to increase the accuracy and reproducibility with which the objectives of current mechanical alignment systems are achieved.

Image-free CAS techniques do not require any special pre-operative planning. The methods surgeons normally use to determine desired frontal and sagittal limb and implant alignment and implant sizes can be used to guide the intra-operative use of the CAS system. Mechanical alignment and CAS techniques use similar approaches for patient positioning and surgical exposure. Leg holders and pneumatic tourniquets which are routinely used with mechanical instrumentation can also be used with CAS.

The initial step in a TKA using CAS is the placement of the screws or pins in the distal femur and proximal tibia to which are attached the trackers (◘ Fig. 4.1b). These are placed outside of the skin incision in a position that avoids injury to neurovascular structures and allows clear visualization of the trackers by the camera. Once the skin incision is made and the distal femur and proximal tibia are exposed, the anatomic landmarks critical for CAS guided navigation are located. The center of the femoral head is determined using a kinematic registration technique (◘ Fig. 4.2a,b). The hip is circumducted in a path guided by the visual cues displayed upon the computer screen. The centers of the knee and ankle joint can be established using kinematic (◘ Fig. 4.2c–f) or surface (◘ Fig. 4.3) registration techniques or a combination of both. The other anatomic landmarks located with a CAS probe are:

- the distal femur (◘ Fig. 4.3d,e);
- the posterior condylar line (◘ Fig. 4.3d,e);
- the anterior femoral cortex (◘ Fig. 4.3f);
- the epicondylar axis; and
- the medial and lateral tibial articular surfaces (◘ Fig. 4.3 g–i).

The pre-surgical frontal and sagittal alignment, medial-lateral laxity in flexion and extension, and range of motion can then be measured and recorded (◘ Fig. 4.4).

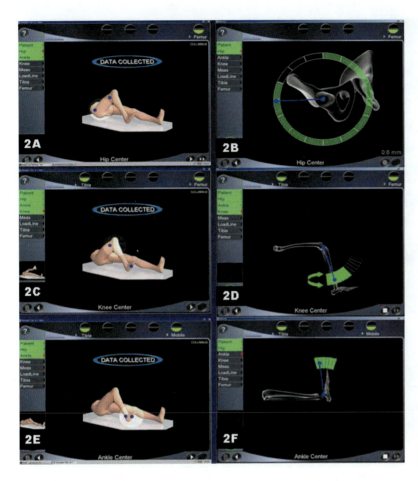

■ **Fig. 4.2a–f.** Computer interfaces illustrating motion necessary to acquire adequate kinematic information to establish location of center of: **a,b** hip joint, **c,d** knee joint, **e,f** ankle joint

Both ligament balancing techniques (similar to those first described by Insall [30]) and anatomic approaches [29] can be used with CAS TKA techniques. As with mechanically-based techniques, the CAS anatomic procedures can begin with either the femoral or tibial preparation. In the example illustrated, the distal femur is first resected by placing a distal femoral cutting block with an attached tracker on the anterior cortex of the femur. The proximal-distal, varus-valgus and flexion-extension position of this block are guided by the CAS system (■ Fig. 4.5). The CAS determination of femoral implant size and anterior-posterior placement can be made using either anterior or posterior referencing techniques. The rotation of the femoral component using CAS can be established using the posterior condylar line, the epicondylar line or the patellar groove (Whitesides' line). A single navigation tool can be used to establish all of these femoral alignment and sizing

objectives (■ Fig. 4.6). The tibial cutting block, to which a tracker is attached, is placed in the desired position of varus-valgus and flexion-extension and at the desired resection level guided by the CAS system (■ Fig. 4.7).

Once the femoral and tibial resections are completed, a trial reduction is carried out. The polyethylene insert that best balances the knee in flexion and extension is selected. The navigation system is used to measure the final alignment of the extremity, the amount of medial-lateral laxity in extension and flexion and the final range of motion. The system can be used to guide the release of tight soft tissues medially, laterally and posteriorly if this is necessary to establish a balanced, well-aligned knee. After the actual implants are inserted, the navigation system is used to measure the final frontal and sagittal alignment of the extremity, the final medial-lateral stability and final range of motion (■ Fig. 4.8).

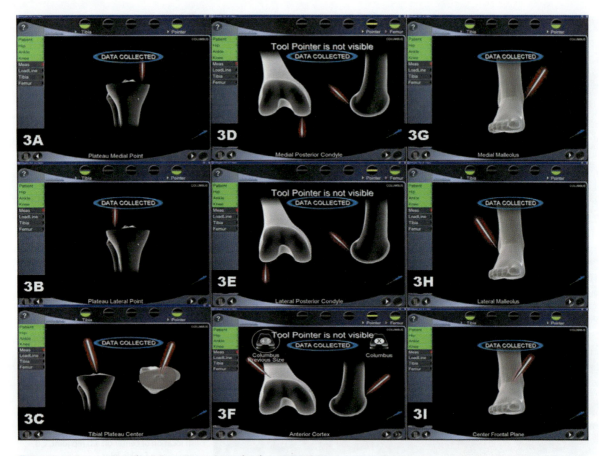

Fig. 4.3a–i. Computer interfaces illustrating position of surface registration pointer necessary to acquire: **a–c** tibial medial and lateral articular surfaces and tibial mid-point, **d,e** location of distal femoral articular surfaces and posterior condylar line, **f** location of anterior femoral cortex, **g–i** location of center of ankle joint

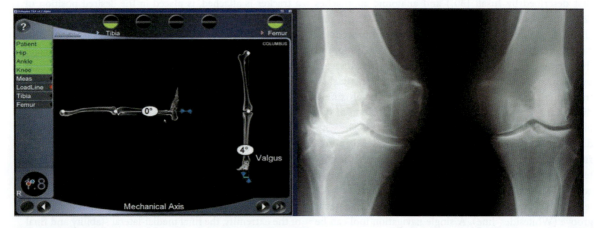

Fig. 4.4. Pre-surgical alignment depicted on computer screen correlates with alignment seen on standing pre-operative X-ray

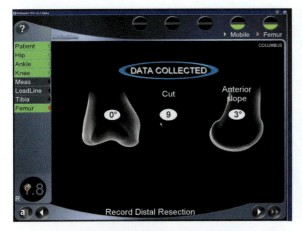

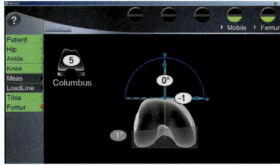

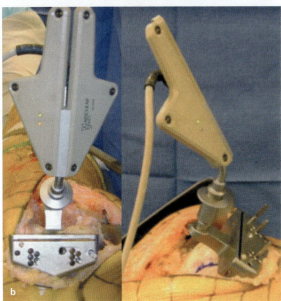

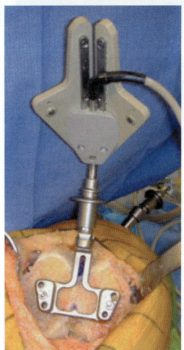

■ **Fig. 4.5a,b.** Resection of distal femur. **a** Computer interface indicating position of distal femoral cutting block with regard to frontal (0 degrees) and sagittal (3 degrees anterior slope) mechanical alignment and depth of resection (9 mm). **b** Frontal and sagittal position of distal femoral cutting block with attached tracker

■ **Fig. 4.6.** Establishing position of 4 in 1 femoral cutting block. Computer interface indicating rotation (0 degrees relative to Whitesides' line) of cutting block and anterior-posterior position of (in this case, the number 5) femoral component (1 mm above anterior cortex). Navigation tool with attached tracker to establish rotation and anterior-posterior position of 4 in 1 femoral cutting block

4

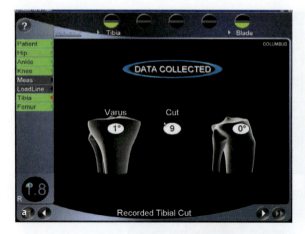

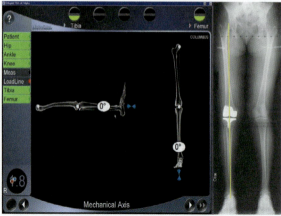

Fig. 4.8. Final frontal and sagittal alignment depicted on computer screen correlates with post-operative standing long x-ray

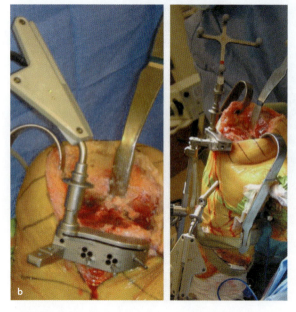

Fig. 4.7a,b. Resection of proximal tibia. **a** Computer interface indicating position of proximal tibial cutting block with regard to frontal (1 degree varus) and sagittal (0 degrees) mechanical alignment and depth of resection from least involved tibial surface (9 mm). **b** Frontal and sagittal position of proximal tibial cutting block with attached tracker

Clinical Results of CAS-MIS for Total Knee Arthroplasty

A prospective study was carried out to compare the effectiveness of CAS-MIS TKA with manually preformed MIS TKA.

Methods

Seventy-eight consecutive TKA were performed by a single surgeon with extensive prior experience in both manual and CAS TKA. Of the seventy-eight TKA, forty were performed with manual instruments and thirty-eight with CAS. The groups were identical with regard to age, sex, BMI, diagnosis, surgical technique, implants, and peri-operative management (◘ Table 4.1). Pre- and post-operative clinical examinations at four weeks, six months, and one year were performed by a physician blinded to the surgical techniques. Pre- and post-operative radiographic measurements of the anterior-posterior mechanical axis and the sagittal tibial and femoral axes were evaluated by an observer blinded to the surgical technique. The Knee Society scoring system was used to assess clinical and functional outcomes relating to measures of range of motion, pain, knee stability, patient mobility, and movement independence. Aesculap Columbus™ cruciate-retaining, condylar implants were used in each patient. The Aescu-

■ Table 4.1. Demographic data

		Unilateral Manual		Unilateral CAS		Total	
# Patients		40		38		78	
Age (years)	(Age range)	64.0	(25.1–87.5)	65.7	(48.0–86.1)	64.8	(25.1–87.5)
Sex (% Male)		43%		37%		40%	
Dx (% OA)		100%		100%		100%	
BMI Avg	(BMI range)	31.5	(19.6–54.8)	33.9	(23.9–44.2)	32.7	(19.6–54.8)
Pre-op Mechanical Axis Alignment	(Alignment Range) Varus (+) Valgus (–)	5.2	(–27–22)	8.9	(–12–20)	6.8	(–27–22)
Pre-op Knee Score	(Knee Score range)	48.1	(17–77)	44.5	(22–79)	46.3	(17–79)
Pre-op Function Score	(Function Score range)	56.7	(35–80)	50.4	(30–80)	53.6	(30–80)
Pre-op ROM	(ROM range)	113.7	(70–140)	112.1	(70–140)	112.9	(70–140)
Pre-op Pain Calculation	(Pain Calculation range)	12.8	(0–30)	12.0	(0–45)	12.4	(0–45)

lap OrthoPilot™ image-free navigation system was used for computer-assisted TKA. This system was selected based on its safety, reliability, and utility as an image-free navigation system. The use of the OrthoPilot for this study was approved by the Institutional Review Board of Northwestern University. The accuracy of the manual instruments used by the surgeon at the beginning of his CAS experience has been previously reported [102].

Results

Clinical and functional scores were not significantly different between MIS-CAS-TKA and manual MIS-TKA patients at one and six months post-operative (■ Table 4.2). The average change in clinical and functional scores from pre-operative to one and six months post-operative was also similar (■ Table 4.3). Pain calculations were slightly higher (less pain) for CAS patients at one month post-operative; however no difference was noted at six months (see Tables 4.2 and 4.3). Range of motion was not significantly different at one and six months post-operative (see Tables 4.2 and 4.3). Mechanical axis, sagittal femoral axis, and sagittal tibial axis radiographic results were not significantly different. (see Table 4.2) The number of units of blood transfused was slightly greater for CAS pa-

tients and tourniquet time was on average, twenty-seven minutes longer for CAS compared to manual TKA (see Table 4.2).

Discussion

Unlike the senior author's initial experience working with CAS [102, 105], this study found no statistically significant radiographic alignment differences between TKAs performed using CAS and manual techniques. This suggests that either external factors such as advancements in implants and mechanical alignment systems have resulted in manual TKA being performed more accurately, or that improvement in manual TKA technique has been realized through more than four years of extensive CAS utilization by the senior author. Although advancements in implants and instruments have been made, mechanical alignment systems still have *inherent* limitations in their ability to accurately determine the location of crucial alignment landmarks [11, 37]. This is further supported by the breadth of studies that have demonstrated superior radiographic alignment outcomes with CAS as compared to manual TKA, suggesting that changes in implants or mechanical alignment systems alone are not sufficient to produce equivalent alignment results [1–6, 8, 9].

▣ Table 4.2. Selected variable results

	Unilateral Manual			Unilateral CAS			Total		
	Avg	Range	Std Dev	Avg	Range	Std Dev	Avg	Range	Std Dev
Knee Score* (Pre-operative)	48.1	(17,77)	15.0	44.6	(22, 79)	13.7	46.3	(17, 79)	14.4
Knee Score (1 Month Post-operative)	69.1	(40, 100)	14.3	75.4	(45, 98)	13.5	72.2	(40, 100)	14.1
Knee Score (6 Month Post-operative)	84.6	(23, 100)	18.3	83.4	(32, 100)	18.5	84.0	(23, 100)	18.2
Function Score* (Pre-operative)	56.7	(35, 80)	17.8	50.4	(30, 80)	12.2	53.6	(30, 80)	12.6
Function Score (1 Month Post-operative)	48.9	(20, 100)	17.8	50.3	(20, 90)	14.9	49.6	(20, 100)	16.3
Function Score (6 Month Post-operative)	62.0	(45, 90)	15.7	64.0	(30, 100)	19.4	62.9	(30, 100)	20.0
ROM (Pre-operative)	113.7	(70, 140)	15.7	112.1	(70, 140)	15.0	112.9	(70, 140)	15.3
ROM (1 Month Post-operative)	103.2	(65, 135)	13.5	105.1	(80, 125)	10.2	104.1	(65, 135)	11.9
ROM (6 Month Post-operative)	116.0	(100, 135)	8.7	117.0	(105, 135)	8.1	116.4	(100, 135)	8.4
Pain Calculation** (Pre-operative)	12.8	(0, 30)	9.1	12.0	(0, 45)	9.7	12.4	(0, 45)	9.3
Pain Calculation (1 Month Post-operative)	25.6	(10, 50)	12.5	29.3	(0, 50)	12.9	27.4	(0, 50)	12.8
Pain Calculation (6 Month Post-operative)	39.5	(20, 50)	10.7	36.5	(0, 50)	15.6	38.1	(0, 50)	13.1
Units of Blood Transfused (units)	.4	(0, 4)	.76	.6	(0, 3)	.82	.48	(0, 4)	1.1
Tourniquet Time (min)	72.9	(47, 110)	13.7	99.6	(60, 131)	16.3	85.1	(47, 147)	19.3
Mechanical Axis (Post-operative Xray) Varus (+) Valgus (−)	−.24	(−6, 8)	3.5	2.1	(−3, 7)	2.7	.80	(−6, 8)	3.1
Femoral Angle (Post-operative)	2.6	(−6, 9)	3.2	2.2	(−2, 7)	2.2	2.5	(−6, 9)	2.6
Tibial Angle (Post-operative)	88.1	(83, 91)	1.7	88.0	(83, 92)	1.9	88.0	(83, 92)	1.8

*Best assessment = 100, ** Max pain = 0, No pain = 50

▣ Table 4.3. Variable change between preoperative, one, and six month follow-up

	Unilateral Manual			Unilateral CAS			Total		
	Avg	Range	Std Dev	Avg	Range	Std Dev	Avg	Range	Std Dev
Knee Score Change Pre-operative – 1 Month Post-operative	20.9	(-18, 64)	21.3	30.8	(-15, 71)	20.6	25.8	(-18, 71)	21.4
Knee Score Change Pre-operative – 6 months Post-operative	36.7	(-26, 76)	26.0	36.9	(-6, 73)	25.7	36.8	(-26, 76)	25.5
Function Score Change Pre-operative – 1 Month Post-operative	-4.4	(-40, 65)	21.0	-2.0	(-35, 55)	22.3	-3.2	(-40, 65)	21.4
Function Score Change Pre-operative – 6 Months Post-operative	4.6	(-20, 35)	14.5	12.7	(-20, 30)	13.5	8.7	(-20, 35)	14.3
Range of Motion Change Pre-operative – 1 Month Post-operative	-10.5	(-57, 38)	16.7	-4.7	(-48, 100)	24.4	-7.7	(-57, 100)	20.8
Range of Motion Change Pre-operative – 6 Months Post-operative	3.3	(-15, 30)	11.6	8.1	(-87, 100)	36.1	5.5	(-87, 100)	25.7
Pain Calculation Change Pre-operative – 1 Month Post-operative	12.8	(-20, 45)	13.7	17.4	(-25, 45)	15.2	15.1	(-25, 45)	14.6
Pain Calculation Change Pre-operative – 6 Months Post-operative	25.5	(0, 50)	15.2	21.5	(-10, 50)	17.9	23.6	(-10, 50)	16.4

This study suggests that it is the intra-operative feedback and training effects realized through extensive use of a navigation system that has enabled the radiographic measures of manual TKA to parallel those of CAS. We believe it is possible for refinements in alignment perception, improvements in intra-operative judgment, and advances in technique to evolve to the point that no significant differences in radiographic alignment are apparent between CAS and manual TKA.

Clinical and patient-perceived functional results were not significantly different for CAS and manual TKA in this study. Outcome measures such as one's level of pain, range of motion, knee stability, mobility, and movement independence, which are measures of greatest importance to the TKA patient, were not significantly different in early follow-up. Thus, even if standard radiographs are not sensitive enough to detect subtle differences in alignment, these differences are not significant enough to influence short-term clinical and functional results. It is important to note the limitations of this study in terms of its duration. The long-term success of TKA is highly dependent upon proper limb and implant alignment, thus it is possible that alignment differences that were too minor to be exposed via standard radiograph in the short-term may become more readily apparent in long-term patient follow-up.

Summary

The widespread interest in minimally invasive arthroplasty surgery is focusing surgeons' attention on the importance of retaining accurate implant and limb alignment as exposure of surgical anatomy is reduced [116]. Techniques using non-frontal resection planes (e.g. the »quadrant sparing« medial approach) are making clear how the position of an implant in one plane critically affects its position in all other planes [105]. CAS systems have the potential for greatly facilitating the evolution of MIS knee surgery. However, the CAS hardware and software must be configured to support safely, accurately and efficiently the MIS systems that are being developed.

References

1. Aglietti P, Buzzi R (1988) Posteriorly stabilized total-condylar knee replacement. J. Bone Joint Surg: 211–216
2. Ayers, DC, Dennis DA, Johanson NA et al. (1997) Common complications of total knee arthroplasty. J Bone J Surg 2 (79A): 278–311
3. Bargren JH, Blaha JD, Freeman MAR (1983) Alignment in total knee arthroplasty: correlated biomechanical and clinical observations. Clin Orthop 1983; 173: 178–183
4. Bathis H, Perlick L, Luring C, Kalteis T, Grifka J (2003) CT-based and CT-free navigation in knee prosthesis implantation. Results of a prospective study. Unfallchirurg 106: 935–940
5. Bathis H, Perlick L, Tingart M, Luring C, Perlick C, Grifka J (2004) Radiological results of image-based and non-image-based computer-assisted total knee arthroplasty. Int Orthop 28: 87–90
6. Berger RA, Crosset LS, Jacobs JJ (1998) Malrotation causing patellofemoral complications after total knee arthroplasty. Clin Orthop Relat Res 356: 144–153
7. Bohler M, Messner M, Glos W, Riegler M (2000) Lcomputer navigated implantation of total knee prostheses: A radiological study. Acta Chir Aust 33 (Suppl): 63
8. Briard JL, Stindel E. Plaweski S et al. (2004) CT free navigation with the LCS surgetics station: a new way of balancing the soft tissues in TKA based on bone morphing. In: Stiehl JB, Konermann WH, Haaker RG (eds) Navigation and robotics in total joint and spine surgery. Springer, Berlin Heidelberg New York Tokyo, pp 274–280
9. Cartier P, Sanouillier JL, Frelsamer RP (1996) Unicompartmental knee artholasty surgery. 10-year minimum follow-up period. J Arthroplasty 11: 782–788
10. Clemens U, Konermann WH, Kohler S, Kiefer H, Jenny JY, Miehlke RK (2004) Computer-assisted navigation with the OrthoPilot system using the search evolution TKA prosthesis. In Stiehl JB, Konermann WH, Haaker RG (eds) Navigation and robotics in total joint and spine surgery. Springer, Berlin Heidelberg New York Tokyo, pp 236–241
11. Currie J, Varshney A, Stulberg SD, Adams A, Woods O (2005) The reliability of Anatomic Landmarks for Determining Femoral Implant = Rotation in TKA Surgery: Implications for CAOS TKA. Presented at the Annual Meeting of Mid-America Orthopaedic Association, Amelia Island, FL
12. Delp SL, Stulberg SD, Davies B, Picard F, Leitner F (1998) Computer assisted knee replacement. Clin Orthop 354: 49–56
13. DeRycke J (2004) Clinical experiences for ACL-Repair with the SurgiGATE System. In: Stiehl JB, Konermann WH, Haaker RG (eds) Navigation and robotics in total joint and spine surgery. Springer, Berlin Heidelberg New York Tokyo, pp 397–399.
14. Dessenne V, Lavallee S, Julliard R et al. (1995) Computer assisted anterior cruciate ligament reconstruction: first clinical tests. J Image Guided Surg 1: 59–64
15. Dorr LD, Boiardo RA (1997) Technical considerations in total knee arthroplasty. Clin Orthop 205: 5–11
16. Ecker ML, Lotke PA, Windsor RE et al. (1987) Long-term results after total condylar knee arthroplasty. Significance of radiolucent lines. Clin Orthop 216: 151–158
17. Eichorn H-J (2004) Image-Free navigation in ACL replacement with the OrthoPilot system. In: Stiehl JB, Konermann WH, Haaker RG (eds) Navigation and robotics in total joint and spine surgery. Springer, Berlin Heidelberg New York Tokyo, pp 387–396
18. Ellis RE, Rudan JF, Harrison MM (2004) Computer-assisted high tibial osteotomies. In: DiGioia AM, Jaramaz B, Picard R, Nolte PL (eds) Computer and robotic assisted knee and hip surgery. Oxford University Press, pp 197–212
19. Fadda M, Bertelli, D, Martelli S et al. (1997) Computer assisted planning for total knee arthroplasty. Proceedings of the First Joint Conference on Computer Vision, Virtual Reality and Robotics in Medicine and Medial Robotics and Computer Assisted Surgery, Grenoble, France. Springer, Berlin Heidelberg New York Tokyo, pp 619–628
20. Fehring TK, Odum S, Griffin Wl, Mason JB, Naduad M (2001) Early failures in total knee arthroplasty. Clin Orthop 392: 315–318
21. Feng EL, Stulberg SD, Wixson RL (1994) Progressive subluxation and polyethylene wear in total knee replacements with flat articular surfaces. Clin Orthop Relat Res 299: 60–71
22. Froemel M, Portheine F, Ebner M, Radermacher K (2001) Computer assisted template based navigation for total knee replacement. North American Program on Computer Assisted Orthopaedic Surgery, Pittsburgh, PA
23. Garbini JL, Kaiura RG, Sidles JA, Larson RV, Matsen FA (1987) Robotic instrumentation in total knee arthroplasty. 33rd Annual Meeting, Orthopaedic Research Society, San Francisco
24. Garg A, Walker PS (1990) Prediction of total knee motion using a three-dimensional computer graphics model. J Biochem 23: 45–58
25. Goodfellow JW, O'Connor JJ (1986) Clinical results of the Oxford knee. Clin Orthop 205: 21–24
26. Hart R, Janecek M, Chaker A, Bucek P (2003) Total knee arthroplasty implanted with and without kinematic navigation. Int Orthop 27: 366–369
27. Hsu HP, Garg A, Walker PS, Spector M, Ewald FC (1989) Effect on knee component alignment on tibial load distribution with clinical correlation. Clin Orthop 248: 135–144
28. Hungerford DS, Kenna RV (1990) Preliminary experience with a total knee prosthesis with porous coating used without cement. Clin Orthop 255: 215–227
29. Insall JW. Surgical approaches to the knee. In: Insall JN (ed) Surgery of the Knee. Churchill Livingston, New York, pp 4–54
30. Insall JN, Binzzir R, Soudry M, Mestriner LA (1985) Total knee arthroplasty. Clin Orthop 192: 13–22
31. Insall JN, Ranawat CS, Aglietti P, Shine J (1976) A comparison of four models of total knee-replacement prosthesis. J Bone Joint Surg 58A: 754–765
32. Insall J, Scott N (2005) Surgery of the knee. Elsevier, Amsterdam
33. Jeffcote B, Shakespeare D (2003) Varus/valgus alignment of the tibial component in total knee arthroplasty. Knee 10: 243–247
34. Jeffery RS, Morris RW, Denham RA (1991) Coronal alignment after total knee replacement. J Bone Joint Surg 73B: 709–714
35. Jenny JY, Boeri C (2000) Computer-assisted total knee prosthesis implantation without preoperative imaging. A comparison with classical instrumentation. Presented at the Fourth Annual North American Program on Computer Assisted Orthopaedic Surgery, Pittsburgh, PA
36. Jenny JY, Boeri C (2001) Implantation d'une prothese totale de genou assistee par ordinateur. Etude comparative cas-temoin avec une instrumentaiton traditionnelle. Rev Chir Orthop 87: 645–652
37. Jenny JY, Boeri C (2004) Low reproducibility of the intra-operative measurement of the transepicondylar axis during total knee replacement. Acta Orthop Scand 75: 74–77

38. Jenny JY, Boeri C (2001) Navigated implantation of total knee prostheses: A comparison with conventional techniques. Orthop Ihre Grenzgeb 139: 117–119

39. Jenny JY, Boeri C (2002) Unicompartmental knee prosthesis. A case-control comparative study of two types of instrumentation with a five year follow-up. J Arthroplasty 17: 1016-1020

40. Jenny JY, Boeri C (2004) Unicompartmental knee prosthesis implantation with a non-image based navigation system, In: DiGioia AM, Jaramaz B, Picard R, Nolte PL (eds) Computer and robotic assisted knee and hip surgery. Oxford University Press, pp 179–188

41. Jiang CC, Insall JN (1989) Effect of rotation on the axial alignment of the femur. Clin Orthop Rel Res 248: 50–56

42. Julliard R, Lavallee S, Dessenne V (1998) Computer assisted anterior cruciate ligament reconstruction of the anterior cruciate ligament. Clin Orthop Relat Res 354: 57–64

43. Julliard R, Plaweski S, Lavallee S (2004) ACL Surgetics: an efficient computer-assisted technique for ACL reconstruction. In: Stiehl JB, Konermann WH, Haaker RG (eds) Navigation and robotics in total joint and spine surgery. Springer, Berlin Heidelberg New York Tokyo, pp 405–411

44. Kaiura RG (1986) Robot assisted total knee arthroplasty investigation of the feasibility and accuracy of the robotic process. Master's Thesis, Mechanical Engineering, University of Washington

45. Kienzle TC, Stulberg SD, Peshkin M et al. (1996) A computer-assisted total knee replacement surgical system using a calibrated robot. Orthopaedics. In: Taylor RH et al. (eds) Computer integrated surgery. MIT press, Cambridge, MA, pp 409–416

46. Kinzel V, Scaddan M, Bradley B, Shakespeare D (2004) Varus/valgus alignment of the femur in total knee arthroplasty. Can accuracy be improved by pre-operative CT scanning? Knee 11: 197–201

47. Klos TVS, Habets RJE, Banks AZ, Banks SA, Devilee RJJ, Cook FF (2004) Computer assistance in arthroscopic anterior cruciate ligament reconstruction. In: DiGioia AM, Jaramaz B, Picard R, Nolte PL (eds) Computer and robotic assisted knee and hip surgery. Oxford University Press, pp 229–234

48. Konermann WH, Kistner S (2004) CT-Free navigation including soft-tissue balancing: LCS-TKA and vector vision systems. In: Stiehl JB, Konermann WH, Haaker RG (eds) Navigation and robotics in total joint and spine surgery. Springer, Berlin Heidelberg New York Tokyo, pp 256–265

49. Konermann WH, Sauer MA (2004) Postoperative alignment of conventional and navigated total knee arthoplasty. In: Stiehl JB, Konermann WH, Haaker RG (eds) Navigation and robotics in total joint and spine surgery. Springer, Berlin Heidelberg New York Tokyo, pp 219–225

50. Koyonos L, Granieri M, Stulberg SD (2005) At what steps in performance of a TKA do errors occur when manual instrumentation is used. Presented at the Annual Meeting of American Academy of Orthopaedic Surgeons, Washington, DC

51. Krackow K, Serpe L, Phillips MJ et al. (1999) A new technique for determining proper mechanical axis alignment during total knee arthroplasty. Orthopedics 22: 698–701

52. Kuntz M, Sati M, Nolte LP et al. (2000) Computer assisted total knee arthroplasty. International symposium on CAOS, Davos

53. Lampe F, Hille E (2004) Navigated implantation of the columbus total knee arthroplasty with the OrthoPilot system: Version 4.0. In: Stiehl JB, Konermann WH, Haaker RG (eds) Navigation and robotics in total joint and spine surgery. Springer, Berlin Heidelberg New York Tokyo, pp 248–253.

54. Laskin RS (1984) Alighment of the total knee components. Orthopedics 7: 62

55. Laskin RS (1990) Total condylar knee replacement in patients who have rheumatoid arthritis. A ten year follow- up study. J Bone Joint Surg 72A: 529–535

56. Laskin RS, Turtel A (1989) The use of an intramedullary tibial alignment guide in total knee replacement arthroplasty. Am J Knee Surg 2: 123

57. Leitner F, Picard F, Minfelde R et al. (1997) Computer-assisted knee surgical total replacement. First Joint Conference of CVRMed and MRCAS. Grenoble, France. Springer, Berlin Heidelberg New York Tokyo, pp 629–638

58. Leitner F, Picard F, Minfelde R et al. (1997) Computer assisted knee surgical total replacement. Proceedings of the First Joint Conference on Computer Vision, Virtual Reality and Robotics in Medicine and Medical Robotics and Computer Assisted Surgery. Springer, Berlin Heidelberg New York Tokyo, pp 630–638

59. Lootvoet L, Burton P, Himmer O, Piot L, Ghosez JP (1997) Protheses unicompartimentales de genou: influence du positionnement du plateau tibial sur les resultants fonctionnels. Acta Orthop Belg 63: 94–101

60. Mahfouz MR, Hoff WA, Komistek RD, Dennis DA (2003) A robust method for registration of three-dimensional knee implant models to two-dimensional fluoroscopy images. IEEE Trans Med Imaging 22: 1561–1574

61. Martelli M, Marcacci M, Nofrini L, LA Palombara F, Malvisi A, Iacono F, Vendruscolo P, Pierantoni M (2000) Computer- and robot-assisted total knee replacement: analysis of a new surgical procedure. Ann Biomed Eng 28: 1146–1153

62. Matsen FA, Garbini JL, Sidles JA (1993) Robotic assistance in orthopaedic surgery. A proof of principle using distal femoral arthroplasty. Clin Orthop Relat Res 296: 178–186

63. Mattes T, Puhl W (2004) Navigation in TKA with the Navitrack System. In: Stiehl JB, Konermann WH, Haaker RG (eds) Navigation and robotics in total joint and spine surgery. Springer, Berlin Heidelberg New York Tokyo, pp 293–300

64. Miehlke RK, Clemens U, Jens J-H, Kershally S (2001) Navigation in knee arthroplasty: Preliminary clinical experience and prospective comparative study in comparison with conventional technique. Orthop Ihre Grenzgeb 139: 1109–1129

65. Miehlke RK, Clemens U, Kershally S (2000) Computer integrated instrumentation in knee arthroplasty: a comparative study of conventional and computerized technique. Fourth Annual North American Program on Computer Assisted Orthopaedic Surgery, Pittsburgh, PA, pp 93–96

66. Nishihara S, Sugano N, Ikai M, Sasama T, Tamura Y, Tamura S, Yoshikawa H, Ochi T (2003) Accuracy evaluation of a shape-based registration method for a computer navigation system for total knee arthroplasty. J Knee Surg 16: 98–105

67. Nizard R (2002) Computer assisted surgery for total knee arthroplasty. Acta Orthop Belg 68: 215–230

68. Noble PC, Sugano N, Johnston JD, Thompson MT, Conditt MA, Engh CA Sr, Mathis KB (2003) Computer simulation: how can it help the surgeon optimize implant position? Clin Orthop 417: 242–252

69. Nuno-Siebrecht N, Tanzer M, Bobyn JD (2000) Potential errors in axial alignment using intramedullary instrumentation for total knee arthroplasty. J Arthroplasty 15: 228–230

70. Oswald MH, Jacob RP, Schneider E, Hoogewoud H (1993) Radiological analysis of normal axial alignment of femur and tibia in view of total knee arthroplasty. J Arthroplasty 8: 419–426

71. Perlick L, Bathis H, Luring C, Tingart M, Grifka J (2004) CT based and CT-free navigation with the BrainLAB VectorVision system in total knee arthroplasty. In: Stiehl JB, Konermann WH, Haaker RG (eds) Navigation and robotics in total joint and spine surgery. Springer, Berlin Heidelberg New York Tokyo, pp 304–310

72. Perlick L, Bathis H, Tingart M, Perlick C, Grifka J (2004) Navigation in total-knee arthroplasty: CT-based implantation compared with the conventional technique. Acta Orthop Scand 75: 464–470

73. Perlick L, Bathis H, Tingart M, Kalteis T, Grifka J (2003) Useability of an image based nagivation system in reconstruction of leg alignment in total knee arthroplasty – results of a propsective study. Biomed Tech (Berl) 48: 339–343

74. Peterman J, Kober R, Heinze, R, Frolich JJ, Heeckt PF, Gotzen L (2000) Computer-assisted planning and robot assisted surgery in anterior cruciate ligament reconstruction. Oper Techn Orthop 10: 50–55

75. Petersen TL, Engh GA (1988) Radiographic assessment of knee alignment after total knee arthroplasty. J Arthroplasty 3: 67–72

76. Piazza SJ, Delp SL, Stulberg SD, Stern SJ (1998) Posterior tilting of the tibial component decreases femoral rollback in posterior-substituting knee replacement. J Orthop Res 16: 264–270

77. Picard F, Leitner F, Raoult O, Saragaglia D (2000) Computer assisted knee replacement. Location of a rotational center of the knee. Total knee arthroplasty. International Symposium on CAOS

78. Picard F, Leitner F, Raoult O, Saragaglia D, Cinquin P (1998) Clinical evaluation of computer assisted total knee arthroplasty. Second Annual North American Program on Computer Assisted Orthopaedic Surgery, Pittsburgh, PA, pp 239–249

79. Picard F, Moody JE, DiGioia AM, Jaramaz B, Plakseychuk AY, Sell D (2004) Knee reconstructive surgery: preoperative model system In: DiGioia AM, Jaramaz B, Picard R, Nolte PL (eds) Computer and robotic assisted knee and hip surgery. Oxford University Press, pp 139–156

80. Picard F, Moody JE, DiGioia AM, Martinek V, Fu FH, Rytel MJ, Nikou C, LaVarca RS, Jaramaz B (2004) ACL reconstruction-preoperative model system. In: DiGioia AM, Jaramaz B, Picard R, Nolte PL (eds) Computer and robotic assisted knee and hip surgery. Oxford University Press, pp 213–228

81. Radermacher K, Staudte HW, Rau G (1998) Computer assisted orthopaedic surgery with image-based individual templates. Clin Orthop Rel Res 354: 28–38

82. Ranawat CS, Boachie-Adjei O (1988) Survivorship analysis and results of total condylar knee arthroplasty. Clin Orthop 226: 6–13

83. Rand JA, Coventry MB (1988) Evaluation of geometric total knee arthroplasty. Clin ORthop 232: 168–173

84. Ritter MA, Faris PM, Keating EM, Meding JB (1994) Post-operative alignment of total knee replacement. Its effect on survival. Clin Orthop 299: 153–156

85. Ritter M, Merbst WA, Keating EM, Faris PM (1991) Radiolucency at the bone-cement interface in total knee replacement. J Bone Joint Surg 76A: 60–65

86. Saragaglia D, Picard F (2004) Computer-assisted implantation of total knee endoprosthesis with no pre-operative imaging: the kinematic model. In: Stiehl JB, Konermann WH, Haaker RG (eds) Navigation and robotics in total joint and spine surgery. Springer, Berlin Heidelberg New York Tokyo, pp 226–233

87. Saragaglia D, Picard F, Chaussard C et al. (2001) Computer-assisted knee arthroplasty: Comparison with a conventional procedure: Results of 50 cases in a prospective randomized study. Rev Chir Orthop Reparatrice Appar Mot 87: 215–220

98. Saragagglia D, Picard F, Chaussard D, Montbarbon E, Leitner F, Cinquin P (2001) Computer assisted total knee arthroplasty: comparison with a conventional procedure. Results of 50 cases prospective randomized study. Presented at the First Annual Meeting of Computer Assisted Orthopaedic SurgeryDavos, Switzerland

89. Sati M, Staubli HU, Bourquin Y, Kunz M, Nolte LP (2004) CRA hip and knee reconstructive surgery: ligament reconstructions in the knee-intra-operative model system (non-image based). In: DiGioia AM, Jaramaz B, Picard R, Nolte PL (eds) Computer and robotic assisted knee and hip surgery. Oxford University Press, pp 235–256

90. Siebert W, Mai S, Kober R, Heeckt PF (2002) Technique and first clinical results of robot-assisted total knee replacement. Knee 9: 173–180

91. Sharkey PF, Hozack WJ, Rothman RH et al. (2002) Why are total knee arthroplasties failing today? Clin Orthop 404: 7–13

92. Sparmann M, Wolke B (2004) Knee endoprosthesis navigation with the Stryker System. In: Stiehl JB, Konermann WH, Haaker RG (eds) Navigation and robotics in total joint and spine surgery. Springer, Berlin Heidelberg New York Tokyo, pp 319–323

93. Sparmann M, Wolke B (2003) Value of navigation and robot-guided surgery in total knee arthroplasty. Orthopade 32: 498–505

94. Stern SH, Insall JN (1992) Posterior stabilized prosthesis: Results after follow-up of 9–12 years. J Bone Joint Surg 74A: 980–986

95. Stockl B, Nogler M, Rosiek R, Fischer M, Krismer M, Kessler O (2004) Navigation improves accuracy of rotational alignment in total knee arthroplasty. Clin Orthop 426: 180–186

96. Strauss JM, Ruther W (2004) Navigation and soft tissue balancing of LCS total knee arthroplasty. In: Stiehl JB, Konermann WH, Haaker RG (eds) Navigation and robotics in total joint and spine surgery. Springer, Berlin Heidelberg New York Tokyo, pp 266–273

97. Stulberg SD, Eichorn J, Saragaglia, D, Jenny J-Y (2003) The rationale for and initial experience with a knee suite of computer assisted surgical applications. Third International CAOS Meeting, Marbella, Spain

98. Stulberg SD (2005) Factors affecting the accuracy of minimally invasive total knee arthroplasty. Presented at the Annual Meeting of American Academy of Orthopaedic Surgeons, Washington, DC

99. Stulberg SD (2005) CAS-TKA reduces the occurrence of functional outliers. Presented at the Annual Meeting of Mid-America Orthopaedic Association, Amelia Island, FL

100. Stulberg SD (2005) Instructional course lecture on computer assisted surgery for hip and knee reconstruction at the Annual Meeting of American Academy of Orthopaedic Surgeons, Washington, DC

101. Stulberg SD, Koyonos L, McClusker S, Granieri M (2005) Factors affecting the accuracy of minimally invasive TKA. Presented at the Annual Meeting of American Academy of Orthopaedic Surgeons, Washington, DC

102. Stulberg SD, Loan P, Sarin V (2002) Computer-assisted naviga-tion in total knee replacement: results of an initial experience in thirty-five patients. J Bone Joint Surg Am 84-A (Suppl 2): 90–98

103. Stulberg SD, Picard F, Saragaglia D (2000) Computer assisted total knee arthroplasty. Operative techniques. Orthopaedics 10: 25–39

108. Stulberg SD, Sarin V (2001) The use of a navigation system to as-sist ligament balancing in TKR. Proceedings of the Fourth Annual American CAOS Meeting, Pittsburgh, PA

104. Stulberg SD, Saragaglia D, Miehlke R (2004) Total knee replace-ment: navigation technique intra-operative model system. In: DiGioia AM, Jaramaz B, Picard R, Nolte PL (eds) Computer and robotic assisted knee and hip surgery. Oxford University Press, pp 157–178

105. Stulberg SD, Sarin V, Loan P (2001) X-ray vs. computer assisted measurement techniques to determine pre and post-operative limb alignment in TKR surgery. Proceedings of the Fourth Annual American CAOS meeting, Pittsburgh, PA

106. Teter KE, Bergman D, Colwell CW (1995) Accuracy of intrmedul-lary versus extramedullary tibial alignment cutting systems in total knee arthroplasty. Clin Orthop 321: 106–110

107. Tew M, Waugh W (1985) Tibiofemoral alignment and the results of knee replacement. J Bone Joint Surg 67B: 551–556

108. Tibbles L, Lewis C, Reisine S, Rippey R, Donald M (1992) Computer assisted instruction for preoperative and postoperative patient ed-ucation in joint replacement surgery. Comput Nurs 10: 208–212

109. Townley CD (1985) The anatomic total knee: instrumentation and alignment technique. The knee: papers of the First Scientific Meet-ing of the Knee Society. Baltimore University Press. pp 39–54

110. Tria AJ Jr (2004) Minimally invasive total knee arthroplasty: the im-portance of instrumentation. Orthop Clin North Am 35: 227–234

111. Vince KIG, Insall JN, Kelly MA (1989) The total condylar prosthesis. 10 to 12 year results of a cemented knee replacement. J Bone Joint Surg 71B: 93–797

112. Wasielewski RC, Galante JO, Leighty R, Natarajan RN, Rosenberg AG (1994) Wear patterns on retrieved polyethylene tibial inserts and their relationship to technical considerations during total knee arthroplasty. Clin Orthop 299: 31–43

113. Wiese M, Rosenthal A, Bernsmann K (2004) Clinical experience using the SurgiGATE system. In: Stiehl JB, Konermann WH, Haaker RG (eds) Navigation and robotics in total joint and spine surgery. Springer, Berlin Heidelberg New York Tokyo, pp 400–404

114. Wixson RL (2004) Extra-medullary computer assisted total knee replacement: towards lesser invasive surgery. In: Stiehl JB, Koner-mann WH, Haaker RG (eds) Navigation and robotics in total joint and spine surgery. Springer, Berlin Heidelberg New York Tokyo, pp 311–318

Bone Morphing: 3D Reconstruction without Pre- or Intra-Operative Imaging

E. Stindel, N. Perrin, J.L. Briard, S. Lavallée, C. Lefevre, J. Troccaz

Introduction

Computer-assisted surgery is an ongoing process that merges pre- and peri-operative data in a so-called PDA loop during which acquisition and perception occurs. Decisions are taken and actions are performed. This process should definitely be seen as a loop, since intra-operative information given by a new generation of sensors can easily be merged with pre-operative data of all modality (geometric, morphologic, kinetics and kinematics etc.) in order to optimize the decision process in real time and therefore modify the planned actions.

These quantitative data have definitely changed the ways of performing surgery, and this was only made possible, thanks to the introduction of computers in the operating room.

A complete description of these basic concepts has been published elsewhere by the authors [1]. In this paper, we focus on the intra-operative acquisition issues. To develop a good guiding system, one needs an accurate and robust model of the patient. It must be obtained, by the surgeon, thanks to an intuitive and fast acquisition protocol. Models vary, and use different kinds of data, as a function of the type of surgery to be performed. If one wants to perform neurosurgery, for instance, one would probably build the model from MR or CT images.

In orthopaedic surgery, models are built using different types of data depending on the procedure itself. We will distinguish between two classes of models: (1) image-based models and (2) non-image-based models. In the first group, the model can be obtain pre-operatively from radiographs or CT scans [2–4], or intra-operatively from fluoroscopic images [5]. In the second group, we will describe two subgroups: in the first one, called a geometric model, the data consist of several landmarks digitized on the patient [6, 7]. In the second group, the 3D shapes of the bones are built from data collected with a 3D optical localizer in relative coordinate systems attached to the bones, using clouds of points and deformable statistical models. This is the bone morphing technology, invented by PRAXIM (patents pending), after several years of research in deformable and statistical modeling performed at Grenoble University (TIMC Laboratory).

Orthopaedic surgery can be defined as a 3D action (the operation) in a 3D space (the operating room) on a 3D object (the patient). Therefore, there is an absolute need for 3D models and we believe that models based on 2D images are of little present-day interest and without promise for the future. While geometric models, based on landmarks only, may be useful in some cases [7], they have several limitations and may not meet the entire surgeon's requirement. Therefore, several applications based on 3D morphologic models have been developed and marketed in the late nineties; however, all these models used CT to provide the data. Building a 3D model from CT has some drawbacks: (1) The high volume of orthopaedic procedures performed each day makes CT scans as routine pre-operative procedures an unacceptably expensive exercise. Also, the radiation burden to the patients would be high. (2) Performing a CT scan takes 20 min per patient. To this has to be added the time it takes to transfer the data to the surgeon's computer or navigation system, and to initiate, check and validate the results of the segmentation/registration process. This procedure, from the raw data to the 3D model, is time-consuming and sometimes cumbersome. Last but not least, because of complex phenomena of error propagation, including segmentation and registration, CT-based navigation is sometimes not as accurate as expected. In 2000, PRAXIM achieved a breakthrough in orthopaedics by the introduction of bone morphing, which can outperform CT in some indications, it has now become a standard and many copies of this technology have been implemented throughout the world. In this paper, we describe the bone morphing technology, and demonstrate its applications in several indications when running the technology on the Surgetics Station (PRAXIM-medivision, La Tronche, France).

Since the first edition of this book was published in 2003, not much has change in the core technology of bone morphing. But the technology itself has spread all over, and many applications have been developed based on this brick, which has now been used in more than 10,000 surgeries.

In research laboratories, this technology and its consequences on the accuracy of systems has been extensively validated over the last two years. In this chapter we will add new validation data which clearly show how the bone morphing approach can outperform landmark based methods or cloud-of-points based methods.

Bone Morphing: 3D Morphologic Data Without Pre-Operative Imaging

In a non-image-based approach, building a 3D model which is specific to the patient's anatomy is quite challenging. This section describes how this goal is achieved in the PRAXIM Surgetics method.

Acquisition of a Random Cloud of 1000 Points

The overall process can be divided into several technical steps. However, for the surgeon, there is only one action to perform: to digitize a cloud of random points on the surface of the bone. After a quick model initialization step, the surface acquisition step is carried out using a pointer with a 1-mm-radius spherical tip instead of using a sharp tip. This enables the surgeon to sweep the pointer quickly and smoothly over the bone and cartilage surfaces. The bone morphing algorithm will then compensate for the radius of the sphere to reconstruct the exact surface. This takes about one minute and thirty seconds for the entire surface of the distal femur, and around one minute for the proximal part of the tibia. If we add the patella (in a TKA procedure), the acquisition step takes only 3 min. After these 3 min, there is nothing else that the surgeon needs to do, the 3D reconstruction is almost real time and perform in a few seconds. This can be even quicker if only a small area has to be modeled, for instance the acetabular fossa during total hip arthroplasty.

3D Statistical Shape Models from Point Data

The second step is to position and deform a statistical model of the bone in order to fit the cloud of points using the algorithm of Fleute et al. [8]. Intra-operatively we use a deformable model, rather than a library of bone models. This 3D deformable shape was built once, and is now used for every surgical procedure. Using the technique described below, PRAXIM have developed several models (acetabulum, tibia, femur, etc.) for use in different applications. However, inside each application there is only one deformable model that will fit small bones as well as very large shapes.

To obtain this 3D statistical shape, three steps are required:
1) Acquisition of training shapes
2) Definition of a point-to-point correspondence with the training shape
3) Statistical analysis

Step 1

A set of n dry human bones is digitized using the OPTO-TRACK 3D localizer (NDI, Waterloo, Canada), resulting in large n sets of non-organized points, randomly distributed on the bone surface. The value n must be sufficient to represent a good variability of the population. Each set of points represents the surface of one bone (femur, tibia, etc.). An additional bone is then digitized with a higher point density. The result of the reconstruction is a triangular mesh of vertices, which is considered as a mean template.

Step 2

Each of the n sets of points is matched to the template in such a way that each vertex of the template mesh is mapped to its anatomically corresponding point on the femur under study. This matching process is based on the result of octree-splines deformation published by Szeliski and Lavallée [9]. The result of this non-rigid 3D to 3D registration is a transformation function T, which maps every point P of the actual data space (the set of points) to a point M of the template in such a way that $M_i = T(P_i)$.

Step 3

After steps 1 and 2 we obtain a collection of n complete 3D reconstructions of the surfaces of the n femurs under study. Each training femur F is then represented by a vector m which describes the vertices of the mesh. The mean shape is then given by: $\overline{m} = \frac{1}{n} E\, m_i$. We then compute the deviations of each training shape from the mean shape using Principal Component Analysis of the deformation field. The final shape is the one which minimizes the necessary deformation to match all the training bones.

Using the statistical process described above using a mean surface and the most significant statistical modes, a new instance of the mean shape is generated by adding a linear combination of the most significant variation vectors to the original mean shape for each bone of the training set. This is achieved by minimizing the residual errors between the reconstructed model and the cloud of random points. It provides the best statistical shape that corresponds to the patient.

Local Deformation to Compensate Pathology Using Octree-Splines

To compensate for deviation of any pathological shape from the statistical shapes, we deform again locally the statistical model adapted to the patient until it fits correctly and precisely the cloud of points using the Szeliski and Lavallée [9] octree-spline algorithm with hierarchical, locally adapted and regularized deformation. A volume embedding the 3D data is created. It is recursively divided into smaller and smaller cubes that create a non-uniform volumetric mesh (not a surface mesh), and each coef-

ficient of the basis functions applied to each point of the mesh is optimized to match the data, whilst the resulting global deformation has regularization properties that make it realistic and stable. This process is more stable and accurate than are simple affine registration methods. Note that steps 2 and 3 are continuous and merged in a single process, so that the user only sees the points before bone morphing is applied at the end of the first step, and then, only two or three seconds later, the 3D model fitted to the points.

This elegant combination of different mathematical techniques makes the result unique. This patented PRAXIM technique is very robust and accurate, as well as extremely powerful in many applications of computer-assisted surgery. In 100% of the cases in which we have been able to test or use this algorithm, it has performed well, exactly as expected.

Clinical Applications of the Bone-Morphing Technique on the Surgetics Station

The chapter of this book is too short to present an exhaustive list of the applications based on the bone morphing technology. In this paragraph we will focus on the first applications that were introduced on the market and which have now been used in more than 10,000 surgeries.

Total Knee Arthroplasty (TKA)

Many computer-assisted protocols are now in use on the Surgetics Station to help surgeons during total knee replacement. A complete chapter of this book is dedicated to the SURGETICS and its use for total knee replacement, covering the bone morphing aspect, and much more. This chapter provides a complete description of the advantages of the bone morphing over other approaches, and of how it can be helpful at various steps of total knee replacement.

ACL Replacement

A specific chapter of this book describes how bone morphing is useful for Surgetics ACL reconstruction, and how it can be used under arthroscopy.

Hip Replacement

During hip-replacement procedures, bone morphing of the acetabulum can be used to

- check and guide reaming,
- give true 3D information on the thickness of the acetabular fossa as it is being reamed, and to determine the size of the acetabular reamer,
- perform a second acquisition per-operatively (which is only possible with the bone morphing technique as CT-scan is no longer available) to check the amount of bone removed by reaming, the sphericity of the acetabulum, and its size,
- help to optimize size choice, thus avoiding over-sizing, and to control the orientation of the cup.

High Tibial Osteotomy (HTO)

High tibial osteotomy is performed through a very small incision. The major challenge in this procedure is to display the 3D anatomy of the upper part of the tibia without any preoperative imaging. Once again, the Bone Morphing technique has helped us to achieve this goal. Most of the points are acquired in the surgical incision, and a few others are collected transcutaneously on the opposite aspect of the tibia. With these two clouds of points, we are able to deform the model to obtain an accurate representation of the actual anatomy. This model is then used in the HTO computer-assisted surgical protocol to plan the cuts in 3 dimensions, thus respecting the constraints of the patient's 3D morphology whilst adjusting the varus and recurvatum angles to correct the deformity. This instantaneous planning is used to guide the saw to perform easy, accurate, and precise surgery.

Unicompartimental Knee Arthroplasty

Bone morphing can be used in unicompartimental procedures in a way similar to total knee replacement. It helps to perform minimally invasive surgery providing a large amount of data with only a small incision. Four areas are digitized through the small incision and several points are directly computed on the model, such as the most distal and posterior points of the condyle. Automatic determination of the femoral component size is performed a by fitting a sphere to the relevant zone of the model. The ideal tibial component size is also computed from the 3D data before the component is automatically positioned by the system (◘ Fig. 5.1).

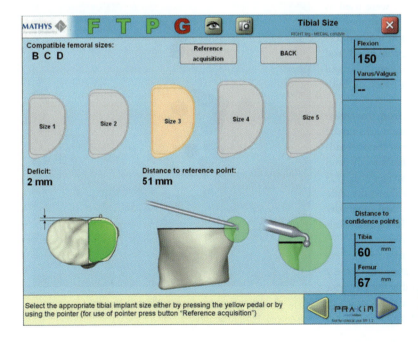

◘ **Fig. 5.1.** Automated planning proposition based on measurement obtain in the 3D model.

Validation Study

As underline above, image-free navigation systems are currently the most widely used systems for total knee arthrosplasty. They rely solely on intra-operative data to plan the placement of the femoral and tibial components for restoring proper alignment and soft tissue balance. Therefore, the way that data are acquired could have a significant impact on the final alignment of the implants. These planning computations can be made either on (1) a set of individual points digitized directly on anatomical landmarks, (2) clouds of points in the area of interest, (3) or a complete 3D model based on the Bone Morphing approach described above.

We recently compared the reproducibility of femoral and tibial implant planning as a function of the acquisition method in computer-assisted TKA. Both landmark-based (i.e direct digitization of anatomic points) and 3D model-based (i.e. bone morphing) acquisition methods were investigated. The study was carried out on a SUR-GETICS system (Praxim-Medivision), using a specific research software. In addition, we analyzed the intra and inter surgeon variability in acquiring by direct digitization alone many commonly used landmarks.

A group of 5 surgeons performed a set of 50 acquisitions (10 per surgeon) on one cadaver. Each acquisition included (a) a set of anatomical landmarks followed by (b) a global 3D cloud of points which were used as input for the Bone Morphing algorithm. We studied (1) the robustness of the landmark acquisition method, (2) the differences between the point-based method and automatic detection of landmarks in 3D models, and (3) the repeatability of implant planning based on both methods [10].

Three main conclusions can be drawn from this study: The reproducibility of directly digitized landmarks can be extremely low if there is not a sharp shape or feature readily identifiable in the local anatomy. This has already been demonstrated by Jenny et al. [11] and de Steiger et al. [12] in the transepicondylar axis, and ◻ Fig. 5.2 shows the same phenomenon at the level of the anterior tibial tuberosity (ATT). ◻ Table 5.1 reports the results of the reproducibility study on five commonly used landmarks.

1) Bone morphing can significantly improve the reproducibility of landmark determination. ◻ Table 5.2 shows the reproducibility in determining the posterior condylar axis using either the landmarks approach or the 3D bone morphing approach. ◻ Figure 5.3 shows

the distribution of two clouds of points. The green one was obtain by direct digitization using a probe, the blue one obtain during iterative computation of the posterior condyle locations based on 3D datasets given by the deformation of statistical model. We can clearly see that the distribution surface covered by points based method is larger than the surface covered by the 3D approach.

2) Bone morphing can not only improve the precision of landmark registration, but can, as a consequence, also improve the reproducibility of implant planning as shown in ◻ Figs. 5.4 and 5.5. These two figures describe the spread of implant planning resulting from a workflow based on a set of few landmarks and a 3D model. We observe a high reproducibility of implant planning in this workflow, except for the tibial axial rotation parameter, which was determined only by a landmarks approach.

As we underline above, bone morphing and landmark-based approaches are not the only systems on the market. In some solutions, a cloud of points is collected in the area of interest and one of these points is selected automatically and labeled as being the landmark (deepest, most

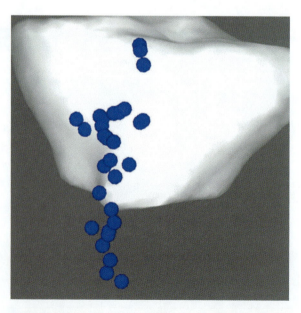

◻ **Fig. 5.2.** Inter-operator reproducibility of landmarks digitization at the Anterior Tibial Tuberosity.

distal, most proximal etc.). These approaches are however less accurate than the bone morphing since they rely only on sparse points or data patches. In the complete 3D approach describe in this paper, a complete 3D surface is build and missing information are added thanks to the existence of the statistical shape model. This improves significantly the robustness of the landmarks computation and provides an accuracy that can reach that obtained with CT reconstructions.

Table 5.2. Reproducibility of the posterior condyle determination using either a pointer (row 1) or an automatic detection in the 3D model obtained with bone morphing technology (row 2). (Results are given in degrees SD)

	A n=8	B n=5	C n=6	D n=10	E n=6	All
Pointer	1.2	1	1.3	2.3	1.7	1.6
Bone morphing	0.9	0.5	1	0.4	1.2	0.9

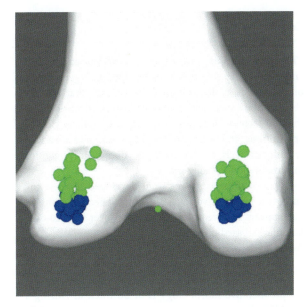

Fig. 5.3. Distribution of landmarks (posterior condyle) digitized manually (*green*) and computed automatically in 3D model (*blue*).

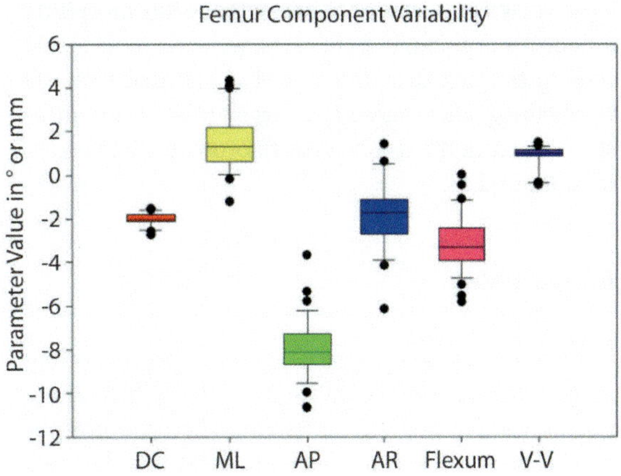

Table 5.1. Reproducibility of anatomical landmarks digitization using a pointer. (n = 35; results are given in mm)

Landmarks	Range	SD
ATT	20.4	4,5
Top of notch	15.5	2,2
Middle of tibial spine	13.43	2,2
Med post. condyle	14.47	3,3
Med epicondyle	23.62	5,0

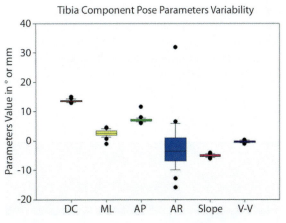

Fig. 5.4. Variability in the femoral planning based on Bone Morphing Data. (*DC* distal cuts, *ML* medio-lateral, *AP* antero-posterior, *AR* axial rotation, Flexum, *V-V* varus-valgus)

Fig. 5.5. Variability in the tibial planning based on Bone Morphing Data. (*DC* distal cuts, *ML* medio-lateral, *AP* antero-posterior, *AR* axial rotation, Slope, *V-V* varus-valgus)

Future Perspectives

Since orthopaedic surgery is moving toward minimally invasive surgery, the ability to acquire 3D data without requiring any skin incision is of high interest. For instance, the HTO procedure described above could benefit from such new techniques. It would be eminently useful if we could capture the entire 3D anatomy of the proximal part of the tibia, instead of the partial acquisition we are doing today. Therefore, some extensions to the actual technique have been developed and are progressively being realized by PRAXIM on the Surgetics Station.

Two new approaches are presented: echo-morphing and fluoro-morphing; in both cases, we use a deformable model. In the first case, this model is matched with 3D data obtained after automated segmentation of ultrasound images. In the second case, fluoroscopic images are used as input data.

Echo-Morphing

In minimally invasive surgery, surgeons are expecting tools that will provide complete 3D data with minimal access or without any skin incisions. The echo-morphing technique has been developed to meet this demand. In this technique, ultrasound images of the bone are acquired with a 2.5 US probe integrated in the Surgetics Station. Theses images are automatically segmented, and a 3D model of the bone is then matched to the points collected during the segmentation process. ◘ Figure 5.6 shows the result of the automatic segmentation of a tibia performed thanks to an algorithm developed by the LATIM, a close scientific partner of PRAXIM-Medivision. The segmentation process is done without any surgeon intervention in real time during surgery.

Fluoro-Morphing

Fluoro-morphing is a new technique developed by PRAXIM (patent pending), which is used for the reconstruction of bone from calibrated fluoroscopic data. Fluoroscopic images are first processed to extract the boundaries of the bone. A specific extended Bone Morphing process is used to deform a 3D statistical model in order to match the original images. This approach gives a true 3D specific model of the vertebra that is being operated on, using transcutaneous acquisition.

Conclusion

The bone-morphing algorithm is a very accurate, fast and easy way to collect 3D shapes during surgery. Based on thousands of acquisitions, one can say that any accessible bony structure can be reconstructed in no more than 90 seconds. It is now routinely use in many clinical applications, and will be followed by even more advanced techniques such as the echo- or fluoro-morphing for minimally-invasive surgery.

These approaches have been developed to meet the surgeons' needs in various situations. The new technology appears to have several advantages over CT and over landmarks-based methods.

Advantages over CT:
1. It is possible to capture the true intra-operative 3D morphology of the bones. In some situations, the 3D preoperative morphology is of no interest. During a TKA, it is necessary to remove the osteophytes BEFORE doing the acquisition, and that is only possible if one can collect 3D shapes intra-operatively, or if one can perform a CT scan DURING the procedure. The situation is the same during an ACL replacement. In

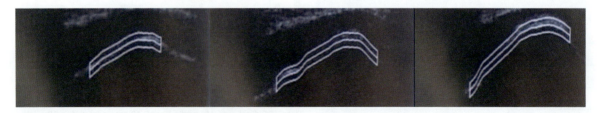

◘ **Fig. 5.6.** Automatic segmentation of ultrasound images at the upper part of the tibia

this case, we sometimes perform a notch plasty. Depending of the location and the size of the plasty, the potential anterior impingement pattern may change or disappear. Therefore, if one wants to plan an accurate graft position, one needs to have a model acquired AFTER the notch plasty. None of this can be achieved with CT; all of this is made possible thanks to the bone morphing technique.

2. The time between the beginning of the acquisition and the final result is less than one minute thirty seconds, which is far faster than CT.

Advantages over landmark-based methods

1. During total knee arthroplasty we need to know where is the 3D prosthesis center, and since all positioning parameters are linked together, we also want to have global planning. This is not possible if one only takes points into account. Visualization of the cuts prior to actual surgery makes it possible to anticipate difficulties and to avoid them, prior to any cuts, which is not possible with landmarks only.

2. During ACL replacement procedures we want to have a 3D representation of the bones on which we can display anisometry maps, and determine targets to guide the drilling of the tunnels. Again, bone morphing meets our needs and a landmark-based method would be much less efficient and more time-consuming.

3. In all cases, the automatic selection of points (such as the most distal point of the condyles) in the model itself is only possible if one has a 3D model of the bones. This decreases the variability that is inherent in manual measurements made by the surgeon.

4. 3D imaging provides a user-friendly interface, and more importantly, a Surgeon-Friendly Interface (SFI). This concept of SFI includes the idea that the friendly interface is based on a friendly surgical protocol. For fast and efficient surgery, a navigation system must provide instantly-comprehensible on-screen anatomical information to guide the surgeon.

5. During the planning stage, the surgeon can be provided with graphical data on the size of the cuts, the amount of bone that will be removed, the bone defect, and so on. None of this can be done if only geometric data are being used.

There is no doubt that making the 3D morphology of bones available to the surgeon during surgery is a real added value. This helps to provide accurate and intuitive

solutions for the surgeons. Simple is not enough. Computer-assisted surgery should appear to surgeon as a mandatory approach, without which operating is simply not possible. 3D true representation of the patient under surgery is the only way of achieving this goal, since it provides robust information in an intuitive environment. Introduced in June 2002, the bone-morphing algorithm is now a standard in medial imaging.

References

1. Stindel E, Briard JL, Merloz P, Plaweski S, Dubrana F, Lefevre C, Troccaz J (2002) Bone morphing: 3D morphological data for total knee arthroplasty. Comput Aided Surg 7: 156–168
2. Kienzle TC III, Stulberg D, Peshkin M, Quaid A, Lea J, Goswami A, Wu CH (1996) A computer-assisted total knee replacement surgical system using a calibrated robot. In: Taylor R et al. (eds) Computer integrated surgery: technology and clinical applications. MIT Press, Cambridge, MA, pp 409–416
3. Nizard R (2001) First experience with the Navitrack system for total knee arthroplasty. In the proceeding of the 21th annual meeting of the Israel orthopaedic association, Israel
4. Taylor RH (1996) An image-directed robotic system for precise orthopaedic surgery. In: Taylor R et al. (eds) Computer integrated surgery: technology and clinical applications. MIT Press, Cambridge, MA, pp 379–396
5. Merloz P (2002) Chirurgie du rachis et visage pédiculaire: navigation à base TDM versus fluoronavigation virtuelle. In: Duparc J (ed) Chirurgie Orthopédique Assistée par Ordinateur 80: 143–149
6. Kunz M., Strauss M., Langlotz F, Deuretzbacher G, Rüther W, Nolte LP (2001) A non-CT based total knee arthroplasty system featuring complete soft-tissue balancing. MICCAI, LNCS 2208: 409–415
7. Saragaglia D, Picard F, Chaussard C, Montbaron E, Leitner F, Cinquin P (2001) Mise en place des prothèses totales de genou assistée par ordinateur: comparaison avec la technique conventionnelle. Résultats d'une étude prospective randomisée de 50 cas. Revue Chirurgie Orthop 87: 18–28
8. Fleute M, Lavallée S, Julliard R (1999) Incorporating a statistically based shape model into a system for computer assisted anterior cruciate ligament surgery. Med Image Anal 3: 209–222
9. Szelisky R, Lavallée S (1996) Matching 3-D anatomical surfaces with non-rigid deformations using octree-splines. Int J Comp Vision 18: 171–186
10. Perrin N, Stindel E, Roux C. Bone morphing vs freehand localization of anatomical landmarks: consequences on the reproducibility of implant positioning in total knee arthroplasty. Computer Aided Surgery, September 2005; 10(5): 1-8.
11. Jenny Y, Boeri C (2004) Low reproducibility of the intra-operative measurement of the transepicondylar axis during total knee replacement. Acta Orthop Scand 75: 74–77
12. De Steiger RN, Leung A (2004) The inter-operative accuracy of the transepicondylar axis using computer assisted surgery. Proceedings of 4th Annual Meeting of the International Society for Computer Assisted Orthopaedic Surgery (CAOS-International), Chicago, IL

The Attraction of Electromagnetic Computer-Assisted Navigation in Orthopaedic Surgery

D.R. Lionberger

Introduction

Navigation in orthopaedic surgery is becoming more accepted as a means of improving and documenting accuracy. Yet, despite the improvements made, the road towards recognition of the capability and versatility of computer-assisted surgery has not always been smooth. Initially, navigation involved imagery, which utilized a localizer to calculate the geometry of the infrared reflective surfaces and light emitting diodes or tracking grids [1]. Image guided procedures utilized patient X-rays and fluoro-imaging obtained prior to or during a procedure as a guide for the physician. However, this was constrained by the necessity of direct, unobstructed line of sight.

Both image-guided and imageless navigation systems require trackers to establish the position of the patient as movement occurs, whereas traditional imageless infrared (IR) navigation eliminates the need for fluoro-imaging while still requiring line-of-sight. Constraints on signal strength as well as a limited arc or azimuth of signal reception hinder its use. Additionally, IR accuracy is proportional to the separation between reflector markers, requiring expansive arrays, which are obtrusive to the surgical field and may injure soft tissue as movement of the extremity is performed.

Due to problems including fixation, signal acquisition, soft tissue trauma, and operative constraints, a technology using a signal that does not require line-of-sight reception was desirable. An electromagnetic computer-assisted surgery (EM-CAS) system has this capability.

Some of the first reports of the use of EM in surgery were in neurosurgical and ENT applications for cranial surgery [2,3]. Other applications of EM technology arose in cardiovascular surgery, where an electromagnetic field was used to guide ferrous-tipped catheters into tortuous vessels that were non-navigable by traditional catheterization techniques. These were tracked by fluoro-imaging yet had the distinction of reversing the role of EM to steer them rather than track them into extremely tight, convoluted vessels [4].

Part of the suspicion about EM technology for orthopaedic applications arises from concerns over the stability of the signal around metallic objects. However, with the advent of multiplex magnetic generators, known as localizers and receiver coils or trackers called dynamic reference frames (DRFs), much of the instability and signal inaccuracy is removed. Precision and accuracy is vastly improved to well beyond the industry standard of ±2 mm and ±2° of angulation. Achieving this level of accuracy allows EM tracking to have equivalent status as traditional line-of-sight IR navigation systems with the added benefit of soft tissue penetration.

The Math Behind Magnets

The heart of the EM system is the localizer coil or field strength generator, which are merely solenoids powered by AC or DC current. There are inherent advantages of both types of technology as there are also disadvantages. For example, the AC system may use one or multiple coil technology, as opposed to the older one coil DC systems with smaller localizers. An AC localizer or generator coil may produce a magnetic field strength in intermittent fashions so as to produce an oscillating radio wave pattern. This magnetic field, generally around one Gauss (0.0001 Tesla), induces an electric current in the coil depending on its orientation to the field. The amount of electric current produced is dependant on both a change in magnetic field as well as its intensity, hence the rationale behind a pulse or oscillating field.

$$EMF = -N\frac{\Delta\Phi}{\Delta t}$$

If the magnetic field is spatially constant across a loop with N turns, the induced electromagnetic flux (EMF) in the coil of N connected loops can be expressed as N times the EMF produced in one loop.

Faraday's law is a relationship derived from *Maxwell's equation*, shown above. This relationship states that the magnitude of the electromotive force (EMF) induced in a circuit is proportional to the rate of change of the magnetic flux that cuts across the circuit.

This also explains how a voltage may be generated when a change in the magnetic field is applied. In other words, these changes could be produced by:

- A change in the magnitude of the magnetic field within the coil.
- A change in the area of the coil, or the portion of that area that happens to lie within the magnetic field (expand the coil or movement out of the field).
- A change in the angle between the direction of the magnetic field and the coil [5, 6].

$$Voltage\ Generated = N\frac{\Delta(BA)}{\Delta t}$$

N= number of turns, Φ = BA = Magnetic Flux, B = external magnetic field, A = area of coil

The coil direction in relation to the field produces the maximum strength; whereas, a 90° polarization negates the electric current produced. The system can then locate and orient the position of the receiver by the electric current it receives from one or more coils. One coil may measure field strength and the direction of the magnetic field, such that the x, y, z position, as well as measuring two of the three Eulerian angles, i.e. pitch and yaw, also known as 5 degrees of freedom. However, the 6th degree, better known as roll, cannot be determined without two

or more receiver coils to obtain this final degree of orientation. This combination of coaxial or tri-axial coils used in a DRF is configured to deliver 6 degrees of freedom, which is mandatory in orthopedic surgery.

Extrinsic Factors in CAS Accuracy

To understand the extrinsic aspects of inaccuracy or precision of CAS systems, one must first look at the hardware performing the measurements.

AC technology uses audio-frequency wave energy to transmit to the receiver DRF. If one uses more than one magnet, a time sequence or frequency multiplexed transmission can create a more consistent and powerful magnetic field that is less susceptible to outside interferences such as metal or environmental factors of other electromagnetic sources. The localizer coil is controlled or driven by the coil array controller, which drives each coil in the transmitter coil array in a time division multiplex or a frequency division multiplex manner. In this regard, each coil may be driven separately at a distinct time or all of the coils may be driven simultaneously with each being driven by a different frequency.

Coils in the DC technology use coils that are usually powered by a direct current source. When the coils are cycled sequentially, they produce a square wave pattern, which are subsequently read by the receiver coil. However, the magnetic fields do not couple energy into loops of wire and, therefore, they require a sensor or flux gate technology. This flux gate technology refers to a larger and more expensive sensor or receiver, which sometimes interferes with navigation issues at a surgical setting. In theory, DC current systems should offer the advantage of less interference from metal and other conductive distortions since a pulsed square wave signal can allow eddy currents to die out before a sample is taken. However, in practice, the effect is a creation of more intense fields from remote metal sources, which actually distort the navigation more than in a pulsed AC system.

Magnetic Signal Distortion

Extrinsic sources of errors seen in both AC and DC-dependant systems occur when metal is in close proximity to the field. Magnetic or electrical fields created by the localizer are capable of inducing errors in DRF coil measurements. These can be classified into two general areas, namely conductive and ferric distortions, which result in »parasitic« eddy currents or bending distortion to the primary localizer field.

Examples of materials, which create conductive distortions, are most steels as well as aluminum or any other highly conductive material. Since titanium is only partially conductive, it remains relatively immune to affecting the field of a nearby coil generation. Even carbon fiber containing Kevlar and other synthetic fiber can create some small conductivity and, therefore, are subject to some small distortions if placed directly in the transmission field.

The second form is ferric distortion, frequently seen with iron-containing alloys. Any object that a magnet is attracted to can be considered ferrous. The stronger the attraction, the more ferrous the metal. Therefore, steels such as the 400 Series and 17–4 stainless, which are highly ferrous, may be expected to disrupt EM signals. Since aluminum and titanium are not as ferrous, they do not »bend« the magnetic field, which can create distortion. Instead, they create electrical aberrant eddy currents, causing field disruption. The effects of ferrous metals are seen in both the AC and DC systems; however AC systems are less affected by remote ferrous interference. As such, it becomes important to ascertain what interference is most damaging to accuracy and how to avoid such interaction.

With the recent advancements in sensitivity and distortion, many of these nuisances (e.g. interference sources) have been eliminated. When the computer senses an externally-generated field or electrical eddy current, the software is designed to turn off the transmission of angular or translational data and flag it as an »off signal.« However, what is in questions is whether or not it can catch this aberration before erroneous values are recorded. Nonetheless, the less disruption the environment can be, the more stable the system.

Intrinsic Factors of Accuracy

There are a number of accuracy measurements CAS can be judged from. The most rudimentary are the mathematical formulas used to generate final angular or translational values. The most basic is suggested by federal and self-imposed industry guidelines that set limits of ±2 degrees of rotation and 2 mm of translation accuracy. An-

other term that is commonly utilized to define accuracy is root mean square (RMS) error. This is the normalization of absolute deviation in values, both positive and negative, obtained by a measure. Center of head measurements are typically expressed in this manner. Therefore, an RMS error of plus or minus 4 mm of the center of the femoral head for kinematic localization should introduce no more than 1° of error to knee axis calculations, which is well within the realm of human hand-held jigs.

Edge of distortion error occurs when signal accuracy is affected such as a metal object placed close to the transmitter or receiver field. Additionally, drift can also occur as fluctuations in the vibrations, voltage, temperature, or circuitry relationships change. Voltage stabilization programs embedded in the software eliminate field fluctuations with most current systems. However, the slow shift of a system's measurements are harder to detect as they may be long term in the form of drift, precision, or delayed value changes over an extended time frame.

As electromagnetic fields are generated in the patient space, they induce currents in DRFs and are delivered to the navigation probe interface through the isolation circuit and then forwarded to the coil array controller. The system must interface with amplifiers, filters and buffers required to assess the signals. Another source of system error is averaging of sampling data. If 10 samples are taken per second, the error may be minimal. However, the figures are still rounded to the nearest degree or millimeter to make navigation more user friendly by eliminating screen clutter. Before issuing 510 K approvals, systems are rounded to the nearest degree and mm, even though many are capable of tighter tolerances [7]. Because the system must make mathematical and trigonometric calculations at high rates, extreme power is necessary to keep intrinsic sampling error to a minimum.

Acquisition speed, or the time required to capture, read, and calculate a receiver, is the culmination of the system's ability in signal generation, sampling frequency, and processing speed of the computer. To improve accuracy, precise detection of outside remote signal errors or interference can be gained by smart instruments, which have defined read only memory (ROM) values. By the computer recognizing a particular distinctive discrete sensor, which has its own ROM chip, the device, when plugged in, is able to be individually calibrated both anatomically as well as specificity to the system without user interaction or formatting to the computer. Despite these industry-stated accuracies, it is important to have clinical as well as bench-tested accuracy of any system to confirm its accuracy as stated by the vendor. Soft tissue shifts, environmental factors of metal or magnetic distortion and surgical tactile accuracy all play a large role in the intrinsic and extrinsic accuracy. The summation of the interplay of all extrinsic and intrinsic effects on accuracy is termed the total system accuracy.

Materials and Methods

There are three basic issues to be addressed in terms of EM acceptability for use in TKR. First, since metal effects can be profound, what does metal interference do to accuracy and how can one avoid these pitfalls? Second, is the EM system accurate in terms of delivering values that can be trusted and are they as accurate as those of IR systems? Third, it must be proven that in a metal-unfriendly environment such as an operating room, clinical accuracy is comparable to traditional IR systems.

Metal Influence

To simulate a metal-free environment, free of vibration or electromagnetic influence, a phenolic surrogate knee on a wooden table was used and pre-testing by Coordinate Measurement Machine (CMM) measurements. The accuracy of the system, Medtronic AxiEM (Louisville, Colorado) with software version 1.1, was certified by the vendors and automatic rounding and averaging was deactivated to provide real assessment of errors and drift of values. To test fundamental accuracy, a common stainless steel mallet was passed into the field to ascertain the location and extent of the edge of distortion (10 cm) for the most significant inaccuracy in distal femoral measurements. Additionally, erroneous distance measurements were assessed to provide a complete algorithm for operative inaccuracy, which may occur with EM in orthopedic applications. By knowing the measurement that was most sensitive to metal, the femoral varus/valgus and translation measurements were used to assess different metal effects. Geometrically matched metal samples of titanium, cobalt chrome, 304 stainless steel, 316 stainless steel, 260 brass, and 6061 aluminum, and 110 copper were then placed into the field at 10 cm from the localizer to obtain RMS deviations of all measured values of a distal femoral cut from the pre-tested angle and translation distance values.

Bench Accuracy

Accuracy assessment was evaluated in a bench study using the above laboratory setting on the same EM machine against a comparable IR system, Medtronic IR (Louisville, Colorado). The same phenolic, surrogate knee previously used was the standard to measure all angular, translational, and gap distance measurements, used in a typical total knee replacement (TKR) procedure. Six runs on each machine were then compared to the other machine using Student's t-test analysis for statistical comparison. An evaluation of drift, stability, acquisition time, acquisition azimuth, and precision was also obtained. The machines were then used to measure accuracy parameters in six runs on fresh, unembalmed cadaver knees in a live OR environment with all systems operational, such as electrocautery, anesthesia, electric hand pieces, and electric OR tables with no reduction in metal mass. Direct comparisons were again made between the EM and IR systems.

Clinical Accuracy

Final evaluation of accuracy was performed clinically in an IRB-approved prospective study of 46 patients, using the aforementioned IR and EM systems. Statistical comparisons for significance were treated similarly by comparing each intra-operative value of all angles and translations obtained against full hip-to-ankle spiral CT data obtained postoperatively. Pre and postoperative knee scores, length of stay, incision length, complications, medication usage, and operative time were compared in a head-to-head IRB-approved prospective trial.

Results

Metal as a Source of Inaccuracy

Edge of distortion measures were seen when a stainless steel mallet was passed within 10 cm of the instrument. The error increased three-fold when tested next to the pointer probe, whereas placing the mallet next to the localizer resulted in negligible error. The EM system was susceptible to metallurgical interference even with the »off-signal« activation alert or clipping safeguard activated. The maximum deflection achieved with a stainless steel mallet close to the pointer probe created as much

6

as 2.7° angular error and 6.3 mm of resection error. This was not replicated when the mallet was placed next to the localizer. This points out potential pitfalls and requires the surgeon to be alert to such errors to prevent them from occurring during surgery.

Resection level measurements from CMM-established translational figures were calculated from all metals. In general, three groups were differentiated in terms of conductive and ferric combined interference. Cold rolled steel induced no error, presumably because of the ferric interference sensor in the system locked down transmission to an »off-signal« before errors could be produced. Titanium proved to have the least effect on EM accuracy followed closely by cobalt chrome (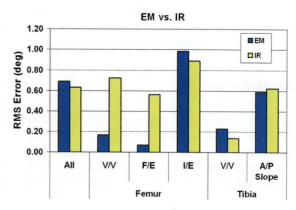 Fig. 6.1). In the second group, ferric interference by any iron-containing alloys proved to show some effect on EM accuracy, but this effect was short-lived as the »off-signal« safeguard activated properly. Surprisingly, ferric interference seemed to play a lesser role in translational errors induced in the EM system than it did in angular errors. The greatest errors from copper and brass did not activate the »off-signal« safeguard [7].

Accuracy in the Lab

In the bench study analysis of accuracy using the EM system against the IR system, all previously measured angles were compared including rotation and femoral to tibia gap distance measurements. The standard deviations of the measurements with the IR system averaged 2.9 times greater than the standard deviations from the EM system. Measurements from both the infrared and electromagnetic surgical navigation systems were accurate within ±1° of the true values (95% confidence interval). Both EM and IR systems showed the most inaccuracy in femoral component internal and external rotation of ±1°. In the remaining measurements, the EM system proved significantly more precise than the IR system.

The variability of the EM system increased more than three-fold when utilized in the operating room compared to the metal-free environment. However, the average of all ten RMS errors between the EM measurements made in the metal free lab and the true values was 0.69°, compared to 0.67° when the system was used in a standard operating room. The greatest error was found in the posterior slope measurement and internal and external rotation measurements. (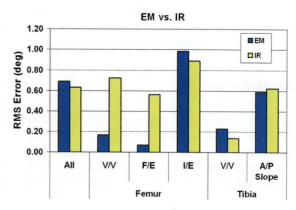 Fig. 6.2) Total system accuracy representing the weighted mean of all possible errors was 0.6°±0.1 for the EM and 0.5°±0.1 for the IR.

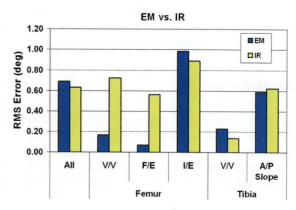

□ Fig. 6.2. Standard deviation of angular errors in IR vs. EM system on the mean of all measurements of varus/valgus of femur and tibia, internal and external rotation of femur and tibia, flexion/extension of femur, and slope of tibia

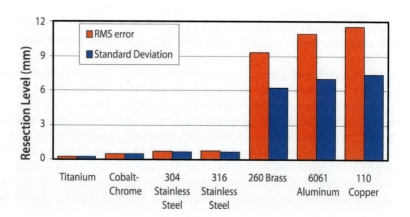

□ Fig. 6.1. Interference caused by different alloys

This comparison showed that the accuracy of the EM system was at least as accurate as the IR with the standard AP and lateral measurements of the femur and tibia, as well as the mechanical alignment. The system was accurate to ±1° with no discernable drift and acquisition time superior to IR [8]. Investigation of acquisition time on a time-expenditure analysis showed that registration time on the EM system to be 58.3% faster than the IR system and a DRF recognition azimuth arc that was 163% larger (field of 360° rather than 137°).

In a similar fashion, the IR system was found to be susceptible to errors in pin bending or rotation during high flexion of the knee as the VMO tethers on the tracker causing as much as 14° error with as little as a 5° rotation in the pin. Pin bending did not produce as much measurable error.

Clinical Head-to-Head Trial of Accuracy

Results of the clinical trials of the head-to-head comparison of EM and IR revealed a number of objective findings similar to that of the bench study in addition to accuracy. Operative time in EM-navigated cases was 7 min greater than that of non-navigated TKR and 5 min less than IR-CAS, even in the inaugural 25 patients [11]. Operative time during the first 25 patients was 71.9 min in the EM group versus 68.3 min in the IR group. This has now improved in the last 100 patients to an asymptote of 55 min in non-complicated medium-sized patients. Time requirements for this system were initially not different than those seen using IR by the author 2 years ago. However, even after adaptation to the IR system, the surgeon had to spend about ten more minutes for tracker mounting, registration and data collection over traditional, non-navigated cases for the first 15–20 cases. As such, the EM system was faster than IR system by eliminating some of the jig reparation and dismantling and included some timesaving steps such as elimination of preliminary cuts, which allowed for corrective recuts without repining saw captures. Operative time using EM is distinctly different thanks to not only increased workflow through better software but from the downsizing of the DRF, which facilitates easier insertion. As previously stated, operative time averaged just 3.6 min (5.2%) greater in EM than our previous experience in IR. Interestingly, the surgeon is able to quickly adapt to the EM system as demonstrated by the slight difference in operative time indicated above even though the surgeon had

had ample time to adapt to the IR system. After 25 cases, the average time for EM is 68 min versus the equivalent adaptation time in IR of 81 min, representing a 20% increase in time expenditure over that of EM.

Accuracy is the litmus test of any navigation system as the final phase of investigation. In a head-to-head trial of the EM versus IR systems, a prospective analysis of alignment accuracy based on spiral CT imaging showed comparable accuracy [9]. Measurements of specific angles and distances recorded intra-operatively during each step proved to be similar with EM tending to be slightly more accurate than IR (● Fig. 6.3) [10]. In addition, the final spiral CT-based calculation of mechanical axis for alignment in the series of patients was found to be within ±3° of neutral alignment in 90% of IR and 93% of EM patients (● Fig. 6.4). When compared to IR, EM accuracy was at least as good when performed in a non-modified traditional operating room maintaining sub-degree accuracy in

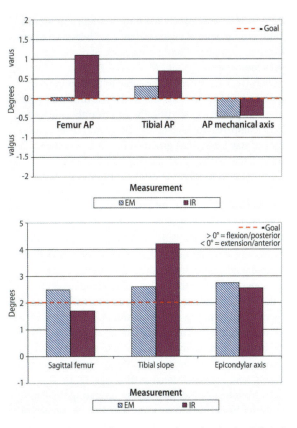

● **Fig. 6.3.** Mean values of measurements from a head-to-head clinical trial of EM versus IR. Data taken obtained from spiral CT images of the hip-to-ankle 16-slice reconstructions

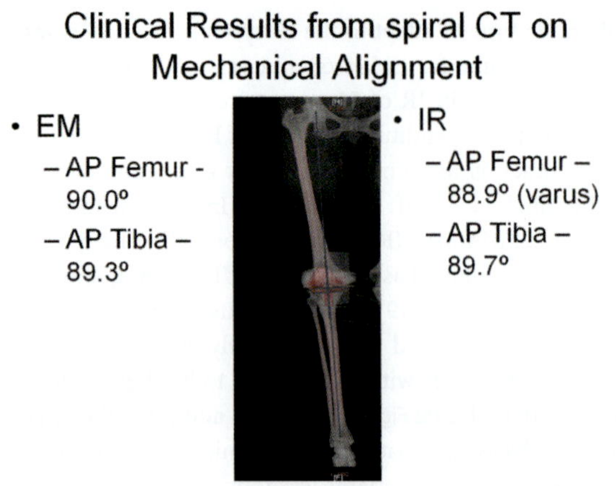

6

Clinical Results from spiral CT on Mechanical Alignment

- EM
  - AP Femur - 90.0°
  - AP Tibia - 89.3°

- IR
  - AP Femur - 88.9° (varus)
  - AP Tibia - 89.7°

Fig. 6.4. EM and IR were both accurate in achieving the 90° goal (p = 0.96). ±3° of ideal mechanical alignment was achieved in 93% of EM and 90% of IR cases

either environment. Functional improvement was similar in both groups, with a slight tendency for better accuracy using the EM system. Considering range of motion at a 6–8 week follow-up, range for EM was 114.2° versus 115.0° in IR. Likewise, knee scores at the same follow-up improved 51 points in EM versus 45 points in IR. The incision length in the EM group was statistically significantly shorter by 1.1 cm compared to that of the IR group. The average length of stay for the EM group was 2.32 days, which was similar to that of the infrared group had 2.54 days.

Clinical Experience in the First Cases

The first 40 cases provided subjective evidence of clinical ease and flexibility over that of IR-CAS. Aside from the rapid adjustment of the surgeon to shorten operative time noted above was the evolution of subtle dependence on the EM's measurements. A previous reliance on a surgeon's ability to cut and maintain the accuracy with traditional cutting instruments has been replaced by a faith in the more analytical and predictive EM system of measurements. Therefore, the EM system became the deciding vote over traditional cutting jigs. Other options made EM more flexible, such as the navigating the femoral cutting block instead of using referencing gauges or preliminary cuts. This flexibility has shaved steps off the procedure while providing the surgeon with predictive screenshots of the progress of TKR preparation.

Discussion

One of the first obvious differences when using the EM system compared to the IR system is the absence of large tracker arrays. Because of the large lever arm on the reflective trackers, ridged bi-cortical fixation is mandatory in IR to assure there is no movement of the tracker array. The arrays are affixed with large, ridged fixation mounts and as a result can cause bone, muscle, and soft tissue trauma. These have been reported to induce scar tissue around pin sites, resulting in arthrofibrosis or fracture, leading to delayed or suboptimal postoperative performance. Use of less obtrusive, down-sized trackers may minimize this complication. Fixation via low profile screws used in EM applications is much simpler and less invasive compared to that of the IR's fixation mounts. This indirect pin complication has been described by other authors and was seen in our series through a higher incidence of arthrofibrosis and range of motion loss, and a need for manipulation. The incision length for EM patients was 1.1 cm statistically significantly shorter than the IR group, and this reflects similar limitations to the recovery from wound trauma for both systems [10, 12].

Therefore, the most important provision EM brings to the table is the ability of navigating minimally invasive surgery. The fact that EM DRF trackers, mounted inboard to the incision, affords a smaller incision in addition to preventing soft tissue trauma to the vastus medialis from external pins that mount IR trackers (■ Fig. 6.5) may explain the subtle difference in enhanced range of motion and improved knee scores in EM over IR. Whether or not one is an advocate of smaller incisions, the invasive destructive nature of four or more bicortical pins negates much of what an MIS total joint surgery can provide. We found that incision length even in the first 40 cases performed conformed to the principles of MIS. The incision did not require modification or extension to accommodate placement of trackers, exceptional guidance. If one believes precision is as important as minimization of tissue trauma, the use of EM appears to be a good marriage of technologies.

Reception of signal in EM is clearly better than IR by 163%. Even in a metal contaminated field, EM reception was possible in a variety of positions. However, because larger cutting jigs are required, localizer position becomes more crucial in the EM setting just as camera angle and distance is in IR. Optimal distance from the DRF is 20 cm, but transmission can occur as distant as 500 cm if no metallic interference is detected. However, in the presence of

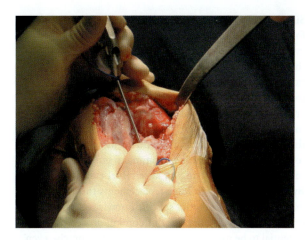

Fig. 6.5. DRF wires are the only visible vestige of an EM-CAS as the incision remains free of imposing tracker arrays, in contrast to that of IR-CAS

metal, the »sweet spot« for reception can shrink to as little as 10–20% of the field. Once a surgeon becomes accustomed to these idiosyncrasies, the versatility and freedom of EM over IR is readily apparent.

Accuracy of waypoint acquisition, whether in EM or IR, is crucial in properly orienting the CAS system. There are points that must be properly identified to ensure that the angular alignment by CAS is valid. Even the most precise machine cannot make up for sloppy landmark identification. Two cardinal waypoints are in the distal femoral center and the tibial spine. If a translation of 2 cm is accidentally digitized as a landmark, this may result in as much as 1.5° of error in varus/valgus measurements. Though not as important, the composite of femoral or tibial articular surfaces or malleoli have less of a mathematical implication to the mechanical axis calculation than the centers of the femur and the tibia.

Metal is to EM what line-of-sight disruption is to traditional IR navigation. One of the most important disruptions comes from ferromagnetic interference. While sensing an induced parasitic field, the machine's default is activated and the readings are turned off momentarily. Although it is imperative to have this type of program to lessen erroneous readings, it can be frustrating when quantifying measurements.

Clearly our studies proved that metals may interfere with reception strength (○ Fig. 6.2). Although aluminum created significant errors, it was also intercepted by an »off-signal« status before interfering with accuracy. Even

though some metals had a surprisingly low interference constant given their iron content, such as the 300-series stainless (303, 316L), they proved to evoke more potential danger of allowing erroneous signals without the software catching them. It behooves the surgeon to maintain a clear field to minimize this error. Cobalt chrome and titanium alloys responded similarly to those found in previous studies of DC current. With refinement for optimal sampling frequency and more modern high speed software in the EM system, the effects of these metals created negligible measurement errors in our bench study [13, 14]. Nonetheless, EM systems mandate the use of inert metal or plastic instruments that do not create interference or dampen response time of measurement. These are the dangerous offenders that the EM »off-signal« safeguard is not able to detect.

The results from our bench and clinical study showed the EM system to be at least as accurate as the IR. The most inaccurate measurements were in the internal and external measurements of the femur. This is one of the more difficult landmarks to obtain due to disagreement in its identification in both the patient and on imaging whether CT or X-ray. Despite this inaccuracy found in both EM and IR, the precision and accuracy of the EM system was equal, if not superior, to IR. Despite this, it may not be entirely fair to hold the CAS system responsible for the skewed results given the plethora of disagreement over accurately identifying the true epicondyles. Nonetheless, both systems were capable of measurements in the operating environment within ±1 mm translational accuracy and ±1° with a 95% confidence interval, which is well below the stated ±2° and ±2 mm quoted by the industry. While the results of the bench study were acceptable, the clinical study also showed that 93% of the patients in the EM group had a mechanical axis alignment within the ±3° range using spiral CT imaging. Since the majority of previous studies have reported 90–95% of patients within this range based on less accurate 36 inch AP weight-bearing films, achieving a figure of 93% certainly compares well with the expected accuracy.

Sampling of magnetic signals created by the localizer were sensitive to movement, just as are their receivers. Therefore, ridged or steady dampening movement during acquisition or measurements was found to improve speed of data registry. If there is any movement in the localizer, the response time on the DRF is lengthened as the computer has to search for the appropriate signals again. Stabilization of rapid motion may be achieved by placing the localizer on a firm platform or support provided in the operating room.

Environmental exposure to magnetism is an age-old debate that has not been completely elucidated [15, 16]. As its uses have transcended application to bone and tissue ingrowth, cartilage generation, or pain relief, there are still no published studies implicating detrimental effects; only studies that speak of the beneficial results have been published. Although a magnetic flux field may temporarily affect proper activation or engagement of the cardiac monitoring and pacemaker capabilities, modern construction of pacemakers have included circuits that are able to tolerate small magnetic fields, which reduces the possible affects of an EM system.

In addition to the aforementioned advantages, the EM-CAS system, like other navigation systems provide the potential to:

1. Reduced outliers for acceptable angulation and alignment for implants.
2. Document pre- and post-surgical kinematics, providing a permanent record or retrievable digital file as a safeguard for the physician.
3. Archiving of screen images for research purposes.
4. Refinement of first cut to a more perfect cut is likely due to a more precise starting point along with instantaneous real-time feedback during the cut.
5. Avoidance of the femoral canal violation, inducing intra-operative pulmonary complication of fat embolisms.
6. Elimination of IM guide inaccuracy from femoral bowing creating flexed femoral components.
7. Anticipation and predictive measures allowing for an intra-operative template of a best fit scenario.
8. Flexion and extension balance through gap distance measurements to optimize range without giving up stability. These real time measurements are obtained dynamically at specific flexion angles and represent a far better solution to balancing isometry and joint line restoration, replacing the »feels right« tensioning.
9. Rotational mating of the prosthesis to the anatomic axis of motion.
10. Femoral axis prioritization by the surgeon of Whiteside's line, functional axis, or posterior condyle, as opposed to a set position defined by the industry or the vendor.

Unfortunately, many CAS systems require added personnel to enter the data or shift on the various screen options.

Simple solutions currently utilized include a wireless or foot-activated mouse or voice activated commands. However, even this requires the surgeon to temporarily take their attention away from the field to the screen. Additionally, some newer programs offer user-specific choices to adapt different procedural sequences and alignment criteria to be customized to the surgeon rather than being proprietarily specific. Similar to the arthroscopist, the surgeon rapidly acquires faith in the system's ability to guide the procedure as a »command guidance« instrument, rather than relying on false visual cues (◘ Fig. 6.6). By shortening steps in knee replacements through smart jigs, drills, and prosthetic- specific knowledge-based programs, knee replacement in this coming decade have the potential to be much easier while being more precise even for the casual joint replacement surgeon.

Inaccuracy begets failure in total knee replacement. To align and mate prosthetic interfaces based on individual patient parameters instead of textbook averages provides the potential to extend the life of prostheses and improve functional outcomes. Rand and his colleagues found that 28% knees failed at 10 years, whereas Jeffery et al. found 24% failing at 8 years if mal-aligned [19, 20]. With revision surgery for total knee replacements increases by 600% as expected by 2030, any reduction of this burden by enhanced accuracy and outcomes has vast economic implications [19]. The question is now, »Can we afford to not be more precise?« If computerization can accomplish in the private healthcare sector the same efficiency it has in the business fields, all of us will benefit. Yet, adoption of new ideas is slow and confounded by preconceived notions, which may or may not be valid or accurate [17].

Through all of the glitz and glamour of bringing a computer to the operating room, we as surgeons have a duty to avoid implying to our patients or colleagues that the computer automatically makes us better surgeons than those not using the technology. Although the literature has clearly implied CAS helps reduce outliers, it does not eliminate them. If nothing more, it gives the surgeon the consolation of a precise and redundant check of what he already should have suspected to be correct. Remaining complacent to new technology has never been a tradition of orthopedic surgeons. Only decades of review will truly tell the result of what this era of computer technology did to improve our understanding of the knee mechanics and whether it translates into more durable and functional knees. Nonetheless, it is an excellent start.

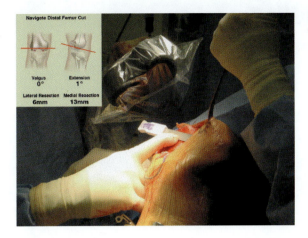

Fig. 6.6. Freshening up unsatisfactory cuts to perfect alignment is easily done without cumbersome correction jigs. The surgeon can maintain constant updates of correction progress without losing reception of navigational signals when the surgeon or assistants are in the way of the receiver

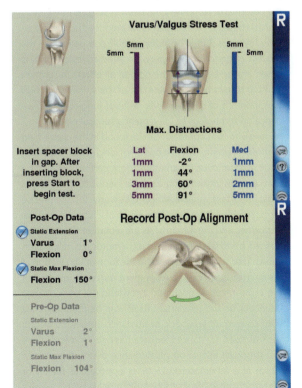

Fig. 6.7. Screen capture of EM program showing typical data available to the surgeon on a real-time basis to aid in intelligent conclusions on tissue balance rather than a »feels right« technique

References

1. Reinhardt H, Meyer H, Amrein E (1988) A computer assisted device for the intra-operative CT-controlled localization of brain tumours. Eur Surg Res 20: 51–58
2. Fried MP, Kleefield J, Gopal H, Reardon E, Ho BT, Kuhn FA (1997) Image-guided endoscopic surgery: results of accuracy and performance in a multicenter clinical study using an electromagnetic tracking system. Laryngoscope 107: 594–601
3. Manwaring KH, Manwaring ML, Moss SD (1994) Magnetic field guided endoscopic dissection through a burr hole may avoid more invasive craniotomies. A preliminary report. Acta Neurochir (Suppl) 61: 34–39
4. Halliday D, Resnick R, Walker J (1997) Fundamentals of physics. Part 3. 5th edn. Wiley, Hoboken
5. Solomon SB, Magee CA, Acker DE, Venbrux AC (1999) Experimental nonfluoroscopic placement of inferior vena cava filters: use of an electromagnetic navigation system with previous CT data. J Vasc Interv Radiol 10: 92–95
6. Sadika MNO (1989) Elements of electromagnetism. Saunders College Publishing, Philadelphia
7. Victor J, Hoste D (2004) Image-based computer-assisted total knee arthroplasty leads to lower variability in coronal alignment. Clin Orthop Relat Res 428: 131–139
8. Lionberger DR, Stevens F (2006) Metal influence on EM Navigation in the OR (in progress)
9. Lionberger DR, Haddad JL, Ho DM, Weise J (2006) How does electromagnetic navigation stack up against infrared navigation in minimally-invasive total knee replacements? (in progress)
10. Lionberger DR, Stevens F, Conditt MA, Kulkarni N, Ismaily SK, Noble PC (2006) Is electromagnetic navigation in total knee replacement reliable? A comparison of accuracy. AAOS 2006
11. Lionberger et al. (2006) Poster. AAOS 2006
12. Wagner A, Schicho K, Birkfellner W, Figl M, Seemann R, Konig F, Kainberger F, Ewers R (2002) Quantitative analysis of factors affecting intraoperative precision and stability of optoelectronic and electromagnetic tracking systems. Med Phys 29: 905–912
13. Milne AD, Chess DG, Johnson JA, King GJ (1996) Accuracy of an electromagnetic tracking device: a study of the optimal operating range and metal interference. J Biomech. 29: 791–793
14. LaScalza S, Arico J, Hughes R (2003) Effect of metal and sampling rate on accuracy of Flock of Birds electromagnetic tracking system. J Biomech 36: 141–144
15. ICNIRP (1998) International Commission on Non-Ionizing Radiation Protection Guidelines for limiting exposure to time varying electric, magnetic and electromagnetic fields (up to 300 GHz). Health Physics 74: 494–522
16. Repacholi MH, Greenebaum B (1999) Interaction of static and extremely low frequency electric and magnetic fields with living systems: health effects and research needs. Bioelectromagnetics 20: 133–160
17. Lionberger HF (1960) Adoption of new ideas and practices. Iowa State University. Press Ames Iowa, pp 107–115
18. Kurtz S, Lau E et al. (2005) The future burden of hip and knee revisions: US Projections 2005 to 2030. Poster. AAHKS Annual Meeting, 2005
19. Rand JA, Coventry MB (1988) Ten-year evaluation of geometric total knee arthroplasty. Clin Orthop Relat Res 232: 168–173
20. Jeffery RS, Morris RW, Denham RA (1991) Coronal alignment after total knee replacement. J Bone Joint Surg Br 73: 709–714

CAOS for Technical Skills Training in Orthopaedic Surgery

P.C. Noble, M.A. Conditt, M.T. Thompson, S.K. Ismaily, K.B. Mathis

Introduction

In recent years there has been a growing recognition of the importance of the functional outcome of orthopedic procedures. This is especially true in total joint replacement, where it has been unequivocally demonstrated that surgical technique is one of the primary factors determining joint function and longevity after the operative procedure. For example, in total hip arthroplasty it is universally accepted that placement of the acetabular and femoral components are critical determinants of post-operative success [1]. Research has shown that many of the parameters describing the function and longevity of an artificial joint such as gait, restoration of leg length, stability, loosening, wear, and osteolysis, can all be impacted by the position and orientation of either the femoral stem in the femur or the acetabular cup in the pelvis [2–4]. Likewise, in the knee it has been shown that the dominant failure mechanisms are related to pre-operative technical factors of component alignment, final overall limb alignment, and ligamentous imbalance [5].

This growing recognition of the importance of surgical technique has led to a need for systematic, validated methods for training and assessing surgical skills. It is increasingly recognized, in virtually all fields of surgery, that practice and skills development must be separated to the extent necessary to prevent undue risk to the patient. While this is true in theory, the tools and systems are not yet in place to adequately train future surgeons. In this context, Computer-Assisted Orthopedic Surgery (CAOS) has much to offer. Computer technology, in some form or other, is universally accepted as a source of simulated reality which is all pervasive in television, advertising, and entertainment. This same technology has made some in roads into education, however, in the orthopedic context, our primary exposure to the potential of computers has been in Surgical Navigation, which is based on the fundamental premise that computer-based systems should be indispensable components of the process of performing surgery. An alternative approach is based on the belief that the goal of all efforts in surgeon training should be empowerment of the surgeon through development of surgical skills, without long-term dependence on technology to implement a surgical plan.

Rationale for this approach can be found in the classic field of motor learning, where it has been long established that, aside from practice, information about performance, in the form of both intrinsic and extrinsic feedback, is the single most important variable affecting outcome [6]. The precise format of this information, how much of it is fed back to the performer, and the timing of its presentation all affect performance and learning. In learning a motor skill, it has been shown that terminal feedback in the form of knowledge of results (feedback on the movement outcome in terms of the environmental goal) and knowledge of performance (feedback on the movement itself) can be more effective than concurrent feedback, or guidance, presented during the task itself. Guidance feedback has been shown to have the strongest effects on performance during the trials in which it is administered [7–9] as opposed to the more permanent changes attributed to motor learning achieved through post-performance feedback [10]. In fact, it has been suggested that a heavily guiding form of feedback (»enabling«) is actually detrimental to learning [11].

Methods of Quantifying Surgical Technique in Orthopaedic Surgery

Technical performance in orthopaedic surgery may be defined by a host of parameters. These parameters attempt to predict the success of the surgeon in achieving mechanical and biological homeostasis through correction of a deformity, removal of diseased tissue, and/or avoidance of residual deficits in function or cosmesis. The simplest parameters to quantify are those defining the spatial and mechanical environment after surgery. These parameters typically describe quantities such as:

1. The alignment of bones on each side of a joint or bony fragments fixed in position after a fracture,
2. the shift in the original position of musculoskeletal tissues (e.g. bones or bony fragments, tendons, or muscles) with respect to their relative position in the healthy skeleton,
3. the laxity of joints under external distracting or shearing loads, or
4. the relative position of bones during joint motion, including the limits of motion imposed by the joints or body tissues.

Based on extensive experience in reviewing the results of each operative procedure, orthopedic surgeons have developed quantitative guidelines for target values of each of these parameters. Through reference to these target values, surgeons are able to gauge their success in achieving the »technical goals« of each procedure.

Although many surgeons agree on the values of each of the parameters defining the technical success of each operative procedure, few tools are available, during the surgical process, to inform the surgeon the extent to which the technical goals of the procedure have been achieved.

A CAOS-Based Training System

To overcome these obstacles, we have taken a different approach than surgical navigation, utilizing similar technology. We have developed a computer-based system that allows the surgeon to train outside the operating room to develop and refine skills specific to a particular surgical procedure. Once these skills have been developed, the surgeon is able to operate freely in the operating room without the expense or the impediments associated with surgical navigation.

This system allows us to measure the technical success of a surgical procedure in terms of quantifiable geometric, spatial, kinematic or kinetic parameters. This process entails calculation of these parameters from data collected during a surgical procedure and then comparing these results with values of the same parameters derived from target values defined by the surgeon, surgical convention, or computer simulation of the same procedure prior to the operation itself (◘ Fig. 7.1).

The measurement procedure is implemented in the following steps:

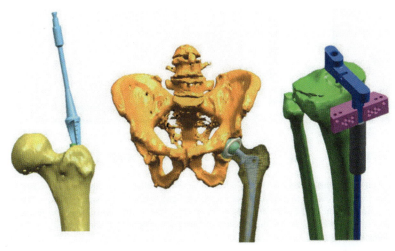

◘ **Fig. 7.1.** 3D representations of instances during surgical procedures showing the relative positions of the patient specific bones and the instruments or components used

7

Step 1: Development of Computer Models

Initially, we create three-dimensional computer model of
- the bony and soft-tissue structures affected by the operation, and
- the instruments and implants utilized during the operation.

Computer models of prosthetic components and surgical instruments are generally available for orthopaedic manufacturers and are relatively easy to integrate into computer-assisted design (CAD) programs. This enables the construction of composite models of implanted components through assembly of device files with individualized computer models of skeletal anatomy derived from diagnostic CT scans. In the event that implant or instrument models are not available from the device manufacturer, it is relatively straightforward to generate computer models by reverse engineering physical components. For many teaching applications, it is not necessary to obtain patient-specific data, as training exercises may be performed on a computer screen, or using plastic replicas of bony anatomy. In this case, generic 3D models can be utilized to show the general effects of specific surgical

strategies, including component placement and the relative performance of different designs (◘ Fig. 7.2).

Step 2: Setting of Target Values for Technical Parameters

For each surgical procedure, the surgeon sets the values of the parameters that form the basis for evaluating his technical performance in performing the procedure. Typically, these parameters will define the three-dimensional position or alignment of bones or bony fragments or devices implanted during the surgical procedure. They may also describe the physiologic motion of a joint (e.g. joint laxity), soft-tissue balance, range of motion. In some instances, the surgeon may simply elect to accept default values for each parameter that have been adopted from published guidelines. In other cases, the surgeon may choose to simulate the surgical procedure within the computer using computer-generated models of bony and soft-tissue structures and the surgical instruments and implants. On the basis of this simulation and, quite possibly, computer routines that predict some parameters describing expected joint function, the surgeon may elect

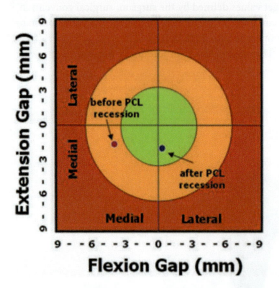

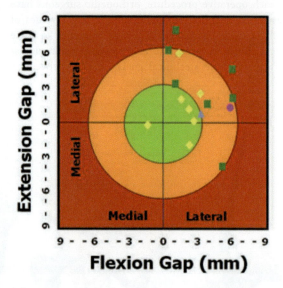

◘ **Fig. 7.2.** Soft-tissue balance performance plots for total knee arthroplasty showing the flexion gap versus the extension gap. The inner circle shows the desired performance target, the concentric circle shows acceptable performance and the outer region shows clinical questionable performance. The left plot is for one surgical procedure and shows the outcome before and after a corrective procedure performed to better equalize the gap balances. The right plot shows the performance of a series of surgical procedures from different surgeons, each with a different cadaver and the same instrument set

to modify the default parameters or may accept their applicability.

Step 3: The Surgical Procedure

Once the surgeon has set the target values for each technical parameter, he or she performs the same surgical procedure on a model, cadaver, or patient. During this procedure, the three-dimensional position and orientation of the surgeon's instruments and/or surgical implants and the bones and/or soft tissues are recorded using an optical tracking system or similar device. During the data collection process the surgeon receives no information regarding his or her technical performance or any differences between the intended position or orientation of each instrument or implant, and the actual position or orientation achieved during the surgical procedure.

Step 4: Calculation of Technical Parameters

The data collected during the operative procedure are processed, allowing calculation of the three-dimensional positions and alignments of the instruments and/or im-

plants and the bones and/or soft tissues and values of all technical parameters.

Step 5: Evaluation of Technical Performance

The output parameters derived from the surgical procedure are compared with the original target values. In the case of many operations, this entails comparing the three-dimensional position and alignment of implanted components after surgery with the intended or target values.

Data Representation

Several different report formats are available to display the results of the system in a way that is most meaningful for the surgeon. One form is a plot in which at least two variables are displayed, e.g. measures of bony alignment and joint laxity. It is also possible to depict the performance of one individual surgeon in comparison with a group of surgeons who have performed the same procedure. Alternatively, parameters or information summarizing the distribution of those values on the plot can be displayed (■ Fig. 7.3).

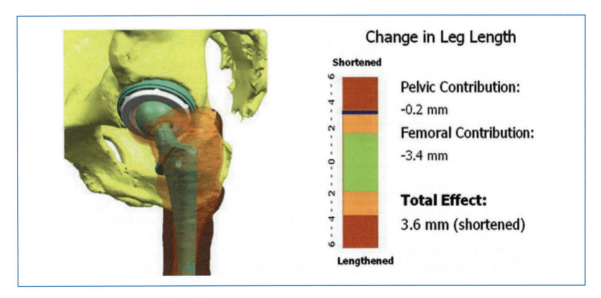

■ **Fig. 7.3**. 3D model of the predicted position of the femur before (transparent), and after (solid) THR. The relative contribution to overall leg length produced by changes in cup and stem position are illustrated. 3D model of the predicted position of the femur before (transparent), and after (solid) THR. The relative contribution to overall leg length produced by changes in cup and stem position are illustrated

Diagnostic Routines

The results of this procedure are displayed on displayed on a computer monitor using visualization routines that allow the surgeon to view:

1. each step of the surgical procedure,
2. the placement of each instrument with respect to each bone, and
3. the consequences of each surgical decision in terms of the final placement of the prosthetic components.

When differences between the intended and achieved results are detected, the system displays the cause of the deviation in terms of each surgical step and variations in the placement and/or alignment of the relevant instruments. The system allows the surgeon to determine the specific errors in surgical technique that have led to the observed deviation of outcome from the original pre-operative goal (⬛ Fig. 7.4).

For example, following a total knee replacement procedure, the system may reveal that the knee has inadequate range of motion in flexion and that this is associated with an osteotomy of the proximal surface of the tibia that has too little posterior slope. The diagnostic routines might then show the surgeon that this error was due to malalignment of the tibial cutting guide in the sagittal plane, and that correct placement required that the distal foot of the guide be elevated by an additional 10 mm above the anterior surface of the tibia.

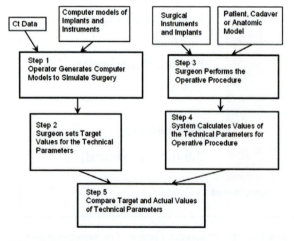

⬛ **Fig. 7.4.** Diagrammatic representation of a bioskills system designed to quantitatively assess surgical performance

Prognostic Routines

The system also enables the surgeon to predict the functional result achieved by the original plan and the actual placement of the components at surgery. Computer routines »exercise« models of the prosthetic components, simulating motion and laxity. These routines allow the surgeon to decide whether a hip replacement will allow adequate range of motion in performing prescribed procedures, or whether a knee replacement can be performed without soft-tissue releases to achieve acceptable gap kinematics.

Discussion

It is widely agreed that the acquisition of surgical skills, like any other highly developed motor-sensory task, requires years of repetitive practice, combined with quantitative assessment and critical feedback. The system described in this chapter is one approach to providing these essential elements using the tools popularized for Computer-Assisted Orthopedic Surgery (CAOS). CAOS-based systems offer an attractive alternative to traditional methods for acquisition and assessment of surgical skills. This approach can be incorporated into the traditional educational environment to augment training of surgeons by »apprenticeship« to experienced mentors. The CAOS-based system allows trainees to develop and rehearse essential surgical skills with individualized feedback which quantifies errors in technique and estimates the magnitude of functional deficits which would arise as a consequence. It is our belief that this approach can reduce the risk of complications from surgical procedures because critical errors in surgical technique may be identified and corrected before trainees progress to real operative procedures.

In previous studies we have utilized the computerized bioskills system to assess the surgical skills of fifteen surgeons and trainees of varying levels of experience. Each of these volunteers performed total knee replacement in a cadaver using a standard set of instruments and implants. Through CAOS surveillance of each procedure it was possible to compare the intended and actual alignment and position of each instrument and the resulting placement of the prosthetic components. The change in position of the joint line, and the femur and tibia were also recorded in addition to joint laxity in flexion and extension during the application of standard distraction forces to femur and tibia. Our results indicated that discrete steps in the surgical procedure make the largest contributions to the ultimate alignment and laxity of the prosthetic joint. In general, the greatest variability was seen in determining the correct rotational orientation of the tibial component, and in achieving matched flexion and extension gaps. Much of his difficulty arose from errors in AP placement of the femoral cutting guide and in obtaining the desired posterior slope during resection of the proximal tibia. As expected, the magnitude of these critical errors and their variability correlated with the experience and years of training of each volunteer.

It may be argued that the widespread distribution of surgical navigation systems, at least in large medical centers, eliminates the need for training of surgeons in more than the operation of the navigation system. It is true that, where available, navigation systems provide the surgeon with immediate measurements of the position and orientation of the implants and instruments. However, the interpretation of the data measured by navigation systems still necessitates the skill and insight of the surgeon, and all but robotic systems guide the surgeon in cutting hard and soft tissues, without performing the surgical procedures itself. In addition, the high cost of navigation systems, the risk of user and system error, and the increased time taken to perform navigated procedures all favor the use of CAOS-based tools to train and prepare surgeons to operate freely and confidently, without dependence on computer-based measurements.

Although surgical navigation is technologically appealing, use of this technology in many operating rooms presents several disadvantages. All navigation systems require additional time and personnel in the operating room to set-up and operate the equipment, to attach markers to the skeleton, to register computer models to the markers, and to collect and interpret data. This leads to longer operations and a significant reduction in productivity for the operating room. As the systems, the markers, and the additional operating room time are all extremely expensive, and as reimbursement for operative procedures is often fixed, utilization of surgical navigation systems is often commercially unattractive. In addition, the computer routines developed for use with surgical navigation systems are specific to each orthopedic procedure. This means that surgeons who are not specialized, and who perform procedures involving different parts of the body (e.g. knee replacement, ligamentous reconstruc-

tion, and fracture reduction) can only gain access to this technology if they operate at large medical centers with the resources to afford the cost of the navigation system and each of the specialized computer programs. In practice, as most surgery is performed in small facilities, most patients will not be able to receive the benefit of the existing navigation technology.

The advantages of a CAOS-based approach to enhancing surgical training is that it is more economical than surgical navigation, and it is less intrusive in terms of the normal speed and productivity of the surgeon. With such a system, training can be performed outside the operating room, at a central location, independent of the size, budget, or surgical facilities present within a surgeon's own hospital. Moreover, using a computerized bioskills training system, surgeons can repeat the same procedure until each technical step is mastered. As part of each training session, a computer-based system can provide an objective, quantitative assessment of the surgeon's success in achieving the goals of the procedure.

At present, we have yet to determine how rapidly lessons learned in the bioskills laboratory are incorporated into surgical practice within the operating room. Previous experiences with surgical navigation suggest that, after relatively few cases, surgeons identify systematic errors in their surgical technique and readjust their perception of correct component alignment and position. A further question which relates to all methods of surgical training is the durability of lessons learned in the simulated environment. In many occupations involving highly skilled psycho-motor tasks (e.g. musicians, pilots, and athletes), constant practice and rehearsal are an essential to keeping skills sharp. This suggests that CAOS may have an additional role in retraining, refreshing and accrediting surgeons through the use of simulation exercises on a regular basis.

References

1. Muller ME (1992) Lessons of 30 years of total hip arthroplasty. Clin Orthop 274: 12–21
2. Lewinnek GE, Lewis JL, Tarr R, Compere CL, Zimmerman JR (1978) Dislocation after total hip-replacement arthroplasties. J Bone Joint Surg Am 60: 217–220
3. Paterno SA, Lachiewicz PF, Kelley SS (1997) The influence of patient-related factors and the position of the acetabular component on the rate of dislocation after total hip replacement. J Bone Joint Surg Am 79: 1202–1210

4. D'Lima DD, Urquhart AG, Buehler KO, Walker RH, Colwell CW Jr (2000) The effect of the orientation of the acetabular and femoral components on the range of motion of the hip at different head-neck ratios. J Bone Joint Surg Am 82: 315–321

5. Berend ME, Ritter MA, Meding JB, Faris PM, Keating EM, Redelman R, Faris GW, Davis KE (2004) Tibial component failure mechanisms in total knee arthroplasty. Clin Orthop Relat Res 428: 26–34

6. Bilodeau IM (1966) Information feedback. In: Bilodeau EA (ed) Acquisition of skill. Academic Press, New York, pp 255–296

7. Annet J (1969) Feedback and human behavior. Penguin, Middlesex, England

8. Holding DH (1970) Learning without errors. In Smith LE (ed) Psychology of motor learning. Athletic Institute, Chicago, pp 59–74

9. Singer RN (1980) Motor learning and human performance, 3rd edn. Macmillan, New York

10. Salmoni AW, Schmidt RA, Walter CB (1984) Knowledge of results and motor learning: A review and critical reappraisal. Psychology Bulletin 94: 355–386

11. Schmidt RA, Lee TL (1999) Motor control and learning, 3rd edn. Human Kinetics, Champaign

7

Cost Analysis of Navigation[1]

C. Lavernia, V.H. Hernández, J.P. Hommen

Introduction

The cost of healthcare in the United States and throughout the world has been increasing at an alarming pace. Total national health expenditures rose by almost eight percent in 2003 and health care spending in the United States reached $ 1.7 trillion which was more than four times the amount spent on national defense.

The Medicare program in the United States is the second-largest social insurance program, with 42 million beneficiaries and total expenditures of $ 309 billion in 2004. One of the principal drivers in health care costs is new technology. Cost utility studies of new technology are scarce and somewhat lacking. Most surgical subspecialties are eagerly embracing new technologies as soon as it becomes available. Computer-Assisted Orthopaedic Surgery (CAOS) has received significant attention in the orthopaedic literature. Development and validation of navigation systems has also been the subject of several publications. It is clear from this literature that these systems help surgeons improve accuracy of implant placement and diminish the variance between procedures.

The cost of a navigation system in the U.S. today varies from $ 55,000 to over $ 300,000 (see Table 8.2). At the time of this writing, the food and drug administration (FDA) panel has approved 14 systems, (Table 8.1) and more than 16 commercial firms in the United States sell or lease the computer equipment and instruments used for computer-assisted orthopaedic surgery. An exhaustive search of the following databases including Medline, Cochrane Database of Systematic Reviews (CDSR), Database of Abstracts of Reviews of Effectiveness (DARE), Cochrane Controlled Trial Register, HealthSTAR, NHS Economic Evaluation Database (AMED), relevant audit databases, and the Worldwide Web demonstrated no published articles on the cost utility of CAOS. These searches were performed in a structured fashion utilizing electronic databases and relevant audit databases between 1998 and 2006, using free text terms to identify papers that evaluated the cost utility or cost effectiveness of CAOS. A few papers casually mentioned the costs of these technologies in their methodology.

Hip and knee arthroplasty has clearly been shown to be cost effective by a number of authors in several countries. The most commonly utilized technique to measure cost effectiveness is the cost utility ratio. This ratio involves the calculation of the impact of a specific intervention on the patient quality of life as well as the costs of that technology intervention. This ratio is then utilized to calculate what the costs per quality year for that particular intervention. Any new or additional expense that the surgeon or industry brings forward must be added on. The total cost must be factored in a calculation of further increases in quality adjusted well years. CAOS faces a significant hurdle as the current cost effectiveness of total hip and total knee arthroplasty is impressive without this new technology.

[1] Ethical Board Review statement: The authors certify that a local IRB has approved this investigation and informed consent was obtained from each participant.

◧ **Table 8.1.** FDA approved orthopaedic navigation systems for TJA

Product	Hip	Knee	Lab	FDA Approved	Device Class
Orthopilot	Yes	Yes	Aesculap/B. Braun	04/27/2005	II
Acumen	Yes	Yes	Biomet	07/08/2004	II
VectorVision	Yes	Yes	BrainLAB	11/02/2005	II
HipNav	Yes	No	Center for Medical Robotics and Computer Assisted Surgery	n/a	
Ci System	No	Yes	Depuy Orthopaedics/J&J	08/12/2003	II
InstaTrak 3500 Plus	No	No	GE Healthcare/General Electric	03/24/2004	II
NaviPro	Yes	Yes	Kinamed	06/03/2002	
StealthStation System	Yes	Yes	Medtronic Navigation	01/25/2002	II
Navitrack	Yes	Yes	Orthosoft	01/14/2005	II
PIGalileo TKR	No	Yes	Plus Orthopedics USA	05/20/2002	II
Surgetics Ortho Kneelogics	No	Yes	Praxim medivision	06/07/2005	
AchieveCAS	Yes	Yes	Smith & Nephew Orthopaedics	n/a	
Stryker Navigation System	Yes	Yes	Stryker	04/21/2005	II
Z-BOX	Yes	Yes	Z-KAT	04/24/2003	II

◧ **Table 8.2.** Costs of purchase options available for systems in joint replacement surgery

Company	System	Purchase Price	Leasing Price	Per Case
Striker	Navigation System II	$ 276,414		
Striker	eNlite	$ 242,468		
Orthosoft	Navitrack	$ 210,000	$ 10,000	$ 700
Medtronic	Stealthstation System	$ 150,000	$ 2100*	$ 850
Plus Orthop	PIGalileo CAS	†	N/A	$ 180
Aesculap	Orthopilot	$ 160,000	N/A	N/A
Smith & Nephew	AchieveCAS	$ 125,000	N/A	$ 250–$ 700
BrainLAB	VectorVision	$ 260,000 ‡	N/A	$ 833
Depuy (J&J)	Ci System	$ 130,000–$ 300,000‡	N/A	$ 150–$ 300

* Fee per case. † Based on a commitment of use his knee implants. N/A: This option is not available. ‡ Depends on the applications chosen.

Materials and Methods

Our unit has navigated over 100 primary hips and knee procedures at the time of the writing of this chapter. There is a number of costs associated with all navigation systems. These include the purchase or lease of the navigation system, the materials and services, as well as the additional surgery and hospital times that have to be consumed when using CAOS. Direct costs include expenditures for materials and services associated with the use of these systems and include tracker devices, instrument trays, the navigation computer, and camera. Indirect costs include the loss of productivity associated with learning the technique as well as the extra time in the operating room utilizing the technique.

As part of our registry all surgical procedures done at our unit are prospectively studied and detailed data collection is done on all associated costs of arthroplasty surgery. A subset of our registry and a cohort of 200 primary knees and hips were used for time comparison. A trained observer measured the individual steps of the procedure from skin-to-skin times, for both the navigated and cohort cases.

Marketing Impact

To measure the potential marketing impact of a navigation system, we recorded the number of calls made to the office two weeks before and two weeks after a web casting of a total knee replacement using EM navigation. Calls for new appointments and questions related to the navigation were compared.

Direct Costs

Direct costs include expenditures for materials and services associated with the use of image guided navigation systems. A crude estimate of the aggregative cost was used to demonstrate the direct cost.

Equipment

Navigation systems share several similar components:
- **Tracker Devices:** Individual trackers for femur, tibia or pelvis, are used to recognize the pelvis, femur or tibia. These can be infrared or electromagnetic, and can be wired or wireless (battery powered). The trackers for TKA and THA navigation systems range in cost from $ 6000 to $ 7000, and $ 6438 to $ 10,385, respectively.
- **Instrument tray:** Specifically designed trackers, jigs, pointers, and guides vary from $ 1500 for the regular instrument tray to $ 5400 for special jigs used for minimal invasive surgery.
- **Navigation Computer and Camera**: There are two forms of technologies to relay data from the patient trackers and surgical instruments to the computer system. Infrared technology requires a mounted stereoscopic camera for signal transmission whereas electromagnetic systems use wires connected directly to the computer. The computer can be a laptop or a CPU device, which contains software for hip or knee navigation. The software itself costs around $ 60,000 dollars for each module (hip or knee).

The total cost of the equipment, including the computer, software, camera, trackers and trays is approximately

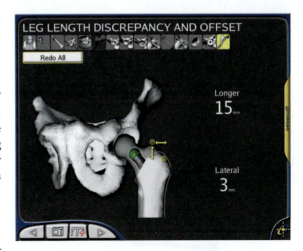

◘ Fig. 8.1. Total Hip Navigation Screenshot (orthosoft)

$ 150,000 for portable systems, and ranges from $ 125,000 to 277,000 for fixed stations (◘ Table 8.2). Some companies have a lease option ($ 10,000 per year), as well as a fee per case option ($ 2100 per case).

The hourly cost for an operating room at our institution is $ 1313 the first hour of surgery and $ 309 for every additional half hour. Anesthesia professional fees are calculated on a point-based system; where one point equals 15 min or $ 40. A structured literature search revealed no previous cost-effectiveness data in CAOS.

Statistical Analysis

SPSS® (v13.0, Chicago, IL) was used for all analyses. And a p value less than 0.05 was considered statistically significant.

Results

To present the potential benefits we tallied the total dollars spent per year as a function of cases performed. A plot was then made of the percent of these costs that were balanced by the economic benefits that a reduction of revisions would yield.

◘ Figures 8.2 and 8.3 show a plot of the relationship between the percent of the total costs, (including initial investment, maintenance and disposables) that are returned

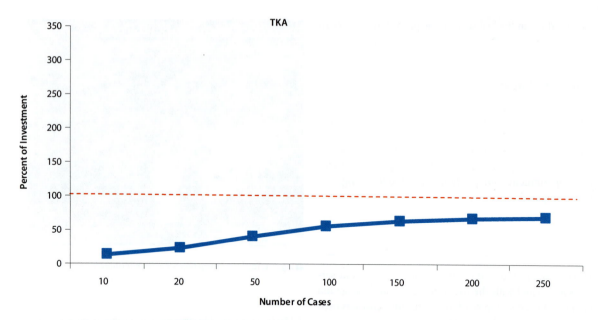

■ **Fig. 8.2.** Percent of the investment covered by the benefits as function of the cases performed per year. (TKA)

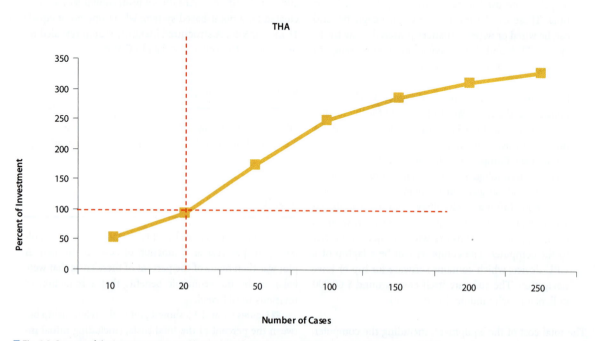

■ **Fig. 8.3.** Percent of the investment covered by the benefits as function of the number of cases done. (THA)

to society by the benefits (reduced revision rates and dislocations) as a function of the number of surgeries. We defined one hundred percent return as that point in which the volume of yearly cases performed yields the reduction in revision and dislocation rates that compensates for the expenses. This is represented in the graphs by the dotted line. This point is the number of cases required for the total expenses to match the benefits in reduced revisions.

Increase in Office Appointments after Marketing

A total of 419 calls, were received in a period of 36 working days. These calls include a total of 168 calls for new appointments before the webcast and 239 after the webcast, the mean numbers of calls per day asking for new appointments before the web casting were 13 ±1.2 S.E and after the web cast were 21 ±1.9 S.E (p=0.002). A total of 12 calls were specifically in reference to the navigation system.

Discussion

The proper positioning of implants in primary arthroplasty has a significant impact on both the short and the long term outcomes of the surgical procedure. The most important factor in early dislocation after total hip replacement has been reported to be component position. Poor component position has also been associated with early loosening from excess wear and impingement in both hip and knee arthroplasty. In addition impingement due to poor positioning of the components has been associated with massive osteolysis. The burden of revision in primary total joint replacement has been reported to be between 8–17%.[12] Improvement in the positioning of implants in primary arthroplasty should reduce these numbers significantly. CAOS has been shown to diminish the variance in both primary hip and knee arthroplasty.[13,14]

Total Hip Replacement

In order to model the potential economic benefits of utilizing CAOS, we assumed that two quantifiable and measurable benefits would be a reduction of the revision rates due to dislocation and aseptic loosening. The burden of revision surgery in total hip replacements is significantly larger than that of total knee replacement. Kurtz et al,[12] reported 17.5% burden of revision on a yearly basis. Malalignment of total hip replacement components has been strongly correlated with premature wear, osteolysis, decreased range of motion as well as dislocation. Von Recum et al,*** demonstrated that an accuracy of 5° for acetabular lateral opening and 6° of anterversion could be obtained by utilizing computer assisted orthopaedic surgery. Bozic et al reported that 18% of the revisions were done due to aseptic loosening and 19.5% due to osteolysis. In order to make our model compatible with contemporary data we assumed that only 75% of the revision cases could be avoided if the implants were positioned appropriately. We further assumed that only half of the osteolysis and revision cases were due to component malposition since fixation modalities and implant design have also been associated with early revision.

An additional benefit that society could garnish from the use of computer assisted orthopaedic surgery in primary arthroplasty of the hip is a reduction in the early dislocations. The dislocation rate in primary hip replacement has been reported to be about 5%.[15] Sanchez-Sotelo et al,[10] reported that the costs of revision surgery for dislocation was 148% that of a primary. In order to model the benefits of the surgical intervention using navigation we assumed that 75% of these dislocations could be avoided by proper position of the components. Our data demonstrates the CAOS is extremely cost effective. A center that performs 25 hips per year would recover the investment in 5 years. If the additional time per case is reduced to 10 minutes, only 20 cases per year are required to have a return in the investment.

Our model neglects some potential benefits that could be obtained by using the current systems. Most of the new systems give the surgeon leg length, femoral offset and medial position of the acetabular component. Leg length is one of the primary causes of lawsuits in orthopedics. In addition there is a potential for decreased wear that could be observed if the offset and medialization of the reconstruction was improved with then use of CAOS.

Total Knee Replacement

In knee replacement surgery the major quantifiable benefit obtainable by improved implant positioning would be a reduction of the revision rate due to aseptic loosening, since dislocations in primary TKR are rare. The proper positioning of TKA components has a significant impact in both, short and long term outcomes. In primary total knee replacement revision rates have been reported to significantly decrease when the alignment is kept within 3° of the normal mechanical axis.[16–18] CAOS has been reported in the literature to decrease the variance of implant placement and improve overall alignment of implants.[19]

The yearly burden of revision TKA is 12%.[12] Almost 45% of this burden has been attributed to component malalignment. Investigators have reported that of those aseptic TKA's that fail within 5 years, 3% are due to joint loosening, 27% from instability, 8% from patellar problems, and 7% from wear. In order to have a somewhat realistic model we assumed that 50% of the aseptic loosening and 50% of the osteolysis could be avoided by proper positioning of the components. Gioe, T. et al stated that 13.75% of these revisions are due to aseptic loosening, 15% are due to osteolysis and 5% from instability. This assumption was made to account for revisions due to failure of fixation as well as design issues. In order to realistically model potential benefits we assumed that only 75% of these revision cases could be eliminated by proper component positioning.

Figure 8.1 shows the break even point for primary TKR. If 250 TKR per year are done only 70% of the investment is returned. However if we assume elimination of all the revisions the investment is returned with 300 surgeries per year.

As noted in these graphs, the hips have a much smaller threshold to the breakeven point than the knees. This is due to the significantly higher revision burden reported for hip surgery when compared to knee surgery. In addition in hip surgery loosening dislocation are reduced while in knee arthroplasty dislocations are extremely rare. In primary knee surgery the benefits do not catch up with the costs when the average reported added time is modeled.

Marketing Impact

Based on our results of a 42% increase in two weeks in new appointments, and 12 additional calls referring to the CAOS technique, an investment in CAOS might be justified. However, as with all of new techniques in technologies there is a diminishing rate of return as they become more commonly used and accepted.

Conclusion

The cost effectiveness of computer assisted surgery has been demonstrated in other surgical fields such as ENT. However, the potential cost-effectiveness in orthopedic surgery remains unknown. CAOS may potentially increase the accuracy of implant placement and the restoration of the normal mechanical alignment, thereby reducing the number of revision TKAs and THAs performed each year. CAOS in hip arthroplasty is cost effective at low surgical volumes. In Knee arthroplasty CAOS does not become cost effective unless the model is changed to assume elimination of all revisions.

References

1. Cossey AJ (2005). The Use of Computer-Assisted Surgical Navigation to Prevent Malalignment in Unicompartmental Knee Arthroplasty. The Journal of Arthroplasty; Vol. 20 No. 1, pp 29–34.
2. Kalairajah Y. (2005). Blood Loss after Total Knee Replacement. Effects of Computer-Assisted Surgery. The Journal of Bone & Joint Surgery (Br); 87-B, pp 1480–82.
3. Sikorski, JM. (2003). Aspects of Current Management. Computer-Assisted Orthopaedic Surgery: Do We Need CAOS?
4. Lavernia, CJ. (1997). Cost Effectiveness and Quality of Life in Knee Arthroplasty. Clinical Orthopaedics & Related Research; 345, pp 134–139.
5. Nogler, M. (2004). Reduced Variability of Acetabular Cup Positioning with Use of an Imageless Navigation System.
6. Delp SL (1998). Computer assisted knee replacement. In: Stulberg SD, Davies B, Picard F, Leitner F. Clinical Orthopaedics & Related Research; 354, pp 49–56.
7. Tria, A. (2006). The Evolving Role of Navigation in Minimally Invasive Total Knee Arthroplasty. A Supplement to The American Journal of Orthopaedics; July 2006, pp 18–22
8. Lavernia CJ (2006). The Increasing Financial Burden of Knee Revision Surgery in the United States. Lee DJ, Hernandez VH. Clinical Orthopaedics & Related Research; 446, pp 221–226.
9. Bozic KJ (2005). Hospital resource Utilization for Primary and Revision Total Hip Arthroplastyy. Katz, P; Cisternas, M; Ono L, Ries M; Showstack The Journal of Bone and Joint Surgery Am. Vol 87 A. pp 570–576.
10. Sanchez-Sotelo J. (2006) Hospital Cost of Dislocation After Primary Total Hip Arthroplasty. Haidukewych G; Boberg CJ. The Journal of Bone and Joint Surgery. Vol 88 A. pp 290–294.
11. Labor UDo. (2006) Consumer Price Indexes. U.S. Department of Labor Bureau of Labor Statistics. http://www.bls/gov/cpi/home.htm.
12. Kurtz, S. (2005) Prevalence of Primary and Revision Total Hip and Knee Arthroplasty in the United States from 1990 through 2002. Mowat, F; Ong K; Chan N; Lau E; Halpern M. The Journal of Bone and Joint Surgery Am. Vol 87 A. pp 1487–1497.

13. Anderson KC. (2005) Computer Assisted Navigation in Total Knee Arthroplasty. Comparison with Conventional Methods. Buehler, K; Markel, D. Vol 20. Suppl. pp 132–138.

14. DiGioia, A. (2002) Comparison of a Mechanical Acetabular Alignment Guide with Computer Placement of the Socket. Vol 17. pp 359–364.

15. Sierra, R (2005) Dislocation of Primary THA Done through a Posterolateral Approach in the Elderly. Raposo J; Trousdale R; Cabanela M. Clinical Orthopaedics & Related Research; 441, pp 262–267.

16. Ritter MA, (1994) Postoperative alignment of total knee replacement. Its effect on survival. Faris PM, Keating EM, Meding JB. Clin Orthop Relat Res 299, pp 153–6.

17. Moreland JR, (1998). Mechanisms of failure in total knee arthroplasty. Clin Orthop Relat Res 226, pp 49–64.

18. Sharkey PF, (2002). Why are total knee arthroplasties failing today? Hozack WJ, Rothman RH, Shastri S, Jacoby SM. Clin Orthop Relat Res 404, pp 7–13.

19. Sparmann M, (2003) Positioning of total knee arthroplasty with and without navigation support. A prospective, randomised study. Wolke B, Czupalla H, Banzer D, Zink A. J Bone Joint Surg Br; 85–6, pp 830–5.

20. DiGioia, A (2004). Computer and Robotic Assisted Knee and Hip Surgery. Oxford University Press, New York, pp

21. U.S Food and Drug Administration. Center for Devices and Radiological Health. Department of Health and Human Services. Approval PMA Database. (2005)

22. National Hospital Discharge Survey (2003). Data obtained from: U.S. Department of Health and Human Services; Centers for Disease Control and Prevention; National Center for Health Statistics

23. American Academy of Orthopaedic Surgeons, Department of Research and Scientific Affairs. (2005)

Validation and Metrology in CAOS

J.B. Stiehl, J. Bach, D.A. Heck

Introduction

Computer-assisted orthopaedic surgery has become an important recent innovation with benefits to many applications as have been explored in this text. We believe that this technology will revolutionize our field, enhancing clinical outcomes in ways yet unrealized. The current development will pave the way for robotic applications, minimally invasive surgery, and »virtual surgery«. An important clinical aspect is »does it work.« Like the advent of many new ideas, the proof or validation follows, often lagging years behind the early use. We propose that any new computer application must be thoroughly evaluated, both from the bench testing that leads to governmental approval, and to clinical bench testing and validation studies, that ultimately will prove efficacy.

From reviewing the current literature in computer-assisted surgery, there is a serious lack of consistency both of terminology for validation and the statistical measures applied. This is not surprising, as the international bodies of engineers and scientists that establish such guidelines are not in close agreement. At the CAOS International Society annual meeting held in Chicago in 2004, a group of leading engineers with a few orthopaedic surgeons sat down to begin the process of writing standardization guidelines. These ASTM standards will be finalized and published, with the long-term idea of eliminating some of the discrepancies. We have organized this chapter to explore system validation from an historical perspective outlining how other fields of medicine and industry are dealing with this problem. Finally, we will make our recommendations as to what and how scientists and clinicians should be reporting out there, so that we all understand what they are talking about.

History

The reasons that the field of measurement as a distinct endeavor has emerged are multiple. However, the principle reason relates to the desire of people to trade and to maximize the value that can be obtained through specialization and economies of scale. Historically, prior to standardization and measurement in communication, the ability to reproduce knowledge through the written word was dependent upon the speed and accuracy of scribes. Scribes would replicate an original work by manually copying the original content onto papyrus, sheepskin scrolls and eventually paper.

The Chinese are believed to have been the inventors of the printing press, which would allow the creation of multiple copies of a single engraving. With the development of the alphabet and standardization in language, Gutenberg was able to extend the value of the printing press through the invention of movable, interchangeable type of standard dimensions. This allowed the more cost-effective production of written works such as the Bible, and is believed to be responsible for the commencement of the Renaissance which has led into the current information age.

An economic study was performed in which it was assumed that a single scribe would take approximately one year to produce a single copy of an important work such as the Bible. Estimates using current United States Labor laws ($ 8.50/hour cost), would lead us to believe that the labor required to produce a single copy would be approximately $ 17,000. The Gutenberg printing shop was able to produce a single work for $ 57.00 or an approximate 300 times reduction in cost. In today's world, as a result of standardization in telecommunication, electronic equipment, software, and interconnecting networking technologies, the incremental costs of downloading a similar volume are less than one cent. We are now living in an age where the impact of standardization is propelling a knowledge revolution based upon the additional cost reduction of approximately 6000 in the reproduction and dissemination of information. (http://cybertiggyr.com/gene/new-age-copyright/)

In the more recent physical world, the concept of standardization, and interchangeability based upon improved measurement and manufacturing was extended to clockworks, firearms and other equipment. The processes developed by gunsmith Honoré Blanc in 1778 were transmitted through Jefferson to Eli Whitney who then partially implemented them in the sale of firearms to the United States about 1808. Thomas Jefferson felt that the standardization of measurement was so important that these powers were specifically outlined in the specified powers of Congress in the Constitution of the United States.

For the government of the United States, the implementation of standardized, interchangeable parts addressed the problems of firearm field maintenance. From a manufacturing perspective, the successful firm was able to reduce production costs by the substitution of lesser skilled and therefore lower cost labor. (http://en.wikipedia.org/wiki/Interchangeable_parts) In an interesting twist of fate, associated with the French revolution, in 1806 they discontinued the process of standardization for »social reasons«. This process of standardization and interchangeable parts was improved by others and eventually became known as the American Method of Manufacturing [9].

The American method of production, including the use of the assembly line, was further refined by the Japanese after World War II. The Japanese combined the concepts of interchangeability and mass production with those of Shewart's statistical process control as communicated through Deming. Shewart had worked in the telecommunications industry and developed manufacturing approaches based upon the use of numerical techniques that resulted in interchangeability, and the efficient mass production of telecommunication equipment. The Shewart techniques resulted in improved product quality, system reliability, lower costs of production and the development of an interoperable telecommunications system. Deming communicated these statistical techniques to both US manufacturers and the Japanese after World War II. The US automobile manufacturers initially ignored the improved systems of quality production and lean manufacturing but they were embraced and extended by the Japanese manufacturing industry. It is currently believed that the failure to incorporate these manufacturing innovations has contributed to the ongoing difficulties of the US automobile industry in meeting the demands of the increasingly competitive marketplace.

How do these historical anecdotes relate to medical and surgical practice? The same basic needs for continually improving quality and cost management are present within our healthcare delivery system (IOM, Crossing the Quality Chasm). Although there are certain differences between the standardized, interchangeable manufacture of objects and the delivery of medical and surgical services, there are many more parallels.

When we walk into an operating room, we rely on standard procedures to assure safety. Our anesthesia colleagues have worked to standardize and improve the safety characteristics of their processes. The development of High Reliability Organizations (HROs) have resulted in a lowered risk of anesthesia-related mortality such that the current risk is now vanishingly small. The corresponding risk of mal-practice judgments and their associated costs have been controlled. The JCAHO in conjunction with organizations such as the AAOS has recently mandated procedures designed to improve safety through systematic approaches to identity management.

The quality of the instrumentation and the devices that we use has improved. Manufacture of orthopaedic devices in the 1980s was associated with process capabilities of 0.6. Currently, process capabilities have improved to approximately 1.3. The electronic components in the computers and cellular telephones that we use are manufactured to process capabilities of 2.0. The overall patient outcomes associated with knee arthroplasty have correspondingly demonstrated a temporal trend of improvement.

Standard Settings Organizations

In today's world, multiple organizations exist that are involved in promulgating standards. In Europe, standard organizations include the International Organization for Standardization (ISO) and the International Electrotechnical Commission (IEC). In the United States, the Institute of Electrical and Electronics Engineers (IEEE), the American National Standard Institute (ANSI), American Society for Testing of Materials (ASTM), Underwriter's Laboratories, the United States Military (Milspec), the National Electrical Code (NEC), the National Electrical Manufacturers Association (NEMA), the National Institute for Standards and Technology (NIST) are some of the major organizations involved in »standard« setting. Unfortunately, as may be expected with the lack of parsimony in the writing of »standards« and the potential economic impacts of compliance or non-compliance with a particular standard that can be related to »quality«; the terminologies and procedures used to allow for determination of errors in measurement are not always consistent.

For example, the term »accuracy« may be reflecting different attributes of a particular measurement. In some circumstances, accuracy may mean the standard deviation of a number of measurements determined from measures of a fixed object. However, unless the distribution of the measures is normal, the calculation of the standard deviation may be misleading to the casual ob-

server. The reporter may then express »accuracy« as a range of measures. Some organizations prefer to use the term »precision« to express this attribute of measurement error (◘ Fig. 9.1).

Alternatively, accuracy may be related to the »closeness« that a particular instrument's mean value is in comparison to a known standard fiducial or »artifact«. In this circumstance, the »accuracy« is reflecting a calibration difference, or bias between the known standard and the instrument performing the measure. Themselves recognizing the need for common procedures and definitions, the standards organizations work to varying degrees to reconcile disparate approaches. The process of standard harmonization can be very lengthy and frustrating. For example, when the ISO was created in 1947, one of their first actions was to harmonize conflicting standards that had been unable to be reconciled since 1924 (◘ Fig. 9.2).

An alliance between the ISO was also created with the IEC with the understanding that the »name and technical procedure of the IEC will be maintained«. Unfortunately, marriage on these terms was problematic and has resulted in difficulties reconciling the worlds of electronics and mechanics to this day. Currently, the ISO is a network of the national standards institutes of 156 countries. Each country has one member. The Central Secretariat in located in Geneva, Switzerland, and works to coordinate the system. The ISO members also include industry and trade

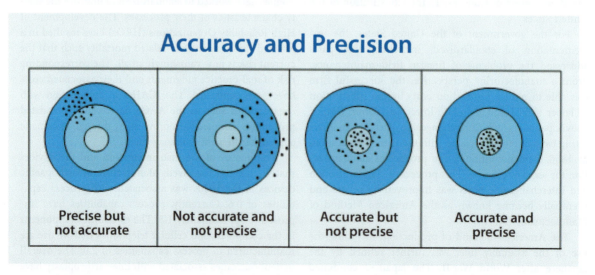

◘ **Fig. 9.1.** Accuracy, precision and stability are relative terms by definition designed to conceptualize performance of a function, in this example target shooting

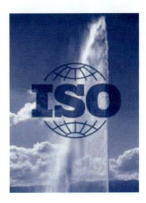

◻ Fig. 9.2. Emblem of the International Standards Organization

therefore offered the opportunity to draft the first standard regarding CAS systems.

The assembled members of the various constituencies (industrial, academic, clinical, regulatory) agreed that CAOS was sufficiently mature that it would benefit from standards. As a result, a committee was formed and tasked with the assignment of drafting a standard regarding reporting of accuracy in CAOS systems. The core membership of this committee consists primarily of researchers and clinicians, though members of CAOS industry have participated as well.

associations. As a result, it acts as a bridge organization between public and private endeavors.

Unfortunately from the perspective of parsimony, the world of computer-assisted surgery crosses the disciplines of electrical engineering, computer engineering, mechanical engineering and metrology as well as research that is conducted transnationally. As a result, it is difficult to currently compare the quality and performance of CAS devices because of the non-standard definitions, surgical applications, testing conditions, as well as analytic approaches.

ASTM Standards Group Effort

As CAOS systems have evolved and more systems have become available, objectively comparing them has become increasingly difficult. Many industries use standards as a way to address such challenges. Standards are necessary to allow end users (in this case, surgeons and hospital purchasing agents) to make informed decisions. The initial decision point is what system to purchase. Once this decision has been made, the surgeon still has options within a particular system. Many systems have both image-based and imageless modalities.

An organizational meeting to establish a committee to develop new standards for CAOS was held in conjunction with the 2004 International CAOS Society meeting in Chicago. At this meeting representatives of ASTM International presented an overview of the standards writing process. While there are other specialties (Neurosurgery, ENT, etc.) that use CAS, none have taken on the task of drafting an ASTM standard. The CAOS community was

Initial Efforts

The first step in drafting the CAS standard was to define its scope. It was decided that a modular approach, starting with a limited generic standard and adding modules for more sophisticated tasks, was most appropriate. The first standard deals exclusively with evaluating the localizer functions of the navigation system. As for the writing of this book this standard is near completion. While the end user will ultimately want to know the accuracy parameters of a system under clinical application, the digitization accuracy must be characterized in order to be able to make sense of the accuracy values under complex surgical procedures

The scope of this first standard is to addresses the techniques of measurement and reporting of basic static performance (accuracy, repeatability, etc.) of surgical navigation and/or robotic positioning devices under ideal conditions. The aim is to provide a standardized measurement of performance variables by which end-users can compare within (e.g. different fixed reference frames or stylus tools) and between (e.g. different manufacturers) different systems. The parameters to be evaluated include the determination of the location of a point relative to a coordinate system, relative point to point accuracy (linear), and the repeatability of single point. These evaluations are to be made at various locations within the measurement volume of the system and with varying tool orientations. A reporting format for the results is provided.

Future Standards

The initial standard will serve as the basis for subsequent standards for specific tasks (cutting, drilling, milling, reaming, etc.) and surgical applications (TKA, THA, IM nailing, plating, osteotomy, etc.). Additional standards addressing imaging modality (fluoroscopy, CT, MRI, ultrasound, etc.) for image based systems, and the software for registering the images or the imageless data to the patient may also follow.

Statistical Measures for Validation

Overview

In general terms the concept of measurement based on current ISO and NIST definitions begins with determining the measurable quantity where the value is generally characterized by a unit of measurement. The »true value« is defined as a given quantity which is obtained from a perfect measurement. True values are considered indeterminant as an infinite number of values are needed to create the true number. Commonly, this problem is solved by creating a »conventional true value« which is considered a better estimate. In some parlance, this could be considered also as the baseline, »ground truth«, or reference value. Measurand is the particular quantity subject to measurement, and could be for example the inclination of the acetabular component compared to the axial plane of the human body. Influence quantity is the sum of measurements that subtly affect the measurand, in this example slight variations in assessing the edges of the acetabular component. Accuracy of measurement is the qualitative assessment of the measured value to the true measured value. This differs from precision which is defined as the closeness of agreement between independent test results obtained under stipulated conditions which encompasses both repeatability and reproducibility. The measure of precision is usually computed as a standard deviation of the test results.

Repeatability is the closeness of measure under the same conditions. Reproducibility is the measure when there is a changed condition of measurement such as using different observers. The error of measurement is the result of the measurement minus the true value of the measurand. Random error is the measurement of a measurand minus the mean after an infinite number of measures. Systematic error is the mean of measurement of the measurand minus the true value of the measurand after an infinite number of measures. Random error is equal to the error minus the systematic error. Systematic error is equal to the error minus the random error. A correction is the value added to the measurement to correct for systematic error. Type A error deals with uncertainties of the statistical measure. Type-B error relates to errors other than those determined by statistical measures.

Descriptive Statistics

For descriptive measures the ISO and NIST recommend the following measures be determined: mean, standard deviation (square root of variance), and the experimental standard deviation.

Mean

$$\overline{x} = \frac{x_1 + x_2 + x_3 + ... + x_N}{N} = \frac{1}{N}\sum_{i-1}^{N} x_i$$

Standard Deviation

$$\sigma = \sqrt{\frac{(x_1 - \overline{x})^2 + (x_2 - \overline{x})^2 + ... + (x_N - \overline{x})^2}{N}}$$

$$= \sqrt{\frac{d_1^2 + d_2^2 + ... + d_N^2}{N}}$$

$$= \sqrt{\frac{1}{N}\sum_{i-1}^{N}(x_i - \overline{x})^2} = \sqrt{\frac{1}{N}\sum_{i-1}^{N} d_i^2}$$

Experimental Standard Deviation

$$\sigma = \sqrt{\frac{1}{N-1}\sum_{i-1}^{N} d_i^2}$$

Process Capability Analysis

Process capability analysis is the approach that is commonly used for process qualification in industrial quality management. In high quality manufacturing, processes are first brought into statistical control. After the process is in control, the process is then characterized mathematically. The process capability index (C_p) is mathematically formulated as:

$$C_p = \frac{(USL - LSL)}{6\sigma}$$

Where USL is the Upper Specification Limit, LSL is the Lower Specification Limit and σ is Standard Deviation. Commonly, purchasers will require that the supplier is able to produce components with capability indices (C_p) of 1.3 or higher. The capability index however is limited in its utility as it is an expression of precision but does not address the problem of accuracy. Six sigma programs, such as that used at Motorola, will frequently require the calculation of the offset capability index or C_{pk}.

$$C_{pk} = \min\left[\frac{(USL - \bar{x}}{3\sigma}, \frac{\bar{x} - LSL}{3\sigma}\right]$$

Where USL is the Upper Specification Limit, LSL is the lower Specification Limit and σ is Standard Deviation. Although it is not clear as to what the specific level of quality is appropriate for a specific medical process, very high quality manufacturing is associated with processes that are capable of producing at levels where the C_{pk} exceeds 2.0.

The most important variable in the process capability analysis is the upper and lower control limits. This requires that you know the target center or the accurately determined value for which you are trying to calculate the precision. For example, a standard target or »ground truth« could be an accurately measured known such as

the mechanical axis of the lower extremity which traverses the center of the hip joint, center of the knee joint and center of the ankle joint. Then you must determine a reasonable or acceptable limit of variation from this target center beyond which an unacceptable result has occurred. For a total knee replacement, one could argue that the prosthetic postoperative leg alignment must be placed within 5° of the normal mechanical axis of the leg. For the six sigma formulas, the upper and lower specification limits would be 5°.

The examples in ◘ Fig. 9.3 demonstrate the effect a large or small standard deviation, and also the effect of a mean that is offset and does not coincide with the center of the target or desired measurement.

We believe the strength of this analysis is the ability to easily compare results from multiple sources or studies with a limited amount of standard data required. The type of values created for the C_p and C_{pk} allow one to compare results with other techniques or technologies. Finally, a basic assumption of the equation is that any isolated value or measurement outside of the specified control limits will cause the C_p or C_{pk} to become unacceptable.

We recently evaluated the available literature for assessment of acetabular component position using the above process capability analysis formulas (◘ Table 9.1). As noted, we used the Lewinnek et al. suggestion for an acceptable upper and lower limit of positioning to be +/- 10° for the target conventional true value [1]. Interestingly, we find that computed tomography performs quite well with the Six Sigma formula which is consistent with prior literature.

◘ **Table 9.1.** Recent literature assessment using process capability analysis. (Upper and Lower Specification Limits: +/-10° for cup inclination and anteversion)

Reference	Modality	Object	N	Control Measurement	Inclination°	Anteversion°	C_p Inclination	C_p Anteverion
Grutzner et al. [3]	Fluoroscopy, Digitizing	Patients	50	CT Measurement	1.5 (SD: 1.1)	2.4 (SD:1.4)	2.22	1.38
Nogler et al. [2]	Imageless	Cadaver	12	Digitizing Arm	-3.86 (SD: 3.4)	-4.89 (SD: 4.55)	0.98*	0.36*
Tannast et al. [5]	Fluoroscopy	Cadaver	14	CT Measurement	0.7 (SD: 2.8)	-6.6 (SD: 6.0)	1.19*	0.55*
Jolles et al. [4]	CT	Plastic Bones	50	Electromagnetic Digitizing	Mean SD: 2.5	Mean SD: 1.5	1.33	2.2
Present study (see below)	Fluoroscopy	Cadaver	24	CT; CMM	0.6 (SD: 0.9)	3.2 (SD: 2.5)	3.7	1.3*

* Denotes below acceptable limits for process capability which is greater than 1.3.

9

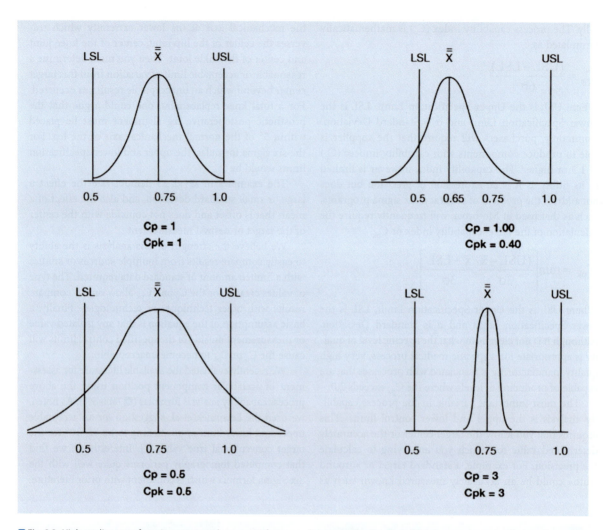

Fig. 9.3. High quality manufacturing process rely on a satisfactory process capability index (C_p >1.3) and offset capability index (C_{pk} >2.0). An important consideration is the upper specification limit (USL) and lower specification limit (LSL) that are determined when the process has been brought into control

Fluoroscopy, when combined with anatomical digitizing methods also offered acceptable precision. However, in our own study as noted below, the precision of fluoroscopy for cup anteversion was not process capable, nor was the one study that evaluated an imageless cup referencing system. These were not the conclusions of the authors in their studies as they did not have a robust tool to compare with other published work. We conclude that process capability analysis will be a powerful tool to compare various systems.

Clinical Bench Testing Methods

For validating the clinical performance of any CAOS application, a simulation of the operative procedure is needed to understand the basic systematic error of a system. The idea is to create a very accurate assessment tool which is basically a phantom or »artifact« that replicates the typical measurements during the operative procedure. The artifact is fabricated in such a way that the length of assessment

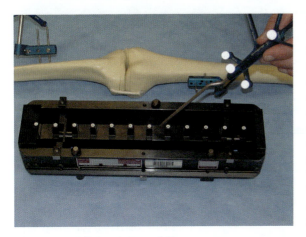

parallels the targeted application, for example the length of the femur or more specifically, various sites on the femur where screws may be inserted. The artifact is calibrated using a coordinate measuring machine, which typically has an accuracy of 0.038 millimeters (0.018 inch). The small holes or divots in the phantom have a known dimension and the touch pointing tool can be placed into these small divots. Additional considerations may include temperature, distance of the optical camera from the target, or small motion of the tracking device attached to the phantom.

We have previously reported our results using a artifacts with traceability to the National Institute of Standards and Technology (NIST), to evaluate the repeatability and linearity of the Medtronic Treon Plus system (Louisville, CO) (**Fig. 9.4). A Weber gage block with equally spaced reference platforms 2.54 cm apart across a range of 25.4 cm was used as the primary artifact. The block was placed first parallel and then perpendicular to the plane of the imaging bar. The perpendicular attitude was established by using a NIST traceable triangular artifact. Each position of the Weber block was referenced using the point indicator six times in a random order with varying probe attitudes. Ambient temperature was constant during the short period of data acquisition.

The Treon Plus system was found to have small but statistically systematic biases in comparison to the fiducial block in both parallel and perpendicular attitudes relative to the imaging bar (**Fig. 9.5a,b, respectively). The mean bias for the parallel condition was 0.26 mm. Regression

analysis demonstrated a fixed bias of 0.52 mm (p=0.00). The mean bias varied inversely according to the distance from the center of the imaging bar. The further the point of measurement from the center of the imaging bar the greater the deviation from the known artifact. The slope of the deviation was small at 20.00232 mm and was statistically different (p=0.01). The mean bias for the perpendicular condition was 0.69 mm. Regression modeling demonstrated a fixed bias of 0.79 mm (p=0.00). The mean bias varied inversely according to the distance from the imaging bar. The further the point of measurement from the imaging bar the smaller the deviation from the known distance. The slope of the deviation was small at 20.00085 mm and was not statistically different from zero (p=0.33).

An example of a phantom that could be utilized for assessing hip CAOS applications is shown here (**Fig. 9.6) This device is constructed to model the human hip joint with the attached femur. Measurements of the hip center, femoral shaft axis offset, and leg length may be done after the phantom has been calibrated with a coordinate measuring machine. This pelvic phantom is 250 mm in relation to the Y axis and 300 mm in relation to the X axis. The femur is 370 mm in shaft length. The ball and socket are articulated with a strong magnet. Finally, holes are placed along the shaft of the device at 15 mm intervals.

Clinical Outcome Studies

We have performed several clinical studies where we have simulated the operating room setting utilizing cadavers to replicate the surgical setting. The object of this assessment is measure as closely as possible the CAOS procedure, and then validate the instrumented cadaver. We have utilized computed tomography and a NIST traceable coordinate measuring machine (accuracy =0.038 mm) to create the conventional true value or »ground truth«.

In the example shown, we have placed an acetabular component into a cadaver pelvis with most of the soft tissue removed, and studied the position of an acetabular component that had been placed at 45° inclination and 17.5° of anteversion. The cadaver specimen was then taken to the operating room where it was secured to the standard operating room table, and the fluoroscopic protocol was used to measure the cup position (**Fig. 9.7). The system studied was the Medtronic Treon Stealth system using an earlier version of flururoscopic software designed for cup navigation (**Fig. 9.8).

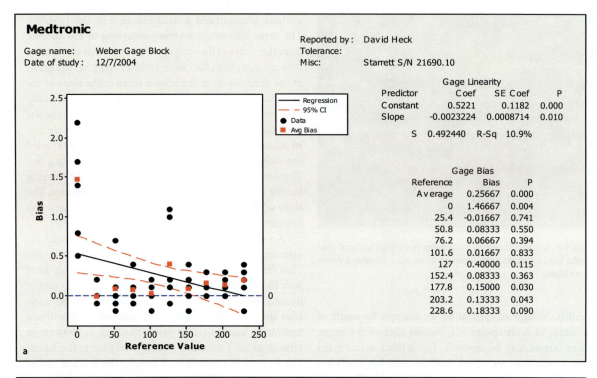

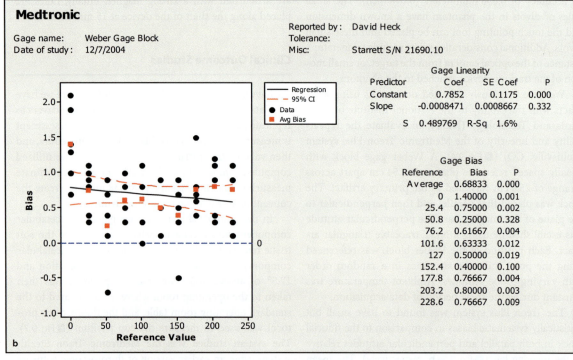

Fig. 9.5. a Assessment of accuracy parallel to the light bar (mm). **b** Assessment of accuracy perpendicular to the light bar (mm)

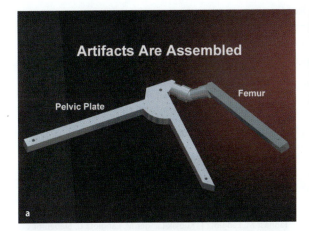

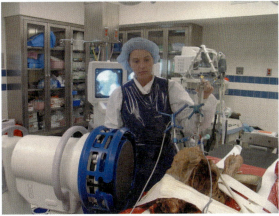

🔲 **Fig. 9.7.** Example of in-vitro testing of a fluoroscopic referencing protocol utilized in computer navigation of acetabular component insertion. Note the cadaver has been positioned in the lateral decubitus position in the operating room to simulate the in-vivo surgical scenario

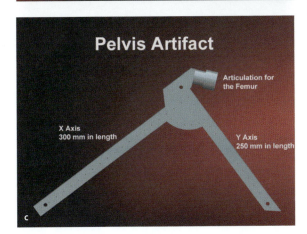

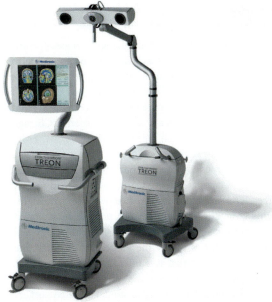

🔲 **Fig. 9.6. a** Phantom or artifact used to assess accuracy of a computer navigation protocol used in total hip arthroplasty. **b** Details of the femoral shaft artifact. **c** Details of the pelvic and acetabular artifact. (Figure contributed by Dr Nicholas Dagalakis, National Institutes of Standards and Technology, Gaithersberg, Maryland)

🔲 **Fig. 9.8.** Example of a »capital« system, with one tower consisting of the computer, video screen, keyboard and storage shelves and the second tower with the optical cameras for the optical line of sight system (Medtronics, Louisville, CO)

The results revealed that the mean CMM abduction measurement of the acetabular cup position was 46.028° (SD=1.075°; range: 43.32°–46.848°). The mean CMM anteversion measurement of the acetabular cup position was15.798° (SD= 0.411°; range: 15.07°–16.38°). Using the fluoroscopic referencing system, repeatability of the acetabular component position was assessed by one surgeon repeating eight trials with complete image acquisition and cup insertion. The mean inclination was 42.88 (SD= 1.5°; range: 39.5°–44.58°). The mean anteversion was 17.58° (SD= 3.0°; range: 14.5°–22.58°). Three surgeons assessed reproducibility using the fluoroscopic referencing technique. Each surgeon performed eight trials in a random fashion (n-24). The mean overall group inclination was assessed as 48.58 (SD= 0.9°; range: 46°–50.8°). The mean overall group anteversion was 17.88° (SD= 2.5°; range: 13.5°–23.58°). If we then apply the process capability Six Sigma formulas as noted above, we calculated that the Cp was 3.7 for cup inclination and 1.3 for anteversion. Our conclusion from this study was that the fluoroscopic system was precise for measuring cup inclination but not for cup anteversion.

Conclusions

The discussion of current methodologies to assess computer assisted surgery has reached an important juncture for we which have provided an interesting viewpoint. The current ASTM guidelines committee has not completed its work though we present the current state of the art that has now culminated from a process that began in Chicago at the CAOS International meeting, June 17, 2004. From the prior work of Deming and others, Six Sigma process capability analysis is not new, but offers a very powerful means to compare technologies from a broad variety sources. Our examples as noted above offered insights for this comparison that were not previously available. Finally, our recommendations for basic terminology and descriptive statistics follow the guidelines of NIST and ISO, and we believe that this offers a sound framework of communication between the surgical and research groups advancing the field of computer-assisted surgery and robotics.

References

1. Lewinnek GE, Lewis JL, Tarr R, Compere CL, Zimmermann JR (1978) Dislocations after total hip replacement arthroplasties. J Bone Joint Surg [Am] 60: 217–221
2. Nogler M, Kessler O, Prassl A, Donnelly B, Streicher R, Sledge JB, Krismer M (2004) Reduced variability of acetabular cup positioning with use of an imageless navigation system. Clin Orthop Relat Res 426: 159–163
3. Grutzner PA, Zheng G, Langlotz U, von Recum J, Nolte LP, Wentzensen A, Widmer (2004) C-arm based navigation in total hip arthroplasty-background and clinical experience. Injury 35 (Suppl 1): S-A90-5
4. Jolles BM, Genoud P, Hoffmeyer P (2004) Computer-assisted cup placement techniques in total hip replacement improve accuracy of placement. Clin Orthop 426: 175–179
5. Tannast M, Langlotz F, Kubiak-Langer M, Langlotz U, Siebenrock K (2005) Accuracy and potential pitfalls of fluorscopy-guided acetabular cup placement. Computer Aided Surgery 10: 329–336
6. Tobias P, Croarkin C. NIST/Sematech Engineering and Statistics Handbook(eVersion). (http://www.itl.nist.gov/div898/handbook/)
7. ISO (1993) Guide to the Expression of Uncertainty in Measurement. International Organization for Standardization, Geneva, Switzerland
8. Taylor BN, Kuyatt CE (1994) Guidelines for evaluating and expressing the uncertainty of NIST measurement results. National Institute of Standards and Technology, Gaithersburg, MD
9. Alder K (1997) Innovation and amnesia: engineering rationality and the fate of interchangeable parts manufacturing in France. *Technology and Culture* 38: 273–311

Part II Total Knee Arthroplasty

Part II A Navigation: Total Knee Arthroplasty

II A

Postoperative Alignment of Conventional and Navigated Total Knee Arthroplasty

W.H. Konermann, M.A. Saur

Introduction

Total knee arthroplasty (TKA) requires attention to the entire complex of knee joint mechanics, active muscle forces and passive ligament structures. Prosthetic component design must accommodate the patients knee anatomy, biomechanical stability, function, and mobility. It is uniformly reported in the literature that the longevity of a knee prosthesis is patient specific, but depends upon correct component design and alignment, implant fixation, soft tissue balancing and a physiological lower extremity axis [1, 12, 15, 17, 22, 24]. One has to appreciate that minimal mal-positioning of intra- or extra-medullary tools may lead to considerable variations of implant positioning. Thus, reconstruction of the correct mechanical lower extremity axis as well as soft-tissue balancing is vital for good results. TKA survivorship of 80% to 95% after 10 years are reported [10, 16, 18, 19, 24] but is significantly reduced in cases with more than four degrees of varus or valgus deformity, as Rand and Coventry reported in their series with 71% and 73%, respectively, compared to 90% in cases, where the component alignment was within the range of 4 degrees [20]. In a similar study of Jeffrey et al the loosening rate after 12 years was 3% in well aligned TKA (less than 3 degrees varus/valgus) and 24% less optimal aligned cases (more than 4 degrees varus/valgus) [8].

Alignment of the Lower Extremity

The mechanical axis of the leg (Mikulicz) is defined as a line that passes the femoral head center, the center of the knee and the center of the ankle joint. Any alteration of that line represents a mal-alignment. In cases of varus deformity the mechanical axis deviates medially and in valgus deformity laterally from that line. The femoral angle between anatomical and mechanical axis ranges from 5 to 9 degrees depending of the neck length. The inner angle of the femoral implant is taken from the tangent to the femoral condyles and the mechanical femoral axis. The inner angle of the tibial implant is taken from the tibial shaft axis, which is identical with the mechanical axis and the tibial plateau plane (implant) on a.p. views. In physiological cases the inner tibia angle measures 87 degrees or 3 degrees varus slope, the inner femoral angle measures 93 degrees. On sagittal views tibial and femoral slope can be measured. The femoral slope is taken from the tangent of the implant and mechanical femoral axis, as is the tibial slope (◘ Fig. 10.1). Position of the patella component (central, lateral, medial, superior, inferior) is calculated off axial and lateral patella views.

All axes are subject to computed calculations [3, 6, 14, 20, 21]. In order to minimize potential errors standardized radiographs with one leg stand are required making sure that central beams are crossing the midline of the patella. Lateral views should fall perpendicular to the joint space so that both implant pegs have the same length. Exact radiographs will require fluoroscopic guidance.

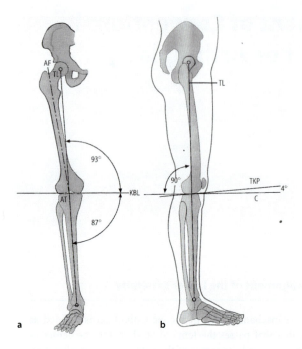

Fig. 10.1 a Anterior-posterior (a.-p.) view of anatomical and mechanical axes and angles. *AF* anatomical axis of femur, *AT* anatomical axis of tibia, *KBL* knee base line, *TL* weight bearing line (Mikulicz). **b** lateral view with mechanical axis and tibia tangent. *TKP* Tangent of tibia plateau, *TL* weight bearing line (Mikulicz), *C* vertical to TL. (Modified from [3])

Alignment of Conventional Knee Prostheses

Rand and Conventry [20] reported a series of 193 TKA with more than 11 years follow-up (1972–1975) in which 83% had moderate or no pain, the revision rate was 20%, and a survivorship of 69% after 10 years. Components with an increased mal-alignment of 3 degrees varus deformity to the mechanical axis (17 of 53) or more than 4 degrees to the tibial axis (21 of 45) show a higher loosening rate. Revision surgery was performed in 20% (39 of 193) of the cases. Indication for revision surgery included 7 cases with component mal-alignment (6 varus, 1 valgus defomity). Jeffrey et al. [8] reported a series of 115 TKA (1976–1981) with a mean follow-up of 8 years in which an aseptic loosening rate of 24% was significantly associated with mal-alignment of more than 3 degrees. In 11 revision cases only 2 cases had proper alignment. There was no correlation between loosening and pre-operative defor-

mity, but high significant correlation between loosening and post-operative deformity.

Ritter et al. [22] observed 421 PFC TKA (1975–1983) of which 56% had varus, 31% had neutral, and 13% had valgus mal-alignment post-operatively. Eight cases required revision surgery due to component loosening, of which 5 cases had varus mal-alignment, 3 cases had neutral mechanical axis.

Delp et al. [2] confirmed the importance of accurate implant alignment for optimal outcome. Their complication rate included aseptic loosening, instability, dislocation, fracture, and infection which counted for 5–8%. Complications such as patello-femoral pain and reduced range of motion ranged from 20 to 40%.

Matsuda et al. [13] examined 20 Miller-Galante TKA with a mean follow-up of 87 months of which 17 were implanted in a mean varus angle of 0.9 degrees (4 valgus to 5 varus). However, Matzuda demands a longer follow-up period for more definitive statement to mal-alignment an loosening.

Schwitalle et al. [23] looked at 248 PFC TKA with a follow-up over 5 years. In 15 (4.5%) cases revision was related with mal-alignment and surgical technique. In their series mal-alignment and not well balanced soft tissues increased the incidence of late complications, i.e. 6 cases (2%) with aseptic and 4 cases (1,3%) with septic loosening.

König et al. [11] reported long-term results of 495 PFC TKA after 5 to 10 years with only 2 aseptic loosening of tibial and femoral components after 5 and 6 years respectively, which were treated successfully with revision surgery. The complication rates of 5.2% after 10 years and revision rate of 2.4% are published [4].

In summary, not all authors consider mal-alignment as a major contributing factor of implant failure. Whereas Jeffrey et al. [8], Rand and Coventry [20], as well as Ritter et al. [22] consider the postoperative angle as a major concern, Tew et al. [25] and Hsu et al. [5] do not. Gomoll et al. [4] investigated a series of 155 PFC TKA after 10 years and found no aseptic loosening and non-progredient radiolucent lines of less than 1 mm in 16%. In another series of 235 TKA with PCL retention 90% did not require surgery 8% had aseptic loosening.

Ranawat et al. [19] investigated 112 TKA after 11 years and found radiolucent lines (RLL) in 60% of the cases with BMI being a factor. The mechanical axis ranged from 3 degrees varus to 10 degrees valgus (10 had 0 to 3 degrees varus, 17 had 0 to 4 degrees valgus, the remaining cases had 5 to 10 degrees valgus). Survivorship after 11 years was 94.1%. Ranawat reported no association with age, sex, diagnosis, cement mantle or mal-alignment, but a significant correlation of RLL and BMI.

Comparison of Alignment in Navigated and Conventional TKA: Literature

Miehlke et al. [15] compared results of 60 OrthoPilot (Aesculap, Tuttlingen, Germany) navigated TKA with 30 conventional TKA. Three months postoperatively mechanical, femoral and tibial axes in anterior-posterior and lateral view were evaluated. With regards to the mechanical axis 61,7% were within 2 degrees of varus or valgus angle, 35% cases had a deviation of 3 to 4 degrees, and 3.3% had more than 4 degrees mal-alignment. In the conventional group more than 4 degrees of mal-alignment was observed in 10% of the cases. The authors state a significantly better alignment in the lateral tibial axis when using the OrthoPilot navigation system particularly with less outliers.

Jenny and Boeri [9] implanted 40 Search Prosthesis TKA with the OrthoPilot navigation system and compared this with a matched group of conventionally implanted Search Prosthesis TKA. In 85% of the navigated cases the axis was within 3 degrees with only 72% in the conventional group. Taking all five axis into account optimal results within 3 degrees were obtained in 62% of the navigated compared with 30% in the conventional group. Janecek et al. [7] using the same system reported 30 cases and compared the results with 30 conventional PFC and T.A.C.K. TKA. Angle of less than 2 degrees were found in 83% of the navigated TKA and only 37% in the other group. Four degrees deviation was found in 17% of the navigated, but in 46% of the conventional group. None of the navigated TKA had more than 4 degrees, but 17% in the other group.

Comparison of Alignment in Navigated and Conventional TKA: Own Series

In the time between 09/1999 and 12/2001, 100 Search Evolution prostheses (Aesculap, Tuttlingen, Germany) were implanted using the OrthoPilot navigation system (Aesculap, Tuttlingen, Germany). A control group underwent conventional implantation using LCS knee prostheses (DePuy Int, Leeds, UK) in the time between 03/2001 to 07/2001. There were 2 surgeon in the navigated group and 6 surgeons in the control group with no significant differences among them. Lateral radiographs in lying position were compared two weeks post-operatively. The error of this method is one degree for individual measurement and two degree for beam position [26]. The following data were encountered: sagittal orientation of the femoral component in relation to distal and ventral (slope) as well as sagittal alignment (slope) of the tibial component. The mechanical axis and alignment of both components in relation to it was measured on standardized one-leg stand views. Demographic data include mean age (70 years), with 75% females. There were no differences comparing both groups.

Radiographic results were separated into perfect, optimal, acceptable, and unacceptable. Categories were defined using deviation from ideal values (◘ Table 10.1).

Mechanical Leg Axis a.p. View

A neutral mechanical axis (0 degree) was achieved in 55% in the navigated group (A) and in 27% in the conventional group (B). Alignment within 3 degrees of varus or valgus was observed in 93% in group A and 77% in group B. Both differences were significant (◘ Fig. 10.2).

◘ **Table 10.1.** Definition of results, deviation from the desired angle

	Coronal mechanical axis	Coronal orientation of the femoral component	Sagittal orientation of the femoral component	Coronal orientation of the tibial component	Sagittal orientation of the tibial component
Perfect	0	0	0	0	0
Optimal	≤3°	≤2°	≤2°	≤2°	≤2°
Acceptable	4°–5°	3°–4°	3°–4°	3°–4°	3°–4°
Unacceptable	>5°	>4°	>4°	>4°	>4°

Femoral Axis, a.p. View

Perfect perpendicular alignment (90 degrees) was obtained in 49% in group A (navigated group) with 95% within 2 degrees varus/valgus deviation. In group B 42% were perfectly aligned with 79% within 2 degrees deviation. Both differences were significant (■ Fig. 10.3).

Femoral Axis, Lateral View

Perfect slope alignment (0 degree) on lateral views was obtained in 39% in group A (navigated group) and in 65% within 2 degrees anterior/posterior deviation. Ideal

value for posterior slope in this design was defined by the manufacturer with 5 degrees. In group B (5 degrees slope considered perfect) only 10% were perfectly aligned (0 degree) and 45% within 2 degrees deviation. Both differences were significant (■ Fig. 10.4).

Tibial Axis, a.p. View

Perfect perpendicular alignment (90 degrees) on coronal views was obtained in 53% in group A (navigated group) and in 98% within 2 degrees varus/valgus deviation. In group B 57% were perfectly aligned and in 86% within 2 degrees varus/valgus deviation. In group

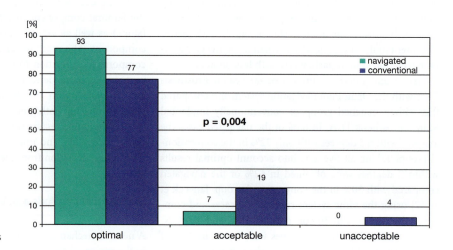

■ **Fig. 10.2.** Coronal mechanical leg axis, comparison of both groups

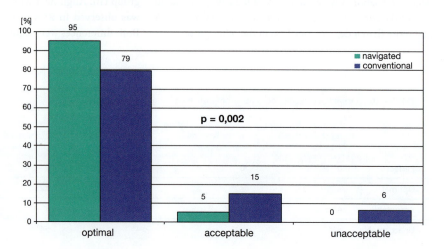

■ **Fig. 10.3.** Coronal orientation of the femoral component, comparison of both groups

B were some outliers. Both differences were significant (◘ Fig. 10.5).

Tibial Axis, Lateral View

Perfect slope alignment (0 degree in group A) on lateral views was obtained in 55% in group A with 91% within 2 degrees anterior/posterior deviation. As described, 5 degrees posterior slope was defined as ideal angle, however, different angles may have been considered intra-operatively from the surgeon due to individual patients' anatomy. Taking 5 degrees as ideal angle, we found in group B (5 degrees slope considered perfect) only 14% perfectly

aligned tibial components with 65% within 2 degrees deviation. Both differences were significant (◘ Fig. 10.6).

Summary of All Five Axes

We defined the following criteria as a acceptable result: mechanical axis within 5 degrees and each other of the four axes within 4 degrees. There were 84% in group A (navigated group), that met these criteria and 61% in group B. An optimal result (mechanical axis within 3 degrees and each other of the four axes within 2 degrees) was observed in 54% in group A and 15% in group B (◘ Figs. 10.7 and 10.8).

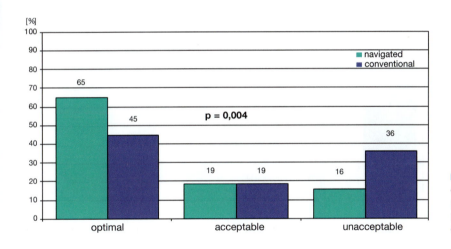

◘ **Fig. 10.4.** Sagittal orientation of the femoral component, comparison of both groups. Planned posterior slope of 5 degrees in conventional group B

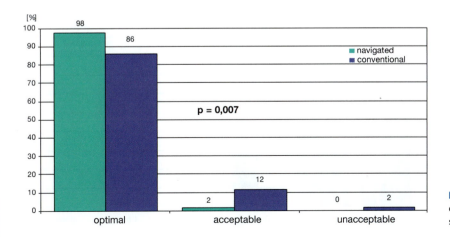

◘ **Fig. 10.5.** Coronal orientation of the tibial component, comparison of both groups

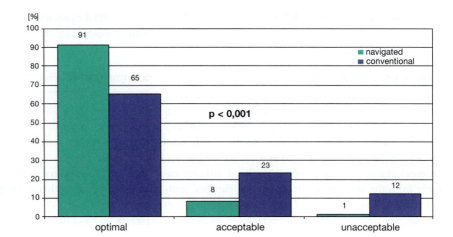

Fig. 10.6. Sagittal orientation of the tibial component, comparison of both groups. Planned posterior slope of 5 degrees in conventional group B

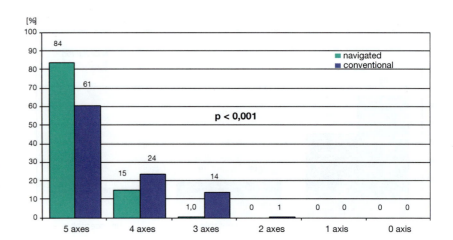

Fig. 10.7. Number of cases with acceptable alignment (mechanical axis: 0 degrees ±5 degrees, each other axis ±4 degrees deviation). Planned femur and tibia slope in the sagittal plane in conventional group was 5 degrees

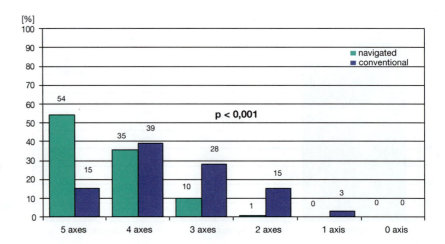

Fig. 10.8. Number of cases with optimal alignment (mechanical axis: 0 degree ±3 degrees, each other axis ±2 degrees deviation). Planned femur and tibia slope in the sagittal plane in conventional group was 5 degrees

Statistical Analyses

The Wilcoxon et al. U-Test was employed for statistical significance. Both groups were compared using the Chi-Square-Test.

Summary

Reconstruction of mechanical axes, perfect component alignment/design, and balancing of the soft tissues are major factors that increase survivorship of TKA. The literature states, that TKA components are implanted significantly more accurately and precise when using computer navigation. In this series, we were able to confirm these data. Current comparative studies, however, focus on radiographic data, but not on clinical outcome. Whether or not more precise aligned TKA components will improve the long-term outcome may be expected, but has yet to be confirmed by future trial.

References

1. Bargren JH, Blaha JD, Freeman MAR (1983) Alignment in total knee arthroplasty. Clin Orthop 173: 178–183
2. Delp SL, Stulberg SD, Davies BL, Picard F, Leitner F (1998) Computer assisted knee replacement. Clin Orthop 354: 49–56
3. Elke R, König A (2001) Präoperative Planung der Knietotalprothese. In: Eulert J, Hassenpflug J (Hrsg) Praxis der Knieendoprothetik. Springer, Berlin Heidelberg New York Tokio, S 33–41
4. Gomoll AH, Schai PA, Scott RD, Thornhill TS (2001) Das PFC-Modular-System. In: Eulert J, Hassenpflug J (Hrsg) Praxis der Knieendoprothetik. Springer, Berlin Heidelberg New York Tokio, S 233–243
5. Hsu HP, Garg A, Walker PS, Spector M, Ewald FC (1989) Effect on knee component alignment on tibial load distribution with clinical correlation. Clin Orthop 248: 135–144
6. Insall JN, Binazzi R, Soudry M, Mestriner LA (1985) Total knee replacement. Clin Orthop Relat Res 192: 13–22
7. Janecek M, Bucek B, Hart R (2001). OrthoPilot (Aesculap) – Computernavigation der Endoprothese des Kniegelenks. Acta Chir. Austriaca 33: 175
8. Jeffrey RS, Morris RW, Denham RA (1991) Coronal alignment after total knee replacement. J Bone Joint Surg 73 B: 709–714
9. Jenny JY, Boeri C (2001) Navigiert implantierte Knietotalendoprothesen – Eine Vergleichsstudie zum konventionellen Instrumentarium. Z Orthop 139: 117–119
10. Knutson K, Lindstrand A, Lidgren L (1986) Survival of Knee arthroplasties, a nation – wide multicenter investigation of 8000 cases. J Bone Joint Surg 68 B: 795–803
11. König A, Gruss J, Kirschner S (2001) Ergebnisse der Press-Fit-Condylar-Prothese (PFC). In: Eulert J, Hassenpflug J (Hrsg) Praxis der Knieendoprothetik. Springer, Berlin Heidelberg New York Tokio, S 226–230
12. Lampe F, Honl M, Wieman R, Hille E (1999) Computergestützte Navigation Gelenkerhalt und Endoprothetik bei Gonarthrose. Erschienen in: Implant 2–1999/Kasuistik. Springer, Berlin Heidelberg New York Tokio
13. Matsuda S, Hiromasa M, Nagamine R, Urabe K, Harimaya K, Matsunobu T, Iwamoto Y (1999) Changes in knee alignment after total knee arthroplasty. J Arthroplasty 14: 566–570
14. Merchant AC, Mercer RL, Jacobsen RH, Cool CR (1974) Roentgenographic analysis of patellofemoral congruence. J Bone Joint Surg 56A: 1391–6
15. Mielke RK, Clemens U, Jens JH, Kershally S (2001) Navigation in der Knieendoprothetik – vorläufige klinische Erfahrungen und prospektiv vergleichbare Studie gegenüber konventioneller Implantationstechnik. Z Orthop 139: 109–116
16. Nafei A, Kristensen O, Knudson HM, Hvid I, Jensen J (1996) Survivorship analysis of cemented total condylar knee arthroplasty. J Arthroplasty 11: 7–10
17. Picard F, Saragaglia D, Montbarbon E, Chaussard C, Leitner F, Raoult O (1999) Computer assisted knee Arthroplasty preliminary clinical results with the OrthoPilot System. 4th International CAOS Symposium, Davos
18. Ranawat CS, Boachie-Adjei O (1988) Survivorship analysis and results of total condylar knee arthroplasty. Clin Orthop Rel Res 226: 6–13
19. Ranawat CS, Flynn WF, Saddler S, Hansraj KH, Maynhard MJ (1993). Long-term results of total condylar knee athroplasty. Clin Orthop 286: 94–102
20. Rand JA, Coventry MB (1988) Evaluation of geometric total knee arthroplasty. Clin Orthop 232: 168–173
21. Rand JA, Ilstrup DM (1991) The accuracy of femoral intramedullary guides in total knee arthroplasty. J Arthroplasty 12: 677–682
22. Ritter MA, Faris PM, Keating EM, Meding JB (1994) Postoperative alignment of total knee replacement. Its effect on survival. Clin Orthop 299: 153–156
23. Schwitalle M, Eckhardt A, Heine J (2001).Ergebnisse der Press-Fit-Condylar-Prothese (PFC). In: Eulert J, Hassenpflug J (Hrsg) Praxis der Knieendoprothetik. Springer, Berlin Heidelberg New York Tokio, S 217–224
24. Scuderi GR, Insall JN, Windsor RE, Moran MC (1989) Survivorship of cemented knee replacement. J Bone Joint Surg 71B: 798–803
25. Tew M, Waugh W (1985) Tibial-femoral alignment and the results of knee replacement. J Bone Joint Surg 67 B: 551–556
26. Wright JG, Treble N, Feinstein AR (1991) Measurement of lower limb alignment using long radiographs. J Bone Joint Surg 73B: 721–723

Computer-Assisted Implantation of a Total Knee Prosthesis without Pre-Operative Imaging: The Kinematic Model

D. Saragaglia

Introduction

Computer-assisted surgery began with stereotactic neurosurgery [1] towards the end of the 1980s. This new technique had for aim to improve the precision of operations, reduce surgical invasiveness, and improve the traceability of interventions.

The history of computer-assisted implantation of total knee prostheses dates back to 1993 when we set up a work group including 2 surgeons (D. Saragaglia and F. Picard), 1 medical doctor/computer scientist (P. Cinquin), 2 computer scientists (S. Lavallée and F. Leitner), and an industry partner, which was at the time I.C.P France (bought-over by Aesculap-AG, Tuttlingen, Germany, in 1994). In our first meeting the senior surgeon, drew up the specifications defining computer assistance for total knee replacement. A pre-operative scan was not needed to guide surgical navigation for several reasons: this was firstly because, at the time, this examination was not part of the pre-operative check-up required for a knee prosthesis, secondly, we felt that an examination of this sort could only complicate the operative procedure, and lastly, this would have added additional cost and a considerable amount of radiation exposure for the patient. We needed to have a reference to the mechanical leg axis throughout the whole operation so that the cutting guides could be placed perpendicular to this axis in a frontal and a sagittal plane. The cutting guides needed to be placed freehandedly without any centro-medullary or extra-medullary rods. Finally, the operation was not supposed to last more than 2 hours (maximum tourniquet time) and the procedure was to be accessible to all surgeons, whatever their computing skills.

The project was assigned to F. Picard, as part of his Postgraduate Diploma in Medical and Biological Engineering, and to F. Leitner, a computer scientist who was completing his training. After 2 years of research, the system was validated by the implantation of 10 knee prostheses on 10 cadaver knees, and the results were published in 1997 [2, 3] in several national and international publications, including CAOS, SOFCOT, and SOBCOT.

After obtaining consent of the local ethics committee on December 4, 1996, the first computer-assisted prosthesis was implanted in a patient, on January 21, 1997 (D. Saragaglia, F. Picard, T. Lebredonchel). The operation lasted 2 hours and 15 minutes and was uneventful.

A prospective randomized study comparing this technique to the conventional technique began in January 1998 and was completed in March 1999. The results were published in several national and international meetings and in a lead article in the French Journal of Orthopaedic Surgery [4]. In March 1999, the prototype that we had used in this study evolved to a final model called Orthopilot™ (B-Braun-Aesculap, Tuttlingen, Germany). Since that time, numerous papers have been published [5–16] confirming that this technique was well founded and more than 35,000 prostheses have been implanted worldwide with Orthopilot™. The software packages have evolved (3.0, 3.2, 4.0, 4.2) but the basic principle has remained the same since the system was created.

Material

The equipment includes a navigation station (■ Fig. 11.1), which allows the markers to be spatially located in real time, as well as an ancillary device adapted to this navigation. The navigation station is made up of a personal computer, an infrared Polaris localizer (Northern Digital Inc.), and a dual-command foot-pedal. The progress of the operative protocol is defined in the software and the surgeon controls this via the pedal and a dedicated graphic interface.

This navigation station also includes ancillary devices, which are the markers and their fixing system.

Markers, also called »rigid bodies«, are a collection of infrared diodes held together rigidly. The localizer knows the position of each of these diodes and therefore the attitude (position and orientation) of the marker itself. All the objects that need to be tracked can have markers attached to them. It is also possible to mark out specific points in space using a metallic pointer linked to a marker (■ Fig. 11.2) whose accurate extremity coordinates are pre-recorded. The markers are attached to the bone using special bicortical screws. We have continued to use active markers that are attached to the navigation station but passive wireless markers are also available.

The ancillary device is made up of cutting guides equipped with markers that are firmly attached to the bone by 3 or 4 threaded pins. These guide the tibial cut (height of cut, valgus-varus, tibial slope) and the femoral cut (height of cut, valgus-varus, flexum, recurvatum). The chamfers cutting guide also allows the anterior and posterior cuts to be made. A distractor guides the ligament balance in flexion and in extension.

Method

The pre-operative planning is exactly the same as for a conventionally-implanted prosthesis: standard X-rays – or even better, pangoniometry – are used to evaluate the axis and the shape of the femur and tibia. Stress X-rays are useless because the computer evaluates deformation reducibility by forced varus or valgus movements.

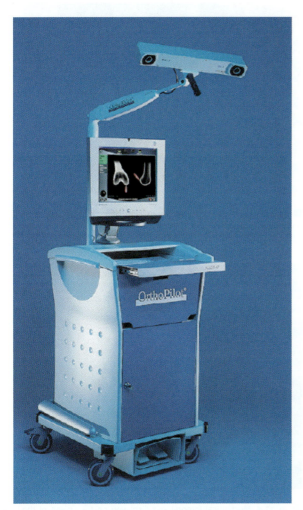

■ **Fig. 11.1.** The Orthopilot™

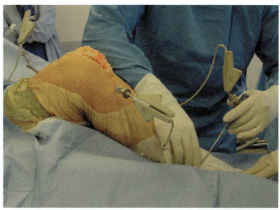

■ **Fig. 11.2.** Metallic pointer equipped with a rigid body

Obtaining the Mechanical Axis

Insertion of the Markers

To reduce the length of the incision, the femoral and tibial markers are inserted percutaneously and are positioned so that they can be seen throughout the whole operation without the need to move the localizer (■ Fig. 11.3).

»Calibrating« the Leg

The limb is calibrated by locating the center of the femoral head (H), the center of the knee (K), and the center of the ankle (A) through appropriate movements of the hip, knee, and ankle.

The center of the femoral head is located by moving the leg in a small circular motion, slowly and progressively, with the knee in extension or in flexion. This lets the localizer track the infrared diodes of the femoral »rigid body« and locate the center of the femoral head.

Locating the center of the ankle is more complicated than locating the center of the hip because there is only one degree of freedom and this means only a rotational axis can be located. To do so, a »rigid body« must be placed at the level of the proximal extremity of the tibia and another placed at the level of the talus neck using a metal plate and an elastic strap, which avoids the need to make an incision on the instep and to insert a screw. Flexion and extension movements and palpation of the malleoli and of the anterior tibio-talar joint midpoint allow the localizer to track infrared diodes and locate the center of the ankle.

It is also relatively complicated to locate the center of the knee because it is an instantaneous center of rotation which moves during flexion. Firstly, flexion and extension movements give the flexion-extension axis; secondly, axial rotation movements of the tibia, when the knee is flexed at 90°, give another axis; the intersection of these two axes gives the center of rotation of the knee. To calculate this center, the localizer will follow the movements of the »rigid bodies« that were first placed on the lower extremity of the femur and on the upper extremity of the tibia.

Palpation Stages

The palpation of the tibial plateau (healthy and damaged) will determine the height of the cut. With the help of a metallic pointer, to which a mobile »rigid body« is attached, the healthy plateau is palpated in the middle (not at the front) to integrate a part of the posterior tibial slope.

The middle of the tibial eminence and the summit of the femoral groove are also palpated to facilitate the search for the center of the knee.

Palpation of the femur (posterior side of the medial and lateral condyles, the most distal point of the medial and lateral condyles, and the anterior cortex of the distal femur just above the upper margin of the trochlea) will determine the size of the prosthesis, guarantee the articular center of the femur, and will give the valgus or varus femoral mechanical axis (■ Fig. 11.4). Palpation of the epicondyles gives an idea of the distal femoral epiphyseal torsion of the femur.

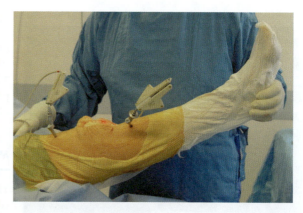

■ **Fig. 11.3.** Rigid bodies percutaneously implanted at the distal femur and the proximal tibia

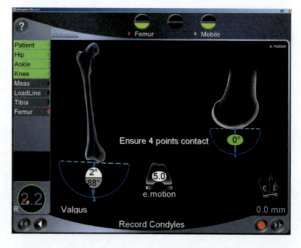

■ **Fig. 11.4.** Mechanical femoral axis displayed on the screen of the computer

Palpation of the ankle allows its center to be integrated, which completes acquisitions made during kinematic calibration. The tip of the medial malleolus, the tip of the lateral malleolus, and the middle of the tibiotarsal joint must be palpated.

The Mechanical Leg Axis

At this stage of the operation, points H, K, and A have been found and their coordinates are in the reference system of the femoral and tibial »rigid bodies«. The mechanical leg axis has therefore been determined and can be compared to the pre-operative pangoniometry. The size of the prosthesis is also known and is displayed on the screen.

Navigation

Using the manual valgus or varus stress given by the surgeon at 10° of flexion, a stress goniometry can be obtained which means reducibility can be tested and it will become clear whether or not the peripheral soft tissue will have to be released. Furthermore, the system allows a dynamic goniometry to be obtained and thus the varus or valgus can be evaluated in flexion at 30° (walking position) or at 90°. This gives an idea of the global femoral rotation [13], a notion that had been completely ignored until now and that is particularly overlooked when, with conventional techniques, systematic external rotation is given to the femoral implant.

Positioning the Cutting Guides

The tibial cutting guide is mounted on a support, which allows the valgus-varus, the height of the cut, and the posterior tibial slope to be measured. We currently prefer to position this cutting guide freehandedly, without any supports, which means shorter cutaneous incisions can be made. This cutting guide is positioned in front of the tibia with its »rigid body« (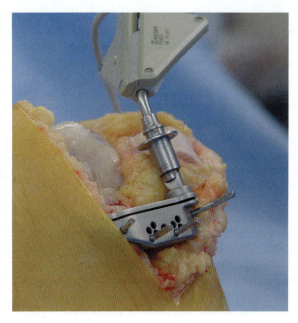 Fig. 11.5) and it is fixed to the bone by 4 threaded pins once the correct measurements are displayed on the screen, which for us are a valgus-varus at 0°, a posterior tibial slope at 0°, and a cutting height of 8 or 10 mm which corresponds to the thickness of the prosthesis tibial plateau. Once the cutting guide is fixed into position, an oscillating saw is used to make the cut.

The femoral cutting guide equipped with its »rigid body« is then placed against the anterior side of the distal

Fig. 11.5. Tibial cutting guide equipped with a rigid body inserted by a reduced incision

end of the femur, with the knee flexed at 90° after the overhang of the femoral trochlea has been resected. An appropriate support can be used or this cutting guide can be fixed freehandedly which means that the initial approach might be less extensive. Then, the surgeon adjusts the valgus-varus of the distal femoral cut (at 0° for us), the posterior slope (between 0 and 2° of flexum to avoid cutting the anterior cortex), and the height of the resection (minimal resection in the convex side of the deformity to reduce ligament imbalance).

At this stage of the operation, the computer has carried out a »bony« alignment of the leg and the prosthesis is then implanted using the classic ancillary equipment especially when making the anterior, posterior, and chamfers cuts.

Implanting the Prosthesis

The implantation of the trial prosthesis enables thanks to computer assistance, to check the mechanical leg axis in extension, in the walking position, and in flexion at 90°. Ligament balance is also controlled by taking stress valgus or varus measurements, and assessing any medial or lateral gaping.

The mechanical leg axis can also be checked when the prosthesis is permanently implanted. This will allow the detection of any excess medial or lateral cement that is liable to change the axis by 1 or 2° (1 mm of cement = 1°).

Rotation of the Femoral Implant

We never systematically apply external rotation of the femoral implant, at least in genu varum. We only apply rotation according to the femoral valgus or varus (◘ Fig. 11.4). If in the case of genu varum, the femur is in a valgus of 3° or more, we believe it is logical to apply external rotation, because it will be necessary to resect more of the distal medial condyle and as a result more of the posterior condyle if we want the ligament to be balanced in flexion [15]. This rotation does not need to be navigated since the ancillary makes it easy to perform. If the femur is in varus, and if the genu varum is hyper-reducible, it is equally logical to apply internal rotation, since less distal medial condyle will be resected and therefore less posterior medial condyle [15]. In the case of genu valgum, external rotation is almost systematic since the femoral valgus is almost constant. We usually apply 1 degree of rotation for 1 degree of femoral valgus and do not exceed 5 to 6 degrees of rotation, to limit the cut in the anterolateral cortex of the femur.

Ligament Balance

There are two ways to proceed: either by working from reducibility of the deformity tests (valgus and varus stress near extension) or by following ligament balance management software. We prefer to use the first method, which enables the surgeon to reflect on and to remain master of his/her decisions.

We proceed in the following way: when the mechanical leg axis appears on the computer screen, before any ablation of osteophytes, we apply manual force in varus and valgus, with the knee at 5 to 10° of flexion, to assess the reducibility of the deformity and the gap in convexity. If the deformity is completely reducible, or even hyper reducible, we are certain that the ligaments will be balanced in extension and that it will not be necessary to release soft tissue in the concavity. The same is true if reducibility gives a hypo-correction of 2 to 3°. If hypo-correction is greater than this, it will be necessary to allow for the progressive release of soft tissue with trial implants, after removing the osteophytes. However, it should be stated that a perfect balance does not necessarily mean that there

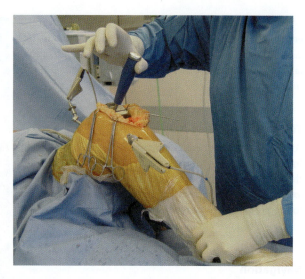

◘ **Fig. 11.6.** Checking of the ligament balance in flexion at 90°

is a symmetrical gap between the medial and the lateral side, since it is known that in a normal knee, the lateral compartment is more lax than the medial compartment. And so we readily accept, in genu varum, a gap of 3 or 4° more for the lateral compartment of the knee.

As far as the management of gaps between extension and flexion is concerned, we never have an imbalance since, on one hand we commonly use a PCL retaining prosthesis which is a good »keeper« of the gaps, and on the other hand the bone resection thickness is identical to the thickness of the implants. Thus, there is no reason for the balance which was adequate before the implantation of the prosthesis to change afterwards.

Finally, the medial-lateral balance in flexion can be controlled without any distractor, since we believe that this is an artificial procedure which does not guarantee an adequate balance; indeed, creating tension between the two sides is subjective and difficult to reproduce from one surgeon to the next. To check this balance, it is sufficient, once the cutting guide for the chamfers has been applied at the distal femur level, to raise the thigh through the use of this supporting point, to manually pull into the axis of the knee flexed at 90 degrees, and to check the parallelism of the cutting guide with the cut of the tibial plateau (◘ Fig. 11.6). In genu varum, parallelism is perfect in most cases and it is not necessary to release soft tissue. Otherwise, above all in genu valgum, it is necessary to progressively release the medial or lateral collateral ligaments.

Results

The results of the prospective randomized study which we carried out with the prototype were published in 2001 in the French Journal of Orthopaedic Surgery [4]. These results showed that the system was reliable, effective, and reproducible. If it did not demonstrate its superiority in a statistically significant manner, with regard to the conventional technique (84% of 180°+/-3° HKA angles versus 75%), it ensured better distribution of axes around 180° and an improved implantation of condylar and tibial pieces (around 90°), in the frontal as well as the sagittal plane. It must be stressed that the study was carried out with a prototype and that several technical errors (»rigid bodies« were not sufficiently anchored, inaccurate ankle palpation, no intra-articular palpation of the knee) probably affected the accuracy of some data.

Another study [9] carried out with the latest generation of Orthopilot™ demonstrated a significant statistical difference in favor of the computer-assisted technique (94% of optimum implantations as opposed to 78%). Other publications also confirmed the relevance of navigation in total knee replacement and Orthopilot™ effectiveness [5–8, 11, 12, 14, 16]. We carried out another study with Orthopilot™, with the aim of assessing computer-aided femoral implant rotation. This series, consisting of 50 cases, showed that 100% of mechanical axes were distributed between 177 and 183° [13].

Discussion

The use of an image-free computer navigation device can today be seen as a reliable technique which allows obtaining a mechanical axis at 180°+/-3° on the frontal plane and an optimal position of femoral and tibial implants on the lateral view, in over 95% of cases.

Orthopilot™ is a navigation system which helps the surgeon during total knee replacement. This device based on kinematic and palpation »calibrating« of the lower limb is different from CT-guided or fluoroscopic-guided navigation. The major disadvantage of image-assisted navigation is the use of a CT-scan to recreate the knee in 3D (100 cuts, each 1 mm apart, are necessary to recreate the knee joint – Delp [17]). The radiation to which the patient is exposed, the additional cost, and the long and fastidious nature of the pre-operative planning are all points which might limit the use of such a system. We do not think that fluoroscopy-assisted navigation is well adapted for prosthetic surgery of the knee, because of supplementary radiation of the surgeon and his/her surroundings and the introduction of 2 more machines in the operating theatre (the image intensifier and its screen!).

The kinematic model is particularly well adapted to minimally invasive surgery since it is not necessary to make a large approach to palpate the intra-articular reference points.

For a trained surgeon, the length of the operation is just 5 min longer than the length of a conventional one, above all if a »light« version of 4.0 or 4.2 software is used and if freehand cutting guides are used with a reduced incision.

The kinematic model could be criticized for the difficulty to obtain a »center« of the knee, when there is major gonarthrosis with rupture of the anterior cruciate ligament, peripheral laxities, and postero-medial or postero-lateral bone loss. Cadaver experiments, in fact, demonstrated that the section of the anterior cruciate ligament and/or the posterior cruciate ligament had little effect on the center of rotation of the knee (establishing a rotational center by looking for the point on the femur which is most equidistant, in the sense of the fewest squares, from a point on the tibia). Moreover, the palpation of conspicuous intra-articular points makes the system notably more robust.

Conclusion

The Orthopilot ™ is the reference kinematic model for computer-assisted Total knee replacement. For almost 10 years, its software has been regularly improved to achieve a remarkable level of reliability in any hand. It is particularly well adapted to minimally invasive surgery since it is not useful to broadly open the knee to locate its center in a reliable and reproducible way.

References

1. Lavallée S (1989) Geste médico-chirurgicaux assistés par ordinateur: application à la neurochirurgie stéréotaxique. Thèse, génie biologique et médical, Grenoble
2. Leitner F, Picard F, Minfelde R, Schultz HJ, Cinquin P, Saragaglia D (1997) Computer-assisted knee surgical total replacement. In: Lecture note in computer science: CURMed-MRCAS'97. Springer, Berlin Heidelberg New York Tokio, pp 629–638

3. Picard F, Leitner F, Saragaglia D, Cinquin P (1997) Mise en place d'une prothèse totale du genou assistée par ordinateur: A propos de 7 implantations sur cadavre. Rev Chir Orthop 83 (Suppl II): 31

4. Saragaglia D, Picard F, Chaussard C, Montbarbon E, Leitner F, Cinquin P (2001) Mise en place des prothèses totale du genou assistée par ordinateur: comparaison avec la technique conventionnelle. A propos d'une étude prospective randomisée de 50 cas. Rev Chir Orthop 87: 18–28

5. Clemens U, Miehlke RK (2003) Experience using the latest Orthopilot software: a comparative study. Surg Technol Int 11: 265–273

6. Decking R, Markmann Y, Fuchs J, Puhl W, Scharf HP (2005) Leg axis after computer-navigated total knee arthroplasty. A prospective randomized trial comparing computer-navigated and manual implantation. J Arthroplasty 20: 282–288

7. Haaker RG, Stockheim M, Kamp M, Proff G, Breitenfelder J, Ottersbach A (2005) Computer-assisted navigation increases precision of component placement in total knee arthroplasty. Clin Orthop Relat Res 433: 152–159

8. Hart R, Janecek M, Chaker A, Bucek P (2003) Total knee arthroplasty implanted with and without kinematic navigation. Int Orthop 27: 366–369

9. Jenny JY, Boeri C (2001) Implantation d'une prothèse totale de genou assistée par ordinateur. Etude comparative cas-témoin avec une instrumentation traditionnelle. Rev Chir Orthop 87: 645–652

10. Jenny JY, Boeri C, Picard F, Leitner F (2004) Reproducibility of intraoperative measurement of the mechanical axes of lower limb during total knee replacement with a non-imaged-based navigation system. Comput Aided Surg 9: 161–165

11. Jenny JY, Clemens U, Kohler S, Kiefer H, Konermann W, Miehlke R (2005) Consistency of implantation of a total knee arthroplasty with a non-image-based navigation system. A case control study of 235 cases compared with 235 conventionally implanted prostheses. J Arthroplasty 20: 832–839

12. Miehlke RK, Clemens U, Jens JH, Kershally S (2001) Navigation in knee arthroplasty: preliminary clinical experience and prospective comparative study in comparison with conventional technique. Z Orthop Ihre Grenzgeb 139: 109–116

13. Saragaglia D, Chaussard Ch, Liss P, Pichon H, Berne D, Chaker M (2002) Contribution of computer navigation in the evaluation of femoral rotation during total knee replacement. In: Troccaz J, Merloz P (eds) Surgetica 2002: computer-aided medical intervention: tools and applications. Sauramps Medical, Montpellier, pp 19–21

14. Saragaglia D, Gorduza D (2006) Résultats de 22 prothèses totales du genou mises en place avec assistance par ordinateur pour déviations en genu valgum. In press

15. Saragaglia D, Rooney B (2004) The rotation of the femoral implant: relevance of computer aided total knee arthroplasty. In: Chambat P et al. (eds) La prothèse du genou. Sauramps Médical, Montpellier, pp 163–168

16. Stulberg SD, Loan P, Sarin V (2002) Computer-assisted navigation in total knee replacement: results of an initial experience in thirty-five patients. J Bone Joint Surg 84A (Suppl 2): 90–98

17. Delp SL, Stulberg, SD, Davies B, Picard F, Leitner F (1998) Computer assisted knee replacement. Clin Orthop 354: 49–57

CAOS in Mobile Bearing »Tibia Cut First« Total Knee Arthroplasty

J.B. Stiehl

Introduction

Mobile bearing total knee arthroplasty was initially introduced by Goodfellow with the concept of allowing greater mobility of the polyethylene insert while maintaining very high articular surface conformity with the idea of producing better wear characteristics. Buechel and Pappas developed the Low Contact Stress mobile bearing design in 1977 developing this concept into a system of devices that allowed for a variety of similar implants and surgical techniques. For many surgeons around the world, this concept has stood the test of time, offering favorable wear characteristics and more adaptable prosthetic knee kinematics. Stiehl et al. have performed a number of kinematic evaluations of mobile bearing total knees finding mobile bearing devices to be typical of all total knee arthroplasties, with a significant variation of condylar surface translations, condylar liftoff and screw-home rotation. Perhaps the most unique aspect of the mobile bearing device is the ability to allow for unrestricted femoral tibial rotation of the polyethylene insert. In addition, uncoupling the modular tibia allows the surgeon to have significant freedom from errors that may arise from mal-rotation of the tibial component, often leading to such problems as patellar subluxation, tibial post wear, and catastrophic posterior medial implant wear.

After total knee arthroplasty, fluoroscopic video kinematic studies have demonstrated that while some cases demonstrate the expected internal rotation with knee flexion, others will actually exhibit paradoxical external rotation with knee flexion. Computer assisted surgical navigation (CAOS) offers a unique opportunity to evaluate tibial rotation along with numerous other parameters such as mechanical alignment, joint flexion, ligamentous balance, and tibial axis alignment in flexion. This chapter describes an experience evaluating the data gathered from a large number of cases where tibial rotation was specifically documented before and after total knee arthroplasty in a group of patients where the »tibial cut first« method was utilized.

Methods

A group of 85 patients underwent primary total knee arthroplasty utilizing the »tibial cut first« technique. Implants utilized where either the LCS mobile bearing prosthesis or the Nexgen LPS Flex prosthesis. The Medtronic Universal imageless navigation system was used in all cases with dynamic reference base markers attached to either the medial proximal tibia or the distal medial femur over the medial epicondyle (◘ Fig. 12.1). The medial femoral 3.2 mm pin placement is made by palpating the anatomical medial epicondyle and then directing the pin parallel to the transepicondylar axis. This placement avoids interference of the intra-medullary rod used in the standard »tibial cut first« method, and places the pin above the intercondylar notch such that implant may be placed without impingement on the pin. The second pin is placed 1.5 centimeters more proximal, medial to lateral anterior to the supra-condylar ridge in the dense cortical bone of the distal femur and

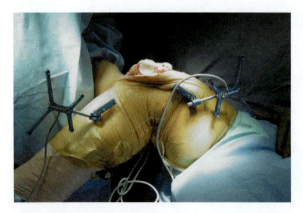

Fig. 12.1. Note medial placement of distal femoral and proximal tibial arrays (see text)

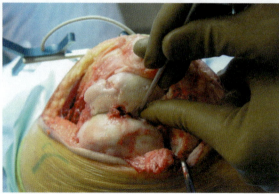

Fig. 12.2. Femoral center reference point selection which is located at the center of the intercondylar notch, and coincides with the AP axis of Whiteside and the transepicondylar axis

posterior to the intra-medullary canal. Prior anatomical studies have verified that this placement avoids neurovascular structures by a wide margin.

Navigation Referencing Protocol

The specifics of the navigation referencing are an important element of the technique and bear detailed description. Hip center determination is done using the kinematic method originally described by Saragaglia. Femoral referencing is done with the two most important points being the femoral center, and the cortical reference of the anterior femoral cortex. For the Medtronic Universal system, the computer definition of the femoral center is a point under the roof of the intercondylar notch that is in the middle of the intercondylar notch and lies in the anterior/posterior axis of Whiteside (Fig. 12.2). From dissections, this point also lies directly on the transepicondylar axis of the distal femur (Fig. 12.3). The surgical epicondyle depression is the reference for the medial epicondyle and the lateral epicondyle is the most prominent point of that landmark.

For the tibial reference, the tibial center is defined as the bisection of the transverse tibial axis. The transverse tibial axis is a line that connects the anterior/posterior midpoints of the medial and lateral condylar surfaces (Fig. 12.4). The tibial center approximates the lateral insertion of the anterior cruciate ligament. The anterior/posterior tibial axis is a perpendicular extension of the tibial center of the transverse tibial axis. This point typi-

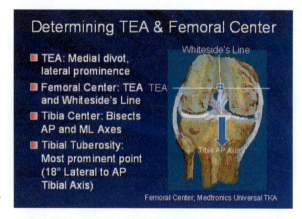

Fig. 12.3. Diagram demonstrates relationship of the AP axis of Whiteside, the transepicondylar axis, and the anterior/posterior tibial axis

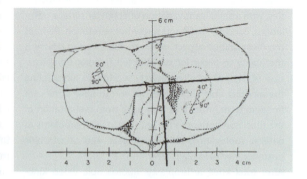

Fig. 12.4. Diagram demonstrates the transverse tibial axis, anterior/posterior axis of the tibia, and the vector from the tibial center to the tibial tuberosity (18°)

cally matches the extension of the femoral AP axis that may be extended onto the anterior surface of the tibia. Great care must be taken to determine the tibial center, as this will affect both coronal and sagital plane measurements. The posterior condylar axis of the tibia is 3–4° external to the transverse tibial axis. The center of the tibial tubercle is typically about 18° external to the AP axis of the tibia. Finally, the transverse tibial axis should nearly approximate the transepicondylar axis in regards to coupled rotation. The center of the distal tibia is determined by picking points that center over the medial and lateral malleoli, the transmalleolar axis. The computer algorithm then picks a point on the transmalleolar axis which is 40% from the most medial point.

»Tibia Cut First« Surgical Technique

The »tibia cut first« method with mobile-bearing total knee arthroplasty follows the original technique of Insall where ligament balancing is done initially in extension before any bone cuts are made. The tibia cut is made perpendicular to the mechanical axis with a 7° posterior slope to the proximal tibia. The anterior distal femoral cut is made precisely at the distal anterior surface of the femur, and the flexion gap is cut with a block that removes the posterior condyles after ligament tensioning is done. Ligament tension is determined either with a gap spacer, or a custom tensioner that adjusts and measures the amount of tension to cut a specific gap (◘ Fig. 12.5). With this technique, the flexion gap is determined by the ligament tension and not a specific anatomical reference such as the posterior condylar axis or the transepicondylar axis. The flexion gap is measured and a distal femoral resection then removes enough distal bone to create a similar gap in extension. For the Nexgen LPS Flex Mobile system, this gap is two millimeters less than the flexion space. Distal femoral chamfer and notch cuts complete femoral preparation.

Tibial component placement is centered on an initial mark on the proximal tibia that was a continuation from the femoral AP axis with the knee held in extension. This is also adjusted to make the spine cam relationship optimal and centered with motion. In general, the femoral AP axis mark matched the optimal position, and a new navigated instrument for tray positioning seeks to match this position which is determined at the beginning of the procedure. Because of the assumed inaccuracy of the

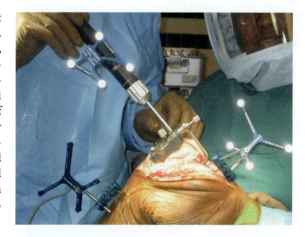

◘ **Fig. 12.5.** Operative example of the anterior cortical reference being established by using computer guidance

transepicondylar axis referencing, all rotational measurements from the computer were considered to be relative. Axial rotation as a nominal measurement was determined at full extension and at 90° flexion and moved either external or internal to the femoral transepicondylar axis. The position of this rotation and the amount was then re-measured after the prosthetic implantation. Finally, the direction of rotation was determined after implantation to determine if this had altered. Following final preparation for femoral implantation, trials are inserted to assess the tension of the gaps that are created. These gaps typically will not have laxity over 3 mm, with a maximum allowed laxity in any plane of 6 mm.

Data Analysis

Alignment was determined by referencing the mechanical axis (MA) and the transepicondylar axis (TEA). Measurements included pre-release mechanical axis, 90° flexion alignment (tibial shaft axis) and tibial rotation. Post-implantation measurements included mechanical axis alignment compared to long-standing radiographs, femoral and tibial component rotation, and final 90° flexion alignment (tibial shaft axis) and rotation related to the TEA. The tibial rotation was defined mathematically by the relationship of the anterior posterior femoral axis which is perpendicular to the transepicondylar axis and measuring the vector to the midpoint prominence of the tibial tubercle (◘ Fig. 12.6) More recently, the Medtronic image-

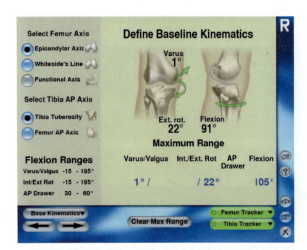

Fig. 12.6. Computer screen image of the 91° flexion measurement, demonstrating the tibial shaft axis to be varus 1° in relation to the transepicondylar axis, and tibial rotation of the tibial tuberosity at 22° external to the AP tibial axis

less reference added the femoral anterior posterior axis of Whiteside as an additional mark to determine femoral rotation eliminating the need for the transepicondylar axis. Standard descriptive statistical analysis was performed.

Results

Pre-release mechanical alignment(MA): 5° varus +/−7° (range: 14° valgus to 20° varus). CAOS post implant MA: 0.7° varus +/− 1.1° (range: 3° valgus to 2.5° Vvarus). Radiographic post MA: 0.3° varus +/− 1.3° (range 4° valgus to 4° varus). Pre-release (tibal shaft axis) 90° flexion: 2.6° varus +/− 5.5° (range: 13° valgus to 19° varus). Post implant (tibial shaft axis) at 90° flexion: 0.1° varus +/− 4.5° (range: 12° valgus to 10° varus). Tibial shaft axis at 90° did not change from baseline to post implant, and was outside the TEA: >5° – 25%; >2° – 50%. Baseline measurement of tibial rotation from 0° to 90° flexion: 4.1° +/− 8.9° of tibial internal rotation (range: 18° external rotation to 23° internal rotation). Post implant tibial rotation from 0° to 90° flexion: 3° +/− 7° of tibial internal rotation (range: 18.5° external rotation to 20° internal rotation). Of baseline group, 41% demonstrated tibial external rotation. After TKA, 37% had tibial external rotation with flexion. When comparing the nominal rotation at 0° before and after TKA, it was noted that the tibial rotation point at 0°

moved more externally in 40% and more internally in the rest but the mean change for the overall group was 2.6° of internal rotation. In 23% of cases there was a change in the direction in tibial rotation from the baseline measurement to the final measurement after total knee arthroplasty. Finally, in 70% of cases, the final tibial rotation measured after TKA was +/− 5° from the starting baseline position.

Discussion

After TKA, alterations from the rotation of the normal knee may be related to anterior cruciate deficiency, prosthetic geometry, and differences in surgical technique in individual patients. Stiehl et al. have studied in-vivo weight-bearing kinematics of mobile-bearing TKA's using the tibial cut first method as used in this study and assessed the amount of screw-home rotation evident with gait [1]. Maximum internal rotation with flexion was 9.6° while the maximum external rotation with flexion was 6.2°. The average tibial rotation for 20 patients was internal rotation of 0.5° with knee flexion but 40% of TKA's demonstrated tibial external rotation with knee flexion.

Dennis et al. evaluated the LCS rotating platform mobile-bearing prosthesis finding that eighteen of 35 knees (51%) had a normal rotation pattern from heel-strike to toe-off, and 30 of 35 knees (86%) had a reverse rotation pattern during at least one analyzed increment (30°). The average amount of axial rotation from heel-strike to toe-off was 0°, and the average maximum amount of axial rotation at any increment during stance-phase was 3°. For gait, the average maximum amounts of normal and reverse rotation for the mobile-bearing PCL-sacrificing TKA study group were 7.3° and −10.1°, respectively. The overall maximum amounts of normal and reverse rotation of any individual TKA for gait, regardless of type, at any increment were 9.6° and −13.3°, respectively. Only 11 of 35 rotating platform total knees (31%) achieved at least 5° of normal rotation, no knees achieved more than 10°, and five of 35 knees (14%) achieved more than −5° of reverse rotation. Comparing the results of all different total knees, patients having a PCL-sacrificing mobile-bearing TKA had, on average, slightly less rotation during a deep knee bend than patients having either a PCL-retaining or posterior-stabilized mobile-bearing TKA, and less than patients with normal knees (p=0.0003). For deep knee bend, the average maximum amounts of normal and reverse rotation for the mobile-bearing PCL-sacrificing

TKA study group were 11.4° and −5.9°, respectively. The maximum amounts of normal and reverse rotation of the overall total knee group at any flexion increment were 21° and −8.4°, respectively. The authors conclude that although average axial rotation values after TKA were limited, review of individual TKA patients revealed a substantial number with high magnitudes (>20°) of both normal and reverse axial rotation that exceeds the rotation limits of most fixed-bearing TKA designs. This may be an advantage for mobile-bearing TKA designs with a rotating platform that can accommodate a wider range of axial rotation without generating excessive PE stresses.

The results of my study were similar to the fluoroscopic studies in that roughly 40% of TKA's demonstrated tibial external rotation with knee flexion. However, the range of rotation was much greater in the CAOS studied patients which could be as much as 20°. This would suggest that the lack of weight-bearing forces in the CAOS TKA's could explain much of this difference. The occurrence of tibial rotation after total knee arthroplasty would appear to be quite variable and there were no factors that predict which patients will externally rotate with flexion.

From the computed tomographic studies of Berger et al., the transtibial axis is defined as a line bisecting the sagittal plane centers of the tibial medial and lateral condyles. The anterior posterior line perpendicular to the transtibial axis is roughly 18° medial to the tibial tubercle center, and closely coincides with the femoral transepicondylar axis if it were translated distally in the coronal plane [2]. Thus, there is a strong reason to couple the femoral anterior-posterior axis with the anterior-posterior tibial axis, and to utilize these points as references in a CAOS system. Preliminary experience with an instrumented tibial tray trial would suggest that matching this placement with the initial computer referencing anterior posterior tibial axis provides a viable option for image guided tibial tray placement. This may have greater application in minimally invasive surgical approaches.

This study confirmed that the CAOS directed component position was within 2° of the optimum MA position in 97% of cases. However, in only a minority of cases did the final femoral component rotation and tibial shaft axis compare to the pre-operative normal transepicondylar axis reflecting a decoupling of flexion tensor spacing with extension space alignment. Tibial rotation findings parallel prior fluoroscopic kinematic analyses. This study suggests that there may be a fixed relationship between the initial baseline tibial rotation and the final tibial component implant position. Further study will be needed to prove if baseline tibial rotation may guide final implant positioning.

References

1. Stiehl JB, Dennis DA, Komistek RD, Crane HS (1999) In-vivo determination of condylar liftoff and screw home in a mobile bearing total knee arthroplasty. J Arthroplasty 14: 293–299
2. Berger RA, Crossett LS, Jacobs JJ, Rubash HE (1988) Rotation causing patellofemoral complications after total knee arthroplasty. Clin Orthop 356: 144–153
3. Berger RA, Crossett LS (1998) Determining the rotation of the femoral and tibial components in total knee arthroplasty: A computer tomography technique. Oper Tech Orthop 8: 128–133
4. Dennis DA, Komistek RD, Mahfouz MR, Walker SA, Tucker A (2004) A multicenter anaylsis of axial femorotibial rotation after total knee arthroplasty. Clin Orthop 428: 180–189
5. LaFortune MA, Cavanagh PR, Sommer III HJ, Kalenak A (1992) Three dimensional kinematics of the human knee during walking. J Biomech 25: 347–357
6. Boldt JG, Stiehl JB, Thuemler P (2002) Femoral rotation based on tibial axis. In: Hamelynck KJ, Stiehl JB (eds) LCS mobile bearing knee arthroplasty. Springer, Berlin Heidelberg New York Tokio, pp 175–182
7. Stiehl JB, Clifford D, Komistek RD Correlation of in-vivo kinematics with retrieval polyethylene insert wear patterns in failed total knee arthroplasty. Clin Orthop (Pending Publication)
8. Vertullo CJ, Easley ME, Scott WN, Insall JN (2001) Mobile bearings in total knee arthroplasty. J Am Acad Orthop Surg 9: 355–364

Total Knee Arthroplasty using the Stryker Knee Trac System

K.A. Krackow

Introduction

This author was in the process of studying the effects of soft-tissue release in managing varus and valgus knee deformities when the possibility of guiding the entire total knee operation became apparent. We were using magnetic spatial tracking equipment in a first stage cadaver study of the effects of sequential soft tissue release on the achievement of proper alignment and ligament balance. The natural step after this preliminary work was to measure similar changes occurring during actual surgical cases. An Optotrak infrared tracking system was purchased (Northern Digital Corp. Ontario, Canada), which required the development of custom software for our application. In planning this software it became apparent that nearly all of the relevant anatomic landmarks for TKA could be indicated to this type of system. The single point having great importance in knee alignment which is out of the field, is the center of the femoral head. Recognizing that the motion of the femur at the hip is about a point in space which *is* that femoral head center, it became immediately apparent that this point could be determined mathematically simply by tracking the motion of the femur.

With this determination it then followed that we could track and measure the displacements occurring during the entire total knee operation. Rather than measuring only relative movement of the tibia in relationship to the femur, similar to the cadaver study, we could determine absolute positions of the femur and tibia in the whole body. In addition to positions of the bones themselves it followed that we could determine the positions of jigs, resulting cuts, and positions of the trial and final prosthetic components. As a result of these realizations, software and hardware were developed to these ends. A study of the accuracy of the femoral head determination was undertaken in cadavers, and this very equipment was used to assist in the performance of the entire total knee procedure. The first fully navigated total knee arthroplasty was successfully done, in our first try, in August 1997. The cadaver study and that case were the subject of a publication which implicitly became the first report of a fully navigated TKR [1].

Material and Methods

The Stryker Knee Trac is an *imageless* navigation system using cordless, battery powered infrared light emitters positioned on a variety of implements. There are a minimum of two »trackers« which are rigidly attached to bone and a third instrument, a pointer (◘ Fig. 13.1). The pointer is a simple pointed rod with trackers at a handle plus finger-tip controls to communicate with the computer via an array of infrared detectors. It is these detectors which triangulate the position of the infrared emitters placed on each instrument or marker in the field of view. There is a very sufficient spherical field of view so that the detector and its associated computer are more than six feet away from the operative field.

In addition to the emitting trackable instruments, there are associated, adjustable mechanical jigs for placing the respective distal femoral and proximal tibial cuts

(■ Fig. 13.2). Other anterior, posterior, and chamfer femoral cuts are made with more standard knee system mechanical instruments. The standard tibial surface preparation instruments from the knee system in use, are employed to guide the placement of tibial component fixation features, e.g. stem preparation, peg holes, etc. Patellar preparation is done with standard mechanical instruments.

The trackers and essentially all aspects of the software are generic, therefore applying to any total knee prosthesis and its additional system instrumentation.

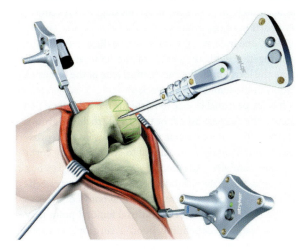

■ **Fig 13.1.** Rigid attachment of femur and tibia »*trackers*«. Pointer collecting data

The designation »imageless« used above in the first sentence of this section signifies that the entire navigation process and essentially all pre-operative planning are done without the requirement of images such as CT scans or intra-operative fluoroscopy. Although, for a variety of obvious reasons, it is not recommended, routine radiographs could be omitted, their use is not, absolutely required.

Surgical Navigation Process

After routine exposure of the knee, trackers are placed in the distal femur and proximal tibia (■ Fig. 13.3). It is this writer's current practice to place these within the exposure incision, but many other surgeon users place them through separate small incisions, stab wounds. It is necessary that both femoral and tibial trackers be far enough away from the joint lines so that they do not interfere with the placement and adjustment of any mechanical instrumentation to be used.

The distal femoral and proximal tibial trackers consist of two major elements each. One is a screw-pin device which is placed with bicortical fixation (■ Fig. 13.1). It is rotationally stabilized by a rotating, ratchet stabilized feature which becomes rigid as the pin is screwed into position. The infrared emitters defining the spatial position of the tracker are arranged on a very generic structure which has a quick-release clamping mechanism. In this way some of the bulk of the bone tracker is eliminated, providing room for associated mechanical instrumenta-

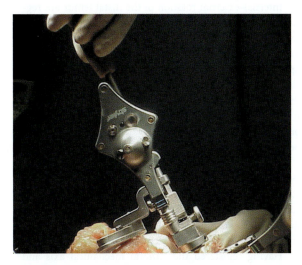

■ **Fig 13.2.** Dedicated adjustable femoral navigation jig

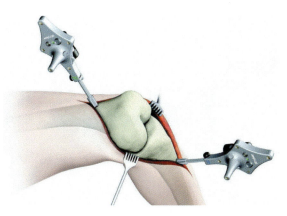

■ **Fig 13.3.** Knee trackers anchored proximally and distally in the knee incision

tion, and not obstructing the surgeon during bone sawing and other observations.

This modular feature also allows the emitter array to be used on other devices, lessening the number of implements involved and also expense (■ Fig. 13.4). Such other devices consist of several different surfaces used to assess the position of a cutting jig, the resulting cut, and the position of both trial and final components. Also, each emitter array can be rigidly attached to the mechanical cutting guides so that the distance and angulation of these cutting jigs can be determined continuously without requiring a member of the team to hold a tracker in place.

The only perishable or disposable items in the entire system are the small batteries, one of which powers each emitter array.

With femoral and tibial trackers in place the registration process is begun. This is the process of indicating to the computer, i.e. the navigation system, the location of points necessary for defining the bony landmarks used in positioning components in proper position. The actual form of any bone is not necessary for this purpose and is never »appreciated« by the system. The determination of certain points leads to the calculation of lines or axes as well as planes which are used for defining rotational and translation positions.

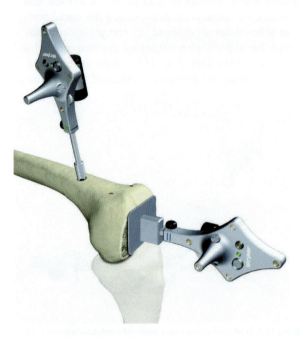

■ **Fig 13.4.** Checking the distal femoral cut

Registration

First the femur is rotated in a nearly random pattern of circles and arcs to locate the center of the femoral head. Most patients undergoing TKR are free of major restrictive hip disease, and so such passive motion essentially is always obtainable. Small effort is made not to move the thigh in a course manner that causes excessive pelvic motion. The software is constantly checking certain calculations which relate to pelvic motion so that the ultimate location of the femoral head center is very consistently and accurately determined. Error messages with temporary abortion of the process will otherwise occur.

Next, one indicates the center of the distal femur. This point together with the center of the femoral head will define the location of the mechanical axis of the femur in relation to the femoral bone tracker.

It is my personal choice to relate the medial-lateral position to the deepest aspect of the distal trochlear groove just above the intercondylar notch. One wants the prosthetic femoral condyles in general to symmetrically cover the bony condyles. Additionally, any intercondylar box encasing a tibial stabilization peg is almost always centered between the respective, remaining bony condyles.

The anterior position of this distal femoral point may be more variable depending upon a surgeon's assumptions, beliefs, and therefore, preferences. An anteriorly placed point will lead to a more extended axis, while a posteriorly placed point directs the femoral mechanical axis to a more flexed orientation.

Internal-external rotation of the distal femur are registered by indicating the medial epicondyle of the femur, then the lateral one, and lastly using the pointer as an axis to indicate the AP or Whiteside axis of the femur. The operating surgeon can customize the software process by eliminating either the epicondylar axis determination or the AP axis determination in the initial set-up scheme. It is alternatively possible to trace the trochlear groove, providing a set of points used to calculate a plane that can be associated with neutral AP femoral rotation.

It is more commonly preferred to use the AP axis of Whiteside in combination with the epicondylar axis. The software rotates one of these axes 90 degrees and the resulting axis is averaged with the other. That is to say, the final rotational position of the femur is registered as a 50–50 combination of the epicondylar and Whiteside axes.

Having registered the femoral mechanical axis and the neutral rotation of the distal femur the location of the femoral joint line is registered by tracing separately the distal surfaces of the respective medial and lateral condyles (□ Fig. 13.1). The overall size of the patient's distal femur is recorded via the anterior posterior dimensions. A separate tracing is performed, using the pointer-tracker applied sequentially to the posterior surfaces of the medial and lateral condyles. The cortical surface of the femur anteriorly is traced, usually collecting the points from the lateral ridge-like aspect just cephalad to the lateral trochlear flare. This is generally the anteriorly most prominent part of the distal femur, where the anterior femoral cut will be made and will exit.

Analogous steps are used to register the tibia. At this time the tibial tracker is in its place and points or data are input with the pointer. A center point is determined at the proximal tibia. For this surgeon this is the medial-lateral center of the sulcus created by the medial and lateral edges of the tibial spines, the attachment or foot-print of the anterior cruciate ligament. Considering the anterior bow of most tibiae, this point is set near the center of this ACL region, which is somewhat to the anterior aspect of the tibial surface.

Neutral rotation of the tibia is determined using the pointer as a line indicator rather than a point indicator. One can inspect the proximal tibial surface and any other geometry he/she prefers and mark or estimate either neutral medial-lateral or anterior-posterior rotation. There are no established landmarks for this axis. And, there is little argument that the bony geometry of the proximal tibial, especially the degenerated one, is highly variable.

It is this writer's preference to start with an axis defined by the attachment location of the posterior cruciate ligament, connected to the »30–35%« region of the tibial tubercle. The latter refers to a point or plane 30–35% of the way from the medial border of the tubercle, 0%, as one considers 100% the lateral border. The respective medial and lateral plateau surfaces are separately traced to register the tibial joint-line. All that remains is to locate the center of the ankle.

One simply points to the center of the ankle after first indicating the intermalleolar axis by sequentially locating the medial and lateral malleoli. One can think of this process as determining an intermalleolar axis and then pointing to that axis so that the perceived center of the ankle is located along the designated intermalleolar line.

It should be apparent at this point that having defined the center of the proximal tibial, the center of the ankle, the surfaces of the tibial plateaus and the neutral AP axis

of the tibia, this registration process provides essentially all of the necessary information to judge jig placement, assess the position of the resulting tibial cut and measure the location of the trial and final tibial component positions.

In addition, the initial alignment and kinematics of the operative knee can be determined.

Results and Observations

Before reporting outcome results, it is appropriate to acknowledge specific findings of interest. This type of instrumentation enables one to assess many aspects of the operative knee as well as the procedure itself that were heretofore unobtainable.

Two basic important pieces of information are obtained immediately after registration. First, one can assess the true point of maximum passive extension, which generally means the existence and degree of flexion contracture. Clearly obesity, tourniquet position and the surgical drapes tend to understate the amount of flexion positioning at the knee.

In addition, there is the situation of combined flexion contracture with either varus or valgus alignment. One can probably accept or suspect that varus and valgus deformities may be overstated in the presence of mild to moderate flexion contracture. It is common for the hip to rotate so that one sees greater axial deformity not appreciating the flexion contracture. It is very obvious early, to the surgeon that what was thought of as varus or valgus mal alignment, to some degree is greater or unsuspected flexion contracture in combination with less varus or valgus deformity. One will see situations in which two-thirds of the suspected deformity is due to flexion contracture and not varus or valgus.

Just as this flexion contracture finding is relevant at the outset, it is just as pertinent during trial reductions toward the completion of surgery. One commonly sees that a tibial insert of thickness chosen to address some collateral laxity, is in fact imparting a flexion contracture state which may be highly undesirable.

In the goal of assessing flexion contracture without navigation, it is a practice utilized by some, probably nowhere published, that compression at the heel, i.e. simulated axial loading, may be used to assess whether the knee is at full extension. The theory here is that a flexed knee pushed from the heel below will see a flexion moment that effectively causes the knee to bend as the axial loading occurs. One immediately sees that this criterion is absolutely invalid. Its validity can only be assumed if there is no frictional resistance at the knee and if there is no weight in the extremity, i.e. vertical force acting at the level of the knee. As these last two features are never realized, the flexed knee, especially with trial components undergoing greater frictional resistance to movement, offers significant resistance to flexion even at angles of 10–15 degrees.

The importance of these accurate assessments is that better understanding of the partition of flexion deformity to varus-valgus deformity allows more intelligent planning of releases and possibly distal femoral resection level.

True Varus-Valgus Deformity

In addition to the proper segmentation of the varus-valgus angulation from the real flexion contracture, navigational equipment allows one for the first time to assess at the outset the true amount of deformity, i.e. varus/valgus deformity which must be addressed. I am referring to the tensor or tension stress concept likely first introduced by MAR Freeman of the U.K. Neither passive correction of a deformity or full measurement of a long-standing radiograph supply the information necessary to determine the actual asymmetry of the soft-tissue sleeve which must be addressed to properly balance the knee in a varus/valgus sense. One is able using computer assistance to determine at the outset the tibio-femoral angle present when the tibia is held distracted from the femur, when the capsular-ligamentous complex is taut on both the medial and lateral aspects. It is this degree of asymmetry which must be adjusted to achieve proper collateral balance.

In the very first fully navigated TKR which we reported, the patient possessed no true varus deformity despite the fact that his long standing radiograph showed a 9 degree varus angulation.

Further, navigational tools display not only the resulting angular positions of the distal femoral and proximal tibial cuts, but the orientation of trial and final components as mentioned repeatedly above. The point of this is that these positions may be different from the cuts themselves. In the case of the femoral component, true position may vary during placement on the bone as the component either comes to a deeper position or remains at a proud position. The former is generally due to bone softness or

defect while the latter, on the femur particularly, is due to incomplete seating from incomplete bone preparation.

The issue of deeper seating into softer bone is so consistent that we routinely navigate the final position of components, particularly during cementation. There is a fairly consistent tendency for both femoral and tibial components to implode into the softer bone present on the convex side of the deformity – the medial compartment in valgus and the lateral side in varus deformities.

Similarly, it is possible to assess any failure to seat anteriorly or more importantly posteriorly at the tibial baseplate. Particularly the posterior lateral corner is difficult to evaluate thoroughly.

Just as may be apparent in conclusional discussion below these occurrences may be difficult or impossible to discern in even the largest studies. A two or three degree anterior tibial slope which could be of great clinical significance, especially when the target was a level, zero degree cut, would represent 0.2–0.3 of a degree difference in the group average with ten patients, and 0.2–0.3 degree difference with a hundred cases. If there were ten such patients in the larger group, the difference in the mean tilt would be only 0.2–0.3 degrees, not likely to be considered of clinical significance. For the individuals, though, this can be very significant. Anterior slopes at the tibia can be associated with abnormal anterior displacement of the femur on the tibia and worse, premature tibial loosening as the baseplate sinks into softer anterior bone, the original joint line sloping posterior.

Some Negative Factors

Navigation equipment costs money, at least for the primary case at hand. There is the cost of the equipment as well as any expendables or disposable items.

In addition, there is some added time associated with placing bone trackers and performing registration. In our own experience, the placement of trackers and performance of the registration may be done in as little as 5 min. Additional time is usually spent adjusting one's cuts and other aspects, based upon the information the system provides. The greatest amount of time is spent *getting it right!* By this is meant finding out that a cut or component position is not right and making the satisfactory adjustments. It is fairly estimated that these aspects will add a minimum of 5 min and a maximum of 30–40 min to one's case. It the jigs wind up in the right position with the cuts also correct, the components seat properly, and the alignment management is correct, the additional time is only the brief elements of checking and verification.

This latter aspect, checking, is actually quite rapid. When inaccuracies are determined, the adjustment and sequential checking of additional attempts to get something correct are individually a lot more rapid than with traditional mechanical instruments. It is much faster to move the plane-probe, i.e. a flat surface with attached tracker, into position to asses the results of additional adjustments.

Clinical Outcome Results

It appears that all full journal publications of the results of navigated total knees show an average diminution in varus/valgus axial mal-alignment of about 50% [2–6]. More importantly when one analyzes the results, the numbers of patients presenting outlier results, e.g. alignment errors greater than 3 degrees, is reduced. While 5 degrees has commonly been used as a dividing line between satisfactory and unsatisfactory, recent analysis suggests that errors in the varus direction of more than 3 degrees are associated with substantially diminished survival leading to early loosening [7, 8].

In terms of pain relief or other subjective, even objective measurements, it is clear that clinical reports to date show no differences *on average* between navigated and non-navigated knees. Again, averages–the numbers tested for statistically significant differences may be misleading. In addition, the functional and subjective aspects of outcome assessment in less than a 5+ year time frame certainly may not reveal what will subsequently prove to be very significant differences for meaningful proportions of patients.

Summary and Conclusions

Additional imaging as provided by CT scans or use of intra-operative fluoroscopy seem not to be necessary.

Navigation systems provide information such as range of motion, particularly the point of maximum passive extension, and the amount of true varus/valgus deformity which have until now been unobtainable.

Navigation permits the assessment of trial component and final component position, also previously unobtainable. This information can permit more accurate component placement and the avoidance of mal-alignment or flexion contracture.

Resistance to the adoption of more expensive, somewhat time-consuming methods exists. It is this surgeon's prediction that widespread adoption of knee navigation will require at least one, possibly two things. First is what may be called a training generation of experience. As residents and fellows see and do total knees both ways, they will come to appreciate and understand the differences and the significant value of computer assistance. The second is the continued improvement in software and hardware so that the entire process of navigation is simpler and less time consuming.

References

1. Krackow KA, Serpe L, Phillips MJ, Bayers-Thering M, Mihalko WM (1999) A new technique for determining proper mechanical axis alignment during total knee arthroplasty: progress toward computer-assisted TKA. Orthopedics 22: 698–702
2. Chauhan SK, Clark GW, Lloyd S, Scott RG, Breidahl W, Sikorski JM (2004) Computer-assisted total knee replacement. a controlled cadaver study using a multi-parameter quantitative CT aSSESS-MENT OF aLIGNMENT (the Perth CT Protocol). J Bone Joint Surg Br 86: 818–823
3. Chauhan SK, Scott RG, Breidahl W, Beaver RJ (2004) Computer-assisted knee arthroplasty versus a conventional jig-based technique. A randomised, prospective trial. J Bone Joint Surg Br 86: 372–377
4. Krackow KA, Phillips MJ, Bayers-Thering M, Serpe L, Mihalko WM (2003) Computer-assisted total knee arthroplasty: navigation in TKA. Orthopedics 26: 1017–1023
5. Sparmann M, Wolke B, Czupalla H, Banzer D, Zink A (2003) Positioning of total knee arthroplasty with and without navigation support. A prospective, randomized study. J Bone Joint Surg Br 85: 830–835
6. Stulberg SD, Loan PB Sarin V (2002) Computer-assisted navigation in total knee replacement: results of an initial experience in thirty-five patients. J Bone Joint Surg Am 84(S): 90–98
7. Ritter MA, Faris PM, Keating EM, Meding JB (1994) Postoperative alignment of total knee replacement. CORR 299: 153–156
8. Sharkey PF, Hozak WJ, Rothman RH, Shastri S, Jacoby SM (2002) Insall Award Paper. Why are total knee arthroplasties failing today? COOR 404: 7–13

Navigated Total Knee Arthroplasty and the OrthoPilot System

R.G. Haaker, M. Senkal, A. Ottersbach, R. Willburger

Introduction

Following its development period from 1993 to 1997 in joint and spinal surgery, the OrthoPilot system has proved its technical efficiency from 1997 onwards in a cadaver study [20] and in subsequent clinical trials.

Moreover, the OrthoPilot navigation system has also shown substantially better results compared with the use of manual instrumentation [4, 9, 17, 24]. It was reported in a multicenter study [3] that a statistically significant improvement in the alignment of the knee prosthesis components in respect of the mechanical leg axis and the femoral and tibial individual axes could be achieved with the OrthoPilot system as opposed to the manual technique.

The superiority of the navigated implantation technique became particularly obvious when the five set parameters of 0±3° for the mechanical axis and 90±2° for the individual axes were observed. Such results, which are to be considered very good, were achieved in 49.6% of cases with the navigated technique, whereas the attainment rate with the manual implantation technique was only 30.8%. In a comparative investigation between 100 navigated and 100 manually inserted cases with the Search Evolution knee, Haaker et al. [7] showed even clearer differences in favor of the navigated technique using the same criteria. With the navigation technique they observed very good results in respect of all five axes in 54% of the cases, whereas this was the case in just 15% of the patients treated with manual implantation technique.

In software versions 1.0 to 2.2 the OrthoPilot system simply navigated the tibial resection and the distal femoral resection planes of a total knee arthroplasty. Versions 3.0 and 3.1 included, in addition, the rotational alignment of the femoral component through acquisition of the transepicondylar axis via the medial and lateral femoral epicondyle. The inaccuracies in defining the femoral epicondyles must be taken into account here. The goal in total knee replacement is not only to create an accurate axis of the leg within ±3° of the Mikulicz' line, but also to balance the soft tissues. This is necessary to prevent unequal polyethylene wear and early implant failure as well as to achieve stability of the knee during the whole range of motion.

Exact positioning of the femoral component in relation to the tibial component in both extension and flexion may be facilitated by recording the data of the flexion and extension gaps. The Galileo system and the VectorVision system [1] also integrate the measurement of extension and flexion gaps. The Stryker Leibinger navigation system [15] uses the distance between femoral epicondyles and the resection on the proximal tibia to arrive at two curves for the medial and lateral side of the knee joint over the entire range of movement. These curves provide information about contractures on the one hand or instability on the other, and in this way make soft tissue management possible. However, inaccuracies exist in the difficulties in exactly determining the femoral epicondyles.

Version 4.0 of the OrthoPilot system uses a special gap spreader to achieve accurate recording of flexion and extension gap data (◙ Fig. 14.1, 14.2). This allows conclusions to be made about a necessary soft tissue release, and thus soft tissue management as a whole.

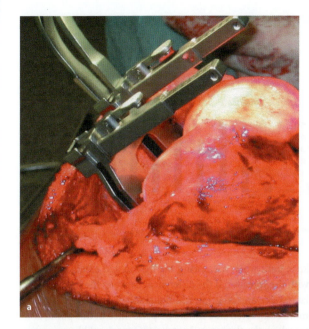

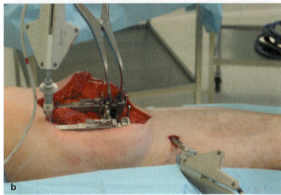

Fig. 14.1 a,b. A special spreader is used to determine the flexion gap (a) and the extension gap (0° position, b)

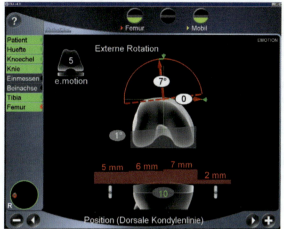

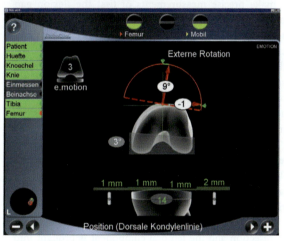

Fig. 14.2. Example of the final matching of medial and lateral flexion and extension gaps as well as rotation of the femoral component and height of the tibial component, a balanced extension gap, flexion gap laterally 7 mm, medially 2 mm

Materials and Methods
(Surgical Technique with Version 4.0)

There are no differences from the previous software versions 3.0 and 3.1 in respect of the distal femoral entry point, intra-operative kinematic analysis with circumduction of the hip to determine the femoral axis which runs through the centre of the femoral head, the definition of the centre of the ankle and knee joints and the acquisition of the knee joint line, the deepest defect point of the

dorsal femoral condyles, the anterior cortex on the distal femur and the malleolar triangle. When the leg axis has been established and displayed on screen following kinematic analysis, the first qualitative information about a necessary soft-tissue release is provided. But Version 4.0 goes further than this limited possibility of performing soft-tissue release. In addition, the more modern system employs a universal alignment guide for both tibial head and distal femoral resection. This guide can be adjusted in all three degrees of freedom, allowing the valgus/varus position, slope and resection height to be adjusted. Only the resection blocks for the tibial and femoral sides are different. The tibial resection block is first fixed into position provisionally on the head of the tibia using the universal alignment guide. Next follows the precise alignment in all planes and final fixation of the block, after which the tibial resection is performed. The tibial resection plane data are subsequently recorded using a tibial template and the accuracy of the resection is checked.

When this has been completed, a femoral plate is placed on the distal femoral condyles, positioned at right angles to the defined femoral axis, and used to record the distal femoral condyle plane, which is important for determining the extent of the distal femoral resection.

The potential size of the femoral component, established by the acquisition of the femoral data, is also continuously displayed on the screen. The next step is to make precise measurements of first the flexion gap and then the extension gap using a special spreader. The measurements are brought together and also indicated on screen. Then the universal alignment guide is provisionally fixed onto the distal femur and aligned in all planes, including the resection height, before being manually fixed into position on the distal femur. The femoral alignment always takes account of the medial and lateral sides simultaneously in their relation to the tibial resection.

The respective value with reference to the resultant height for the tibial polyethylene component is also given. This is followed by distal femoral condyle resection. The data of the distal femoral condyle resection are recorded with the femoral navigation template.

Now the femoral template is laid onto the distal femoral resection and the femoral component is brought into rotational alignment with the tibial resection plane. During this procedure the effects of the rotation of the femoral component on the flexion and extension gaps can be directly observed, as can the effects on the flexion and extension gaps of changing the size of the femoral component. In addition, the system informs the surgeon on screen about the anterioposterior position of the component, to avoid notching of the anterior femoral cortex (◻ Fig. 14.3).

When properly balanced conditions of the medial and lateral side in flexion and extension have been achieved, after the correct size of femoral component has been selected and rotational alignment performed, the locating points for the four-in-one resection template are drilled through the femoral template. Then the remaining femoral bone resection is carried out using the four-in-one cutting block.

In practice, a difference of more than 5–6 mm should not be tolerated between the medial and lateral side of the

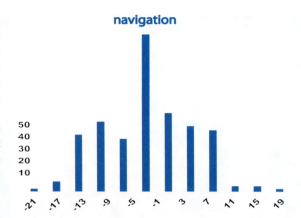

◻ Fig. 14.3. Pre-operative leg axis in 150 TKAs

knee joint when measuring the flexion and extension gaps with the spreader. If the differences between the medial and lateral side are too great, additional soft-tissue release on the more contracted side should be performed at this point, after which the flexion and extension gaps should be re-measured. This procedure helps to ensure that no unrealistic values for the femoral component occur during subsequent rotational alignment. Version 4.0 of the OrthoPilot system also contains a module that, following tibial resection, gap measurement and distal femoral condyle resection, permits the surgeon to simulate the conditions that would exist if potential femoral and tibial components were used.

After all the bone resections have been completed, the trial components are implanted and the final axial conditions achieved are displayed on screen. The bones are prepared for the femoral and tibial anchoring mechanisms and the knee endoprosthesis is implanted, including a patella component if required. After implantation the data for the definitive position of the endoprosthesis components are recorded (◻ Fig. 14.3).

Method and Results

Version 4.0 of the OrthoPilot knee navigation system is used in combination with the e.motion and Columbus knee prostheses. The e.motion knee endoprosthesis system offers a prosthesis that maintains a high surface congruence between the femoral component and the tibial polyethylene component between 5° hyperextension and 90° flexion, with the help of a rotational gliding platform. The authors' clinical experience was gained using the e.motion knee endoprosthesis system. 550 navigated implantations of e.motion knee endoprostheses have been carried out to date. Complete data records are available for the first 150 cases. We performed TKR type e.motion in 89 women and 61 men. The preoperative leg axis differed from –11° of valgus to 21° of varus. Using the same assessment criteria cited by Clemens et al. [3] and Konermann and Saur [13] the results were as follows: a very good result was achieved for the mechanical axis in 134/150 cases (81%, ◘ Fig. 14.4).

Outliers were present in 16/150 (19%) in respect of the mechanical axis. Certain weaknesses can still be found in the femoral alignment in the lateral plane which results in a slide varus in those outliers.

To judge the soft-tissue balancing and especially the external rotation of the femoral component according to the soft tissues in up to 9°, we looked for the alignment of the patella in the tangential 45° radiographs. The lateralization and the patella tilt have been compared with the preoperative situation. The results are shown in ◘ Table 14.1 and 14.2.

Discussion

The accuracy of the measuring angles on single long leg views is 2°, therefore, the long leg views are more precise than short leg radiographs (5°) [16]. Additional disadvantages of short leg views include errors from 1.6° to 1.9° [4, 19], oblique errors, and rotational errors as much as 2°, which mimic increased valgus in internal rotation and increased varus in external rotation [9, 17]. Interobserver error is reported with 1.1° rotation and intraobserver error with 0.9° rotation.

In the literature the accuracy of the mechanical axis in conventional TKAs has been within 3° of Miculicz line in

40 to 50% [6, 12, 24]. Jeffrey et al. reported revision rates of 3% in cases with optimal recreated mechanical axes and 24% in cases with suboptimal recreated mechanical axes (>3° out of Miculicz line) within 8 years [10]. But in summary, not all authors consider mal-alignment as a major contributing factor of implant failure. Whereas Jeffrey et al. [10] Rand and Coventry [22] , as well as Ritter et al. [23] consider the postoperative angle as a major concern, Hsu et al. [8] do not.

Ranawat et al. [21] investigated 112 TKA after 11 years and found radiolucent lines (RLL) in 60% of the cases with BMI being a factor. The mechanical axis ranged from 3 degrees varus to 10 degrees valgus (10 had 0 to 3 degrees varus, 17 had 0 to 4 degrees valgus, the remaining cases had 5 to 10 degrees valgus). Survivorship after 11 years was 94.1%. Ranawat reported no association with age, sex, diagnosis, cement-mantle or mal-alignment, but a significant correlation of RLL and BMI.

So by now it is not proven that higher accuracy using the navigation system leads us to extended standing times of TKAs. Precision in recreating the mechanical axis is independent from the experience of the surgeon. As Mahaluxmivala et al. reported, senior surgeons created the same numbers of outliers as young surgeons [16].

All resection planes were created using a manual oscillating saw with its known inaccuracy, particularly with soft and sclerotic bone. Therefore, we recommend a navigational double-check of all resection planes by putting a plate through the slot in the resection blocks while it is not fixated. However, this was not done in the current

◘ **Table 14.1.** Patella alignment according to the lateralisation of patellar bone pre-operative and post-operative

	Pre-operative	Post-operative
0 mm	39%	74%
1–2 mm	25%	15%
3–5 mm	22%	8%
>5 mm	14%	3%

◘ **Table 14.2.** Patella alignment according to the tilt of the patellar bone preoperative and postoperative

	Pre-operative	Post-operative
0°	44%	54%
1–5°	30%	34%
>5°	26%	12%

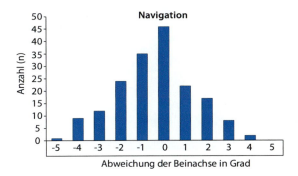

◘ **Fig. 14.4.** Postoperative alignment in 150 navigated TKAs

patients. The cementing technique is an additional error regarding definite component alignment.

Intra-operative identification of the femoral axis is difficult because of the soft tissues and tourniquet. Laskin reported a 4-cm error of the surgeon identifying the femoral head center [15]. Intra-medullary alignment however, has potential errors including a wide or deformed femur and an incorrect entry point.

In addition, the plane of the femoral reference osteotomy, which has to be oriented relative to the mechanical axis of the femur, cannot be defined exactly just by using the intra-medullary rod, as this only permits detection of the anatomical axis. Cutting is usually performed according to measurements in two-dimensional radiographs quantifying the discrepancy of both axes. Moreover, numerous studies showed that differing radii of femoral curvature are responsible for incoherency of the anatomical axis with the one suggested by the intra-medullary rod and that just by inconstant choice of the point of insertion variations up to 8.3° are possible [18].

Although increased surgery time was expected in the navigated group, there was only a mean of 10 min additional time including the learning curve. In the future the operating time will increase when femoral component rotation and AP positioning and soft tissue tension in flexion and extension are navigated. However time is saved because of the decreased need for considerable time consuming correcting maneuvers using the intra-medullary instruments. There was a decreased need to correct soft tissues when navigation was used.

There is concern about fat embolization with intra-medullary techniques. In addition to concerns about the accuracy of intra-medullary instrumentation, the introduction of rods into the canal has been shown to increase the intra-medullary pressure and produce embolization of fat particles into the circulation. In the extreme situation, this has resulted in respiratory symptoms with changes observed on chest radiographs, neurologic symptoms and even death [5]. The development of techniques and equipment for computer-assisted total knee surgery allows accurate implant positioning without instrumentation of the intra-medullary canal [9, 11, 20, 23, 25].

If there is to achieve a better patella alignment with extended external rotation of the femoral component cannot be judged by now. We have realized a reduction of lateralization of patella and patella tilt in comparison to preoperative situations. If this leads to reduced anterior knee pain after TKA needs further clinical investigations.

At least a wrong femoral component rotation (internal rotation) with its bad influence on anterior knee pain shown by Kienapfel and coworkers [12] can be prevented easily using this navigation system.

Conclusion

To sum up, the latest OrthoPilot software version, integrating soft-tissue balancing, shows excellent overall results. The instruments to use it minimal invasive are available just now (◘ Figs. 14.5, 14.6).

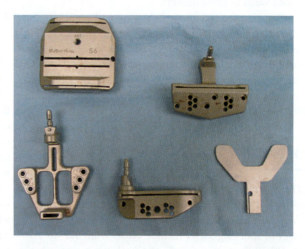

◘ **Fig. 14.5.** Minimal invasive instruments

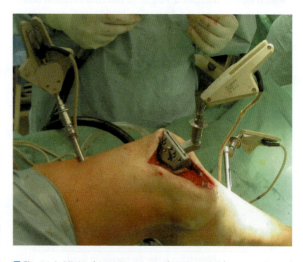

◘ **Fig. 14.6.** Minimal invasive approach using a mid-vastus snip and the mini-4-in-one Cutting block

References

1. Bäthis H, Perlick L, Grifka J (2004) Alignment in total knee arthroplasty. A comparison of computer-assisted surgery with the conventional technique. J Bone Joint Surg Br 86: 682–687

2. Bonnici AV, Allen PR (1991) Comparison of long leg and simple knee radiographs in assesment of knees prior to surgery. J Bone Joint Surg 73B (Suppl 1): 65–69

3. Clemens U, Miehlke RK, Kohler S, Kiefer H, Jenny JY, Konermann W (2003) Computer-assisted navigation with the OrthoPilot system using the search-evolution TKA prothesis – Results of a multicenter study. In: Stiehl JB, Konermann WH, Haaker RG (eds) Navigation and robotic in total joint and spine surgery. Springer, Berlin Heidelberg New York Tokio, pp 234–241

4. Delp SL, Stulberg, SD, Davies B, Picard F, Leitner F (1998) Computer-assisted knee replacement. Clin Orthop 354: 49–57

5. Dorr LD, Merkel C, Mellman MF, Klein I (1989) Fat emboli in bilateral total knee arthroplasty. Clin Orthop 248: 112–118

6. Fehring TK, Odum S, Griffin WL, Mason JB, Nadaud M (2001) Early failures in total knee arthroplasty. Clin Orthop 392: 315-318

7. Haaker RG, Stockheim M, Kamp M, Prof G, Breitenfelder J, Ottersbach A (2005) Computer navigation increases precision in component placement in TKA. Clin Orthop 433: 152–159

8. Hsu H, Garg A, Walker PS, Spector M, Ewald FC (1989) Effect of knee component alignment or tibial load distribution with clinical correlation. Clin Orthop 248: 135–144

9. Jenny JY, Boeri C (2001) Computer-assisted implantation of total knee prostheses: a case control comparative study with classical instrumentation. Comp Aided Surg 6: 217–220

10. Jeffrey RS, Morris RW, Denham RA (1991) Coronal alignment after total knee replacement. J Bone Joint Surg 73B : 709–714

11. Jeffery JA (1999) Accuracy of intramedullary femoral alignment in total knee replacement: Intraoperative assessment of alignment rod position. Knee 6: 211–215

12. Kienapfel H, Springorum HP, Ziegler A et al. (2003) Effect of rotation of the femoral and tibial components on malalignment in knee arthroplasty. Orthopaede 32: 312–318

13. Konermann W, Saur MA (2004) Postoperative alignment of conventional and navigated total knee arthroplasty. In: Stiehl JB, Konermann WH, Haaker RG (eds) Navigation and robotic in total joint and spine surgery. Springer, Berlin Heidelberg New York Tokyo, pp 219–225

14. Krackow KA, Serpe L, Philips MJ, Bayers-Thering M, Mihalko WM (1999) A new technique for determining proper mechanical axis alignment during total knee arthroplasty: Progress toward computer assisted TKA. Orthopedics 22: 698–702

15. Laskin RS (1984) Alignment of total knee components. Orthopedics 7: 62–67

16. Mahaluxmivala J, Bankes MJK, Nicolai P, Aldam CH, Allen PW (2001) The effect of surgeon experience on component positioning in 673 press fit condylar posterior cruciate-sacrificing total knee arthroplasties. J Arthroplasty 16: 635–640

17. Miehlke RK, Clemens U, Jens J-H, Kershally S (2001) Navigation in knee arthroplasty: Preliminary clinical experience and prospective comparative study in comparison with conventional technique. Z Orthop 139: 109–116

18. Olcott CW, Scott RD (1999) The Ranawat Award. Femoral component rotation during total knee arthroplasty. Clin Orthop 367: 39–42

19. Patel DV, Ferris BD, Aichroth PM (1991) Radiological study of alignment after total knee replacement: Short radiographs or long radiographs? Int Orthop 15: 209–210

20. Picard F, Leitner F, Saragaglia D, Cinquin P (1997) Mise en place d'une prothèse totale du genou assistée par ordinateur: A propos de 7 implantations sur cadavre. Rev Chir Orthop 83 [Suppl II]: 31–36

21. Ranawat CS, Boachie-Adjei O (1988) Survivorship analysis and results of total condylar knee arthroplasty. Clin Orthop 226: 6–13

22. Rand JA, Coventry MB (1988) Ten-year evaluation of geometric total knee arthroplasty. Clin Orthop 232: 168–173

23. Ritter MA, Faris PM, Keating EM, Meding JB (1994) Postoperative alignment of total knee replacement: Its effect on survival. Clin Orthop 299: 153–156

24. Saragaglia D, Picard F, Chaussard C, Montbaron E, Leitner F, Cinquin P (1997) Mise en place des prothèses totale du genou assistée par ordinateur: comparaison avec la technique conventionelle.A propos d´une étude prospective randomisée de 50 cas. Rev Chir Orthop 87: 18–28

25. Sharkey PF, Hozack WJ, Rothman RH, Shastri S, Jacoby SM (2000) Insall Award Paper: Why are total knee arthroplasties failing today? Clin Orthop 404: 7–13

CT-free Navigation including Soft-Tissue Balancing: LCS Total Knee Arthroplasty and VectorVision System

W.H. Konermann, S. Kistner

Introduction

The specific challenges in total knee arthroplasty are sufficiently well known. In order to obtain excellent long-term results, the following criteria have to be considered:

- General criteria:
  - patient selection
  - Correct indication
  - Peri-operative management
- Specific criteria:
  - Prosthetic design
  - Surgical technique, implantation technique
  - Reconstruction of the mechanical leg axis
  - Reconstruction of the joint line
  - Ligament balancing

Mal-alignment of either leg axes or implant components and the imbalance of the soft tissues reduce the longevity of knee implants [5, 9].

The advantages of navigated versus conventional surgery were presented in one of the largest multi-center studies worldwide [3, 4]. Results were based on an optimal alignment of the prosthesis with respect to the reconstruction of the mechanical leg axes.

Buechel [1, 2] reported on specific data relevant for the LCS knee implant, e.g. the optimal ligament balancing and an equal flexion and extension gap. Besides the correct alignment of the prosthesis, an optimal ligament balancing is of utmost importance for excellent long-term results.

Konermann and Saur based their prospective study on 100 patients with a conventionally implanted LCS prosthesis compared to 100 patients with the Search Evolution prosthesis placed using the OrthoPilot navigation system. The authors found an optimal alignment with maximal aberrance of 3° from the mechanical leg axis (varus, valgus) in 77% of conventional cases versus 93% in navigated cases [6] (see chapter 10).

Concept of the VectorVision CT-free Knee Navigation System

The VectorVision CT-free knee navigation system (BrainLAB AG, Germany) assists in achieving a correct alignment of the prosthesis, the reconstruction of the joint line as well as in implementing an optimal balance of the ligaments and an equal extension and flexion gap.

The camera arm and computer workstation are integrated into the VectorVision compact navigation system. The navigated instruments are tracked passively via reflective marker spheres. The spheres reflect infrared-light, emitted by the camera, which enable the tracking of surgical instruments in the operating room. There are no bothersome cables in the surgical field. The system is controlled by the surgeon via touch screen monitor. Reference arrays are attached to both the femur and tibia using a bicortical Schanz pin or two K-wires.

Steps in a Navigated Procedure

The points, acquired through pivoting of the hip joint and with a pointer, are utilized for the patient registration and are at the same time the basis for the planning of the implant position. After acquisition of the registration points, a generic model from the database is morphed to the acquired points. This model then has to be verified using relevant points on the tibia as well as on the femur. It has to be taken into consideration that this model can only offer an additional 3-D orientation. The correct planning of the implant position is based on the collected points and clouds of points, which are acquired by dragging the tip of the pointer along defined areas of the bone surface.

Registration

1. The first step is to define the center of the femoral head by pivoting the femoral head in the acetabulum. The

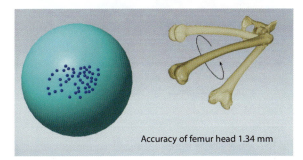

Accuracy of femur head 1.34 mm

Fig. 15.1. Femoral head calculation

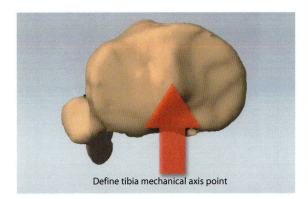

Define tibia mechanical axis point

Fig. 15.2. Define tibia mechanical axis point

center is defined as the average value of three calculated rotational centers. The indicated error value is the deviation of these centers to each other (Fig. 15.1).
2. In the next step the center of the distal endpoint of the mechanical tibia axis is defined by identifying the medial and lateral malleolus with the pointer.
3. Definition of the proximal point of the mechanical tibial axis (Fig. 15.2).
4. Definition of the tibial size.
   The tibial size is defined by defining the most medial, lateral, anterior and posterior point on the tibia with the pointer. The points should be acquired in the area where the resection level is planned to be and will be utilized to define the size of the tibial implant component (Fig. 15.3).

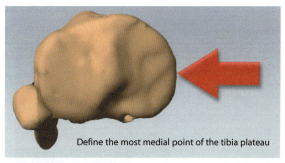

Define the most medial point of the tibia plateau

Fig. 15.3. Define tibial implant component

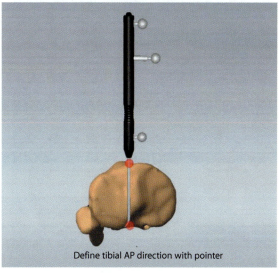

Define tibial AP direction with pointer

Fig. 15.4. Define a-p direction of the tibia

5. Definition of the A-P direction of the tibia.
   The A-P direction of the tibia is defined with the VectorVision pointer as it is essential to define the neutral rotational alignment of the tibial implant component. The A-P direction is also the basis for the alignment of the posterior slope, which is defined along the medio-lateral direction (90° to the A-P direction) (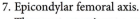 Fig. 15.4).

6. Acquisition of landmarks on the tibia (bone morphing).
   A series of landmarks are collected on the tibial bone surface by dragging the tip of the pointer along three defined areas: the anterior cortex, and the medial and lateral tibia plateaus. The deepest point is calculated from the points acquired on the medial and lateral tibia plateaus, which is then used as the reference for the resection level (■ Fig. 15.5).

7. Epicondylar femoral axis.
   The most prominent medial and lateral point of the femoral epicondyles are acquired on the bone surface. The line connecting these two points is one of the reference lines for the femoral rotation and influences the implant position accordingly (■ Fig. 15.6).

8. Definition of the femoral sulcus.
   The femoral sulcus determines the exit point of the anterior resection plane and has an important impact on the sizing of the prosthesis. A correct definition avoids anterior notching (■ Fig. 15.7).

9. Femoral mechanical axis.
   The most distal end point of the femoral mechanical axis is defined, which influences varus and valgus position (■ Fig. 15.8).

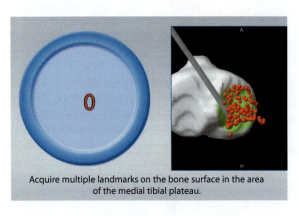

Acquire multiple landmarks on the bone surface in the area of the medial tibial plateau.

■ **Fig. 15.5.** Define medial tibia plateau (bone morphing)

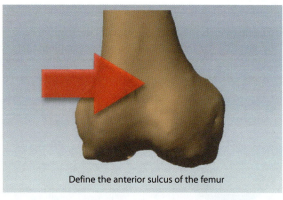

Define the anterior sulcus of the femur

■ **Fig. 15.7.** Define anterior femoral sulcus

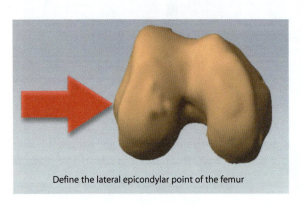

Define the lateral epicondylar point of the femur

■ **Fig. 15.6.** Define Lateral Epicondyle

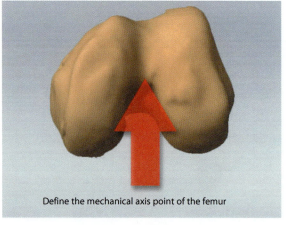

Define the mechanical axis point of the femur

■ **Fig. 15.8.** Define femoral mechanical axis

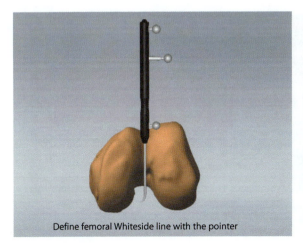

Define femoral Whiteside line with the pointer

Fig. 15.9. Whiteside line

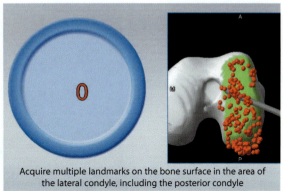

Acquire multiple landmarks on the bone surface in the area of the lateral condyle, including the posterior condyle

Fig. 15.10. Define lateral femoral condyle (bone morphing)

10. Whiteside line.
The Whiteside line is defined with the VectorVision pointer and is one of the reference lines for the femoral rotation (■ Fig. 15.9).
11. Acquisition of landmarks on the femur (bone morphing).
Multiple points are acquired on the medial and lateral femoral condyles and the anterior area of the femur. The resection level of the distal femur will be calculated from the most prominent distal point. This has an impact on the implant size as well (■ Fig. 15.10). The posterior condylar line is the third line of the reference lines for the femoral rotation.
12. Model Morphing.
An integrated anatomical knee joint database enables a generic 3D model to be morphed to the actual patient anatomy.
13. Verification of the femur and the tibia.
A specific point on the tibia and the femur (e.g. drill hole point) are defined with the VectorVision pointer. These points are used to check the accuracy of the system e.g., if a Schanz pin is loose.

Planning

Based on the data acquired intra-operatively, the system automatically calculates an initial optimal implant posi-

tion. The implant position is displayed on the monitor in a comprehensive planning overview.

Fine-Tuning of the Femoral Implant

After the implant size and position are calculated by the system, the implant components can be fine-tuned by the surgeon. The following fine-adjustment features are provided:
1. Resection level
2. Anterior-posterior alignment of the implant
3. Medial-lateral alignment of the implant
4. Anterior-posterior slope
5. Medial-lateral slope
6. Internal and external rotation
7. Implant size (■ Fig. 15.11)

Fine-Tuning of the Tibial Implant

The same adjustments can be applied to the tibia:
1. Resection level
2. Anterior-posterior alignment of the implant
3. Medial-lateral alignment of the implant
4. Anterior-posterior slope
5. Medial-lateral slope
6. Internal and external rotation
7. Implant size (■ Fig. 15.12)

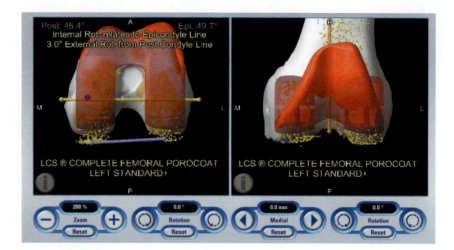

■ **Fig. 15.11.** Confirm position of femoral implant

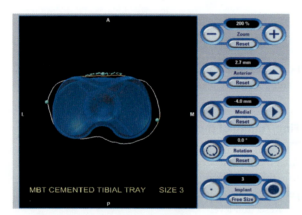

■ **Fig. 15.12.** Confirm position of tibial implant

The system's toolbox enables the calculation process to be influenced. The treatment planning allows basic alignment parameters to be pre-defined, such as:

1. Determination of tibia resection (in relation to the deepest point on the affected or healthy plateau)
2. Selection of the rotational axes (posterior condylar axis, epicondylar axis, Whiteside line)
3. Selection of the implant alignment (posterior alignment, anterior alignment)

Additionally, the toolbox provides the possibility for:

1. A re-registration
2. The acquisition of additional reference points
3. The selection of the implant (cemented, non-cemented, rotating platform, a-p glide inlay, etc.)

Navigation and Verification

The ligament balancing function as well as the navigation and verification of the bone cuts enable a continuous adaption and optimization of the LCS implant position. Tibia and femur are not adapted one after the other, but alternating step by step. Adhering to the conventional surgical technique, the distal femoral cut and the tibial resection level have to be parallel when the knee joint is in full extension.

The VectorVision software determines the tibial slope based on the antecurvature of the anterior femoral cortex and therewith against the femur implant position. The limits of the slope range from a maximal 10° to a minimal 5°.

1. **Calculation of the sagittal angle between the distal femoral anatomical axis and the mechanical axis.**
   To define the femoral antecurvature the LCS-yoke is placed on the anterior cortex of the distal femur. The angle between the femoral mechanical axis and the tangent on the distal anterior femur is defined. The position of the LCS-yoke is navigated using the LCS navigation adapter and stored (■ Fig. 15.13, 15.14).

2. **Calculation and verification of the tibial slope.**
   Within a specific range (5°–10° posterior slope) the software recommends a tibia slope depending on the calculated antecurvature of the femur. The value of the tibia slope – regardless of the recommendation – can be adjusted by the user (■ Fig. 15.15).

3. **Navigation of the tibial resection.**
   The resection level can be referenced either from the highest or lowest tibial plateau. The slope is defined through the previous calculation. The tibial cutting

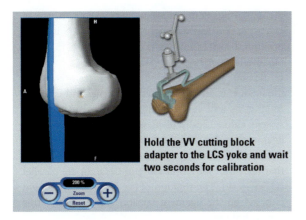

Hold the VV cutting block adapter to the LCS yoke and wait two seconds for calibration

◧ **Fig. 15.13.** Calculate anterior alignment

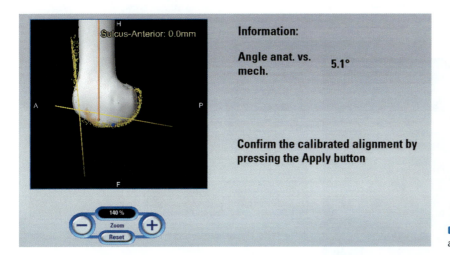

Information:

Angle anat. vs. mech.   **5.1°**

Confirm the calibrated alignment by pressing the Apply button

◧ **Fig. 15.14.** Confirm anterior alignment

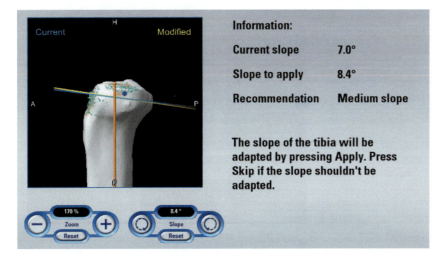

Information:

Current slope   **7.0°**

Slope to apply   **8.4°**

Recommendation   **Medium slope**

The slope of the tibia will be adapted by pressing Apply. Press Skip if the slope shouldn't be adapted.

◧ **Fig. 15.15.** Verify tibia slope

block is navigated to the planned position and fixed with 3 or 4 drill pins. The bone cut is performed and verified. The performed cut is updated and displayed. Deviations to the planned resection level on the tibia (varus/valgus, slope and height) are displayed allowing for additional navigation and resection if necessary (◘ Figs. 15.16, 15.17).

4. **Ligament balancing in extension.**
   In extension a defined force is transferred to the joint with a specific spreader tool. Flexion, extension and the size of the joint gap are calculated by the navigation system and displayed. If deviations (varus/valgus) from the mechanical leg axis (0°) are displayed on the monitor, appropriates soft tissue management should be performed to achieve the proper mechanical leg axis and joint stability. The system recalculates and displays the actual ligament values and the extension gap in extension. For further calculation of the LCS implant position the extension gap is essential (◘ Fig. 15.18).

5. **Ligament balancing in flexion.**
   In flexion again a defined force is transferred to the ligaments and the maximal internal and external rotation as well as the flexion gap is calculated. The system automatically displays the actual data of the ligament tension and the flexion gap dimension. The rotational alignment of the femur is then calculated so that the posterior femur cut and tibia cut are parallel (◘ Fig. 15.19). The rotation of the femoral component is based on the ligament tension and we prefer this gap-technique.

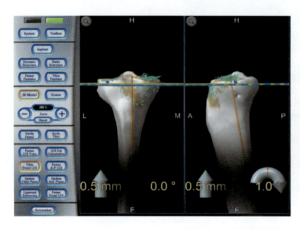

◘ Fig. 15.16. LCS tibial plane navigation

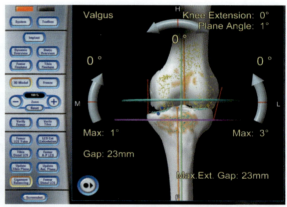

◘ Fig. 15.18. Ligament balancing in extension

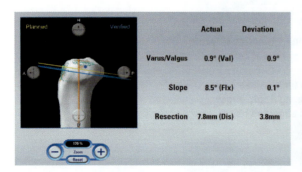

◘ Fig. 15.17. Verify tibial plane

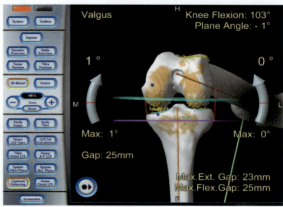

◘ Fig. 15.19. Ligament balancing in flexion

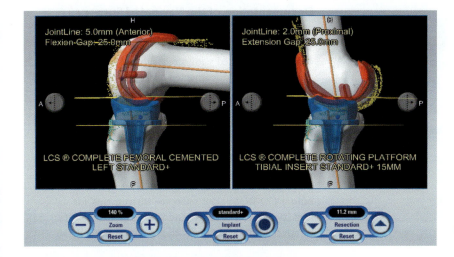

Fig. 15.20. Confirm LCS component optimization

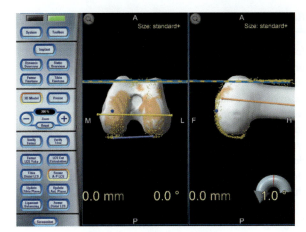

Fig. 15.21. Navigate LCS anterior cutting block

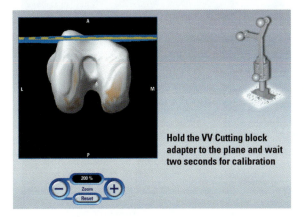

Hold the VV Cutting block adapter to the plane and wait two seconds for calibration

Fig. 15.22. Verify femoral anterior cut

6. **Calculation of the femoral LCS implant position.**
Based on the information stored from the ligament balancing, the VectorVision system calculates the ideal position and size of the femoral component as well as the required size of the inlay, so that flexion and extension gap will be identical. The surgeon can find a compromise between retaining the joint line and having an equal flexion and extension gap by modifying the distal resection level or changing the implant size. All variables for implant position are fully accessible to allow for an ideal result (Fig. 15.20).

7. **Navigation of the anterior and posterior femoral cut.**
Rotation and the position of the anterior and posterior resection level are defined by the previous calculations. The A-P femoral cutting block is navigated to the planned position and fixed with two drill pins. The anterior and posterior cuts are performed. By verifying the performed cuts the femoral data are updated. If the actual cuts deviate from the planning (rotation, slope) the surgeon has the opportunity to perform corrective navigated cuts (Figs. 15.21–15.23).

8. **Navigation of the distal femoral cut.**
The distal femoral cut is performed based on the verified anterior cut. This ensures an ideal preparation of the bone and results in an ideal implant-to-bone fit. The distal femoral cutting block is navigated to the planned position, fixed with drill pins and the cut is performed. By verifying the cut, the information on the femur is updated and visualized on the monitor. Any deviations to the treatment plan can be intra-operatively detected and immediately corrected (Fig. 15.24).

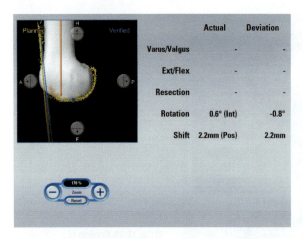

Fig. 15.23. Femur plane deviations

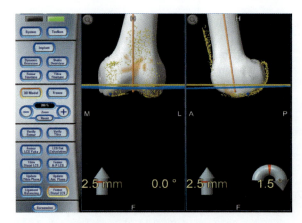

Fig. 15.24. Navigate LCS femur distal cut

9. Additional cuts.

The final preparation (chamfer cuts and lug holes) of the femur is performed using the conventional cutting template.

Implantation

After performing the cuts, assisted by the navigation system, the prosthetic components are implanted in the same way as during a conventional surgery. In this step a correct rotational alignment of the tibial component in respect to the tibial resection level is essential (e.g. parallel to the holes of the k-wires).

Documentation of the Navigated Surgery

During navigation every phase of the surgical procedure can be documented with screenshots. All performed cuts are automatically documented by the VectorVision system.

After implantation the achieved leg axis can be checked with support of the navigation system. The stability of the leg can be controlled by bringing the leg in full flexion and extension as well as positions in-between. The documentation of the displayed values is performed with screenshots (◘ Fig. 15.25). A navigation report includes all parameters of the patient and the screenshots are copied onto a CD-ROM. The reference instruments for navigation (two reference arrays and Schanz pins or K-wires) are removed and the wound is closed conventionally.

Results

In this prospective study 50 patients were operated on primary TKA using the CT-free navigation system. The surgeries were done by one surgeon, who has experience in over 500 computer-assisted surgeries. Measurements were made by one independent observer two weeks after surgery based on a lateral fluoroscopy with the patient lying supine. The slope of the femoral component was defined in relation to the distal anterior femur cortex. The slope of the tibial component was defined in relation to the proximal posterior tibial cortex.

The mechanical leg axis was measured using an AP long leg x-ray. The frontal orientation of the femoral

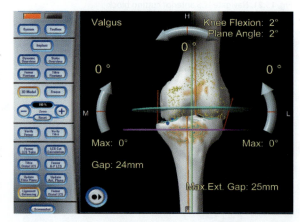

Fig. 15.25. Documentation of the implanted LCS Prosthesis in extension

component in relation to the femoral mechanical axis and the frontal orientation of the tibia component in relation to the tibia were measured as well. The long leg x-ray images were acquired in a strictly standardized method, the central x-ray was adjusted to the patella, which is defined as centric between the femoral condyles.

The values determined using the X-ray images contain a human error of 1° and a positioning error of 2° for the radiological measurements.

Mechanical Leg Axis

The mechanical leg axis was measured as 0° in 60% of the cases. If a deviation of ≤3° varus/valgus for the mechanical leg axis is defined as a very good result and the potential radiological measurement error is taken into consideration, then 100% of the navigated prostheses were placed with good results.

Femoral A-P Axis

The inner angle of the femoral prosthesis in the frontal plane was measured to be the ideal 90° in 50% of the navigated cases. 100% achieved a good result when considering a deviation of ≤2° varus/valgus.

Lateral Femoral Axis

The flexion-extension aligment of the femoral component was 11,2° flexion slope (± 1,6° range: 9,8°–13,2°). The design of the LCS prosthesis is such, that the distal femoral cut is not perpendicular to the saggital anterior/posterior femoral cuts, but in 105°. This means that the femoral curvation is not 11,2° average but 3,8° to the saggital femoral mechanical axis.

Tibial A-P Axis

In 52% of all navigated tibia prostheses an exact alignment to the frontal tibial axis, defined as having an inner angle of 90°, was achieved. Very good results were achieved for 100% of all navigated knee joints accepting a ≤2° deviation in varus/valgus alignment.

Lateral Tibial Axis

The posterior slope of the tibial component was 6,2° (±1,4° range: 4,8°-7,6°). The recommended posterior slope of the LCS prosthesis is 7°.

Comprehensive Overview on 5 Axes

Summing up the result for all 5 axes and by defining a ≤3° deviation of the mechanical axis and ≤2° for all 4 axes as an excellent result, then 100% of all navigated prostheses meet this goal.

Conclusions and Visions

Based on our actual experiences the VectorVision CT-free knee navigation system in conjunction with the LCS prosthesis enables an optimization of:
1. the reconstruction of the mechanical leg axis,
2. the implant position,
3. the ligament balancing,
4. the flexion and extension gap,
5. the reconstruction of the joint line.

Another advantage is the user-friendly workflow of the VectorVision software, that can be considered as easy to use as well for surgeons who are not enthusiastic on new technologies [7]. The navigation system is adapted to the surgical technique and the surgeon does not have to change his conventional handling for example with the spacer or cutting blocks. The disadvantage of all navigated methods is the extension of the surgery (10–15 min). The mean time of the surgery is 73 min (55–90 min.) This additional time is tolerable in routine surgery.

The inaccuracy of the cuts, e.g. caused by deflection of the saw blades treating sclerotic bones, initially are not taken into account by navigation. The verification of the bone cuts after resection with navigation now provides relevant data on the accuracy of the cuts and they can be intra-operatively corrected by re-resection. However, surgeons would need new cutting or milling tools or possibly new minimally-invasive robots to further improve resection accuracy.

Once again it has to be stated that the navigation system as a more accurate technology currently is evaluated in conjunction with a measuring instrument, the fluoroscopy, that is accompanied with an inaccuracy of 3°.

For the future the integration of pressure sensors [8, 10] (see chapter 23) is suggested, which should be inserted during different surgical steps and being integrated in to the trial prosthesis as well as the implanted inlay.

For the femoral rotation the surgeons use different procedures: the femoral component can be oriented according to the transepicondylar axis, to the posterior condyles or to the Whiteside line. The fourth technique is the gap technique based on the ligament tension, which achieves a perfect balanced flexion and extension gap. In the presented technique we only use the gap technique.

Utilizing the data, further optimization of the ligament balancing can be achieved. Pressure on the medial and lateral implant components can be measured in full extension and different flexion levels. The surgeon would be able to create a navigated fine tuning release to achieve perfect ligament balancing in any stage of the surgery.

Navigation opened new horizons and ways to go in the last eight years. Constant and worldwide exchange of ideas on both surgeons and engineers sides enabled the development of minimally-invasive surgical techniques providing innovative approaches and new designs of the prosthesis. Thanks to the navigation we are stepping into a new age of total knee replacement surgery. Primarily this will bring decisive advantages for our patients.

References

1. Buechel FF, Stiehl JB (2004) Total knee arthroplasty. In Stiehl JB, Konermann WH, Haaker RG (eds) Navigation und robotic in total joint and spine surgery. Springer, Berlin Heidelberg New York Tokyo, pp 175–179
2. Buechel FF, Pappas MJ (1986) The New Jersey low-contact-stress knee replacement system: biomechanical rationale and review of the first 123 cemented cases. Arch Orthop Traum Surg 105: 197–204
3. Clemens U, Miehlke RK, Kohler S, Kiefer H, Jenny JY, Konermann W (2002) Computerassistierte Navigation mit dem OrthoPilot-System und der Search-Evolution-Knieendoprothese. In Konermann W, Haaker R (Hrsg) Navigation und Robotic in der Gelenk- und Wirbelsäulenchirurgie. Springer, Berlin Heidelberg New York Tokio, pp 207–216
4. Clemens U, Konermann WH, Kohler S., Kiefer H, Jenny JY, Miehlke RK (2004) Computer-assisted navigation with the OrthoPilot system using the Search Evolution TKA prosthesis – results of a multicenter study. In: Stiehl JB, Konermann WH, Haaker RG (eds) Navigation und robotic in total joint and spine surgery. Springer, Berlin Heidelberg New York Tokyo, pp 234–241
5. Jeffrey RS, Morris RW, Denham RA (1991) Coronal alignment after total knee replacement. J Bone Joint Surg 73 B: 709–714
6. Konermann WH, Saur MA (2004) Postoperative alignment of conventional and navigated total knee arthroplasty. In Stiehl JB, Konermann WH, Haaker RG (eds) Navigation und Robotic in Total Joint and Spine Surgery. Springer, Berlin Heidelberg New York Tokyo, pp 219–225
7. Konermann WH, Kistner S (2004) CT-free navigation including soft-tissue balancing: LCS-TKA and VectorVision systems. In: Stiehl JB, Konermann WH, Haaker RG (eds) Navigation und robotic in total joint and spine surgery. Springer, Berlin Heidelberg New York Tokyo, pp 255–265
8. Mortier J, Zichner L (2002) Computerassistierte Druckmessung im patellofemoralen Gelenk mit elektronischen Drucksensoren. In: Konermann W, Haaker R (eds) Navigation und Robotic in der Gelenk- und Wirbelsäulenchirurgie. Springer, Berlin Heidelberg New York Tokio, S 425–428
9. Rand JA, Coventry MB (1988) Evaluation of Geometric total knee athroplasty. Clin Orthop 232: 168–173
10. Wasielewski RC, Galat DD, Komistek RD (2004) Computer-assisted ligament balancing of the femoral tibial joint using pressures sensors. In: Stiehl JB, Konermann WH, Haaker RG (eds) Navigation und robotic in total joint and spine surgery. Springer, Berlin Heidelberg New York Tokyo, pp 197–203

Navigated Total Knee Arthroplasty and the Surgetics Bone-Morphing System

E. Stindel, J.L. Briard, C. Plaskos, J. Troccaz

Introduction

Total knee replacement is a challenge that aims at achieving a pain free, stable, and mobile joint. Both mobility and stability are essential for long term survivorship of the implants and this can only be achieved if the implants are properly aligned with the mechanical axis of the lower limb and if two ligament complexes are perfectly managed: the tibia-femoral and patello-femoral ligament complexes. From a mathematical point of view, performing a knee joint replacement is therefore a rather complex optimization problem in which the best compromise must be found in order to allow a full range of motion with perfect mobility/stability in both the femoro-patellar as well as the tibio-femoral joint. In this paper we describe our approach for solving this optimization problem thanks to the integration of several innovative bricks of technology into a so called »Computer Assisted Surgical Protocol«, or *CASP*.

It is worth noting that solutions developed today must be compatible with less invasive surgery; we believe that the recent tendency towards MIS in orthopaedics is warranted because it corresponds to a strong need expressed by patients. The current situation is challenging however since we do not believe that MIS techniques and implants as they exist today are sufficient to address the needs of the majority of surgeons. MIS results in reduced access and visibility. It is difficult to perform as well in such conditions. Some experienced surgeons have performed and developed MIS techniques without navigation. However, disseminating the skills, the know-how and the knowledge seems to be an overwhelming challenge. Appropriate technology is therefore required.

Performing surgery under conventional fluoroscopic guidance solves part of the visualization problem since it provides real-time images. However, it is only a 2D projection which has to be integrated mentally to 3D. This is known to be another difficult task. In addition, introducing a C-arm for routine hip or knee surgery raises several issues that many surgeons might not accept: manipulation of C-arm is not easy in the OR, the C-arm device must always be available, an assistant is often needed to manipulate the C-arm to obtain satisfactory images, the risk of infection increases, x-ray radiation for the staff and the patient is a serious concern, and working several hours with lead protection against x-rays adds an additional burden that would be nice to avoid. Navigated C-arms that are often used in traumatology eliminate partially the 2D problem since one can work on several projections at the same time. But the other issues remain. More recently, 3D navigated C-arms such as the ISO-C 3D of Siemens have been connected to Praxim navigation systems [8], thus offering intra-operative 3D data in the OR. But it is unlikely that such sophisticated and expensive devices will be used for routine hip and knee procedures all over the world. Thus, we strongly believe that the Echo Surgetics solution that we propose in this chapter is the ultimate solution for routine MIS hip and knee procedures.

This innovative technique in 3D modeling will be the foundation on which computer assisted surgical protocols will rely to interact with »universal«, »open« and »intelligent« instrumentation. Given the new constraints of emerging

MIS techniques, surgical navigation tools will clearly become more and more critical for routine practice. Links will be created between instruments and software through a new generation of sensors that will be able to provide quantitative data, such as distances and forces, which will be used with dedicated algorithms to steer active tools. Our strong assumption is that the future of MIS will be limited without CAOS.

In this chapter we will describe the CASP specifically developed by Praxim for the LCS knee implant (DePuy Orthopaedics Inc., Warsaw, IN, USA), as well as some novel and innovative bricks of Praxim technology which currently are being integrated into the Surgetics Station (PRAXIM SA, La Tronche, France). The Surgetics Station is an open platform navigation system offering CT-free hip and knee applications that provide geometric AND morphologic 3D data without any preoperative or intra-operative images (no CT, no MR, no fluoroscopy). The method uses data collected intra-operatively with a 3D optical localizer in relative coordinate systems attached to the bones, which is the core Bone Morphing technology (PRAXIM patents pending). These data are used to solve the optimization issue, described above, thanks to well-adapted algorithms that interact with open and universal instrumentation.

Aims

As in any optimization case, many parameters must be taken into account. None of them are independent and all interact on each other. The main objective for the developer is, firstly, to define a set of goals that must be achieved at the end of the procedure. From a mathematical point of view, theses goals will be seen as the output of the optimization loop.

Concerning the Praxim CASP developed for the DePuy LCS implant, we wanted to be able to:

- control the alignment of the implants with respect to the mechanical axis, this means to be able to control and plan any tibial and femoral cut in 3D (level and orientation),
- control stability, which requires a soft tissue registration algorithm, under correct alignment,
- manage both soft tissue compartments (femoro-patellar as well as femoro-tibial),
- perform automatic and efficient sizing of the implants,
- perform accurate cuts thanks to intelligent instruments,
- include quality control at each step.

Moreover, we wanted a Surgeon Friendly Interface (S.F.I.). More than a User Friendly Interface, the concept of a S.F.I. which we introduced in the previous edition of this book in 2003, includes the notion that the CASP must be *surgeon* friendly and expressed on the screen through a User Friendly Interface. For additional background information on computer aided systems and interfaces, see for example reference [14].

The software also runs on the *NanoStation* from PRAXIM-Medivision. This new navigation station embodies a very compact and easy-to-use design. Thanks to its small size it can be easily displaced from one O.R. to another and even from one clinic to the other since it can be folded into a standard airline-sized case equipped with wheels.

The software relies on 3D geometric and morphologic data. Geometric data may be sufficient for controlling the alignment of the components [11, 13, 18, 20], but they do not provide a complete representation of the knee. An important drawback of these methods is that they provide only an approximate knee center, by direct digitization or by kinematics analysis of the pathological knee joint, which is rather controversial. Conversely, 3D morphologic data obtained by the bone-morphing technique are very useful to visualize in real time and in three dimensions prior to any real cut: the bone defects, the planned surgical cuts, the choice of the implant size, position and rotation with respect to the bone cortical surfaces, the distances between bones and components. Any of those parameters affects directly the implant position during the planning phase, and all those parameters are linked together. For instance, changing the size of the implant will have immediate impact on its position and knee balancing, which is why only a global planning strategy makes sense. The morphological data also provides a lot of information to control or even automate the location of the points digitized by the surgeon. Therefore, the challenge is really geometric AND morphologic. 3D morphologic data are also very important for the concept of S.F.I introduced above. The visualization of the real 3D morphology of the epiphysis is an important part of the system, for allowing the surgeon to control the planning to achieve and to simulate different options in alignment, bone cuts, and their consequences on stability. In previous systems, 3D data were collected through CT acquisition followed by 3D reconstructions. Apart from the problem of the accuracy of the reconstruction, CT scans are very costly with respect to time, money, and irradiation to the patient. These drawbacks are no longer necessary thanks to the Bone Morphing technology introduced by PRAX-IM-Medivision. For more information on the technical approach we recommend reading the specific chapter on Bone Morphing included in this book.

The Computer-Assisted Surgical Procedure (CASP)

The first step of any CASP is to fix a reference system to each bone or tool we want to track during the surgery. For TKA, one reference system (DRB) is fixed on the tibia, one on the femur, and one on the patella (optional). The fixation to the bone must be perfectly rigid and stable, even in osteoporotic patients, since they will be used as reference systems to build a global and specific geometry of the patients' limb.

The second step consists of collecting 3D locations of points in order to create the anatomical reference planes (frontal, axial, sagittal) and to build the mechanical axis. To address the issues of alignment as well as ligament balance and patellar tracking, several key points have to be registered:

The Center of the Hip

In TKA procedures, the hip is outside the operating field; therefore the detection of the center of the joint H is based upon a kinematic method. There is no need of a rigid body on the iliac crest. Once, the femoral rigid body is placed, the surgeon performs a circular motion with the lower limb with the knee in full extension. During this motion the subsequent positions of the femoral rigid body are stored by the computer in the localizer reference system. Noise must be taken into account because of the non spheroid shape of the femoral head, the motion of the pelvic bone, and the limits of the accuracy of the optical localizer. Therefore, the center of the hip is not unique, and is always in motion. Any method of detection which would not take this into account will be inaccurate. In our approach the algorithm searches for a point in 3D space C_h that optimizes some criteria based on the minimum of a function

$$F(c) = \sum_{i=1}^{i=100} \left\| c_{i-1} - c_i \right\|^2 ,$$

where i is the position of the femur at time t and C_i is the corresponding calculated center. The resulting center can be

seen as the point in 3D space attached to the femur with the smallest trajectory during the acquisition motion [23, 25].

The Center of the Knee

During TKA procedures, the knee joint is more-or-less open so the digitization of geometric points (landmarks) is relatively easy. Accurate determination of the knee center is difficult because there is no precise definition that applies to the pathological knee [4, 6, 16]. However the direct localization of an approximation of the center of the pathological knee K_0 is easy using the optical probe. Such a point will *not* be used to define the HKA angle during the planning phase; it is only an indication to compute an approximation of the pathological axes of the patient pre-operatively. In the Surgetics approach using bone morphing, the knee center K_p is the center of the knee prosthesis that is planned along each step of the CASP. This definition corresponds exactly to what we expect post-operatively. Planning the implant position on the bone is therefore the only way to accurately define and control the post-operative knee center and HKA angle.

The Center of the Ankle

The purely morphological approach that we choose is based on the digitization of two points on the bones. Using the same probe used for the knee joint, the surgeon digitizes one point each on the lateral and medial malleoli. The system computes the middle of the segment defined by these two points. This approach has been extensively investigated and found to be sufficiently accurate and quick to perform [24, 25].

A few other points are recorded such as two points on the anterior femoral cortex in order to compute the ideal antero-posterior location of the femoral implant. Some points will then be used to build the femoral and the tibial axis. This step depends strongly on the chosen CASP running on the Surgetics Station and adapted to the prosthesis and to the surgical technique. For instance, in the Surgetics CASP applied to the LCS prosthesis of DePuy, we have chosen to use the two most posterior points on the femoral condyles in combination with the hip center to define the frontal plane. The tibial sagittal plane, which is probably one of the most important to define, is given by the ankle center and two points digitized on the tibia: the first one is on the tibial tuberosity, the second is between the medial and the lateral tubercle of the intercondylar eminence. Importantly, for any point for which a mathematical definition exists, the system uses the Bone Morphing surfaces and geometric axes to compute a new point that is more accurate and repeatable than the surgeon selected point. The surgeon selected point is then used only to check unlikely gross errors of the automated and refined bone-morphing points. This is an iterative and complex process that depends on each point and that benefits from the bone morphing described in the next section.

The Bone Morphing

From the surgical point of view, the bone morphing technique consists of collecting two clouds of points with the probe (one for the femur and one for the tibia). These points are gathered by sliding the spherical tipped probe on the articular surfaces. During this sliding motion the localizer records the 3D location of the probe tip. This process takes about 1 min 30 for each volume. This point cloud is then matched to a unique deformable model included in the system (see [7, 26] or the specific chapter in this book for a more technical description). The output of this deformation process is an accurate representation of the epiphysis of the bone at surgery. Its accuracy can be checked intra-operatively by the surgeon. The mean error between the model and the actual bone is usually below 0.5 mm.

Morphologic and geometric data will help to optimize the tibial and femoral cuts (location and orientation) in order to solve the complex optimization issue of properly implanting a total knee joint prosthesis. This issue will be solved in a three step procedure:

Optimization Loop

Step 1 – Optimization of the Tibial Cut

This is the first step of the planning process. The level of the tibial cut is important in order to have good and long lasting fixation of the implant and to avoid an unnecessarily thick tibial insert. This level is computed after recording the relative position of the tibia with respect to the femur at 97° of flexion. The level of the joint line is optimized to fit an implant with the smallest polyethylene

component (10 mm) and to obtain the best fitting implant for the femoral side based on data collected from the bone morphing model. The tibial cut is then performed: neutral in the coronal plane, with 7° slope in the sagittal plane, and centered at the computed level.

The bone morphing allows visualization of the cut and a possible bone defect due to wear. Once performed, the accuracy of the tibial cut is registered and will be used for further planning.

Step 2 – A New Approach to the Ligament Balance Issue: Integration of Intelligent Tools and Active Software

Precise soft tissue balancing is considered by many TKA surgeons as one of the most challenging tasks to realize, therefore a global solution had to be designed to steer the surgeons in this difficult task and to avoid misalignment as they are frequently reported in the literature with intra- and extra-medullary devices [10, 27].

In the previous edition of this book [5] we introduced the notion of AVS (Adjustable Variable Spacer) commonly called spacer blocks. These spacer blocks are assembled intra-operatively by the surgeon, inserted into the joint and then fine-tuned using quantitative data provided by the SFI on the compromise between gaps and mechanical alignment. In manual surgery, the adjustments in the size of this asymmetric spacer were made intuitively by the surgeon in a sometimes cumbersome mental optimization loop.

To speed up this process the authors and the PRAXIM-Medivision developers designed a totally new generation of software that steers the surgeons in the difficult task of ligament balancing. This software is now used with the original static spacer blocks, but in the future the process will be completely automated using miniature intelligent instruments that act as a dynamic or active spacer system.

If a pre-operative flexum deformity is noticed, an optional loop is performed during which the HKpA is assessed successively at 20 and 0 degrees of flexion. If a significant difference is noticed in the alignment, this indicates the existence of retraction of the posterior capsule. In such a case a posterior release will be necessary.

In all other cases the optimization loop starts by a »traction test« during which the collateral ligaments are put under tension by the surgeon (◘ Fig. 16.1). The software gives immediate data on the components that must

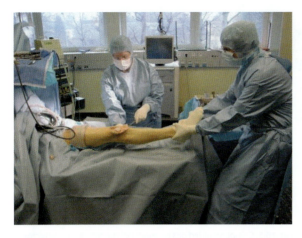

Fig. 16.1. First step of the ligament balance optimization: the traction test

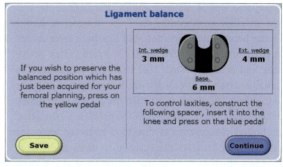

Fig. 16.2. Graphic User Interface of the LCS® software. Measurement provided to the surgeon to build the adjustable spacer block

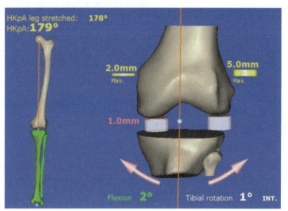

Fig. 16.3. Graphic User Interface of the LCS® software. Real time quantitative data on the residual gap during the varus-valgus stress test (*in red*). Maximum of laxity achieved during the test (*yellow*). On the left side of the screen, the value of HKpA angle is displayed to reach the best compromise between balance and alignment

be used to assemble the spacer (◘ Fig. 16.2). Based on these data, the surgeon builds immediately the appropriate spacer and inserts it into the joint.

The residual laxities (internal and external) are then assed during a varus/valgus stress test. At this step the SFI provides real-time information on the medial and lateral gaps, and records the maximum amount of laxity achieved during the test (◘ Fig. 16.3).

Maximum laxities are then compared to a threshold defined by the designers of the implants. If the amount of residual laxity is above this threshold, the software advises the surgeon to modify the spacer and indicates which component to add (◘ Fig. 16.4) on each side of the spacer in order to reach the threshold between alignment and balance. If the compromise between balance and axes can not be obtained a concomitant release of the soft tissue can be performed. In specific cases a condylar osteotomy may be added, though, this situation and specific problem is beyond the scope of this paper.

When the appropriate compromise is achieved the user graphic interface provides the amount of accepted laxity to the surgeon and stores the relative position of the tibia and femur.

This optimization cycle will soon be improved by the integration of a miniature intelligent tool that has been invented to help surgeons perform the technically demanding task of soft tissue balancing and implant planning. [17]. Although technically advanced in design and implementation, this system will provide a global, automatic and simple solution for surgeons, allowing them

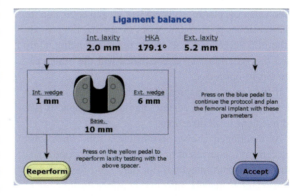

Fig. 16.4. Results of the varus-valgus stress test. Automatic proposition for the construction of new spacer block

to easily and almost instantaneously characterize the soft tissue envelope surrounding the knee in order to better plan the best implant position and ligament releases for that particular patient. The device is based on an active spacer and sensing system that has been engineered to be small enough to fit entirely inside the knee joint (after making the tibial plateau cut) with the patella completely reduced (◘ Fig. 16.5). This avoids the problems associated with biased measurements due to a reflected extensor mechanism, and allows the surgeon to asses and incorporate into the plan the femoro-patellar joint at the same time as the femoro-tibial joint.

The device is hydraulic, using fluid-filled pouches to elevate each plateau from a base height of ~6 mm, ensuring compatibility with virtually any TKA implant size (◘ Fig. 16.6). A controller embedded into the Praxim navigation platform precisely regulates the volume and flow rate through each pouch, and provides independent force read-outs to the surgeon. This device can be used in many different control modes according to a selected strategy to reach a trade-off between balancing and geometric alignment, all of them running on PRAXIM-Medivision platforms and applications.

The global concept presented here, is in its final development phase and, may be integrated on any platform, with any implants. It may therefore impact the field far beyond the unique issue of the LCS prosthesis address in this paper.

Step 3 – Optimization of the Femoral Cuts

Based on the soft-tissue constraints measured in step 2, the femoral planning can then be achieved. A second optimization loop is used, and a set of femoral cuts is proposed when the planning gives a flexion gap equivalent to the extension gap. Therefore, one can say that the priority of the LCS Surgetics CASP is soft tissue balancing. Only when this criterion has been satisfied will the others parameters be optimized.

If the surgeon disagrees with the proposition, he or she may use the touch screen to adjust the implants size and positions in all directions.

As mentioned above, performing a total knee joint replacement is equivalent to solving a complex optimization problem that integrates not only tibio-femoral data but also femoro-patellar information, since the location of the femoral implant has direct impact on the kinematics of both the patellar and tibial joint compartments.

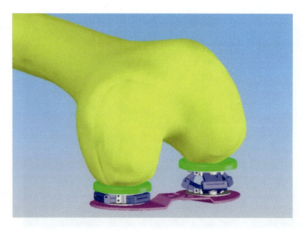

◘ **Fig. 16.5.** Computer aided design model of the robotized distractor

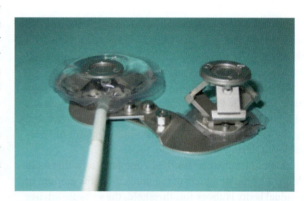

◘ **Fig. 16.6.** Hydraulic prototype shown with fluid-filled pouch and parallel plateau mechanism

Tracking of the Patella

To take the patella into account in the optimization loop we developed as an option a patella tracker which can be attached to the anterior surface of the patella (◘ Fig. 16.7). The kinematics of the patella, its shape, and a few anatomical landmarks are registered at the beginning of the procedure before the medial arthrotomy.

The femoral planning can then be adjusted using this data since the system displays in real time the distances between the posterior surface of the patella and the virtual femoral implant as the knee is flexed, indicating the predicted intensity of the contact between the patella and the femoral components. Thus, before making any femoral cuts, adjustments in the femoral implant position can be made to optimize patellar tracking.

16

In a preliminary study, we have been able to demonstrate that, as they are performed today, total knee replacements introduce an important perturbation in the kinematics of the patella [21]. To describe this phenomenon we report two cases out of fifteen during which we measured the kinematics of the patella pre and post operatively (◘ Figs. 16.8, 16.9). These post-operatively compiled curves represent the difference in the rotation of the patella with respect to the femur before and after replacement of the femur. They are presented as a function of the flexion angle, in the three fixed directions of the femoral reference frame: Y axis – posterior condylar axis (i.e. medio-lateral); Z axis – normal to the plane defined by the Y axis and the femoral center (i.e. proximal-distal); X axis – normal to Y and Z (i.e. antero-posterior). Note that the patella was not resurfaced in these patients and the changes observed are therefore only a result of the femoro-tibial replacement. If the TKR had no consequences on the patello-femoral joint kinematics the three lines would be centered about the zero axes. Although the magnitude of the changes in rotation were typically <10°, both of these two figures show important differences in the patellar kinematics for the three directions.

Introduced in computer-assisted surgery by Praxim in 2002, the femoro-patellar compartment remains an important issue for knee surgeons. The quality of the results and the well being of our patients implies that the integration of the femoro-patellar joint in the planning optimization loop is warranted.

A New Way to Design Workflows

To speed up the adoption of navigation, developers should take into account that any surgical procedure can be achieved trough several workflows. Even in conventional surgery, surgeons have their own habits, tricks, and ways to succeed.

Depending on the implants or the technique, some surgeons will perform a tibial cut first, others will perform the femoral cut first. Some will prioritize alignment instead of ligament balance and vice-versa. For some surgeons, the patella tracking is not an issue as long as the rotation of the femoral component is well managed.

In the past, two types of workflows have been introduced on the market, linear workflow or net-like workflow in which you can come back to any step at any time of the procedure.

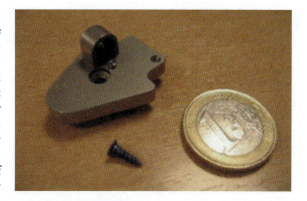

◘ **Fig. 16.7.** Mini-fixation for the patella tracker

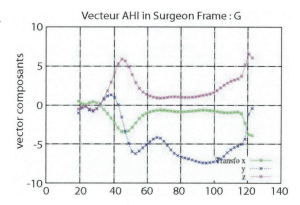

◘ **Fig. 16.8.** Differences between pre and post-operative kinematics of the patella. Amount of rotation around the 3 axis of the surgical reference system a flexion extension motion

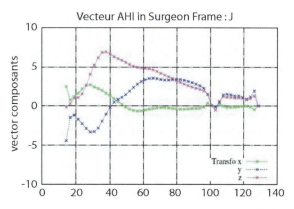

◘ **Fig. 16.9.** Differences between pre and post-operative kinematics of the patella. Amount of rotation around the 3 axis of the surgical reference system a flexion extension motion

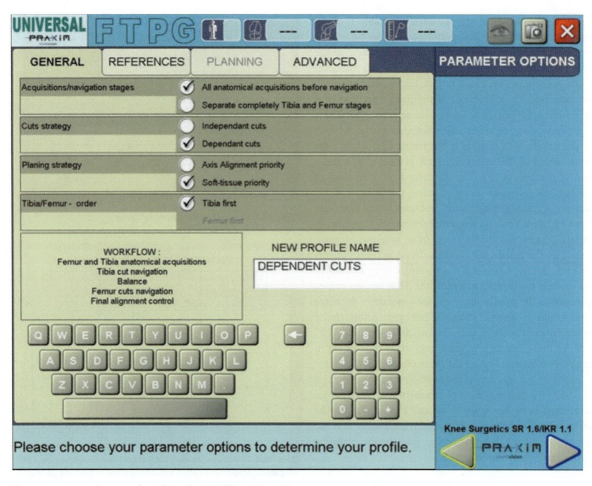

Fig. 16.10. Graphic user interface of KneeSurgetics SR 1.6: the next step in automatic workflow generation

16

For the LCS knee in the Depuy application we used a linear workflow since we believe in its simplicity and efficiency in the OR.

To fulfill the diverse needs of surgeons, the next generation of workflows will be more surgeon oriented. Therefore, Praxim have introduced new applications in which the workflow is designed by the surgeon and stored under his own user profile name. He or she can therefore select any desired option at the beginning of the surgery, and store this configuration in the system so that it is available for the next case. ■ Figure 16.10 shows the graphic user interface of KneeSurgetics SR 1.6. The upper part of the screen displays a list of options that can be selected. The final workflow is summarized below and

the profile can be saved under a new profile name, in this case »DEPENDENT CUTS«.

The remainder of this chapter describes two additional advanced technologies for computer assisted knee arthroplasty that have been specially developed to address the particular needs of MIS surgeons.

Universal and Open Intelligent Instrumentation

Named after the famous Greek sculptor, Praxiteles® is a miniature universal tool for precise milling of the five femoral cuts in TKA, for any implant size or shape. The advantages of this Praxim system is not only improved precision, but also a significant reduction in the number of instruments and trays occupying the valuable space around the OR table. The cost of cleaning, sterilization, and storage is also reduced for the hospital, not to mention the high cost of the numerous instruments themselves.

The Praxiteles system embodies the following features:
- compact, bone-mounted,
- hybrid passive/active architecture,
- automatic guide positioning for each cut,
- manual cutting by surgeon,
- milling or sawing,
- MIS compatible,
- easy-to-use.

A miniature bone-mounted system has been selected instead of a table or floor mounted one to increase the space available to the surgeon in the operating room. In order to minimize the size and weight of the device, a hybrid passive/active architecture is employed, with a miniature manual alignment mechanism for precision adjustment of varus/valgus and internal/external rotation, coupled with two parallel motorized axes in the sagittal plane (◘ Fig. 16.11). This unique architecture (patent pending) permits automatic control of the following variables:
- global flexion-extension implant alignment,
- global anterior-posterior implant positioning,
- global proximal-distal implant positioning,
- any implant size,
- any implant design.

A robot controller is connected to the Praxim Navigation platform. Guide positioning is automated for all of the five cuts to increase speed during surgery – once the device is aligned the guide can be positioned from one cut to the next in just a few seconds. Cutting is carried out manually by the surgeon using a milling or sawing tool, milling being performed with a passive guide that allows the tool to rotate and slide in the cutting plane. An optimized milling technique has been developed to minimize the cutting-force response and to maximize stability and safety, and an integrated irrigation supply that directs water directly at the cutting zone ensures cutting temperatures remain below the necrosis limit.

Incision of the quadriceps and reflection of the patella is not required with this system, and there is no need to immobilize the leg to the operating table since the robot is mounted directly on the medial side of the bone. This allows the MIS surgeon to place the leg in various degrees

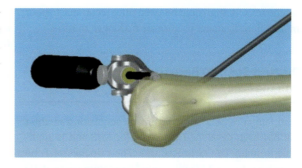

◘ **Fig. 16.11.** Computer aided design model of the Praxiteles milling robot, shown milling the anterior femoral plane

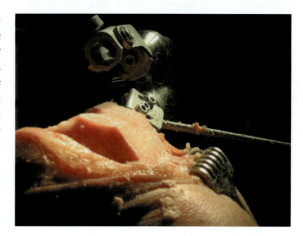

◘ **Fig. 16.12.** Cadaver experiment in open surgery showing femoral cuts milled with the robot

of flexion to access each of five cuts through the »mobile window«. A side-milling approach also facilitates access through the small opening. Because MIS does not only mean to reduce the trauma to the soft tissues, but also to the bone itself, however, we incorporated an attachment for the femoral reference frame directly on the base of the robot. Thus both navigation and execution is performed with only two bone pins placed within the MIS incision.

The precision and usability of the device has been evaluated with a group of expert surgeons in both conventional (◘ Fig. 16.12) and MIS approaches [3, 19, 22]. These tests have shown that sub-degree precision is possible in both open and MIS surgery with negligible increase in operating time to conventional navigation. With perfect implant planning based on bone-morphing and soft-tissue balancing, and fast automatic guide positioning and optimized cutting techniques, OR time could be saved since recuts due to poor implant fit or ligament balance are no longer an issue.

The Next Step: 3D Reconstruction with the *Echo Surgetics* System

Echo Surgetics® is a powerful image acquisition method that has been developed especially for MIS and is applicable to many CAOS procedures. The principle of Echo Surgetics is to use 2.5D ultrasound to acquire relevant 3D bone surface and point data transcutaneously, in order to perform minimally invasive computer assisted surgical protocols on the Surgetics Station. The concept has been implemented in 3 technologies: Echo Point® which enables the surgeon to collect well-identified anatomical landmarks transcutaneously, Echo Matching® which performs automated registration of pre-operative CT images with the patient coordinate system without any additional incisions, and Echo Morphing® which combines 2.5D ultrasound image acquisition with statistical deformable models to build a complete 3D bone surface [15].

An ultimate goal in CAOS is to have an acquisition means that has the following capabilities:

-   no pre-operative imaging,
-   no radiation,
-   3D reconstruction,
-   unlimited volume,
-   compatible with MIS,
-   quick and easy-to-use.

In this section we will focus on the Echo Morphing imaging solution which has the potential to meet all these requirements.

Description of Basic Technology

Echo Surgetics uses an ultrasound system embedded into the PRAXIM navigation platform in which the probe is localized with a rigid body. This principle of 2.5D ultrasound acquisition was introduced in CAOS for the first time in 1993 by the Grenoble research group to register pre-operative CT vertebral images to the patient coordinate system in computer assisted spine surgery [2]. This method was also employed by the Pittsburgh CAOS group for hip surgery [1]. The basic idea is that the ultrasound probe acts like a transcutaneous digitizing probe, by using »specular reflection« on bone surfaces (the echo time in a given area is proportional to the distance between the transducer and the bone surface). An important requirement is to have the ultrasound system embedded into the navigation system in order to access the image parameters (depth, focus, etc.) and to prevent any change of those parameters between the time of calibration and acquisition. The Echo Surgetics system is fully automated and has no visible parameters to adjust; it is intended for the orthopaedic surgeon and not for the radiologist.

The Echo Morphing application, the most advanced of the three Echo Surgetics technologies, is detailed in ◘ Fig. 16.13. ◘ Figure 16.13a depicts the ultrasound system embedded in the Surgetics Station, and ◘ Fig. 16.13b shows the principle of acquisition. The surgeon simply scans over the bone with the ultrasound probe and when a reasonably clear interface between the bone and soft tissues is seen on the screen, the surgeon presses the footswitch pedal to save the image. The computer then automatically detects and segments the bone surface interface, if any, on the saved ultrasound images. This process is repeated for a minimum of 6 images before the bone morphing method is applied on the interface points. If necessary, the surgeon can acquire additional images in a continuous »scanning« mode and the operation is repeated. The screen always shows a 3D view of the ultrasound image plane in comparison with the current reconstruction of the bone for any position of the probe (◘ Fig. 16.13c). In addition, the intersection of the ultrasound plane with the 3D model is computed and overlayed on the ultrasound image (◘ Fig. 16.13d). This feature provides immediate feedback on the robustness and accuracy check of the system for each patient

Echo Morphing accuracy is in the range of 1.5 mm. Echo Morphing has been successfully tested on cadavers and volunteers and has been shown to be a very flexible and powerful means to acquire 3D data very easily and quickly. Accuracy on patients is dependent on 2 factors:

1) the number of ultrasound image acquisitions selected by the surgeon. There is no limit in the iterative process we propose;
2) the distance between the transducer on the skin and the bone surface. Because of variations of the speed of sound, an error of 3% is possible [9, 12]. Therefore, if the distance is 50 mm it can lead to an error of 1.5 mm. However, since the ultrasound probe is typically pressed up against the soft tissue to obtain a good quality image, distances between the transducer and the bone surface are usually small even for obese patients.

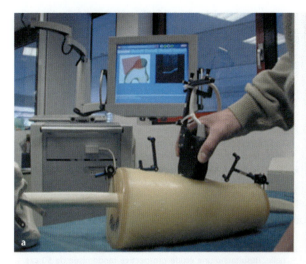

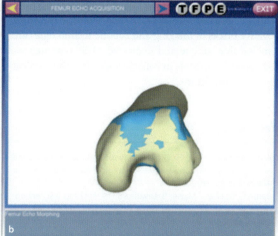

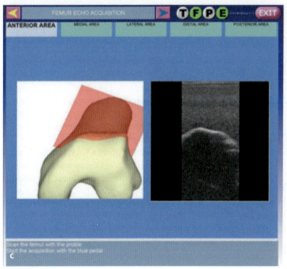

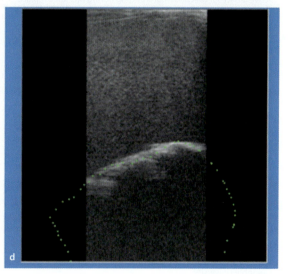

Fig. 16.13a–d. Echo Morphing setup on a femoral phantom. **a** Ultrasound system embedded in the Surgetics Station. **b** Image of acquisition of a plane. **c** Reconstruction of echo morphing: the blue area indicates where the data was acquired. **d** Testing accuracy after reconstruction: the intersection of the ultrasound plane with the reconstructed model is computed and displayed on the 2D ultrasound image

Conclusion

Up to now Computer Assisted Orthopaedic Surgery (CAOS) methods have not been entirely successful in meeting the challenges of Minimally Invasive Surgery (MIS). The PRAXIM family of innovative miniature robotic tools and sensors for precision actuation and data collection has been specially developed to address the needs of MIS surgeons. Following several years of scientific research, engineering, clinical research and validation, we present a line of breakthrough technologies for MIS EchoMorphing, soft tissue balancing and implant planning, and precision bone-milling in TKA, all of them running on PRAXIM navigation platforms (Surgetics Station™ or Praxim NanoStation™).

These technologies are part of the general concept of Minimally Invasive Surgetics. In this concept the most innovative bricks of imaging and robotic technologies are assembled into unique and dedicated MIS computer-assisted surgical protocols in collaboration with the surgical architects of the future.

References

1. Amin DV, Kanade T, DiGioia AM 3rd, Jaramaz B (2003) Ultrasound registration of the bone surface for surgical navigation Comput Aided Surg 8: 1–16
2. Barbe C, Troccaz J, Mazier B, Lavallee S (1993) Using 2.5D echography in computer assisted spine surgery, Proc. IEEE EMBS, San Diego, pp 160–161
3. Bauer A, Plaskos C (2006) Cadaver study: a bone mounted semi-active device for precise femoral cutting during MIS knee replacement. Accepted to the International Conference on Computer Assisted Orthopaedic Surgery
4. Bonnel F (1988) Organisation architecturale et biomécanique de l'articulation fémoro-tibiale. In: Bonnel F (ed) La gonarthrose. Masson, Paris, pp 1–11
5. Briard JL, Stindel E, Plaweski S et al. (2003) CT Free Navigation with the LCS Surgetics Station: A new way of balancing the soft tissues in TKA based on bone morphing. In: Stiehl JB, Konermann W, Haaker R (eds) Navigation and robotics in total joint and spine surgery. Springer, Berlin Heidelberg New York Tokyo, pp 274–280
6. Cazalis P (1994) Diagnostic et traitement d'un genou douloureux. Editions techniques. Encycl Méd Chir 14–325-A-10: 1–16
7. Fleute M, Lavallée S, Julliard R (1999) Incorporating a statistically based shape model into a system for computer assisted anterior cruciate ligament surgery. Med Image Analysis 3: 209–222
8. Grutzner PA, Hebecker A, Waelti H, Vock B, Nolte LP, Wentzensen A (2003) Clinical Study for Registration-Free 3D-Navigation with the SIREMOBIL Iso-C3D Mobile C-Arm. Electromedica 71: S1
9. Ionescu G (1999) Segmentation and registration of ultrasound images by using physiological and morphological knowledge. Grenoble University
10. Jefferry RS, Morris RW, Denham RA (1991) Coronal alignment after total knee replacement. J Bone Joint Surg 73-B: 709–714
11. Jenny JY, Boeri C (2001) Computer-assisted implantation of total knee prostheses: a case-control comparative study with classical instrumentation. Comput Aided Surg 6(4): 217–220
12. Kowal J, Amstutz CA, Nolte LP (2001) On B-mode ultrasound-based registration for computer assisted orthopaedic surgery. Comput Aided Surg 6: 47
13. Kunz M, Strauss M, Langlotz F, Deuretzbacher G, Rüther W, Nolte LP (2001) A non-CT based total knee arthroplasty system featuring complete soft-tissue balancing. MICCAI LNCS 2208, pp 409–415
14. Lavallée S, Bainville E, Bricault I (2000) An overview of computer-integrated surgery and therapy. In: Udupa (ed) 3D Imaging in Medicine. CRC Press, Boca Raton, pp 207–263
15. Lavallee S, Merloz P, Stindel E, Kilian P, Troccaz J, Cinquin P, Langlotz F, Nolte LP (2004) Echomorphing: Introducing an intra-operative imaging modality to reconstruct 3D bone surfaces for minimally invasive surgery. International Conference on Computer Assisted Orthopaedic Surgery
16. Mansat CH (1988) Indications chirurgicales de la gonarthrose. In: Bonnel F (ed) La gonarthrose. Masson, Paris, pp 56–61
17. Marmignon C, Lemniei A, Cinquin P (2004) A computer-assisted controlled device to guide ligament balancing in TKA. International Conference on Computer Assisted Orthopaedic Surgery, pp 65–66
18. Mielke RK, Clemens U, Jens JH, Kershally S (2001) Navigation in knee endoprosthesis implementation – preliminary experiences and prospective comparative study with conventional implementation technique. Z Orthop Ihre Grenzgeb 139(2): 109–116
19. Rit J, Plaskos C (2006) Développement d'une plate-forme micro-robotisée pour la pose naviguée d'endoprothèses de genou: Projet PRAXITELES. Symposium for Minimally Invasive Procedures, Monaco
20. Saragaglia D, Picard F, Chaussard C, Montbaron E, Leitner F, Cinquin P (2001) Mise en place des prothèses totales de genou assistée par ordinateur: comparaison avec la technique conventionnelle. Résultats d'une étude prospective randomisée de 50 cas. Revue de Chirurgie Orthopédique 87: 18–28
21. Stindel E, Guillard G, Briard JL, Perrin N., Savean J, Roux C (2005) Consequences of the femoro-tibial replacement on the femoro-patellar kinematics:an intra-operative in-vivo study. In: Langoltz F, Davies BL, Schlenzka D (eds) Proceedings of the CAOS symposium, International Society for Computed Assisted Orthopedic Surgery. Helsinki, pp 437–439
22. Stindel E, Plaskos C, Cinquin P, Lavallée S, Hodgson AJ (2005) A robotic milling-guide positioner for improved resection accuracy in minimal access total knee arthroplasty. 1ères Journées De Navigation. Hanche – Genou. Lyon, France
23. Stindel E, Gil D, Briard JL, Merloz P, Dubrana F, Lefevre C (2002) Detection of the center of the hip in ct less based system for TKA navigational guidance. An evaluation study of the accuracy and reproducibility of the Surgetic's algorithm. CAOS Symposium, International Society for Computed Assisted Orthopedic Surgery. Santa Fe
24. Stindel E, Gil D, Briard JL, Plaweski S, Dubrana F, Lefevre C (2002) The center of the ankle in CT less based navigation system. What is really important to detect? CAOS Symposium, International Society for Computed Assisted Orthopedic Surgery. Santa Fe
25. Stindel E, Briard JL, Merloz P, Plaweski S, Dubrana F, Lefevre C, Troccaz JL (2002) Bone morphing: 3D morphological data for total knee arthroplasty. Comp Aided Surg 7(3): 156–168
26. Szelisky R, Lavallée S (1996) Matching 3-D anatomical surfaces with non-rigid deformations using octree-splines. Int J Comp Vision 18(2): 171–186
27. Tetter KE, Bergman D, Colwell CW (1995) Accuracy of intramedullary versus extramedullary tibial aligment cutting systems in total knee arthroplasty. Clin Orthop Rel Res 321: 106–110

Modern Navigated Ligament Balancing in Total Knee Arthroplasty with the PiGalileo System

P. Ritschl, F. Machacek, R. Fuiko

Introduction

Ligament balancing of the knee is one of the cornerstones for the function and longevity of a knee endoprosthesis. »Size and shape of the flexion gap should be equal to the extension gap« as Insall [1] put it. In Insall's concept the gaps should be rectangular for the same ligament tension at the medial and lateral side. The decisive point of the gap technique is that it is oriented towards the status and condition of the soft tissue. During the process the posterior cruciate ligament is resected [2]. Reconstruction of the joint line is not taken into account. No data regarding the measure of the ligament tension are provided. The gap technique then met some competition from the »Measured Resection Technique« [3]. The principle of this implantation philosophy consists in the measurement of the resection being replaced by the corresponding implant thickness, both at the femur and the tibia. Unlike the gap technique, the posterior cruciate ligament is preserved in this process. The joint line can consequently largely be preserved and reconstructed. For knee joints that are not significantly deformed, it is thus possible to restore the original conditions of the ligaments. Ligament tension in the joint compartments themselves results from the selected thickness of the implant, and is thus determined by subjective assessment of the surgeon.

The LCS Total Knee Arthroplasty according to Buechel and Pappas [4] simultaneously integrates the rotation of the femur component when determining flexion gap and ligament tension. During this, following the tibial incision, the rotation of the femoral resection level and the width of the flexion gap for evenly stretched ligaments in flexion are initially simultaneously determined through a spacer block. The thus obtained height of the flexion gap is subsequently transferred to the extension gap. In this implantation technique as well, the extent of the ligament tension is determined by subjective assessment of the surgeon. Little significance is attached to the reconstruction of the joint line.

What all these methods have in common is the fact that ligament tension in flexion and extension is defined through individual subjective assessment of the surgeon. No special attention is given to any external influences, such as that of an everted patella, especially in flexion, or the use of a thigh tourniquet. Such subjective assessment of ligament tension is frequently the source of complications. Major revision statistics indicate instability as the reason for a revision in 1/5 – 1/3 of revision operations [5, 6]. As revision operations are usually only performed where clinically particularly abnormal instabilities are present, it must be assumed that the estimated number of unknown cases of sub-clinical instable knees is high.

Using surgical navigation systems, it is possible to quantify and thus objectify factors that have conventionally been determined through subjective assessment, such as ligament tension and joint stability. Software modules to support both implantation techniques are usually available. »Bone referencing« modules are oriented towards the »Measured Resection Technique« and are used for »straight forward« knees, i.e. for knees without any major bone or ligament deformities. In addition to landmark-oriented navigation, »ligament-based« modules, in particular those of the PiGalileo Systems (Plus Orthopedics Aarau, Switzerland), also offer the possibility of force-controlled recording of ligament tension using a ligament balancer, and integrating it in the operative implantation management. Those integrative operation steps comprise for the flexion gap:

— determination of ligament tension,
— determination of femur rotation, and
— implant planning with joint line optimising.

The thus determined flexion gap is then transferred to the extension gap.

In the following, the individual operation steps will be presented and described, and first clinical results will be reported on. Finally, future aspects involving individual ligament tension measurement will be discussed.

Method

The PI-Galileo system is an optical landmark-based navigation system. The navigation camera (Axios 3D, Oldenburg, Germany) has a precision of 0.2 mm and offers the possibility to accurately record forces and distances through differentiation measurements. A computer-controlled, motor-operated two-axis positioning unit of the (»five in one«) femoral incision gauge is an integral part of the navigation system (◘ Fig. 17.1a). Ligament tension and gap size are measured using a ligament balancer with force and distance scale (◘ Fig. 17.1b).

In the following, only the operation steps that are relevant to ligament tension will be described.

Step 1: Visualization of Preoperative Deformity and Stability

Following digitalizing of the femoral and tibial landmarks and calculation of the three-dimensional position of the short and long axes, the existing mal-position and ligament stability/instability are visualized.

During pre-operative measurement, 2 parameters are evaluated on the display:

Deformity in Extension, Flexion and Over the Full Range of Motion

It is clearly visible that the deformity in this case (◘ Fig. 17.2) is present mainly in extension, but not in flexion. The minor valgus deviation in flexion was attributable to a cartilage defect of the lateral-dorsal condyle.

Extent of Instability

Point cloud distribution covers 7° (2°–9°) in extension. In flexion the knee is considerably more stable. The point cloud shows significantly lower deflection.

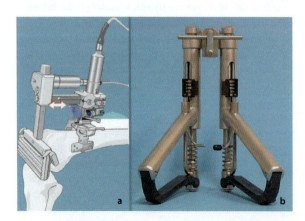

a   b

◘ **Fig. 17.1. a** The computer-controlled motor unit drives a five-in-one cutting block into the pre-calculated position for the femoral cuts. **b** The »double spring« ligament balancer comprises a scale for measuring the force in Newton

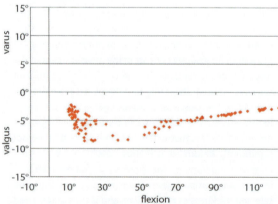

◘ **Fig. 17.2.** Pre-operative leg-axis measurement reveals an obstructed extension of 10° and an average valgus deformity of 6°. Instability ranges from 2° to 9° in maximum extension. In flexion, taut ligament control is present. Bone deformity is responsible for a valgus deformity of 2° and 3°

17

The extent of the instability is due to ligament laxity as well as the cartilage/bone defect.

Following visualization of the deformity, it must be concluded that a soft tissue release is only required in extension, but **not** in flexion.

Step 2: Ligament Balancing in Extension

Following osteotomy of the tibial plateau and removal of the osteophytes, ligament tension is initially determined in extension. For this a strictly repeating algorithm is used:

1. Positioning of the ligament balancer *without* clamping it
2. Alignment of the extremity along the visualized mechanical axis
3. Tensioning of the ligament balancer at 100 Newton in extension and determination of any possible malposition of the axis.
4. If any mal-position is present, execution of a sequential release in extension.

The result of this step is a knee, which is axis-corrected in extension and balanced with 100 Newton both medially and laterally (◘ Fig. 17.3).

Step 3: Ligament Balancing in Flexion and Determination of the Rotation of the Femur Component

Ligament tension in flexion is determined using the same algorithm as describe above. The patella is not everted, but rather held in a laterally subluxed position. Once the ligament balancer has been positioned without clamping and the leg position and femoral rotation in flexion have been checked on the screen, the balancer is clamped at 70–80 Newton, both medially and laterally (◘ Fig. 17.4).

On the display, the flexion gap appears as a rectangular or trapezoidal bar. The target position is a rectangular flexion gap for correct femoral rotation. Rotation of the femur relative to the 3 rotation landmarks (a.p.-line, epicondyle line, dorsal condyle line) is displayed on the screen in real time. Minor adjustment to obtain a rectangular gap can be carried out by changing the rotation at the PI-Galileo motor unit, while observing the rotation landmarks.

The rectangular shape of the bar (and thus of the flexion gap) might also be impaired because of a strong lateral constraint of the extensor apparatus, in particular when the patella is everted. In such a case the preoperatively determined ligament condition (◘ Fig. 17.2) will be helpful to decide whether a soft tissue release is necessary. Before carrying out the dorsal femoral cut, size and position of the femoral prosthesis component must be planned and polyethylene thickness must be determined.

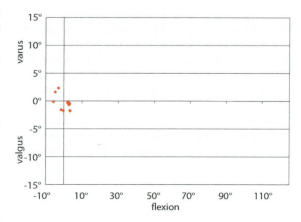

◘ **Fig. 17.3.** Following ligament balancing in extension, symmetric stability with correct axis orientation is obtained in spite of any femoral bone defects

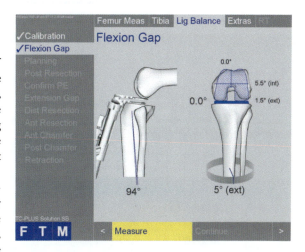

◘ **Fig. 17.4.** Following alignment of the extremity in rotation and flexion, the ligament balancer is positioned and clamped at 70 to 80 Newton on the medial and lateral side. Rotation of the dorsal femoral cut is determined in consideration of the bony landmarks. The blue bar symbolizes the flexion gap which is rectangular in this case

Step 4: Selection of the Prosthesis Components to Optimize Joint Line and Ligament Stability

Based on the data provided, the computer calculates the femoral prosthesis size and the respective polyethylene height. The objectives are the reconstruction of the joint line and the correct resection height of the dorsal condyles. This results in a balanced flexion gap so that the entire implant can be positioned with the desired flexion stability. Since the number of prostheses sizes is limited a fine tuning by the surgeon might be necessary. Such adjustments can be made by changing the prosthesis size, the polyethylene thickness or by an a.p.-shift of the femur component in steps of 0.5 mm. It is thus possible to achieve an ideal prosthesis position with controlled stability, optimized joint line and the best fitting component sizes (◘ Fig. 17.5).

Once all of these parameters have been determined, the motor unit will drive the cutting block to the pre-calculated position, and the surgeon will cut the dorsal condyles.

Step 5: Transfer of the Flexion Gap to the Extension Gap

Following the dorsal femoral cut and removal of dorsal osteophytes, the polyethylene height under the determined ligament tension is checked once again. Removing larger dorsal osteophytes occasionally causes widening of the flexion gap, which can be compensated for by increasing the polyethylene height. Once the definitive polyethylene height has been confirmed, the size and configuration of the flexion gap is determined.

The height of the flexion gap is then transferred to the extension gap. After the ligament balancer has been positioned, the extremity is aligned according to the mechanical axis (screen controlled), the ligament balancer is clamped at 100 Newton and the orientation of the axis is checked for a second time. This second evaluation of the stable axis in extension serves as a control measure following any release in flexion that might have occurred.

The rectangular configuration and width of the extension gap appears on the screen. After confirmation, the motor unit drives the cutting block into the pre-calculated position for the distal cut, which is performed now. The height of the distal femoral resection is shown on the screen, and it is possible to shift the distal cut in half-millimeter steps in proximal or distal direction whenever individual adjustment is desired.

Thereafter, the motor unit drives to all the remaining femoral resection positions (anterior and chamfer cuts) and the resections are carried out. Following positioning of the trial implants, the reconstructed joint line is checked once again and the result with regard to ligament tension is visualized (◘ Fig. 17.6).

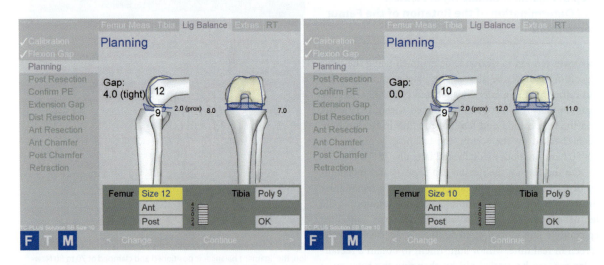

◘ Fig. 17.5. The planning step initially shows a flexion gap that is too narrow by 4 mm for a femur size of 12. Femur size is reduced to 10 after which the flexion gap has the ideal size for the implants used. Changing the femur component does not change the joint line, however, the resection of the dorsal condyles increases

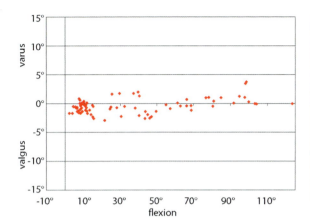

Fig. 17.6. Checking of the operation result with the achieved stability and axis orientation: For varus and valgus stress, the resulting ease of opening is 2.5° over the entire ROM. The axis is correct and the leg is almost fully extended

Table 17.1. The postoperative outcome showed a better function and knee score in the group with ligament balancing technique

	Knee Society Score	Function Score
Preoperative		
A	40	57
B	48	55
16 months follow up		
A	89.3	89.4
B	87.7	83.6

Clinical Results

In a group comparison, the effect of the ligament tension measurement was evaluated. The same implant (TC Plus-SB, Plus Orthopedics, Rotkreuz) and the same implantation technique with the PI Galileo system were used for both groups. All patients were operated by one surgeon.

- Group A with ligament tension technique comprised 61 patients (average age 71.1)
- Group B without ligament tension technique consisted of 60 patients (average age 74.4).

Evaluation was done using the American Knee Society Score. The time of post-operative observation was 15.7 months for Group A, and 17.2 months for Group B.

Both with regard to the function score and the knee score, the group comparison showed better results in Group A with ligament tension measurement.

For almost the same pre-operative initial value, in Group A (ligament tension measurement) the average function score is higher by 5.8 points and the knee score by 1.6 points (Table 17.1).

Discussion

The PI-Galileo system is the first method to implement the principle of quantitatively force-controlled ligament balancing. Existing concepts use spacer blocks or ligament balancers for ligament balancing, on which, however, the applied force cannot be determined as they do not include a scale. Knee stability is therefore subjectively assessed by the surgeon. This can constantly result in sub-clinical, and sometimes also clinically manifested instabilities [5–7]. The forces that are specified for a sufficient ligament stability range from 140 to 160 Newton in flexion (70–80 Newton both medially and laterally) and about 200 Newton in extension (100 Newton both medially and laterally) [8].

Ligament balancing begins in extension. Initially, the pre-operative ligament deformity is determined and visualized on the screen. During this the extent of laxity of the knee joint as well as cartilage and bone defects become visible over the full range of motion. Once the tibial resection has been performed, ligament tension measurement is carried out according to a specially defined algorithm. (step 2). This algorithm is important in order to exclude or to minimize any interfering lever effects on ligament tension measurement.

If the pre-operative ligament tension measurement does not reveal any deformity for 90° flexion, it is not necessary to carry out a release in flexion. However, if a ligament deformity is present also for 90° flexion, a ligament release must be carried out during ligament tension measurement. The subluxed patella is another factor, that has an effect on ligament tension and its influence can currently only be estimated.

The concept of this »load depending gap balancing« has been integrated into the principle of »Measured Resection Technique«. With the help of navigation femoral and tibial resection heights are accurately determined. The achievable joint line, axis orientation, and resection heights for the defined ligament tension can be seen on the display. By adjusting planning steps it is possible to plan an optimal composition of the prosthesis in terms of size, polyethylene height, ap prosthesis position and joint line, as well as tension of ligaments, and to implement these factors during the individual operation steps.

However, the influence of some factors such as the contribution of the laterally subluxed patella on ligament tension in flexion is still uncertain. Furthermore, there are uncertainties with regard to the correct ligament tension in flexion and extension for the individual patient. Individual factors such as gender, size, age, level of activity, individual ligament characteristics in terms of stiffness of the ligaments, etc. have not quantitatively been described to date. Computerized analysis of the individual ligament tension should therefore be aimed at. During such a process the individual stability point of the individual patient knee has to be determined through corresponding calculation steps.

References

1. Insall JN (1988) Presidential address to The Knee Society. Choices and compromises in total knee arthroplasty. Clin Orthop Rel Res 226: 43–48
2. Insall JN, Easley ME (2001) Surgical techniques and instrumentation in total knee arthroplasty. In: Insall JN, Scott WN (eds) Insall & Scott Surgery of the Knee, 3rd edn. Churchill Livingstone, New York, pp 1553–1620
3. Hungerford DS, Krackow KA (1985) Total joint arthroplasty of the knee. Clin Orthop Rel Res 192: 23–33
4. Büchel FF (2002) Surgical technique of the LCS. In: Hamelyneck KJ, Stiel JB (eds) LCS mobile bearing knee arthroplasty. Springer, Berlin Heidelberg New York Tokyo, pp 121-135
5. Fehring TK, Odum S, Griffin WL, Mason JB, Nadaud M (2001) Early failures in total knee arthroplasty. Clin Orthop Rel Res 392: 315–318
6. Sharkey PF, Hozack WJ, Rothman RH, Shastri S, Jacoby SM (2002) Insall Award paper. Why are total knee arthroplasties failing today? Clin Orthop Rel Res 404: 7–13
7. Wasielewski RC, Galat DD, Komistek RD (2004) An intraoperative pressure-measuring device used in total knee arthroplasties and its kinematics correlations. Clin Orthop Rel Res 427: 171–178
8. Himstedt S, Friedrich N, Freudiger S, Moser W (2003) In-vivo-Messungen der elastischen Eigenschaften des Kapsel-Band-Apparates bei Knieprothesenpatienten: Verfahren, Bedeutung für die Praxis und erste Ergebnisse. 7. Kongress der Union Schweizerisch Chirurgischer Fachgesellschaften, Lausanne

17

Navigated Total Knee Arthroplasty with the Navitrack® System

T. Mattes, R. Decking, H. Reichel

Introduction

Correct mechanical leg axis, coronal and rotational alignment, as well as balanced soft tissues are important factors in TKA [3, 5, 9, 12]. Deficiency in conventional instruments and limited measurability in manual surgery techniques are known and induced development of navigation systems in different orthopedic procedures [1, 6].

AT present most experiences are available in TKA navigation. Different studies could show reliable and reproducible results for mechanical leg axis in TKA using navigation [2, 4, 7, 8].

In TKA meanwhile imageless, kinematic systems are standard. CT-based systems may be helpful for special scientific questions.

We use the Navitrack® TotalKnee™ (Orthosoft Inc., Montreal, Canada) with the imageless application since January 2002 for Implantation of the Natural Knee II® System (Zimmer, Warsaw, IN, US) and the Innex™ knee system (Zimmer, Warsaw, IN, US) with specialized software applications for each implant. In December 2005 we tested generic software with new instruments as a further stage in knee navigation.

System Components and Surgery Technique

The navigation System is working with a standard PC and a passive optoelectronic tracking system (Polaris, Fa. Northern Digital Inc., Waterloo/Canada). Bone references and instruments are marked with reflecting spheres. The computer realization of surgical tools and anatomic objects follows the principle of dynamic referencing (tracking). To operate the system from the sterile area, a footswitch and a draped remote control is used.

All necessary data are collected intra-operatively using kinematic analysis or probing anatomical landmarks.

Axis and Surface Model

The hip center results out of kinematic analysis, the knee center and ankle center and also axis definition for femoral rotation are determined digitizing landmarks on the tibia, fibula and femur (◘ Fig. 18.1). The axis points in the knee are mainly comparable with the entrance points of intra-medullary rods in conventional technique. The middle of the ankle joint is calculated by digitizing the malleoi transcutaneously. For tibial rotation alignment, the medial third of the tibial tuberosity and tibial insertion of the PCL are digitized. For the femoral rotation of the Natural Knee we probe the posterior condyles, the epicondylar line or »Whiteside line«, which is similar for the Innex™ knee system. After complete probing, the axis model is shown on the system monitor.

With the mosaic pointer (◘ Fig. 18.2) resection levels and landmarks for system validation can be digitized and give a virtual image of the patient's anatomy, exactly related to the intra-operative determined axis.

Principally, by digitizing infinite surface points a nearly 1:1 image of the real anatomy is possible, for practical

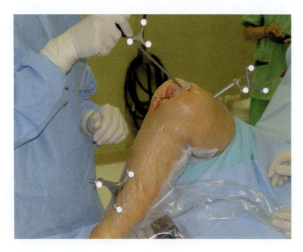

◻ Fig. 18.1. Intra-operative situs probing axis points

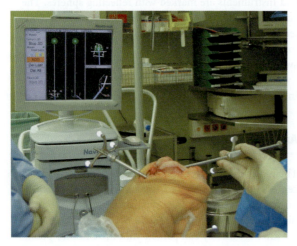

◻ Fig. 18.2. Intra-operative situs probing for mosaic model femoral joint surface

work a few points are sufficient, e.g. for the Natural Knee the anterior femoral cortex to prevent anterior notching, the posterior condyles fore sizing and rotational alignment and the highest and lowest level of the tibial joint line. In severe deformities maybe more mosaic points give a better impression of the patients anatomy and give information for possible profit for augmentation devices.

For better differentiation the size and color of the mosaic points are variable. Therefore, it is possible to focus on very few points in special areas, depending on surgery technique and 3-D imagination of the surgeon,

A validation point, for control of the system is digitized on the medial tibial tuberosity and the medical femoral epicondyle. The bone is there marked e.g. with the electro coagulation. By probing these points with the pointer at any point of surgery the conformity of the virtual model and the real anatomy can be checked. Problems with loosening of registration, e.g. because of movement of the rigid bodies (see below) can be detected.

Surgical Technique

Before collecting data for the axis model fixation of the dynamic reference base (DRB), with 2 pin fixation is done, femoral within the skin incision of the midline approach to the knee, tibial midshaft. Using the optoelectronic tracking system the position of the DRBs must be chosen in the line of sight of the camera and also in adequate distance from the joint line, preventing an interference with the markers from the instruments. On the tibial side, it must be also considered that the DRB is far enough below from the impactor and the tibial stem. We use a tourniquet and an anterior approach. A prolongation of the surgery caused by the calibration can be avoided by doing the tool calibration (pointer, mosaic pointer, universal positioning block – UPB) by the nurse or the assistant while the surgeon does the initial exposure. The pointer and the mosaic pointer are calibrated with an automatic calibration tool. The UPB for the Natural Knee II® -System NK is calibrated automatically, the one for the Innex™ knee system by probing drill-holes on its surface.

In the new generic applications all instruments are calibrated automatically.

Ongoing steps after performing the approach are kinematic acquiring of hip center, digitizing landmarks for knee midpoint, ankle midpoint and rotational axis of femur and tibia, also as probing necessary surface points.

After successful registration a validation based on the clinical aspect is mandatory. If validation is good navigated positioning can start. Depending on the preferred surgery technique (tibia first or femur first) a poly-axial screw is fixed on the proximal tibia, used for the Innex™ knee system or in the distal femur first, Natural Knee II® system. Initial soft tissue balancing may be done before making cuts and is in some cases mandatory. Especially in the Innex™ knee system after tibial bone resection a well-controlled soft tissue balancing is possible with a special developed hydraulic tensor (◻ Fig. 18.3).

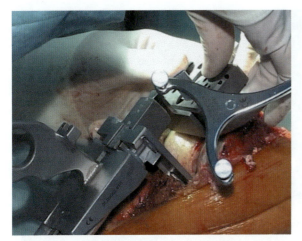

Fig. 18.3. Soft tissue balancing with hydraulic tensor

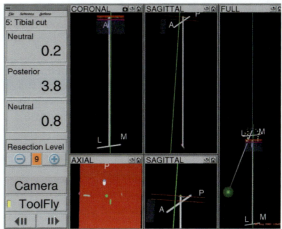

Fig. 18.5. Monitor view tibial alignment

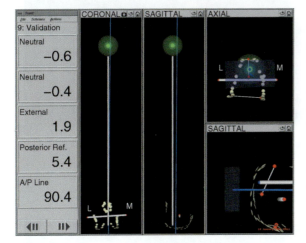

Fig. 18.4. Monitor view femoral alignment and sizing

Based on axis and mosaic model data positioning of the virtual cuts are possible and can be controlled by graphical and numerical data given by the navigation system as shown in **Fig. 18.4** for femoral alignment.

The determination of the femoral implant size results in the lateral view portrayal of the posterior condylar cuts. The pointer can be used for validation of the correct anterior level.

The conventional cutting guide for the posterior condylar resection is attached, the resection level for a standard resection will be adjusted, and the UPB will be removed allowing the bone resection to be done using the oscillating saw. Bringing up the UPB on the resection plane allows a validation and if necessary (e.g. deviation of the saw in sclerotic bone) a correction can be done.

Before final bone preparation, a probing of the validation point should be mandatory in the procedure of navigated surgery, sense to validate the registration and determine possible errors, like movement of the DRBs.

If the distal cut and validation gives no error the femoral rotational alignment and final sizing is done with the UPB on the distal cut, respecting the level of the anterior cortex. In the correct position again two pins are fixed over the UPB. Then the UPB can be removed and the conventional drill guide can be attached to the pins and the femoral holes can be drilled. Over the holes the conventional cutting guide for the a.p., posterior and oblique cuts brought in and bone resection again is done with the oscillating saw. NK II specific grooving is done conventionally with the chisel.

All important angles are shown in the monitor. For tibial alignment a.p.- and sagittal angle is shown **Fig. 18.5**. Posterior slope, therefore, is not given by the system but can adjusted on implants and the patients needs well controlled with additional information of »natural slope« of the patient. The resection level can be adjusted in millimeter steps screwing down the UPB. The positioning again is done by attaching the UPB on the poly-axial screw. In the final position pins are brought in over the UPB (**Fig. 18.6**). Afterwards the UPB and the poly-axial screw must be removed and the conventional tibial cutting guide is attached to the pins. Bone resection is done with the oscillating saw. For validation and controlled correction of cutting errors, the same steps as shown in the femur are possible.

The trial implants are then applied and mechanical alignment is shown by the system. A navigation supported soft-tissue balancing is now possible using the deviation angles under varus and valgus stress. Also a range of motion analysis and documentation is possible. Functional rotational alignment philosophy of the Innex™ knee system is possible with integration of soft tissue balancing using a hydraulic tensor under navigation control.

In the generic application standard jigs can be position as shown in ▫ Fig. 18.7.

The preparation of the patella is conventional in all applications. After implantation of the final components data of final axis, maximal extension and flexion are stored for documentation.

Results

In a randomized clinical trial we compared the navigation controlled alignment (group 1) with the standard instrumentation (group 2) for the Innex™ knee system and the Natural Knee II® system. 24 male and 46 female patients, mean age 67,18 years (50–88 y) were included in the study. Indication for TKA was in all cases primary or posttraumatic osteoarthritis.

Maximum valgus deformity in the manual group was 172°, varus 192°, in the navigated group 162° for valgus and 194° for varus.

Post-operative measurement showed same means in a.p. mechanical axis with 181,2° in group 1 an 18,01° in group 2. In the navigated group 76% of the patients showed post-operatively a good result within 0°–2°, in the manual group 60%, outliners with a.p. axis deviation more than 4° showed 6,6% in group 1 and 13,3% in group 2 (▫ Fig. 18.8).

Functional scores as KSS and WOMAC where similar in both groups 3 month post-operatively. Peri- and post-operative blood loss was not significant different in both groups, surgery time was increased in the navigation group by mean of 18 min. Complication rate was not different except one pin breakage in group 1.

For the new generic application study data are not present at this time.

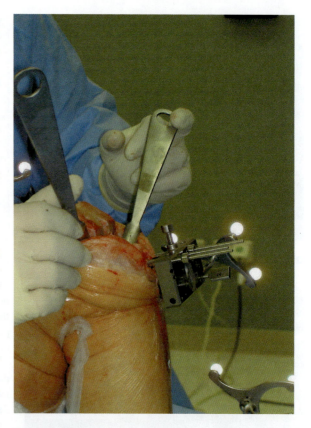

▫ **Fig. 18.6.** Tibial positioning with UPB fixed on poly-axial screw

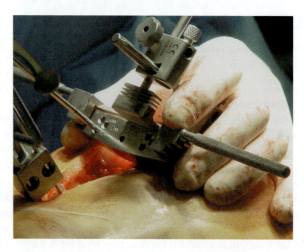

▫ **Fig. 18.7.** Femoral positioning generic application for Natural Knee II

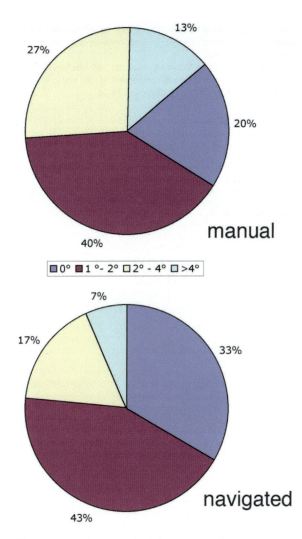

13%

27%

20%

manual

40%

☐ 0° ■ 1 °- 2° ☐ 2° - 4° ☐ >4°

7%

17%

33%

navigated

43%

▣ **Fig. 18.8.** Distribution mechanical axis measured in post-operative long bone X-rays manual versus navigated positioning

Discussion

Navigated TKA with the Navitrack™ system gives reproducible and reliable results concerning correct axis alignment. Experienced surgeons potentially will have in mean similar results in manual techniques like shown with this and other systems [2, 5, 9]. However, a significant reduction regarding outliners and scattering is shown using navigations systems.

A main factor for good results in TKR, beside the correct alignment are well-balanced soft tissues. The new generic software allows functional rotational alignment and well-controlled soft-tissue balancing more than the past software versions. To what extent this will influence functional outcome independent of alignment must be investigated in further studies. Furthermore long term studies are necessary showing possible effects of gained accuracy in TKR using navigation systems.

Early after operation there are no significant differences in functional outcome and life-quality scores between navigated and manual instrumentation in TKA for experienced surgeons, studies for less or inexperienced surgeons may improve theirs learning curve, which must be respected for either navigated or manual procedures, as seen by other groups using navigation systems [4, 7]. Manual experience is mandatory to recognize possible errors of the navigation procedure and correct them.

CT free navigation, with intra-operative acquisition of the axis and surface anatomy is fast and easy to perform. Mosaic points facilitate 3-D imagination of the anatomy too many points may be confusing. Surface morphing based on anatomical atlases is in our opinion abdicable, in defect situations potentially dangerous.

The goal of CT free navigation is a more precise positioning of cutting guides than can be done with conventional intra- or extra-medullary rods [10, 11].

With the Navitrack™ system we could show a precise implant positioning with low expense.

The easy use with intra-operative mosaic model enables an adaptation of the system to different surgical techniques and implants. With the new generic application a personalization to the individual technique of a surgeon is possible and a step to modular navigation system is done.

Analysis of navigated TKR showed several reasons for minor deviation of ideal position. There may problems intrinsic to the surgical technique or conventional instrumentation utilized. Additional problems may arise from bone cuts made on dense sclerotic bone or from areas where the bone is too soft. The implant companies must manufacture and adapt the instruments to the high standard of precision of the navigation system. Manufacturing tolerances for the instrument must decrease.

Conclusion

The Navitrack™ system enables an experienced knee surgeon reliable navigated TKR with or without pre-operative image data (CT scan). The modular concept with implant adapted software and instruments and a generic version allows a universal use.

The CT free Navitrack™ application shows significant reduction of outliners and improves mean alignment in greater collectives.

To justify the expense of navigation, in time of reduced budgets in healthcare systems, of course the benefit is still not calculable, apart from costs of extreme outliners with need of early revision.

Long term effects must be demonstrated in prospective randomized studies.

A further evolution of the navigation systems to expand the usability beyond the primary applications currently used in total hip and total knee replacement is desirable. Minimal invasive procedures and revision cases probably profit more than primary standard cases from navigation.

References

1. Amiot LP Lang K, Putzier M, Zippel H, Labelle H (2000) Comparative results between conventional and computer-assisted pedicle screw installation in the thoracic, lumbar, and sacral spine. Spine 25: 606–614
2. Bathis H, Perlick L, Tingart M, Luring C, Perlick C, Grifka J (2004) Radiological results of image-based and non-image-based computer-assisted total knee arthroplasty. Int Orthop 28: 87–90
3. Ewald FC (1989) The knee society total knee arthroplasty roentgenographic evaluation and scoring system. Clin Orthop 248: 9–12
4. Gill GS, Mills DM (1991) Long-term follow-up evaluation of 1000 consecutive cemented total knee arthroplasties. Clin Orthop 273: 66–76
5. Jenny JY, Boeri C, Picard F, Leitner F (2004) Reproducibility of intraoperative measurement of the mechanical axes of the lower limb during total knee replacement with a non-image-based navigation system. Comput Aided Surg 9: 161–165
6. Jeffery RS, Morris RW, Denham RA (1991) Coronal alignment after total knee replacement. J Bone Joint Surg Br 73: 709–714
7. Honl M, Schwieger K, Gauck CH, Lampe F, Morlock MM, Wimmer MA, Hille E (2005) Comparison of total hip replacements cup orientation and position using different navigation systems and the conventional manual technique. Orthopade 34: 1131–1136
8. Kiefer H, Langenmeyer D, Schmerwitz U (2001) Computerunterstütze Navigation in der Knieendoprothetik. Eur J Trauma Suppl 1: 128
9. Krackow KA, Bayers-Thering M, Phillips MJ, Bayers-Thering M, Mihalko WM (1999) A new technique for determining proper mechanical axis alignment during total knee arthroplasty: progress toward computer-assisted TKA. Orthopedics 22: 698–702
10. Lotke PA, Ecker ML (1977) Influence of positioning of prosthesis in total knee replacement. J Bone Joint Surg 59: 77–79.
11. Teter KE, Bregman D, Colwell CW Jr (1995) Accuracy of intramedullary versus extramedullary tibial alignment cutting systems in total knee arthroplasty. Clin Orthop 321: 106–110
12. Teter KE, Bregman D, Colwell CW Jr (1995) The efficacy of intramedullary femoral alignment in total knee replacement. Clin Orthop 321: 117–121
13. Windsor RE, Scuderi GR, Moran MC, Insall JN (1989) Mechanisms of failure of the femoral and tibial components in total knee arthroplasty. Clin Orthop 248:15–19; discussion 19–20

Experience with Navigated Total Knee Replacements with CT-Free and CT-Based VectorVision® BrainLAB Navigation System

C. Lüring, H. Bäthis, M. Tingart, J. Grifka, L. Perlick

Introduction

Total knee replacement (TKR) has become a standard operative procedure in the past decades [3, 6]. Although, implant design and operative procedure have been optimized, aseptic loosening of prosthesis is still the major problem in TKR. As some authors point out, axial alignment of prosthesis and reconstruction of leg axis is one of the most interesting factors in TKR to gain a long living implant and a highly satisfied patient [20, 21]. Optimal reconstruction of leg axis can be achieved via exact bony resection and optimal balancing of the peri-articular structures, such as the medial and lateral collateral ligament and the posterior capsule [5, 17]. As we know from current literature a correct alignment of the prosthesis is achieved in only 75% of cases, even if they are performed by experienced surgeons [1, 7]. Some authors pointed out that an alignment out of the range of ±3° varus/valgus in anterior-posterior direction results in earlier failure of prosthesis [20, 21]. This fact gains even more interest as the costs for health care management explode in the industrial states and revision surgery should be avoided via best possible primary implantation. Beside this financial point of view the surgeon should try hard to optimize the implantation for the sake of his patient.

The development of navigation systems in total knee replacement has been improved during the recent five years not only because of the mentioned difficulties. Up to now the available navigation systems have a precision of 0.5 mm and 0.5° in clinical routine. They measure leg axis and gap size intra-operatively in real time and some of them support the surgeon within a ligament balancing modus.

Krackow and Co-workers published the first report about computer assisted total knee replacement [12]. The so-called Optotrack® System (Northern Digital Inc.) allowed visualizing the leg axis and the resection planes intra-operatively. The soft- and hardware have been continuously improved during the past years and up to now most of the current systems allow the intra-operative measurement of leg axis, gap size and component rotation [1, 19].

Technical Aspects

CT-Free Software

The clinical routine has shown, that image free systems are most easily to introduce in the operative procedure. They come near to a »plug and play« workflow. The VectorVision® system is very compact, due to the integration of the camera and computer in one unit. This fact allows using the system under conditions with limited space like in most operation rooms. It is an optical (cable free) system which detects the reflecting marker spheres by an infrared camera. The software is controlled by touch screen so that foot switches or additional cables are not necessary (◘ Fig. 19.1).

The CT-free version does not require any pre-operative image sets or planning time. With this technique, reference arrays with passive marker spheres are rigidly

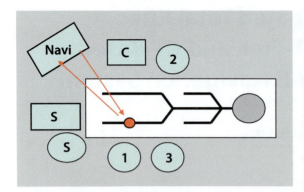

◘ Fig. 19.1. Intra-operative setup: *1* Surgeon, *2* 1st assistant, navigator, *3* 2nd assistant, *S* Nurse, *C* computer

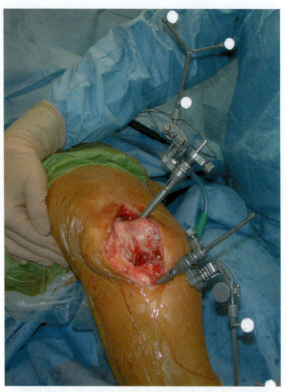

◘ Fig. 19.2. Intra-operative Setup with two reference arrays rigidly attached to both the femoral and the tibial bone

attached to both, the femoral and the tibial bone. At the beginning of the surgical procedure landmarks are needed for navigation. Information about the bone surface is given to the system by sliding a pointer above the tibial plateau and the femoral condyles using a fast and user-friendly algorithm. Then, the system creates an adapted bone model of the specific patient's anatomy and offers the surgeon an automatic planning of the implants. This default planning can be modified depending on surgeon's preferences regarding component size and orientation. To avoid ventral femoral notching a special routine for controlling the ventral femoral plane has been integrated (◘ Fig. 19.2).

Before any cuts are performed, the surgeon has the opportunity to examine and document the preoperative leg axis and to test ligament tension when applying varus and valgus stress. Then usually the tibial cutting jigs can be adjusted according to the planning and are usually fixed by two screws, before resection of bone is performed. After resection, the cut can be controlled with a special tool and possible cutting errors can be detected and corrected (◘ Fig. 19.3).

For rotating the femoral component, the system offers different opportunities. As it is one major goal to achieve a perfect-balanced extension and flexion gap, the femur component can be orientated according to the posterior condyles, to the transepicondylary axis or based on the ligament tension the so-called gap-technique.

As the authors have now experience with over 1100 computer assisted TKR up to now, we prefer this ligament balanced technique for different reasons. Previous studies (e.g. [18]) indicate that a 3° external rotation of

the femoral component according to posterior condylar line only creates a rectangular flexion gap in about 70%. A similar problem has been found in a study by Bäthis et al. [2] as well. As Bäthis found out, 30% of all knees which are operated on in the standard posterior technique might be instable in flexion postoperatively. Although Olcott and Scott defined the transepicondylary axis as most consistently for creating a balanced flexion gap, the study of Jerosch et al. [9] demonstrated a poor reproducibility in defining the transepicondylary axis, even for experienced surgeons with a deviation of up to 23°. Therefore we prefer using the gap-technique for rotational alignment of the femoral component.

When having performed the tibia cut, the distal femur cut is performed navigation controlled using the conventional cutting jigs. Then the achieved planes are checked and documented by a verification function of the navigation system. Afterwards, a ligament balancing is

19

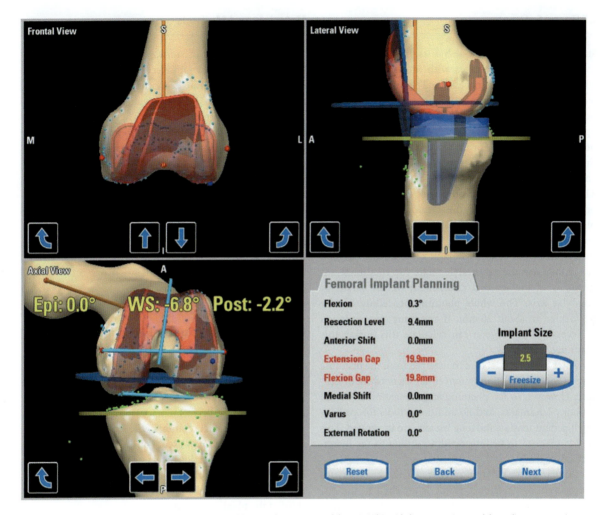

Frontal View   S

M   L

Lateral View   S

A   P

Axial View   A

Epi: 0.0°   WS: -6.8°   Post: -2.2°

P

Femoral Implant Planning

Flexion	0.3°
Resection Level	9.4mm
Anterior Shift	0.0mm
Extension Gap	19.9mm
Flexion Gap	19.8mm
Medial Shift	0.0mm
Varus	0.0°
External Rotation	0.0°

Implant Size

−   2.5   +
Freesize

Reset   Back   Next

▪ **Fig. 19.3.** Rotation of the femoral component is possible according to epicondylar axis, Whiteside line, posterior condyles or ligament tension.

performed using a spreader tool, to achieve a rectangular extension gap. Gap size and deviation of the leg axis are displayed by the navigation system. It is now necessary to perform adequate ligament balancing according to the degree of deformity. Every release step can be controlled and documented by the system. If a rectangular extension gap is created, the knee is flexed to 90°. Again, the spreader tool is inserted between the tibia and the posterior femoral condyles. The navigation system stores this position and recommends the optimal femoral-component orientation to achieve a balanced, rectangular flexion gap. If there are any deviations between the flexion and extension gap, re-

sizing of the femoral component or a modification of the distal femur cut can be performed. The expected values for the extension and flexion gap are notified. Then, the anterior and posterior femoral cuts are prepared by placing the conventional 4-in-1 cutting block.

After insertion of the trial implants it is possible to check the range of motion, the achieved leg axis and joint stability applying stress examination. Every parameter can be documented intra-operatively. Afterwards adjustment of the tibial tray can be performed either by using the navigation system or by dynamic self-adjustment of the trial component.

CT-Based Software

Still, the CT-based technique has its privilege in clinical routine for the severe cases with immense bone loss, where augmentation is necessary. The advantage of this technique is the preoperative CT-scan and the combined possibility to plan the surgical procedure the day before operation. Necessary step or wedge augmentation is possible and helpful. For logistical reasons we perform the CT-scans of the leg (femoral head, knee, ankle) according to a standard protocol the day before operation. Then an automatic preplanning can be performed, based on 3D-surface-images or the original CT-scans. This planning allows a precise orientation of the prosthetic components, representing an optimal alignment to the mechanical limb axis. As default settings, the surgeon can either use the epicondylar axis for rotational adjustment of the femoral component or the posterior condylar axis. The whole planning procedure can be performed in about 20 min. If any bony augmentation is necessary the surgeon can calculate this during this planning session.

After planning, data are transferred from the planning station to the navigation system either via network or ZIP-disc. However, so far, planning and navigation are based on bony-landmarks, and no additional tools for evaluating ligament tension and long leg axis are integrated. This tool is planned to be integrated according to the manufacturer at least.

Similar to the CT-free software, at the beginning of the operation, a reference frame is attached to the distal femur or the proximal tibia, respectively, instead of intra-medullary femoral reaming using a bicortical pin. In contrast to the CT-free version the surface matching process, is performed by the surgeon who has to digitize up to 20 points of free choice on the bone-surface of both, the femur and tibia to match CT-scan and patients anatomy. Next, the conventional cutting blocks of the knee system are orientated in real time visualization, using the navigation system, for the distal femur and 4-in-1 cutting block.

A similar procedure is performed for the proximal resection of the tibia and the orientation of the tibial tray. After resection, the planes can be checked by a verification function. As mentioned above no ligament balancing tool is integrated, the femoral component has to bee orientated according to the posterior condyles or the epicondylar axis.

Materials and Methods

To prove both types of software, we performed a prospective study, with two unselected groups of 65 patients each which were operated on primary TKA using either a computer-assisted CT-free navigation system or the CT-based implantation technique [1]. These 130 consecutive patients were randomized to each group. Patients in both groups were comparable regarding age, gender and preoperative leg deformity. In the CT-free group, 33 female and 17 male patients were included. The mean age was 69.7 ± 8.4 years (range: 51 to 88 yrs.) and the mean preoperative deviation of leg axis was 7.8 degrees $\pm$ 4.8 degrees (range: 18° varus to 21° valgus). In the CT-based group, 40 female and 10 male patients were included. The mean age was 66.1 ± 9.9 years (range: 30 to 80 yrs.) and the mean preoperative deviation of leg axis was 7.6 ± 5.1 degrees (range: 18° varus to 22° valgus).

Computer-Assisted Surgical Technique

The navigation-system used in this study (VectorVision®, BrainLAB) was used in both groups. For the CT-based surgeries, preoperative CT-scans of the hip, knee and ankle region were performed according to the standard protocol. For the axial rotation of the femoral component, the epicondylar axis was used. For the proximal tibial resection plane the resection level was set to 8 mm from the deepest point of the higher tibia plateau level. Rotational alignment of the tibial tray was orientated to the medial third of the tibial tuberosity.

The average time of pre-operative planning and data transfer took 23.2 minutes ($\pm$ 6.5 min).

After performing a standard approach for TKA, two reference arrays with passive marker spheres are rigidly attached to both, the femoral and the tibial bone in both techniques. For the CT-based module this is followed by a surface matching process, where the surgeon has to digitize up to 20 points on the bone-surface of both, the femur and the tibia.

The CT-free operation procedure has been mentioned above. For both techniques the femoral and tibial cutting blocks are orientated to the bone in real time visualization on the navigation system. After resection, all planes were checked by the verification tool of the navigation system.

Radiological Evaluation and Statistics

The axial limb alignment and the component orientation were evaluated on standardized pre- and post-operative full length weight-bearing radiographs by two independent observers three times on different days. The Kolmogorov-Smirnov test was used to evaluate, if axial limb alignment followed a normal (Gaussian-shaped) distribution and no significant departures were identified. Limb alignment between both groups was compared using unpaired t-tests. Level of statistical significance was determined for p<0.05. The coefficient of variation was calculated to determine intra- and inter-observer variability. The intra-observer variability for limb axis determination was less than 3% and the inter-observer variation was less than 4%.

Results

Leg Axis

In the CT-based group, the average deviation from the neutral leg axis was 1.7 degree (±1.3°, range: 5° valgus to 4° varus) and in the CT-free one, it was 1.3 degrees (±1.1° range: 5° valgus to 4° varus) (◘ Fig. 19.4).

92% (46/50) of TKAs in the CT-based group and 96% (48/50) in the CT-free had a leg axis within a range of ±3 degrees (varus/valgus). The maximum deviation from the neutral leg axis was 5 degrees in both groups (CT-based: 2 cases; CT-free: 1 case) (p=0.525).

Component Alignment

Frontal Plane Alignment

The frontal plane alignment of the femoral component (center of the femoral head to center of component) was found within a range of ±3 degrees in 96% (48/50) of cases in the CT-based group and 94% (47/50) of patients in the CT-free group (p= 0.285).

98% (49/50) of patients in both groups had a varus/valgus alignment of the tibial component within a range of ±3 degrees (p=0.654).

Sagittal Plane Alignment

In the CT-based group, the flexion-extension alignment of the femoral component was 5.2 degrees (±2.3° range: 0° to 13°), while in CT-free group it was 7.3 degrees (±3.3° range: 0° to 15°).

In the CT-based group, the posterior slope of the tibial component was 2.6 degrees compared with 2.0 degrees in the CT-free group (standard deviation: 2.2 degrees in both groups.

Surgical Procedure

In both groups no conversion from computer assisted procedure to the conventional technique was required. The mean time for surgery (skin to skin) was 81 min ± (16 min) for the CT-based group and 78 min ± (12 min) for the CT-free group.

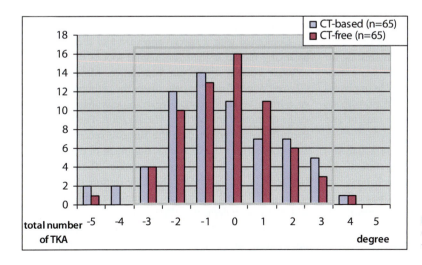

◘ **Fig. 19.4.** Leg axis alignment. Conventional versus computer-assisted technique.

Discussion

VectorVisison® System

The VectorVision System used in our department consists of passive reflecting marker spheres for instruments and reference arrays. From our experience of over 1100 computer assisted implantations, these passive marker spheres guarantee a good visualization during the whole surgical procedure regardless of the leg position. Moreover, no additional cables or footswitches have to be used, which makes the operation theatre clearly arranged. In our point of view this is an advantage compared to active (LED-based) reference arrays. Former problems with contamination of marker spheres with blood have been solved with detachable arrays without loss of accuracy.

Still it has to be recognized that additional operating time is needed when using navigation systems in total knee arthroplasty. However, according to the cited prospective studies, mean duration of the surgical procedure is prolonged by 10–15 min after an initial learning curve. As far as we are concerned this additional time is tolerable in clinical routine even under the daily cost pressure.

Daily Routine

These advantages lead to the fact that computer assisted surgery has become a routinely used operative procedure in total knee replacement in many orthopaedic departments over the past years. Since a post-operative leg alignment within the range of ±3° varus/valgus in the a.p. plane is one critical factor for the longevity of knee prosthesis and the amount of implanted prostheses worldwide is about 500.000 per year, it is quite reasonable that computer-assisted surgery becomes even more interesting for various companies in the future. Besides this, many studies could demonstrate that a lack of accuracy in implantation leads to an earlier aseptic loosening of the prosthesis and results in a revision operation for the patient and increasing costs for the insurances.

Although, knee replacement has become a standard procedure, it is still a highly demanding operation with many difficulties such as the anatomic approach, bony cuts and ligamentous stability [10, 11, 24]. As all these difficulties can end in an early aseptic loosening of the prosthesis; a new technology such as CAS has to support the surgeon in all these aspects to optimize the postoperative result.

Current Literature

As many studies up to now point out and as we could demonstrate in a review of the literature, five out of six current prospective and comparing studies concerning computer-assisted total knee replacement showed that outliners according to the post-operative leg axis and component orientation can be reduced by the use of navigation [1, 4, 8, 13, 23]. Nevertheless, it has to be discussed that for determination of post-operative leg axis and component orientation all authors used conventional weight-bearing long leg X-rays, which can have a calculational error of ±2° – ±4° [8, 22, 24]. Therefore, all values have to be judged critically. Up to now, there is no study which calculates the post-operative leg axis with a standardized CT scan due to ethical problems.

Ligament Balancing

It is commonly accepted that optimal ligament balancing is one critical factor in TKR and can achieve a stable knee over the full range of movement. The surgeon has to be aware of the different effects of ligamentous releases during the operation. A stable knee in extension might be instable in flexion, if for example the posterior cruciate ligament is insufficient. Therefore, the VectorVision® software has been extended with a special ligament balancing modus where the system visualizes the medio-lateral gap size in extension and in flexion and on the same screen the leg axis is shown as well. By using this procedure, the surgeon can see the effect of necessary release steps immediately and can carefully optimize the ligamentous stability by sequential release steps [15].

Combined with a special spreader tool the ligament balancing modus is the most helpful tool of the current software release, up to our experience. Moreover, the CT-free VectorVision® system offers the orthopaedic surgeon important information regarding axis alignment and range of motion in real time visualization. Furthermore, it can be easily adjusted to the surgeon-specific preferences concerning the rotational alignment of the femoral component and level of bone resection. Therefore this is at least in our institution the daily routine navigation, whereas CT-based navigation remains for difficult cases with sever bony deformity (▪ Fig. 19.5).

Up to now, the CT-based software, does not offer the opportunity for visualization of ligament balancing, since

19

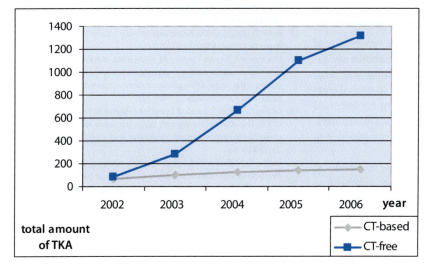

Fig. 19.5. Development of computer assisted total knee replacements over the past four years in the Orthopaedic Department of the University of Regensburg, Germany

Table 19.1. Current prospective randomized studies comparing conventional versus computer assisted technique

Author	(n)	Deviation femur shield frontal plane ≤3°	Deviation femur shield sagittal plane ≤3	Deviation tibial tray frontal plane ≤3°	Deviation tibial tray sagittal plane ≤3°
Mielke et al. 2001 [16]	60	–	–	–	–
Jenny et al. 2001 [8]	100	+	–	+	+
Sparmann et al. 2003 [23]	240	+	+	+	–
Bäthis et al. 2004 [1]	160	+	+	+	+
Chauhan et al. 2004 [4]	70	+	+	+	+

the femoral and tibial navigation can not be performed simultaneously. To date this is still a limitation of the CT-based version compared with the CT-free software. Nevertheless this functionality is under construction.

One major advantage of the ligament balancing modus is the more of information. These aspects led to several experimental studies which focus on optimal handling of soft tissues. The implementation of the ligament balancing modus in our experimental setup led to studies where we could show that the anatomic approach has an influence on the intra-operatively measured leg axis and therefore may falsify the postoperative result [14]. Moreover, it became obvious that the position of the patella

(everted vs. subluxed) influences the leg axis during ligament balancing as well [13].

However, up to now the current literature lacks of studies which show significant differences between the conventional and the navigated technique according to clinical and functional parameters. In a first matched pairs analysis (unpublished data) with 100 patients (conventional vs. navigated technique) two years after TKR we could not find any differences regarding patients satisfaction, WOMAC Score and Knee Society Score, but a superiority of postoperative collateral stability. Nevertheless, to prove this new technology we have to perform more studies which focus on the postoperative mid- and long term results.

Conclusion

The CT-based navigation system offers the opportunity of preoperative planning and correct intra-operative navigation of cutting blocks. Particularly, in situations with large bony defects this planning is helpful. But, additional costs and the time consuming CT-scan have to be discussed critically. For these reasons, we perform CT-based navigation only in cases with severe bony deformities due to trauma or severe rheumatoid arthritis.

As many current studies as ours show, the results of the CT-free systems are very promising not only because the ligament balancing is integrated into the software. The axial alignment and the alignment of the components is superior to the conventional technique. According to our experience with over 1100 computer assisted TKR we can strongly recommend this technique even for experienced surgeons in daily routine.

Literature

1. Bäthis H, Perlick L, Tingart M, Lüring C, Perlick C, Grifka J (2004a) Radiological results of image-based and non-image-based computer-assisted total knee arthroplasty. Int Orthop 28(2): 87–90
2. Bäthis H, Perlick L, Tingart M, Lüring C, Perlick C, Grifka J (2004b) Flexion gap configuration in total knee arthroplasty following high tibial osteotomy, Int Orthop 28: 366–269
3. Bäthis H, Tingart M, Perlick L, Lüring C, Anders S, Grifka J (2005) Total knee arthroplasty and high tibial osteotomy in osteoarthritis – results of a survey in traumatic surgery and orthopedic clinics. Z Orthop Ihre Grenzgeb 143(1): 19–24
4. Chauhan SK, Scott RG, Breidahl W, Beaver RJ (2004) Computer-assisted knee arthroplasty versus conventional jig-based technique. A randomised, prospective trial. J Bone Joint Surg Br 86: 372–377
5. Engh GA (2003) The difficult knee. Severe varus and valgus. Clin Orthop 416: 58–63
6. Font-Rodriguez DE, Scuderi GR, Insall JN (2003) Survivorship of cemented total knee arthroplasty. Clin Orthop 345: 79–86
7. Hood RW, Vanni M, Insall JN (1981) The correction of knee alignment in 225 consecutive total condylar knee replacements. Clin Orthop 160: 94–105
8. Jenny JY, Boeri C (2001) Computer-assisted implantation of a total knee arthroplasty: a case-controlled study in comparison with classical instrumentation. Rev Chir Orthop Reparatrice Appar Mot 87: 645–652
9. Jerosch J, Peuker E, Philipps B, Filler T (2002) Interindividual reproducibility in perioperative rotational alignment of femoral components in knee prosthetic surgery using the transepicondylar axis. Knee Surg, Sports Traumatol, Arthrosc 10: 194–197
10. Kienapfel H, Springorum HP, Ziegler A, Klose KJ, Georg C, Griss P (2003) Der Einfluss der Femur- und Tibiakomponentenrotation auf das patellofemorale Versagen beim künstlichen Kniegelenkersatz. Orthopäde 32: 312–318
11. Kohn D, Rupp S (2000) Knieendoprothetik – Operationstechnische Aspekte. Orthopäde 29: 697–707
12. Krackow KA, Bayers-Thering M, Phillips MJ, Mihalko WM (1999) A new technique for determining proper mechanical axis alignment during total knee arthroplasty: progress towards computer-assisted TKA. Orthopedics 22: 698–702
13. Lüring C, Hüfner T, Kendoff D, Perlick L, Bäthis H, Grifka J, Krettek C (2006) The effect of medial soft tissue release in total knee arthroplasty: A navigation controlled cadaver study. J Arthroplasty 2006; 21(3): 428–34
14. Lüring C, Hüfner T, Kendoff D, Perlick L, Grifka J, Krettek C (2005) Eversion or subluxation of patella in soft tissue balancing of total knee arthroplasty? Results of a cadaver experiment. Knee 13: 15–18
15. Lüring C, Hüfner T, Kendoff D, Perlick L, Grifka J, Krettek C (2005) Influence of the surgical approach in total knee arthroplasty on ligament tension A navigation-controlled cadaver study. Unfallchirurg 108: 274–278
16. Mielke RK, Clemens U, Jens JH, Kershally S (2001) Navigation in der Knieendoprothetik – vorläufige klinische Erfahrungen und prospektiv vergleichende Studie gegenüber konventioneller Implantationstechnik. Z Orthop 139: 109–116
17. Mihalko WM, Whiteside LA, Krackow KA (2003) Comparison of ligament-balancing techiniques during total knee arthroplasty. J Bone Joint Surg (Am) 85: 132–135
18. Olcott CW, Scott RD (1999) Femoral component rotation during total knee arthroplasty. Clin Orthop 367: 39–42
19. Perlick L, Bäthis H, Lerch K, Lüring C, Tingart M, Grifka J (2004) Navigated implantation of total knee endoprostheses in secondary knee osteoarthritis of rheumatoid arthritis patients as compared to conventional technique. Z Rheumatol 63: 1–7
20. Rand JA, Coventry MB (1988) Ten-year evaluation of geometric total knee arthroplasty. Clin Orthop 232: 168–73
21. Ritter MA; Faaris PM, Keating EM, Meding JB (1994) Postoperative alignment of total knee replacement. Its effect on survival. Clin Orthop 299: 153–156
22. Saragaglia D, Picard F, Chaussard C, Montbarbon E, Leitner F, Cinquin P (2001) Computer-assisted knee arthroplasty: comparison with a conventional procedure. Results of 50 cases in a prospective randomized study. Rev Chir Orthop Reparatrice Appar Mot 87: 18–28
23. Sparmann M, Wolke B, Czupalla H, Banzer D, Zink A (2003) Positioning of total knee arthroplasty with and without navigation support. A prospective randomised study. J Bone Joint Surg Br 85: 830–835
24. Stulberg SD, Loan P, Sarin V (2002) Computer-assisted navigation in total knee replacements: results of an initial experience in thirty-five patients. J Bone Joint Surg Am 84: 90–98

19

Navigated Revision Total Knee Arthroplasty, CT-Free Navigation with VectorVision System

L. Perlick, C. Lüring, M. Tingart, J. Grifka, H. Bäthis

Introduction

Total knee arthroplasty (TKA) has been established as reliable treatment for pain relief and restoration of joint function in arthritic knees [18, 26, 30]. Historically, the most common cause for revision TKA is aseptic loosening of the tibial component [7, 13]. This mode of failure may result from technical errors during primary TKA, such as bone preparation and leg alignment [20, 28]. On the other side, knee instability after primary TKA has been discussed as an important factor for TKA-failure. This instability might be due to inequality of flexion and extension gap, inadequate correction of sagittal plane deformities or medial/lateral compartment dysbalance [7, 32].

Recognizing the rising number of primary TKA over the last decade one may assume even a rising number for revisions after a certain time delay. Meanwhile revision total knee arthroplasty represents between 5%, and in some series as many as lo%, of all total knee replacements performed [4, 11].

The primary challenge in revision TKA remains the restoration of an adequate joint line and joint stability. However, this might be complicated by a loss of bone stock and difficulties in identifying relevant bony landmarks [10, 11, 19, 22]. Furthermore, the ability to achieve longitudinal alignment in revision knee arthroplasty is critical to the success of the revision procedure [3]. Therefore, revision total knee arthroplasty (TKA) poses a variety of technically challenging problems.

In the last years navigation systems have been developed to increase the accuracy of prosthesis implantation and component alignment in TKA. So far, several studies have been published, reporting the results of computer-assisted primary TKA [2, 33]. Therefore, it seemed worthwhile to evaluate the benefits of the computer-assisted technique in revision TKA and compare the alignment results with the conventional technique.

Materials and Methods

Study Design and Patients

In March 2002, we started a prospective study to evaluate the patients undergoing revision arthroplasty. Until March 2005, 120 patients were operated on for revision TKA either using a CT-free navigation system (n=60) or the conventional technique (n=60). Patients were assigned to these groups by the day of operation. The study was limited to revisions of type I or II defects [9] after removal of the components, uncontained defects were excluded.

Patients in both groups were comparable regarding age, gender and preoperative leg deformity. 38 female and 22 male patients were included in the study group. The mean age was 71.6 years (range: 55 to 81 years). The most common indications for revision TKA were: Loosening of the tibial component (n=21), loosening of femoral and tibial component (n=10), loosening of femoral component (n=6), inlay wear (n=8) and instability (n=15).

36 female and 24 male patients were included in the control group (average age of 72.8 years, range: 60 to 84 years). Revision TKA was performed because of loosening of the tibial component (n=19), loosening of femoral

and tibial component (n=14), loosening of femoral component (n=5), inlay wear (n=6) and instability (n=16).

Pre-operatively, the average Knee Society Clinical Score was 41 (range: 20 to 53) in the study group and 42 (range: 21 to 58) in the control group.

Operative Technique

In both groups the modular DePuy P.F.C-Sigma™/TC-3 (Warsaw, USA) knee system was used. The tourniquet inflation pressure was set to 350 mmHg in all patients.

In the control group, prostheses were implanted in a conventional »surgeon-controlled« technique as described by the manufacturer. The flexion-extension gaps were precisely balanced with a spreader device before implantation of the components.

In the study group, revision TKA was performed using the CT-free version of BrainLAB's (Munich-Heimstetten, Germany) VectorVision-System®. This type of software module gathers all information during the operation and avoids time-consuming pre-operative data transfer and planning.

At the beginning of the operation, a reference frame was attached to the distal femur and the proximal tibia, respectively. The important bony landmarks and the surface data were gathered in the way which has been described in the chapter for primary TKA. Because the system has been build to perform primary TKAs the surface points were acquired with the old prosthesis in place to enable the system to create a suitable model and to gain information about the prior joint line. In the next step, error analysis was performed by controlling the stability of the knee in extension, mid-flexion and flexion. Furthermore the component-angles were documented.

The tibial cutting block was orientated in real time visualization and adjusted in a way that only a minimal bone resection was necessary to achieve a good bony covering of the tibia tray. The tibial slope was set to 0°, as advised by the manufacturer. In cases which needed augmentations, a parallel cut was performed on the desired high. Then the distal femoral cutting block was adjusted. By placing the pointer on the medial epicondyle respectively the fibular styloid the surgeon is informed about the distance to the cutting plane which can be used for determination of the joint line.

Ligament balancing was performed until a rectangular extension gap was gained. The rotational alignment of the femoral component was adjusted by using the gap technique [5]. After each resection, the planes were checked by the verification tool of the navigation system.

When using a cementless stem for the femoral or the tibial component, the alignment of the component would be determined by the intra-medullary channel. However, this might interfere with the alignment given by the navigation system, which uses the mechanical axis as reference; therefore cemented stems were used in all operations.

Case Presentation

A 61 year old female patient suffering from loss of the right leg and a posttraumatic gonarthrosis on the left side (■ Fig. 20.1) presented with a loosening of a prosthesis which was implanted two years ago. The pre-operative X-rays showed an extra-articular deformity of the femur (■ Fig. 20.2) which prohibits the use of an intra-medullary instrument.

After opening of the knee, the instability resulting from the subsidence of the tibial tray was obvious (■ Fig. 20.3). Femur and tibia were suited with the standard reference

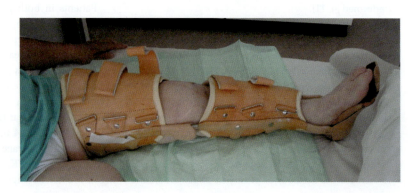

■ **Fig. 20.1.** Pre-operatively, the patient was only able to walk using the splint due to the instability resulting from subsidence of the tibial component

20

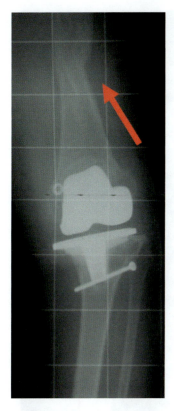

frames and the surface data were acquired like in a primary case with the old prosthesis in place. Care was taken to determine the points for the long axis (ACL-insertion point and notch point) correctly to avoid errors resulting from an asymmetric placement of the old prosthesis. In the next step the stability was documented by screen shots and the prosthesis was removed.

On the tibial side an augmentation with a step of 10 mm was necessary. This was done by performing a marginal cut on the lateral side and placing the block 10 mm below on the medial side with the help of the navigation system (◘ Fig 20.4). On the femoral side the system

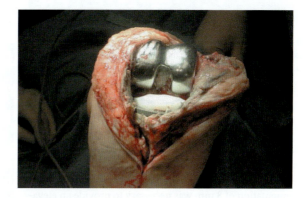

◘ **Fig. 20.2.** The pre-operative X-rays showed a subsidence of the tibial tray and a extra-articular deformity of the femur

◘ **Fig. 20.3.** The intra-operative situs showed an instability in extension and flexion

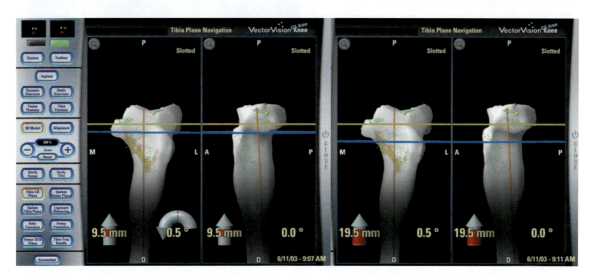

◘ **Fig. 20.4.** The tibia plateau was prepared by a conservative cut on the lateral side. The medial cut was done by shifting the cutting block 10 mm under control of the navigation system

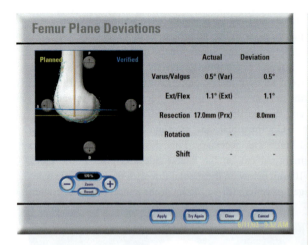

Fig. 20.5. The surgeon is informed about the resection line in comparison to the prior joint line. In this case 8 mm have to be augmented to recreate the joint line

informed us that overall a cut of 17 mm was necessary to get a good bony base for the component. That means with a thickness of 9 mm of the femoral component a distal augmentation of 8 mm was necessary to provide an elevation of the joint line (■ Fig. 20.5). Because of the highly demanding biomechanical situation both the femoral and the tibial component were suited with stems.

The post-operative X-rays showed a precise reconstruction of the leg axis (■ Fig. 20.6).

Post-Operative Evaluation of Radiographs

The axial limb alignment was evaluated on standardized pre- and post-operative full length weight-bearing radiographs by two independent observers three times on different days. The intra-observer variability for limb axis determination was less than 4% and the inter-observer variation was less than 5.5%.

For determination of the joint line the method of Figgie et al. [10] was used. They defined the level of the joint line on lateral X-ray as the distance between the articulating surface and the highest point of the tibial tuberosity.

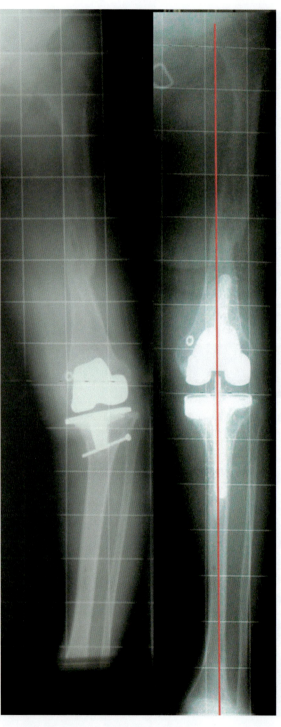

Fig. 20.6. The post-operative X-rays showed a precise reconstruction of the joint line

Results

Component Alignment

Frontal Plane Alignment
Mechanical Leg Axis

In 95% (57/60) of cases the leg axis was within a range of ±3 degrees in the computer assisted group compared with 80% (48/60) in the conventional group (**□** Fig. 20.7). In the computer assisted group, 3 outliners were seen, which exceeded +/- 3 degrees of varus/valgus deviation (maximum 4°) compared with 12 cases in the conventional group (maximum 6°). Out of this 12 cases, 4 cases had a mechanical leg axis deviation of more than ±5 degrees.

Component Alignment

The mean a.p.-deviation of the femoral component was 1.1 degree (±1.3°, range 3° valgus to 2° varus) in the computer assisted group and 2.0 degrees (±1.8° range: 3° valgus to 5° varus) in the control group.

For the tibial component the mean deviation from the neutral position was 1.1 degree ±1.2 degree (computer assisted group) and 1.4 degree ±1.5 degree (conventional group).

Sagittal Plane Alignment

In the computer-assisted group, the flexion-extension alignment of the femoral component was 3.6 degrees (±3.1° range: −1° to 7°), while in the control group it was 6.5 degrees (±4.3° range: 2° to 12°).

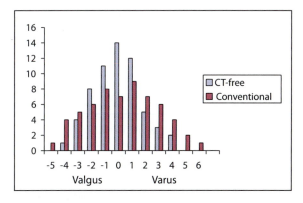

□ Fig. 20.7. Focusing on the achieved leg axis, the values are more closely distributed in the study group (n=60). In the conventional group (n=60) 12 patients (20%) exceeded the range of ±3° valgus/varus deformity, compared with 3 patients (5%) in the study group

In the study group, the posterior slope of the tibial component was 1.8 degrees (±2.1° range: 0° to 5°), while in the control group it was 3.9 degrees (±2.5° range: 1° to 8°) (p>0.05).

Joint Line

Alterations of the joint line were determined by using the technique of Figgie et al. [10]. 78% of cases (47/60) in the computer assisted group and 55% of cases (33/60) the conventional group had an elevation of the joint line of less than 4 mm. In 13 cases (22%) in the computer-assisted and in 22 cases (37%) in the conventional group an elevation between 4 and 8 mm was found. While no patient in the computer-assisted group showed an elevation of more than 8 mm, this was observed in 5 cases (8%) in the conventional group.

Surgical Procedure

No conversion from computer-assisted surgery to the conventional technique was required in the study. The mean time for surgery (skin to skin) was 98 min (±17 min) for the study group and 90 min (±15 min) for the control group.

Discussion

Revision TKA is a technically difficult procedure. Already the Exposure can be difficult because of stiffness and adhesions. In addition, there is often instability due to ligamentous laxity and the bone stock may be poor. Not surprisingly, Robertsson and Co-workers found that only 78% of the cases were satisfied with their knee after revision [29].

The primary goals of revision TKA is to re-establish the correct joint line and the axial alignment. The tolerable limits for postoperative leg alignment in TKA are still controversially discussed in the literature, but the majority of the current studies propose a secure window of +/-3° [16, 25, 27].

We found a significantly better post-operative limb axis for navigation-based revision TKA compared with the conventional technique. Our findings for computer assisted revision TKA are comparable with the data reported by other authors for primary TKA [1, 17, 33].

Different reasons might be relevant for deviation of the mechanical leg axis even if using a navigation system. In all imageless systems, the accuracy of navigation depends on the quality of surface-point acquisition. Another reason for variations of the leg axis is the deviation of the saw blade in dense or weakened bone stock. Plaskos [23] reported cutting errors of 0.6° to1.1° in varus-valgus and 1.8° in flexion/extension. Other factors are variations in cementing the prosthetic components; stem-related deviations as well as inaccuracies in determining the leg axis on post-operative weight-bearing long leg radiographs. However, an important advantage of navigation systems is that some of the errors discussed before can be verified and corrected intra-operatively.

Principles of successful revision TKA include restoration of the joint line to a normal position [24]. Several studies focused on defining useful landmarks and relationships. To our knowledge, only two studies focused on determination of the joint line in revision TKA [22]. Partington et al. [22] used the method described by Figgie et al. [10] for primary TKA. They defined the level of the joint line on lateral X-ray as the distance between the articulating surface and the highest point of the tibial tuberosity. The average distance before TKA was 16 (±5.3 mm), after primary TKA 17 mm (±9.4 mm) and after revision TKA 24 mm (±8.4 mm). In contrast, Noda et al. [21] found a mean distance of 22.3 mm (±2.8 mm) in untreated knees.

Griffin and co-workers [12] analyzed 104 consecutive routine knee MRI scans to define useful landmarks and relationships. On the coronal view the medial epicondylar sulcus-to-joint line distance averaged 27.4 (±2.9 mm, range: 21.0–35.5 mm) from the medial joint line. They reported a significant difference between females (26.3 mm, ±2.5 mm, range: 21.0–34.2 mm) and males (29.2 mm, range: 23.1–35.5 mm). Stiehl and Abbot [34] found a mean distance of the medial epicondyle to the joint line of 30.8 mm and a mean distance of the lateral epicondyle to the joint line of 25.3 mm.

Elevation of the joint line more than 8 mm has been associated with an inferior patients outcome [22], although Scuderi [31] and Insall [15] stated that the joint line could be elevated by 10 mm without significant clinical effect [6]. Similarly, lowering the joint line position excessively may be associated with retropatellar pain and increased risk of patellar subluxation [14].

In consideration of the high standard deviations for each parameter and the limit of 8 mm proposed by Par-

tington et al. [22] it remains questionable if a single parameter will fit for each patient. In cases with lacking information about the untreated knee or the contralateral knee all three parameters mentioned above as well as the meniscal scar should be taken into account.

In this study we used the CT-free version of BrainLAB's (Munich-Heimstetten, Germany) VectorVision-System®, which has been designed for primary TKA. So far, measurement of distances between anatomic landmarks and the joint line can be only performed indirectly, however, a specific revision module is under development. Nevertheless, we noticed a tendency towards a better restoration of the joint line (less than 4 mm) in the computer assisted group (78%) compared the conventional group (55%).

Additional operating time is needed when using navigation systems in revision TKA. However, as a result of our study, an average it took only 16 min longer to perform the navigation-based surgical procedure. In the future, additional time needed might be even further reduced by improvement of the navigation workflow and development of navigation-adapted instruments.

Conclusion

The use of a CT-free navigation system provides a significant improvement of prosthesis alignment in revision TKA. Alignment, range of motion and ligament situation as well as each step of bone resection can be verified and documented during surgery. Particularly, information about the joint line, the size of the flexion and extension gap and the ligament situation is very useful during surgery. In future, the development of specific revision modules should offer the opportunity of exact intra-operative joint line calculation and planning of step-augmentation.

References

1. Bathis H, Perlick L, Tingart M, Luring C, Perlick C, Grifka J (2004a) Radiological results of image-based and non-image-based computer-assisted total knee arthroplasty. Int Orthop 28: 87–90
2. Bathis H, Perlick L, Tingart M, Luring C, Zurakowski D, Grifka J (2004b) Alignment in total knee arthroplasty. A comparison of computer-assisted surgery with the conventional technique. J Bone Joint Surg Br 86: 682–687
3. Bertin KC, Freeman MA, Samuelson KM, Ratcliffe SS, Todd RC (1985) Stemmed revision arthroplasty for aseptic loosening of total knee replacement. J Bone Joint Surg Br 67: 242–248

4. Bourne RB, Crawford HA (1998) Principles of revision total knee arthroplasty. Orthop Clin North Am 29: 331–337

5. Buechel FF, Pappas MJ (1986) The New Jersey Low-Contact-Stress Knee Replacement System: biomechanical rationale and review of the first 123 cemented cases. Arch Orthop Trauma Surg 105: 197–204

6. Cope MR, O'Brien BS, Nanu AM (2002) The influence of the posterior cruciate ligament in the maintenance of joint line in primary total knee arthroplasty: a radiologic study. J Arthroplasty 17: 206–208

7. Dorr LD (2002) Session V: Revision total knee replacement: an overview. Clin Orthop 404: 143–144

8. Dorr LD, Boiardo RA (1986) Technical considerations in total knee arthroplasty. Clin Orthop 205: 5–11

9. Engh GA, Ammeen DJ (1999) Bone loss with revision total knee arthroplasty: defect classification and alternatives for reconstruction. Instr Course Lect 48:167–175

10. Figgie HR III, Goldberg VM, Heiple KG, Moller HS, III, Gordon NH (1986) The influence of tibial-patellofemoral location on function of the knee in patients with the posterior stabilized condylar knee prosthesis. J Bone Joint Surg Am 68: 1035–1040

11. Gofton WT, Tsigaras H, Butler RA, Patterson JJ, Barrack RL, Rorabeck CH (2002) Revision total knee arthroplasty: fixation with modular stems. Clin Orthop 404: 158–168

12. Griffin FM, Math K, Scuderi GR, Insall JN, Poilvache PL. Anatomy of the epicondyles of the distal femur: MRI analysis of normal knees. J Arthroplasty 15: 354–359

13. Hofmann AA, Bachus KN, Wyatt RW (1991) Effect of the tibial cut on subsidence following total knee arthroplasty. Clin Orthop 269: 63–69

14. Insall J, Goldberg V, Salvati E (1972) Recurrent dislocation and the high-riding patella. Clin Orthop 88: 67–69

15. Insall J, Lachiewicz PF, Burstein AH (1982) The posterior stabilized condylar prosthesis: a modification of the total condylar design. Two to four-year clinical experience. J Bone Joint Surg Am 64: 1317–1323

16. Jeffery RS, Morris RW, Denham RA (1991) Coronal alignment after total knee replacement. J Bone Joint Surg Br 73: 709–714

17. Jenny, Mielke RK, Kohler S, Kiefer H, Konermann K, Boeri C, Clemens U, Ratayski H (2003) Total knee prosthesis implantation with a non image based navigation system - A multicentric analysis. Proceedings 70th Annual Meeting AAOS, American Academy of Orthopedic Surgeons New Orleans 96

18. Laskin RS (1976) Modular total knee-replacement arthroplasty. A review of eighty-nine patients. J Bone Joint Surg Am 58: 766–773

19. Laskin RS (2002) Joint line position restoration during revision total knee replacement. Clin Orthop 404: 169–171

20. Lotke PA, Ecker ML (1977) Influence of positioning of prosthesis in total knee replacement. J Bone Joint Surg Am 59: 77–79

21. Noda T, Yasuda S, Nagano K, Takahara Y, Namba Y, Inoue H. Clinico-radiological study of total knee arthroplasty after high tibial osteotomy. J Orthop Sci 5: 25–36

22. Partington PF, Sawhney J, Rorabeck CH, Barrack RL, Moore J (1999) Joint line restoration after revision total knee arthroplasty. Clin Orthop 367: 165–171

23. Plaskos C, Hodgson AJ, Inkpen K, McGraw RW (2002) Bone cutting errors in total knee arthroplasty. J Arthroplasty 17: 698–705

24. Rand JA (1998) Modular augments in revision total knee arthroplasty. Orthop Clin North Am 29: 347–353

25. Rand JA, Coventry MB (1988) Ten-year evaluation of geometric total knee arthroplasty. Clin Orthop 232: 168–173

26. Riley LH Jr, Hungerford DS (1978) Geometric total knee replacement for treatment of the rheumatoid knee. J Bone Joint Surg Am 60: 523–527

27. Ritter MA, Faris PM, Keating EM, Meding JB (1994) Postoperative alignment of total knee replacement. Its effect on survival. Clin Orthop 299: 153–156

28. Ritter MA, Montgomery TJ, Zhou H, Keating ME, Faris PM, Meding JB (1999) The clinical significance of proximal tibial resection level in total knee arthroplasty. Clin Orthop 360: 174–181

29. Robertsson O, Dunbar M, Pehrsson T, Knutson K, Lidgren L. Patient satisfaction after knee arthroplasty: a report on 27,372 knees operated on between 1981 and 1995 in Sweden. Acta Orthop Scand 71: 262–267

30. Scott WN, Rubinstein M, Scuderi G (1988) Results after knee replacement with a posterior cruciate-substituting prosthesis. J Bone Joint Surg Am 70: 1163–1173

31. Scuderi G, Insall JN (1992) Total knee arthroplasty. Current clinical perspectives. Clin Orthop 276: 26–32

32. Sharkey PF, Hozack WJ, Rothman RH, Shastri S, Jacoby SM (2002) Insall Award paper. Why are total knee arthroplasties failing today? Clin Orthop 404: 7–13

33. Sparmann M, Wolke B, Czupalla H, Banzer D, Zink A (2003) Positioning of total knee arthroplasty with and without navigation support. A prospective, randomised study. J Bone Joint Surg Br 85: 830–835

34. Stiehl JB, Abbott BD (1995) Morphology of the transepicondylar axis and its application in primary and revision total knee arthroplasty. J Arthroplasty 10: 785–789

Navigated Total Knee Arthroplasty and the ORTHOsoft Navitrack System

M. Bolognesi

Introduction

The Navitrack® TotalKnee™ (Orthosoft, Montreal, Quebec, Canada) imageless application from ORTHO*soft* allows the surgeon to determine mechanical and rotational axis of a patient's leg during total knee replacement surgery. The Navitrack TotalKnee imageless application does not require any CT images prior to surgery nor does it require any intra-operative fluoroscopy images. All required data is registered with the system intra-operatively. As with most systems available today, this system continues to evolve with regard to software applications, instrumentation and workstation design.

Methods

This system consists of a computer workstation (▪ Fig. 21.1), an optical tracking system, surgical instruments, and tracking devices. There are tracking devices affixed to the universal positioning block (UPB), also known as the Navitrack Positioning Block (▪ Fig. 21.2), and the pointing instrument, which allow these instruments to be tracked and displayed real time on a monitor. Intra-operatively, fixed trackers are attached to the femur and to the tibia. The lower extremity is held in extension during placement of the femoral trackers. Pins are then placed in a unicortical fashion barely engaging the second cortex of the femur. Similar technique is used on the tibia and a specific tracker is attached to these pins at each site.

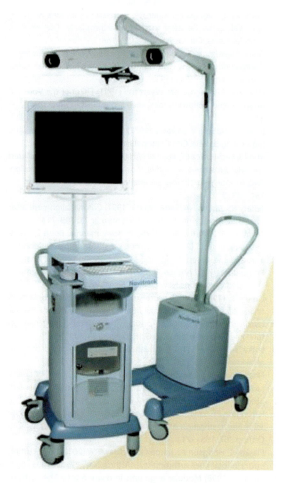

▪ **Fig. 21.1.** The Navitrack computer navigation workstation

The hip then is taken through a range of motion to establish the center of rotation of the femoral head. Fourteen points are documented during this motion analysis to compute the location of the center of the femoral head. This registration is based on cadaveric data from ORTHO*soft* that demonstrates accuracy within 2 mm. The knee then is exposed and the pointing instrument is used to digitize and to reference multiple bony landmarks on the distal femur and the proximal tibia. The landmarks on the femoral side include the intercondylar notch, medial and lateral epicondyles, and the trochlear groove. The universal positioning block with the claws attached is placed on the distal femur to reference the posterior condyles. On the tibial side the landmarks include the center of the tibia, medial 1/3 of the tibial tubercle, the posterior cruciate ligament (PCL), the most medial and lateral points on the plateau, and the medial and lateral malleoli. Once these points are entered, the intra-operative deformity can be determined and evaluated. The varus-valgus deformity as well as flexion-extension deformity can be saved on the system. At this point the surgeon also can make an evaluation of how correctable the deformity is in order to plan soft tissue balancing strategies.

Femoral preparation then is initiated. The poly-axial screw to hold the UPB is placed in the distal femur with no entry into the femoral canal. No intra-medullary rod is placed. The UPB is positioned on the screw with the posterior condyle claw attached. The surgeon then dials in rotation, flexion-extension, and varus-valgus orientation by manipulating the position of the UPB. The goal for flexion is between 3.0° to 5.0° to account for the anterior bow of the femur. The UPB is dialed down medially or laterally to set a neutral varus-valgus block position using the intact condyle as a pivot point. A standard distal femoral cutting block then is applied to the UPB (see Fig 21.2), holes for this cutting block are drilled, and pins are placed to stabilize the block and the femoral lugholes are drilled through the UPB. The drilling of the lug holes sets the rotation. The size of the femur is determined using the pointer. After the distal femoral resection, the UPB is placed flush against the distal cut for validation (Fig. 21.3). The remainder of the femoral preparation is done using standard technique and cutting blocks using the drilled lugholes.

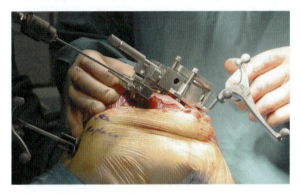

 Fig. 21.2. The Universal Positioning Block is applied to the distal femur to allow navigation of the femoral resection

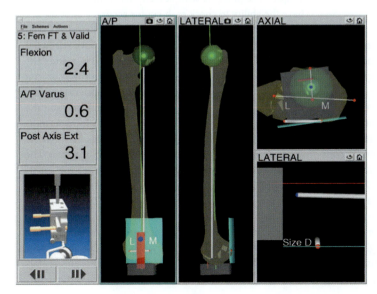

 Fig. 21.3. This screenshot depicts the values obtained after distal femoral resection for flexion, varus-valgus, and rotation

The pointer then is used to identify the most posterior points on the plateau medially and laterally for a more accurate determination of proper tibial rotation. The least involved portions on the plateau medially and laterally are digitized to allow for determination of the natural varus or valgus present at the tibial plateau. An attachment device is impacted into the proximal tibial plateau at the remnant of the anterior cruciate ligament (ACL) insertion site and the UPB is set on the device. The rotation, slope, and varus-valgus orientation are established by positioning the UPB. Once these values are adjusted to the desired positions, the depth of resection is set and drill holes are made through the UPB to allow pin placement. The standard tibial cutting guide then is placed over the pins and the proximal tibia resection is made.

Trials can be placed and the navigation system can evaluate flexion and extension of the knee and overall alignment axis. Again the surgeon can evaluate the soft tissue balancing. The ROM of the knee and overall hip knee ankle alignment can be documented using the system at the time of trial reduction and at the time of final component placement. When a cemented technique is used fine-tuning can be done during cement setup. This allows for further adjustment of varus-valgus alignment and flexion-extension relationships. All of this information can be saved on the system as data points to determine how effectively the deformity was corrected. The pins are removed from the femur and the tibia at the time of wound closure

Results

ORTHOsoft has performed an internal prospective randomized study of 159 patients in 5 European centers, using the Navitrack TotalKnee imageless application, with 83 patients operated with conventional technique compared to 76 patients operated with navigation. This study showed a statistically significant reduction of alignment errors greater than 3 degrees. Overall, 87% of patients operated with navigation had an HKA alignment within 3° compared to 65% of patients operated with conventional surgery (p<0.002). There was an average error of 1.7° between intra-operative displayed measurements compared to the HKA value at 6 months on standing long-leg X-rays.

More recently a study was performed using the Navitrack system to compare the results of a single surgeon using a navigated technique and a standard instrumentation technique [1]. In this study 50 consecutive cases were

performed with the computer and compared to 50 cases performed with standard technique. When the navigation system was used 98% (49/50) of all femoral components were placed within ±3 degrees of the radiographic and clinical goal position and 100% (50/50) of all tibial components were placed within ±3 degrees of 90 degrees for valgus knees and 92 degrees for varus knees relative to tibial anatomic axis. There was a decrease in accuracy in the standard technique group on both the femoral side (five outliers – 90%–45/50, p=0.013) and the tibial side (four outliers – 92%–46/50, p=0.16). There was a similar decrease in accuracy in the standard group for overall tibio-femoral alignment. There were five outliers (45/50–90%) in the computer-assisted group and seven outliers (43/50–86%) in the standard group (p=0.003). There were no complications associated with the trackers in the computer assisted group. The average increase in tourniquet time was 11 minutes in the computer-assisted group.

Discussion and Conclusion

The Navitrack Total Knee imageless application is quick and easy to follow from one step to another. Short animations show key tasks to be performed at each given step. The application aims to streamline the surgical procedure in hopes of adding little time and improving patient outcomes.

The anatomical points that the system requires are simple to acquire. As with other systems the surgeon does have the ability to check each cut for accuracy after the cut is performed. This may minimize the misalignment seen following total knee arthroplasty that some have attributed to movement of pins, inaccuracy in standard jigs, and saw-blade deflection [2–7]. This system does allow the surgeon to choose from three rotation parameters (posterior condylar axis, anterior-posterior axis or Whiteside's line and the epicondylar axis) to make their own decision for determining implant rotation. This information is particularly useful in cases where bony landmarks are damaged or absent. The anterior posterior axis may be of more use for the valgus knee while the posterior condyles may be of more use for a varus knee barring any severe condylar deficiency.

The system does allow for some assessment of soft tissue balancing. After the knee is exposed the surgeon can assess if the coronal deformity is correctable. In a varus knee the surgeon would apply a valgus stress after entering all required anatomical landmarks to see if the deformity will correct. This gives the surgeon the ability make further releases as desired. The surgeon can also place trial components or spacer blocks after performing bone resection and visualize the correction of the deformity on the system. Again, further releases can be made after trials or blocks are placed.

As is the case for most systems, ORTHOsoft's software flow and design has continued to evolve as has its associated instrumentation. Screenshots from the new ORTHO*soft* Knee 2.0 – Universal software application are seen in ◘ Figs. 21.4 and 21.5. This software application allows for more surgeon customization and a more simplified screen display. The actual workstation itself has also evolved to a smaller, more portable unit as seen in ◘ Fig. 21.6. This certainly seems to be the trend for most systems. The actual instrumentation for placement of resections blocks and determining bone resection has also been redesigned in order to fit in smaller exposures as seen in ◘ Fig. 21.7. Efforts are also underway to retrofit

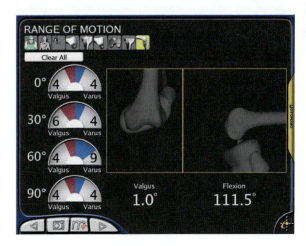

◘ **Fig. 21.4.** The current version of this software allows depiction of pre and post operative range of motion as well as the extent of deformity throughout the range of motion

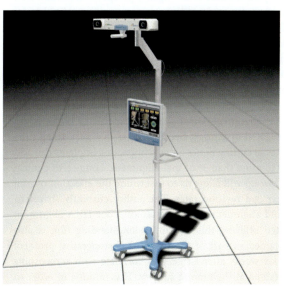

◘ **Fig. 21.6.** The most current system from ORthosoft is smaller and lightweight which allows for easier transportation to different operating room sites

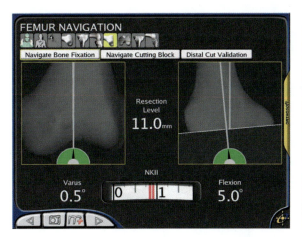

◘ **Fig. 21.5.** Distal femoral resection, varus-valgus position and flexion can all be visualized in a easy to read screenshot with the current software

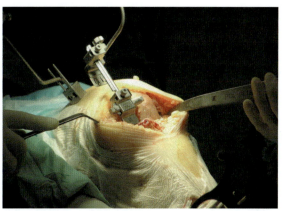

◘ **Fig. 21.7.** Modifications in the instrumentation will allow for navigating total knee arthroplasty with minimally invasive approaches

21

pre-existing instrumentation so that it may be navigated. This would grant surgeons that might be hesitant to part from their standard instrumentation the ability to gain the potential benefits associated with a navigated technique while not being required to abandon familiar instrumentation [1, 8–11].

This system appears to be effective and has been utilized in over 35,000 cases per the company that developed the system. There is an ongoing prospective, randomized multi-center study comparing a computer-assisted technique to a standard technique using this system for implantation of the Natural Knee from Zimmer. This study will enroll over 400 patients and will hopefully further substantiate the system's accuracy, reproducibility, and safety profile.

No system has yet achieved 100% in achieving overall HKA alignment. Once a certain experience is gained on navigated systems, it becomes clear that very small mistakes in cutting bones or even impacting implants can add up to more than 3° of mal-alignment. Long-term clinical follow up will allow us to determine the effect on overall wear and revision rates. The author currently strives to avoid alignment errors outside of 3° for HKA alignment when utilizing this system. A longstanding film is also obtained as part of the standard postoperative protocol at six weeks after surgery to correlate with screenshots obtained at the time of surgery. This in done in order to confirm that the data obtained at the time of surgery continues to correlate with what is seen in the clinic at time of radiographic follow-up.

References

1   Bolognesi MP, Hofmann AA: Computer Navigation versus Standard Instrumentation for TKA: A Single-Surgeon Experience. Clinical Orthopaedics & Related Research. Clin Orthop Relat Res 440:162-169, 2005.

2   Macdonald W, Styf J, Carlsson LV, Jacobsson CM. Improved tibial cutting accuracy in knee arthroplasty. Med Eng Phys. 26(9):807-12, 2004.

3   Toksvig-Larsen S, Ryd L. Surface characteristics following tibial preparation during total knee arthroplasty. J Arthroplasty. 9(1):63-6. 1994.

4   Otani T, Whiteside LA, White SE. Cutting errors in preparation of femoral components in total knee arthroplasty. J Arthroplasty. 8(5):503-10, 1993.

5   Teter KE, Bregman D, Colwell CW: Accuracy of intramedullary versus extramedullary tibial alignment cutting systems in total knee arthroplasty. Clin Orthop 321: 106-10, 1995.

6   Teter KE, Bregman D, Colwell, CW: The efficacy of intramedullary femoral alignment in total knee replacement. Clin Orthop 321: 117-21, 1995.

7   Tillett ED, Engh GA, Petersen T: A comparative study of extramedullary and intramedullary alignment systems in total knee arthroplasty. Clin Orthop 230: 176-81, 1988.

8   Bathis H, Perlick L, Tingart M, Luring C, and Grifka J: CT-free computer-assisted total knee arthroplasty versus the conventional technique: radiographic results of 100 cases. Orthopedics 27(5): 476-80, 2004.

9   Bathis H, Perlick L, Tingart M, Luring C, Perlick, C, et al: Radiological results of image-based and non-image-based computer-assisted total knee arthroplasty. Int Orthop 28(2):87-90, 2004.

10 Hart R, Janecek M, Chaker A, Bucek, P: Total knee arthroplasty implanted with and without kinematic navigation. Int Orthop 27(6): 366-9, 2003.

11 Sparmann M, Wolke B, Czupalla H, Banzer D, Zink A: Positioning of total knee arthroplasty with and without navigation support. A prospective, randomised study. J Bone Joint Surg Br 85(6): 830-5, 2003.

Navigated Total Knee Arthroplasty with the Fluoroscopic Medtronic System

J. Victor

Introduction

Total knee arthroplasty has become a predictable and reliable surgical procedure.

Correct positioning of the components is a key factor in this success. Component mal-position can cause pain [14], limited range of motion [6], instability [22], polyethylene wear and loosening of the implant [11, 30]. In the earlier days of total knee arthroplasty, much attention was given to the correction of limb alignment as the detrimental effects of remaining mal-alignment were obvious and well documented, both clinically [1, 2, 11, 13, 16, 22– 24, 28, 33, 37] and bio-mechanically [3, 12, 15].

With the improvement in surgical training and better instrumentation systems, correct positioning of the components evolved to a routine procedure. Over the last decade, alignment issues received less attention in the orthopaedic literature, but remains a threat to the patient undergoing TKA.

A round table and multi-centre evaluation of the French orthopedic community concluded that 31% of the patients with major pre-operative coronal mal-alignment displayed a deviation of the mechanical axis of more than 5° post-operatively.[7]

Jeffery et al. [17] noted good post-operative coronal alignment (mechanical axis deviation of less than 3°) in 2/3 of their total knee arthroplasties. In 1/3 of the operated knees, mechanical axis deviation in the coronal plane was found. These knees had a mechanical loosening rate of 24% at eight years, as opposed to 3% mechanical loosening for normally aligned knees.

Sharkey et al. [30] showed recently that mal-alignment and mal-position of components still play a significant role in the failure mechanism of modern knee prostheses. A new factor was recently introduced. Increasing interest in minimally invasive surgery (MIS) dramatically reduced the surgical exposure. Surgeons undergo pressure from peers, industry and patients to follow this new trend [8]. The reduction of the surgical exposure limits the ability of the surgeon to find the usual anatomic landmarks that are used for component positioning. Also, as the soft tissues are less spread, positioning and fixation of the cutting blocks can be tedious. It is clear that MIS carries the risk of increased surgical error, even in the hands of experienced surgeons.

Computer assisted surgery was developed before the big wave of MIS hit the orthopaedic community. Two mainstream technologies prevailed: image-less CAS and image-based CAS, the latter being most often combined with fluoroscopy in total knee surgery. The typical characteristic of image based CAS is that the system can create the spatial link between the image and the anatomical landmarks, the defined virtual points, planes and axes. This extra information under the form of a fluoroscopic image allows the surgeon to double check the information relating to the important reference planes and axes. However, these systems do have a significant disadvantage. The image intensifier is an alien tool in total knee arthroplasty. It is bulky, needs draping and poses a potential risk for microbiological contamination. It also increases surgical time and carries a potential radiation hazard. The image-less systems do not have these disadvantages: they are cheaper, easier to use, less bulky, and create no radiation hazard.

22

Both image-less and image-based systems have been evaluated and results of prospective randomized trials showed better coronal and sagittal alignment for the patients operated with CAS than for patients operated with conventional instruments [5, 9, 31, 36]

With the help of a fluoroscopy based CAS system we assessed two variables. We checked the accuracy of the calculation of the kinematic centre of rotation of the hip and compared the outcome between the patients that underwent TKA with and without image based computer assistance [36].

Materials and Methods

A total of 100 patients were included. Randomization was performed in permutation blocks of four. The study was performed on a consecutive series of primary TKA's where every operating day included two conventional and two CAS cases.

Pre-operative assessment included IKS knee and function score, measurement of range of motion (ROM) and radiological examination including digital standing full leg films, antero-posterior (AP), lateral, skyline and condylar radiographs (Philips easyvision 4.2). All patients were operated using a standardized operative technique. The prosthesis used was the Genesis II* (Smith & Nephew Inc., Memphis, Tn), in a cruciate retaining or posterior stabilized version. All patients underwent resurfacing of the patella and all components were cemented. In the conventional group, extra-medullary alignment jigs were used on the tibia and intra-medullary jigs on the femur. The full leg standing films were used for pre-operative planning. The angle between the femoral mechanical axis (FMA) and femoral anatomical axis (FAA) was calculated and used on the distal femoral cutting jig. In the CAS group, a fluoroscopy based spatial navigation device, using active and passive reference frames (hardware: iON*, Medtronic SNT, Louisville CO – software: FluoroKnee, Smith & Nephew, Memphis, TN & Medtronic SNT, Louisville, CO) was used. This system includes the use of a fluoroscopic C-arm with a calibration frame to allow for positional calibration of the fluoroscopic image. A touch screen was positioned on the side of the operating table and covered with a sterile transparent plastic bag to allow the surgeon to control the software (Fig. 22.1). In order to obtain ideal stability for the kinematic determination of the centre of the hip, the patient was stabilized on

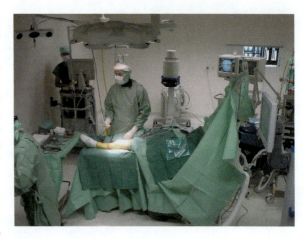

 Fig. 22.1. Operating theatre set-up with fluoroscopic C-arm and touch screen

the operating table using two padded posts, positioned against the iliac crests. No reference frame was attached to the iliac crest. Dual, bicortical pin fixation was chosen to eliminate the potential of insufficient rotational stability of the reference frame and to allow the frames to be positioned outside of the operating field.

At the beginning of the procedure a calibration shot was made with the C-Arm and all instruments were validated. The fluoroscopic images were acquired (AP and ¾ of the hip, AP and lateral of the knee, AP and lateral of the ankle) and labeled. The limb was then moved in a circular fashion to obtain exact definition of the spherical motion that was described by the femoral reference frame. The computer calculated the kinematic centre of rotation and positioned this calculated centre on the obtained fluoroscopic image of the hip.

The surgical approach was identical as for the conventional group. The intra-articular reference points in the knee and the medial and lateral malleolus were defined with the use of a pointer with passive reflecting spheres. The femoral mechanical axis and the tibial mechanical axis were shown on the image and the coronal alignment of the limb was computed and stored.

The bone cuts were made on femur and tibia, based upon the positional information given by the computer system. The resurfacing of the patella was performed using traditional, standard instrumentation. With the trials in place, maximum extension and flexion, and the final coronal plane alignment were determined and noted. The final components were cemented and the tourniquet released.

Hemostasis, wound closure and rehabilitation protocol were identical for both groups.

At six weeks, the patients were seen in the clinic and standard digital radiographs (AP, lateral, skyline) and digital full leg standing X-rays were obtained. All standard X-rays were made using fluoroscopic control for achieving correct orientation in the lateral and coronal plane. In those patients who did not yet achieve full extension at six weeks, the full leg standing X-ray was taken at three months post-operatively. At this stage, International Knee Society (IKS) scores and range of motion measurement was performed on all patients.

On the fluoroscopic images of the hip with the superimposed calculated kinematic centre of rotation that were obtained during surgery, the distance between the anatomic centre of the hip and the calculated centre of rotation was measured for every patient (■ Fig. 22.2). Angles of femoral and tibial component position were noted on AP and lateral X-Rays. The reference on the lateral radiograph was the posterior tibial cortex for the tibial component and the posterior femoral cortex for the femoral component. Overall mechanical coronal alignment was measured on the full leg standing X-rays.

Results

The intra-operative coronal alignment values, as computed during surgery by the CAS system before any bone cuts were made, and the measured pre-operative coronal alignments on the full leg standing films were plotted against each other and are displayed in ■ Fig. 22.3.

The mean distance between the computed kinematic centre of rotation and the anatomic centre of the femoral head was 1.6 mm (range 0–5 mm, standard deviation 1.46). The mean angular mistake on the femoral mechanical axis was 0.19° (range 0–0.71°).

The tourniquet time was longer in the CAS group than in the conventional group (72 min versus 60 min, $p<0.0005$) as was the skin-to-skin time: 93 min versus 73 min ($p<0.0001$). The mechanical axis in the coronal plane was divided into three groups: 0°–2°, 3°–4°, and >4°. In the CAS group all knees (N=49) scored within 0°–2°. In the conventional group (N=48), 73.5% of the knees fell within 0°–2°, and 26.5% within 3°–4°. No knees displayed a mechanical axis deviation of more than 4° (■ Fig. 22.4). The difference in variance between the CAS and the Conventional groups is significant: p (Fisher's exact test) <0.0001. That means that the post-operative alignment in the conventional group tends to be more variable than the post-operative alignment the CAS group.

IKS Knee score at three months post-operatively was 86 in the conventional group versus 87 in the CAS group.

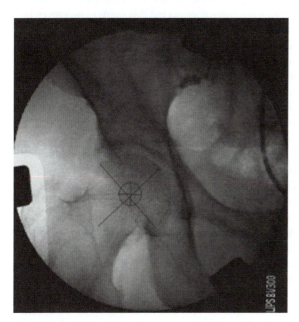

■ **Fig 22.2.** Kinematic centre of the hip as calculated from mathematical algorithm (centre of small circle). The crossing of the two black lines represents the anatomic centre of the hip

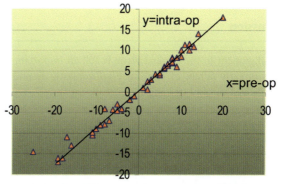

■ **Fig. 22.3.** Plot of the pre-operative coronal alignment measurements on full leg standing radiographs (X axis) versus the intra-operative coronal alignment measurement by the image based CAS system (Y axis). Positive angular values represent mechanical axis varus alignment, negative angular values represent mechanical axis valgus alignment. Pearson correlation index R=0.987

22

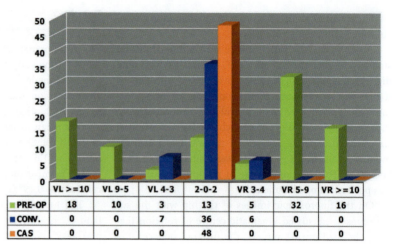

	VL >=10	VL 9-5	VL 4-3	2-0-2	VR 3-4	VR 5-9	VR >=10
PRE-OP	18	10	3	13	5	32	16
CONV.	0	0	7	36	6	0	0
CAS	0	0	0	48	0	0	0

Fig. 22.4. Distribution of pre-operative, conventional post-operative and CAS post-operative mechanical alignment, as measured on full leg standing films

IKS function score was 68 at three months post-operatively in both groups.

Mean flexion at three months was 116 (100–125) in the conventional group versus 114 (90–125) in the CAS group. Fixed flexion contracture was present pre-operatively to an extent of >10° in 4 patients, 5°–9° in 49 patients and <5°, in 44 patients. Post-operatively this was reduced in the conventional group to 1 patient, 7 patients and 41 patients, respectively, and in the CAS group to 0 patients, 4 patients and 44 patients, respectively (Table 22.1).

Mean fluoroscopy time was 21 s (9–34 s), corresponding with a mean radiation of 0.19 Gy/cm^2.

Discussion

Mal-alignment in the coronal plane is still an important cause of early failure of total knee arthroplasty, despite of improved surgical training and instrumentation [7, 17, 26, 30].

The cause of post-operative mal-alignment is most often incorrect bone cuts. The error in performing this bone cut can be analyzed into a *'reference error'* and a *'execution error'*. Conventional instrumentation uses bony references (anatomical landmarks) or ligament references. Reference errors with anatomical landmarks occur because the references are not visible (as with the femoral head), are virtual in nature (as with the femoral mechanical axis) or are variable (dysplasia, bowing of long bones, morphotype variability). The recent popularity of less in-

vasive exposures for total knee arthroplasty will certainly not decrease the incidence of reference errors. Ligament referencing is not an alternative for this problem and will avoid these mistakes as the tibial bone cut is used as a base reference and because the ligaments as such may be shortened or damaged during surgery.

One might assume that the use of computer assistance will rule out surgical errors but this needs to be proven in controlled trials. The *total error* in CAS TKA will consist of the sum of the *camera error,* the *algorithm error,* and the *'execution error'*. The latter will be similar to the situation with conventional instrumentation and is caused by displacement of the blocks during pinning or sawblade inaccuracy. The advantage of CAS is that block displacement can be detected prior to cutting and that the bone cut can be checked afterwards.

The *camera error* and *algorithm error* are specific for the hard- and software used and were subject of this study. The first aim was to assess the accuracy of the kinematic determination of the centre of rotation of the hip. Many navigation systems are used in current orthopedic practice today and most of them use a mathematical algorithm to define this centre. Several in vitro tests have been carried out, mainly by the manufactures but little was published on the clinical performance [36].

The set-up of this study allowed to do this as both kinematic and spatially linked radiographic data were available. The accuracy was excellent. The mean deviation between kinematic and radiographic centre was 1.6 mm (range 0–5 mm). The second arm of the described study was a differential outcome analysis between the two groups. The limits of this study lie in the use of full leg standing radiographs as an outcome tool for measuring alignment. Full leg radiographs are far more reliable for measuring coronal alignment than the 14×17inch films that are often used for this purpose [20, 32], the reason being that the angle between the femoral mechanical and femoral anatomical axis is variable [35]. One needs to see the femoral head before the femoral mechanical axis can be accurately determined. Full leg radiographs have been used in previous studies [29] without correlation between the pre-operative measured values and the intra-operative computed values.

We were able to validate the use of full leg standing radiographs for measuring coronal alignment in this study. The measured value on the film was compared to the computed intra-operative value, before the bone cuts were made. The figures matched exactly (1° or less) for 82% of the knees, as witnessed by the correlation index (◘ Fig. 22.3). Only 2 knees had a mismatch of more than 3 degrees between the measured pre-operative value and the calculated intra-operative value. These patients had severe pre-operative fixed flexion contracture (>15°), explaining the inaccuracy of the pre-operative full leg standing radiograph. As these fixed flexion contractures were corrected after surgery, one can conclude that the post-operative full leg radiographs were reliable for measuring post-operative coronal alignment.

Image-based navigation systems are often criticized because they are more cumbersome to use, take more space and time and carry a radiation hazard. However, the additional visual information provides extra control during the procedure (◘ Fig. 22.5). Every reference point for

◘ **Table 22.1.** Demographic data and pre-operative distribution of variables

	CAS		Conventional	
	mean	range	mean	range
Age [years]	72	56–85	70	40–83
Weight [kg]	76	50–102	78	52–92
Length [m]	1.64	150–176	1.64	149–178
Male/Female	13/37		13/37	
Varus/Valgus	29/21		32/18	
Deformity [°mech. axis]	8.4	0–16	7.5	0–19
Flexion	110	80–120	111	90–125
Ext. Deficit	16	10–20	17	10–20
PS/CR	18/30		23/26	

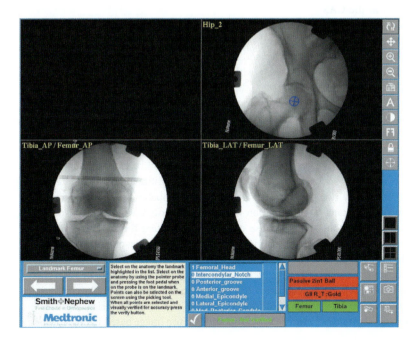

◘ **Fig. 22.5.** Typical screen shot showing the femoral head and a AP and Lateral view of the knee joint. Real time appearance of instruments on the knee image is available during surgery.

coronal and sagittal alignment can be double checked on the screen. This extra control reassures the surgeon who does not like to follow blindly the computer information. The benefit is shown in our results positioning every single patient within the ideal coronal alignment. Previous studies on imageless systems did not report equally good results. Saragaglia et al. [29] took a wider error margin (0–3°) and scored within this margin for 84% of the knees that were operated with computer assistance (Orthopilot®, Braun Aesculap, Tuttlingen). Two out of twenty-five knees were »big« outliers: 5° varus and 7° valgus in the mechanical axis. In the conventional group the results are comparable to ours: they reported 75% of the knees the 0–3° margin, versus 73.5% within 0–2° for our series. Mielke et al. [25] compared 30 navigated cases (Orthopilot®) to 30 matched patients that were treated conventionally. In the CAS group they reported 61.7% within 0–2°. 6.7% in this group had a deviation of more than 4°. Two knees were »big« outliers: 5° and 7°varus. In the conventional group, 10% of the knees displayed a deviation of more than 4°. Jenny and Boeri [18] compared 40 navigated cases (Orthopilot®) against 40 matched conventional cases. The error margin was defined between 0–3°. 95% of the CAS knees scored within this range, versus 85% of the conventional knees. Bäthis et al. [5] performed a randomized trial on 160 patients with the Brainlab Vector Vision® system and achieved good mechanical alignment in the coronal plane (0–3°) for 97% of the patients in the CAS group versus 74% in the conventional group

Sparmann et al. [31] studied the outcome of the use of an imageless navigation system (Stryker Howmedica Osteonics, Allendale, New Jersey) prospectively on a big cohort of 120 navigated cases versus a control group of 120 conventional cases. 97.5% (117/120) in the CAS group displayed a mechanical alignment between 0–2°, versus 77.5% (93/120) in the conventional group. The CAS group had no outliers greater than 3°.

Image-based CAS systems turn out to be particularly interesting in combination with MIS.

CAS systems contribute to the nature of MIS by not using an intra-medullary rod. The intra-medullary canal is not violated. Although we have not been able to demonstrate significantly less blood loss, other authors have done so [21]. Also, the risk of pulmonary complication decreases. In addition, evaluation of stability and ligament balance is possible and can be compared to reference values [34].

With the reduction of the surgical exposure in MIS, anatomical landmarks are harder to locate. Especially

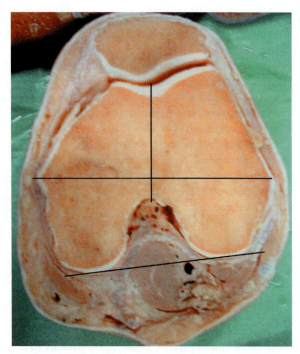

Fig. 22.6. Rotational landmarks of the knee shown on a cross section of the distal femur. Location of these landmarks is easier on a CAT image than on the knee in vivo

the lateral tibial plateau, the posterior part of the femoral condyles and the epicondyles can not be pinpointed as accurately with MIS than with a conventional exposure (□ Fig. 22.6). In imageless systems, location of these reference points is mandatory and is a main determinant for the accuracy of the procedure. It is our fear that accuracy of imageless CAS systems will decrease if used in combination with MIS. Image-based systems have the great advantage that reference points can be chosen or controlled on the X-ray images. This additional information can be extremely valuable and is probably the best way to go in combination with a radical reduction of the exposure.

The use of fluoroscopy offers the advantage of real-time acquisition and virtual merge of the images with reality, as the reference frames are in place at the time that the picture is taken. On the other hand, this real-time acquisition has an important downside: it takes operating time and poses a wound contamination risk. A possible way to avoid this and still use image based CAS is to work

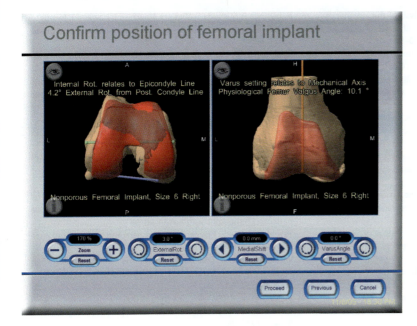

■ **Fig. 22.7.** Virtual imaging of femoral implant in CAT-based CAS application with control of rotational alignment (Brainlab system)

with previously taken images. This technique demands matching of image and reality at the time of surgery. With the use of CAT images this can done. The CAT scan can be made prior to surgery and the operative procedure can be performed virtually (■ Fig. 22.7). The reliability and accuracy of this technique has been demonstrated in a cadaver [27] and in a clinical setting [4]. The added value of CAT for rotational alignment of the femoral component cannot be underestimated. Experimental and clinical studies have shown that there is great inter- and intra-observer variability in the definition of the rotational landmarks. [10,19] The additional information of the CAT data can be of great help, especially in complicated cases with pre-existing congenital or acquired deformities.

Conclusion

There is ample evidence in the literature that computer assistance reduces the incidence of outliers in coronal and sagittal alignment after TKA. In general, the accuracy of image-based systems is a little higher, probably because of the availability of a visual »double check« by the surgeon. We have shown in our study that it is feasible to work with a real time fluoroscopy based technology and

that alignment results are excellent in the coronal and sagittal plane.

The main downsides of image-based systems are irradiation and time issues. This explains why those systems have not been widely accepted in the orthopaedic community. With the advent of minimally invasive surgical exposures for knee arthroplasty it will be more difficult to ensure correct positioning of the implants. Image-based systems offer the greatest added value in these conditions. Despite of the current limitations and draw-backs, 3D image-based technology holds the promise of break-through in our operating theatres.

References

1. Agglietti P et al. (1988) Posteriorly stabilised total condylar knee replacement: three to eight years follow-up on 85 knees. J Bone Joint Surg Br 70: 211–216
2. Bargren JH et al.. (1983) Alignment in total knee arthroplasty. Clin Orthop 173:178–183
3. Bartel DL et al. (1982) Performance of the tibial component in total knee replacement. J Bone Joint Surg Am 64: 1026
4. Bäthi L, Tingart M, Lüring C, Zurakowski D, Grifka J (2004) Alignment in total knee arthroplasty. A comparison of computer assisted surgery with the conventional technique. J Bone Joint Surg 86-B: 982–987

5. Bellemans J et al. (2002) Fluoroscopic analysis of the kinematics of deep flexion in total knee arthroplasty. Influence of posterior condylar offset. J Bone Joint Surg Br 84/1: 50–53

6. Brilhaut J et al. (2003) Prothèse totale de genou et grandes déviations axiales. Les Annales Orthopédiques de l'Ouest 35: 253–288

7. Callaghan JJ (2005) Internet promotion of MIS and CAOS in TKA by members of the Knee Society. Presented at the Knee Society Interim Meeting, NY

8. Chauhan SK, Scott RG, Breidahl W, Beaver RJ (2004) Computer-assisted knee arthroplasty versus a conventional jig-based technique. J Bone Joint Surg 86-B: 372–377

9. Fuiko R, Kotten B, Zettl R, Ritschl P (2004) The accuracy of palpation from orientation points for the navigated implantation of knee prostheses. Orthopäde 33: 338–343

10. Gibbs AN et al. (1979) A comparison of the Freeman-Swanson (ICLH) and Walldius prostheses in total knee replacement. J Bone Joint Surg Br 61: 358

11. Green GV et al. (2002) The effects of varus tibial alignment on proximal tibial surface strain in total knee arthroplasty. J Arthroplasty 17: 1033–1039

12. Hamilton LR (1982) UCI total knee replacement: a follow-up study. J Bone Joint Surg Am 64: 740–744

13. Hofmann S et al. (2003) Rotational malalignment of the components may cause chronic pain or early failure in total knee arthroplasty. Orthopade 32(6): 469–476

14. Hsu HP et al. (1989) Effect of knee component alignment on tibial load distribution with clinical correlation. Clin Orthop 248: 135–144

15. Insall JI et al. (1979) The total condylar knee prosthesis: a report on two hundred and twenty cases. J Bone Joint Surg Am 61: 173–180

16. Jeffery RS et al. (1991) Coronal alignment after total knee replacement. J Bone Joint Surg Br 73: 709–714

17. Jenny JY et al. (2001) Computer-assisted implantation of a total knee arthroplasty: a case-controlled study in comparison with classical instrumentation. Rev Chir Orthop Reparatrice Appar Mot 87: 645–652

18. Jenny JY, Boeri C (2004) Low reproducibility of the intra-operative measurement of the transepicondylar axis during total knee replacement. Acta Orthop Scand 75: 74–77

19. Jessup DE et al. (1997) Restoration of limb alignment in total knee arthroplasty: evaluation and methods. J Southern Orthop Ass 6: 37–47

20. Kalairajah Y, Simpson D, Cossey AJ, Verall GM, Spriggins AJ (2005) Blood loss after total knee replacement: effects of computer-assisted surgery. J Bone Joint Surg Br 87:1480–1482

21. Kumar PJ et al. (1997) Severe malalignment and soft-tissue imbalance in total knee arthroplasty. Am J Knee Surg 10: 36–41

22. Laskin RS (1990) Total condylar knee replacement in patients who have rheumatoid arthritis. A ten year follow-up study. J Bone Joint Surg Am 72: 529–535

23. Lotke PA et al. (1977) Influence of positioning of prosthesis in total knee replacement. J Bone Joint Surg Am 59: 77–79

24. Mielke RK et al. (2001) Navigation in knee endoprosthesis implantation – Preliminary experience and prospective comparative study in comparison with conventional technique. Z Orthop Ihre Grenzgeb 139: 109–116

25. Moreland JR et al. (1987) Radiographic analysis of the axial alignment of the lower extremity. J Bone Joint Surg Am 69: 745–749

26. Nabeyama R, Matsuda S, Miura H, Mawatari T, Kawano T, Iwamoto Y (2004) The accuracy of image-guided knee replacement based on CT. J Bone Joint Surg Br 86: 366–371

27. Ritter MA et al. (1994) Postoperative alignment of total knee replacement. Clin Orthop 299: 153–156

28. Saragaglia D et al. (2001) Computer assisted knee arthroplasty: comparison with a conventional procedure. Results of 50 cases in a prospective randomized study. Rev Chir Orthop Reparatrice Appar Mot 87: 18–28

29. Sharkey PF et al. (2002) Why are total knee arthroplasties failing today? Clin Orthop 404: 7–13

30. Sparmann M et al. (2003) Positioning of total knee arthroplasty with and without navigation support. A prospective, randomised study. J Bone Joint Surg Br 85/6: 830–835

31. Stulberg SD et al. (2002) Computer-assisted navigation in total knee replacement: results of an initial experience in thirty-five patients. J Bone Joint Surg Am 84: 90–98

32. Tew M et al. (1985) Tibiofemoral alignment and the results of knee replacement. J Bone Joint Surg Br 67: 551–556

33. Vandamme G et al. (2005) What should the surgeon aim for when performing computer-assisted knee arthroplasty? J Bone Joint Surg, 87A: 52–58

34. Victor J et al.. (1994) Femoral intramedullary instrumentation in total knee arthroplasty: the role of pre-operative X-ray analysis. Knee 1: 123–125

35. Victor J et al.. (2004) Computer-assisted surgery: image-based computer-assisted total knee arthroplasty leads to lower variability in coronal alignment. Clin Orthop 428: 131–139

36. Windsor RE et al. (1989) Mechanisms of failure of the femoral and tibial components in total knee arthroplasty. Clin Orthop 248: 15–19

Computer-Assisted Ligament Balancing of the Femoral Tibial Joint Using Pressure Sensors

R.C. Wasielewski, R.D. Komistek

Introduction

Many variables contribute to successful total knee arthroplasty (TKA) including patient factors, implant design, and surgical technique. Patient factors, such as bone quality, weight, compliance, and activity level, are difficult to mitigate. Implant design factors that optimize implant longevity (such as large contact areas and high conformity) have been defined and implemented. But surgical technique has been more difficult to quantitatively evaluate because it is more subjective and surgeon dependent. Consequently, advances in surgical technique that lead to improved implant longevity have been difficult to define. Soft-tissue balancing requires correct limb alignment and simultaneous release of contracted ligaments around the knee. When balance is optimized, medial and lateral compartment pressures should be approximately equal. However, an easy and accurate method of measuring these pressures has been difficult to develop. To address this issue, an intra-operative, computer-instrumented tibial insert trial that measures knee compartment pressures through a passive range of motion was developed [1]. Results from this sensor help quantify ligament balancing. It is then possible to compare compartment balance with what the surgeon feels and with postoperative kinematic function. Real-time evaluation of ligament balancing via measurement of compartment pressures may allow surgeons to better optimize implant function and longevity. It may also lead to a better understanding of polyethylene bearing wear on TKA retrievals [2, 3].

Materials and Methods

Thirty-eight patients with knee osteoarthritis (OA) underwent a posterior cruciate sacrificing (non-ps) LCS total knee arthroplasty (TKA) by the same surgeon (Dr. Ray Wasielewski) using a »balanced gap« technique. This technique involves using an extra-medullary alignment jig to cut the tibia perpendicular to its long axis. The knee compartments were balanced in extension with appropriate ligament releases. The knee was then flexed, and a rectangular flexion gap was created by rotating the femoral cutting guide about a femoral intra-medullary guide until parallel to the cut tibia. The flexion gap dimension was measured, and the distal femur was cut to create an extension gap of the same size. With gaps of equal size and dimension in both flexion and extension, the final femoral and tibial preparations were made.

After placement of the femoral and tibial baseplate trial implants on the cut bone surfaces, a computer-instrumented tibial insert trial was placed. This device measures pressures within the compartments of the knee using an FDA approved pressure-sensing matrix array (Novel® Electronics, Inc., Munich, Germany) that is incorporated into a TKA trial polyethylene insert (◘ Fig. 23.1). After the sensing device was placed in the knee, the quadriceps mechanism was re-approximated with three sutures. With trials and sensor in place, the knee was taken through a passive range of motion from 0 to 120 degrees. The magnitude and distribution of medial and lateral compartment pressures were documented throughout this range while video footage was gathered (◘ Fig. 23.2).

Computer-generated pressure nomograms were created from data gathered by the intra-operative pressure sensor for all thirty-eight patients enrolled in the study. These nomograms provided information on force (N), area of force distribution (cm^2), and pressure (N/cm^2) in both the medial and lateral knee compartments in flexion and extension. Differences in pressure magnitude and distribution between the medial and lateral compartments were appreciated from the pressure nomograms. When pressures were greater in one compartment compared with the other or when contact areas were not equal, knees were presumed to be unbalanced.

Optimal compartment pressures, between 10–40 N/cm^2, appeared blue on the pressure nomograms. High pressures of greater than 130 N/cm^2 and greater than 160 N/cm^2 appeared red and pink, respectively.

To subjectively assess compartment balance, the surgeon performed intra-operative stress testing at 0, 15, 60, and 90 degrees. After the pressure data were obtained and the stress testing was complete, the device was removed from the knee and the arthroplasty was completed. Data from the pressure sensors were compared with stress testing to establish correlations.

Post-operative mechanical axis radiographs were obtained for all patients. Sixteen patients agreed to undergo deep knee bend kinematic analysis at three months post arthroplasty. Correlation of the intra-operative compartment pressure data to the occurrence of liftoff during deep knee bend and the influence of the mechanical axis were determined. Also, pressure patterns observed intra-operatively were compared to wear patterns on archived retrievals. These data in combination show the influence of good ligament balance on kinematic function and possibly insert wear.

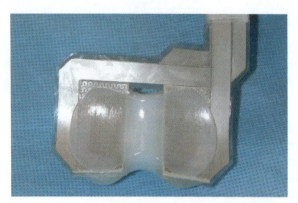

◼ **Fig. 23.1.** The pressure-sensing device is a modification of a Novel pressure matrix array attached to the upper surface of a tibial polyethylene insert trial. It is sandwiched between the insert trial and a protective low molecular weight polyethylene covering

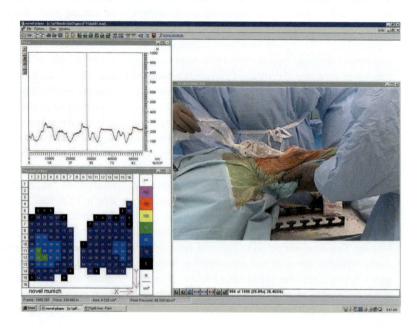

◼ **Fig. 23.2.** An intra-operative sensor data shows force and pressure measurements and video footage for a knee in extension. This knee is well balanced in extension; the sensor shows similar pressure and area measurements for the medial and lateral compartments

Results

Nine of the thirty-eight patients had maximum pressures in the red and pink ranges (>130 N/cm^2 and >160 N/cm^2). Six patients had maximum pressures in these ranges in extension and three in flexion. Five patients had a pattern of increased pressure in the anteromedial aspect of the medial compartment in extension (Fig. 23.3). All of these patients had extensive surgical release of the superficial and deep medial collateral ligaments (MCL), leaving the dynamic pes muscle insertions intact to medially stabilize the knee in extension. All five had pressures greater than 100 N/cm^2, and one patient had a maximum pressure greater than 150 N/cm^2. No patient with this pattern experienced loss of pressure in one or both compartments with early flexion (15–30 degrees), nor did any patient enrolled in this study (i.e., no patient experienced midstance instability). The posterior and medial insertions of the semi-membranosus muscle was never violated.

For every case that the surgeon detected a compartment imbalance during intra-operative stress testing, the sensor revealed a similar compartment pressure imbalance and/or abnormality. In addition, the sensors detected subclinical compartment abnormalities not detected by the surgeon in twelve cases – four in extension (0 degrees) and eight in flexion (90 degrees).

Condylar liftoff correlated with sensor pressure distributions for the sixteen patients undergoing fluoroscopic kinematic analysis. Of the sixteen patients, three had femoral condylar liftoff – one in extension (at 0 degrees) and two in flexion (at 90 degrees). For all three patients, the sensor detected a compartment pressure imbalance at the same joint angle that liftoff occurred. All three patients with medial compartment condylar liftoff had less pressure in the medial compartment relative to the lateral (p=0.05 for patients with liftoff in flexion (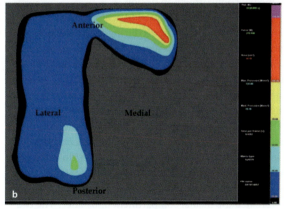 Fig. 23.4); p=0.125 for patient with liftoff in extension (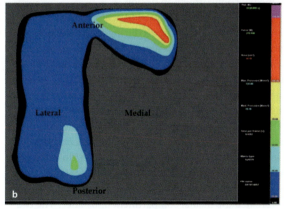 Fig. 23.5), fisher exact test).

Liftoff was 1.01 mm for the patient with liftoff in extension. During TKA, the surgeon noted that this patient's medial compartment was loose in extension, presumably owing to slight over-release of the MCL. Postoperatively, mechanical axis alignment was two degrees of valgus.

One of the two patients with liftoff in flexion had 0.97 mm of liftoff at ninety degrees. During TKA, the surgeon noted looseness in the medial compartment and tightness in the lateral compartment when the knee was flexed. Slight over-rotation of the femoral implant prob-

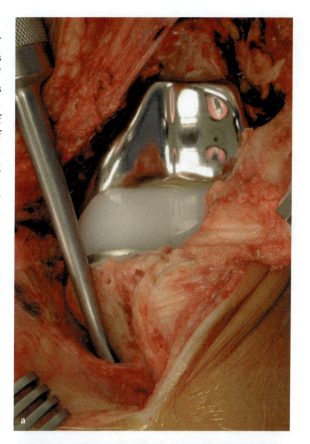

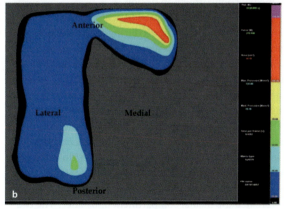

Fig. 23.3. a Knee with implants in place. The superficial medial collateral ligament has been elevated, and the pes anserinus musculature remains. The Cobb elevator shows where the superficial MCL has been taken off the bone, and anterior to this, the pes insertion can be seen. **b** The corresponding pressure nomogram for a knee in extension shows higher pressures anteriorly and medially secondary to the dynamic stabilizers still being in place and creating increased pressure

23

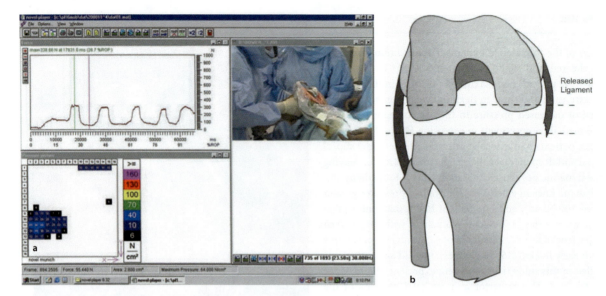

Fig. 23.4. a The intra-operative sensor data for a knee in flexion shows no pressure in the medial compartment. **b** The corresponding schematic demonstrates over-release of the medial collateral ligament with loss of pressure in the medial component with flexion. In this situation, less bone is taken from the posterior medial condyle than from the lateral, resulting in femoral component internal rotation

ably caused this flexion imbalance. For the other patient with liftoff in flexion, liftoff was 1.08 mm at ninety degrees. This patient's pressure nomogram displayed normal pressures in the lateral compartment and no pressures in the medial compartment in flexion.

None of the other thirteen patients exhibited more than 1.0 mm of condylar liftoff during fluoroscopic kinematic analysis. The sensors detected similar compartment pressures throughout the range of motion in nine of these patients but compartment pressure imbalances in the other four (two in extension and two in flexion). One of the two patients with an extension imbalance without liftoff had less pressure in the medial compartment; the other had less pressure in the lateral compartment. In both cases, mechanical alignment was such as to close the lax compartment with weight-bearing. On the other hand, in the one case of liftoff in extension, slight valgus alignment exacerbated the medial compartment imbalance. The two patients with flexion imbalances without liftoff had less pressure in the medial compartment. A mechanical axis or rotational abnormality was not apparent in either of these patients.

Several pathognomonic compartment pressure distributions were associated with balancing. When an extensive medial release was done to address a severe varus de-formity, the superficial and deep MCL and the proximal 1 cm of the semi-membranosus were released but the pes musculature (dynamic medial stabilizers) was retained. This left a characteristic anterior medial tightness on the nomogram (Fig. 23.3b). Over-release of the MCL or over-rotation of the femur left decreased pressure areas medially in flexion (Fig. 23.4b).

Many of the intra-operative pressure distributions were similar to patterns of wear on retrieved inserts in archive (Figs. 23.6 and 23.7). Carbon poly inserts are shown because they more clearly demonstrate the wear patterns seen on all types of inserts.

Discussion

Other attempts have been made to measure knee compartment pressures with some success. Takahashi et al. [4] reported improved varus-valgus stability with intra-operative assessment of compartment pressures using pressure-sensitive film and sequential ligament releases based upon the resultant stress pattern. Wallace et al. [5] were able to balance compartment pressures via PCL release after quantifying knee compartment pressures with an electronic pressure transducer. Morris et al. [6] re-

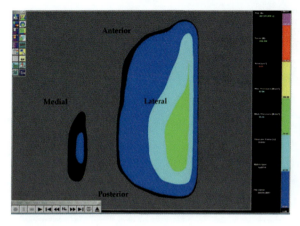

Fig. 23.5. A pressure nomogram displays a loose medial compartment in extension. Good pressures, areas, and distribution appear in the lateral compartment

ported the use of an instrumented tibial component with transducing load cells located between the tibial tray and polyethylene insert. The device used in the present study has several advantages over these previous pressure-sensing devices. The Novel® sensor matrix array was highly conformable to curved articular surfaces. This enabled placement of the transducers within the insert surface equidistant from the femoral implant counter-surface. This increased the sensitivity of the device in measuring contact areas and pressure distributions. In addition, the device allowed real-time feedback of both absolute and relative compartment pressure data.

The device's computerized pressure outputs provide the surgeon quantitative feedback on gap balance and ligament tension. After calibration, the device was capable of measuring absolute force and pressure values. But the absolute pressures measured by the device are probably different from those that will occur in vivo post-operatively. The final components will be subjected to the patient's weight and musculature and to loading conditions with daily living activities [7]. Thus, the device likely functions as a relative measure of in vivo pressure differences, providing the surgeon with additional insight into the adequacy of knee balance, component position, and alignment.

In all cases, the instrumented insert successfully measured compartment pressures throughout the range of motion during trialing. Intra-operative varus and valgus stress testing with the sensing device in place confirmed that real-time increases and decreases in compartment pressures were being detected. In every case that surgeon stress testing detected a compartment imbalance, the sensors also recorded a compartment pressure imbalance and/or abnormality. In addition, the sensors detected twelve cases (eight in flexion and four in extension) of subclinical compartment abnormalities not appreciated with stress testing. Thus, the pressure readings were more sensitive than surgeon feel, especially in flexion, where variables including tourniquet placement, patient size, and stability of setup can make qualitative assessment of ligament balance difficult.

The sensors provided important pressure nomogram data depicting contact area patterns and pressure differences between the compartments. In all patients, the contact areas were relatively large, which corroborated the theoretical advantages of the mobile-bearing knee (a highly conforming articulation of large contact areas and low stresses [8]). Decreased contact areas in extension were most commonly due to over-release medially or from pathological medial or lateral laxities (e.g., valgus and varus knees, respectively). The most common cause of decreased area in flexion was over-release medially in extension, causing a slight concomitant medial laxity in flexion. Additionally, in some cases, slight femoral component over-rotation resulted in decreased area in the medial compartment in flexion. This slight femoral component over-rotation may be attributed to the use of the tensor to balance the knee in flexion. When using the balanced gap technique, the tensor applies pressure to the compartments of the knee in flexion and the AP cutting guide rotates about an intra-medullary guide the appropriate degree in order to create a rectangular flexion gap. When too much tension was applied with the tensioning device, femoral component over-rotation occurred. If the gap was over-distracted more than 4 mm over the final gap size, too much posteromedial distal femoral bone was resected. Consequently, the final flexion gap was not rectangular but slightly trapezoidal. This caused the trial femoral component to be slightly over externally rotated, creating a medial laxity in flexion apparent on the sensor nomogram. Additionally, a falsely tight lateral compartment due to the everted patella results in over-resection of the posterolateral condyle. On the other hand, when just enough tension was applied to distract the flexion gap, the proper amount of bone was resected, allowing correct femoral component rotation, a rectangular flexion gap, and approximately equal medial and lateral compartment pressures.

The sensors gave insight into knee balance by demonstrating certain pressure distributions and patterns. Anteromedial tightness was seen in five of the thirty-eight patients. This pattern was characterized by a relatively high-pressure region of low contact area in the anteromedial corner of the medial compartment (◻ Fig. 23.3). These patients had severe pre-operative varus deformities requiring extensive release of the medial collateral ligament (MCL) while leaving the pes anserinus muscle insertions intact to serve as the dynamic medial stabilizers of the knee in extension. The semi-membranosus muscle insertions were also left undisturbed. None of these patients experienced midstance instability. The retained pes musculature is presumed to create this pattern of pressures, as it does feel tight to the surgeon after component placement (but being tendons, not ligaments, they can lengthen with varus correction). However, it remains unclear whether these anteromedial forces from the dynamic medial compartment stabilizers will create unacceptable wear patterns on retrievals. Although these pressures were almost two orders of magnitude less than the yield point of the polyethylene, they may contribute to accelerated wear. These in vivo stresses will likely be amplified by loading conditions. Only at explantation will these questions be answered.

Comparisons of pressure magnitudes and distributions to wear patterns on insert retrievals (from our retrieval lab) raised interesting questions (◻ Figs. 23.6 and 23.7). Clearly, retrieved inserts with abnormal wear had loading and kinematic conditions resulting in these patterns. If a compartment is left tight intra-operatively, it may remain tight throughout the life of the replacement. Kinematics alone or in combination with balance abnormalities could also result in these wear patterns. It is hoped that as retrievals from our patients are correlated to compartment balance and kinematics, a better understanding of insert wear will be achieved.

Of the three patients with liftoff, one patient had liftoff in extension and two in flexion. The one patient with liftoff medially in extension had decreased medial compartment pressure and a slight valgus mal-alignment (2 degrees of valgus mechanical axis alignment). Two of the thirteen patients without liftoff had abnormal compartment pressures in extension. In both cases, the mechanical axis alignment resulted in loading of the lax compartment with weight-bearing. One of these patients had slight valgus (7 degrees, loose in lateral compartment) and one had slight varus mal-alignment (4 degrees, loose

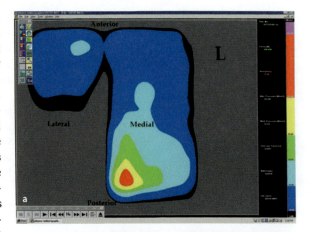

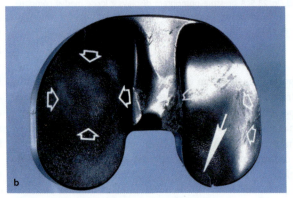

◻ **Fig. 23.6. a** A pressure nomogram demonstrates increased pressures posteriorly and medially. **b** An insert retrieval demonstrates posterior and medial insert wear that may have been caused by the pressures seen in the nomogram

in medial compartment). These data suggest that liftoff may require both a compartment pressure imbalance and abnormal alignment that tends to exacerbate the laxity with physiologic loading. Therefore, it may be important for surgeons to accurately balance and align the limb to mitigate liftoff and optimize implant kinematic function.

Conclusion

The instrumented insert accurately recorded magnitude, location, and dynamic imprint of the pressures in the medial and lateral compartments. These data were more

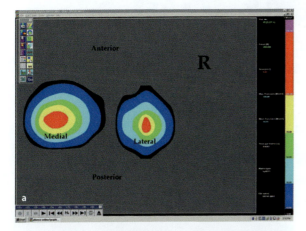

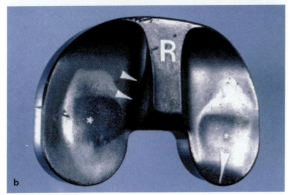

□ **Fig. 23.7. a** A pressure nomogram displays abnormally high compartment pressures in flexion. **b** An insert retrieval has significant wear in the medial and lateral compartments in a distribution similar to that seen on the nomogram. This type of wear pattern could result from the high pressures seen on the nomogram

References

1. Wasielewski RC, Galat DD, Komistek RD (2004) An intraoperative pressure-measuring device used in total knee arthroplasties and its kinematics correlations. Clin Orthop Relat Res 427: 171–178
2. Wasielewski RC, Galante JO, Leighty RM, Natarajan RN, Rosenberg AG (1994) Wear patterns on retrieved polyethylene tibial inserts and their relationship to technical considerations during total knee arthroplasty. Clin Orthop Relat Res 299: 31–43
3. Wasielewski RC (2002) The causes of insert backside wear in total knee arthroplasty. Clin Orthop Relat Res 404: 232–246
4. Takahashi T, Wada Y, Yamamoto H (1997) Soft-tissue balancing with pressure distribution during total knee arthroplasty. J Bone Joint Surg 79B: 235–239
5. Wallace AL, Harris ML, Walsh WR, Bruce WJ (1998) Intraoperative assessment of tibiofemoral contact stresses in total knee arthroplasty. J Arthroplasty 13: 923–927
6. Morris BA, D'lima DD, Slamin J et al. (2001) e-Knee: Evolution of the electronic knee prosthesis: telemetry technology development. J Bone Joint Surg 83A: 62–66
7. Komistek RD, Stiehl JB, Dennis DA, Paxson RD, Soutas-Little RW (1998) Mathematical model of the lower extremity joint reaction forces using Kane's method of dynamics. J Biomech 31: 185–189
8. Heim CS, Postak PD, Greenwald AS (1996) Factors influencing the longevity of UHMWPE tibial components. Instructional Course Lectures 45:303–312

accurate than surgeon feel. This sensor provided objective evaluation of ligament balancing. It also helped confirm the importance of accurate surgical technique and compartment balancing in achieving good total knee arthroplasty function. We hope that the data provided by this sensor will allow surgeons to better understand the aspects of surgical technique that directly affect implant kinematic function, insert wear, and longevity. When implant retrievals are obtained from these patients, a better understanding of the importance of compartment pressures may finally be achieved.

Computer-Assisted Total Knee Arthroplasty Using Patient-Specific Templates: the Custom-made Cutting Guides

M.A. Hafez, K.L. Chelule, B.B. Seedhom, K.P. Sherman

Introduction

The success of TKA is dependent on surgical techniques [7, 8, 34] that require accuracy and reproducibility. Current surgical techniques rely on plain radiographs for preoperative planning and standardized conventional instrumentation (CI) systems for performing the procedure. Plain radiographs have limited accuracy [1, 14, 17, 21, 22, 25, 28, 29]. Ten degrees of knee flexion and 20° of external to 25° of internal rotation can cause significant differences in knee alignment measurements [25]. Conventional instrumentation systems have been reported to have limitations that affect the ultimate accuracy of surgery, especially bone cutting and implant alignment [4, 18, 23, 35]. In addition, CI systems are based on average bone geometry, which may vary widely between patients. Nagamine, Miura et al. (2000) reported several anatomical variations in 133 Japanese patients with knee osteoarthritis (OA). Other authors [36, 37] reported that significant mal-alignment errors (>3°) resulted from using extra-medullary and intra-medullary (IM) rods. The accuracy of using CI for sizing is also questionable [15]. Conventional instrumentation systems are relatively complex tools with numerous jigs and fixtures. Their assembly is time consuming and may lead to errors. Their repeated use carries a theoretical risk of contamination. The use of alignment guides involves the violation of IM canals. This can lead to a higher risk of bleeding [3, 19], infection [26, 27], fat embolism [20] and fractures [5]. Each TKA prosthesis has its own instrumentation. In the United Kingdom, there are more than 30 TKA prostheses and it is common to have different prostheses used in the same hospital [24]. This may overload hospital inventory, sterilization services, nurses' learning curves, and operating room time. Although conventional surgical instrumentation have been repeatedly modified, it appears that further refinements are unlikely to overcome their inherent drawbacks such as the multiplicity of instruments and the medullary canal perforation.

Material and Methods

Authors introduced a new concept of using computer-assisted pre-operative planning to provide patient-specific templates (PST) that can completely replace conventional instruments [10]. Computed-tomography-based planning was used to design two virtual templates. Using rapid prototyping (RP) technology, virtual templates were transferred into physical templates (cutting blocks) with surfaces that matched the distal femur and proximal tibia. The PST technique was applied to 45 TKA procedures using 16 cadaveric and 29 plastic knee specimens. Six out of the 29 PST procedures were included in a comparative trial against 6 cases of TKA using conventional instrumentations [11]. We used the PFC prosthesis (DePuy/Johnson and Johnson, Leeds, UK). The manufacturer provided us with computer aided design (CAD) files of different sizes for the femoral and tibial components, including the polyethylene tibial inserts. Patellar replacement was not considered for this study.

Patient Specific Templating Technique

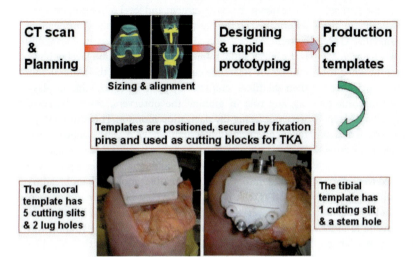

Fig. 24.1. Technical steps for the PST technique

The pre-operative planning (**❑** Fig. 24.1) comprised the following steps: 3-D reconstruction of computed tomography (CT) scan data, sizing and alignment of the prosthetic components, surgical simulation, templates designing, and production of patient specific templates using the rapid prototyping technology. CT scanning was performed for the knee joint, distal tibia and proximal femur, with 1 mm thick slices and 1 mm spacing, which is the minimum requirement for accurate reconstruction of the joint. The femoral and tibial shafts were scanned with 5 mm thick slices and a scan space of 5 mm. This protocol optimized the image quality of the bone for areas of interest around the knee joint, as well as the proximal femur and distal tibia. CT scan images were imported to Materialise software and were displayed in coronal, sagittal and transverse planes. The images were processed using a threshold value to differentiate the areas of interest in both femur and tibia, which could then be segmented from the soft tissue. Similar to conventional techniques, component sizing was initially determined by measuring the anteroposterior (AP) dimension of the distal femur and the contour of the proximal tibia. This allowed the selection of an exact or closely matched size of the femoral and tibial implants from the CAD files. Then, the selected component was superimposed over the bone and visualized in 3-D to confirm the accuracy of sizing and exclude overhanging of the implant on one side of the bone or

notching of the anterior femoral cortex. The interactive 3-D manipulation of images allowed translation and rotation of the prosthetic components individually, until satisfactory prosthesis alignment was achieved. Standard anatomical landmarks and long axes of the femur and tibia were used as guides for proper alignment, rotation and placement of the prosthesis. Virtual positioning of the implants over the bone was visualized in 3 planes and allowed the identification of the volume of bone that needed to be removed. This step was similar to surgical simulation and it was used to evaluate implant placement and the intended bone cutting. Errors could be identified and corrected at this stage, until satisfactory planning was achieved.

To design templates, the 3-D models of the femur and tibia, with aligned prosthetic components in situ, were imported to the CAD component of the Materialize software. One femoral and one tibial template were designed, each in the form of cutting blocks to allow bone preparation based on preoperative planning. This was achieved by creating slits in the templates to allow five flat bone cuts in the distal femur and one cut in the proximal tibia. Lug holes and openings for the fixation stem and the keel were also created. The templates were designed to match the surface geometry of the distal femur and proximal tibia, so that they could only allow the templates to be placed in a unique and secure position (patient specific).

24

The templates were cannulated to allow the passage of the fixation pins providing additional stability to the templates over the bone. The final design of the patient-specific templates was transferred electronically to the RP machine that produced the physical templates. Once manufactured, the templates were autoclaved to simulate clinical circumstances. These templates were designed for single use. The CAD files of the selected sizes of prosthetic components were also transferred to the RP machine to produce physical models of the components. These non-metallic duplicates were meant to prevent artifacts that may occur from metallic implants during post-operative CT scanning.

The rapid prototyped templates were used to perform TKA procedures on both cadaveric and plastic specimens. The femur was rigidly held in a special leg holder that allowed the knee joint to move from full extension to more than 90° of flexion. The standard medial para-patellar approach was used for all of the cadaveric cases. The femoral and tibial templates, one at a time, were uniquely positioned over the respective bone, matching their unique geometry. Fixation pins were inserted into the bone through the cannulated locators to stabilize the templates during bone cutting. Traditional saw blades and drill bits of the appropriate diameter were used to make the various bone cuts and holes for lugs, stem, and keel (◘ Fig. 24.2). MAH performed all surgical procedures except 4 cadaveric TKA procedures that were done by (KPS).

The computer-assisted analysis was performed for six randomly selected postoperative CT scans to evaluate the accuracy of sizing, alignment, and bone cutting (outcome measures). The six specimens were cadaveric and had the non-metallic prosthesis in situ during scanning. The reconstructed post-operative images were superimposed in 3-D planes (coronal, sagittal, and transverse) over the corresponding pre-operative images that represent pre-planned cuts. This made it possible to determine the amount of deviation of the operative performance (bone cutting) from the preoperative plan. The outcome measures were alignment, rotation, and level of bone resection (joint line level).

A reliability test was performed at the Institute for Computer Assisted Orthopaedic Surgery, The Western Pennsylvania Hospital, Pittsburgh, PA, USA, to test the accuracy and repeatability of positioning the templates by 5 observers [12]. The experiment was conducted using only one plastic knee specimen. The planning for TKA and the production of PST was similar to what was de-

scribed above for the PST technique. The knee specimen was held rigidly in a specific leg holder. The primary outcome measure was alignment and level of bone cutting, as determined by the position of the templates. A navigation system VectorVision (BrainLab, Heimstetten, Germany) was used as a tool to measure alignment and level of bone cutting for reference cuts, while placing the femoral and then the tibial templates by each observer, without playing any role in guiding the observers, since observers were not facing the navigation monitor. The routine steps for using navigation systems in TKA were adopted. Two tracking pins were inserted into the distal femur, about a handbreadth from the knee joint and another 2 pins were inserted into the proximal tibia about 2 handbreadths from the knee joint. The tracking pins were 2 mm each and they served as rigid bodies to which one femoral and one tibial tracker were inserted. Surface registration was performed as per routine. A tracking plate that could be tracked by the camera was inserted one at a time into the slits of the templates that corresponded to the reference bone cuts. This step is typically performed during navigated TKA, where the tracking plate is inserted into tibial, distal femoral and anterior femoral slits of the conventional cutting blocks to measure alignment and level of bone cutting, before actual bone cuts are performed.

Each observer was asked to position the tibial templates one at a time, with the tracking plate in-situ (◘ Fig. 24.3). The navigation system continuously tracked the position of the tracking plates and subsequently measured alignment (coronal and sagittal) and level of bone cutting, which were displayed on a computer monitor in real time. When the observer was satisfied with the template position, an independent assessor recorded the measurements that were displayed on the navigation monitor. These measurements were done before bone cutting, as is typically performed, when using navigation systems in TKA. The same process was repeated for the femoral template positioning, with 5 observers and 5 times each. However, in this case there were 2 reference cuts and the template was first positioned, with the tracking plate inserted into the distal femoral slit and then positioned again, with the tracking plate inserted into the anterior femoral slit. The distal femoral slit was meant to measure alignment (coronal and sagittal) and level of bone cutting and the anterior slit was for femoral rotation.

Quantitative analysis was performed using Fredman's repeated measure non- parametric analysis of variance (ANOVA) and Kruskal Wallis analysis of variance (ANO-

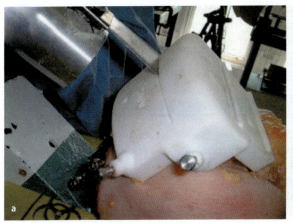
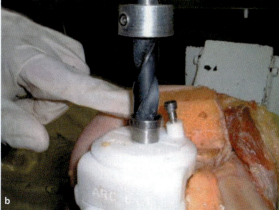

Fig. 24.2. TKA using only a femoral (**a**) and a tibial (**b**) templates (cutting blocks)

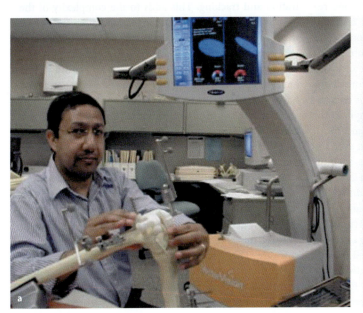
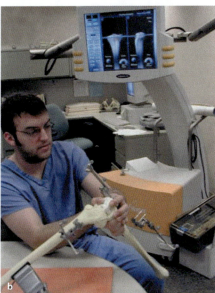

Fig. 24.3. Testing the reliability of positioning the femoral (**a**) and the tibial (**b**) PST by multiple observers using a navigation system as a measurement tool

VA). The recorded measurements from all observers were compared to a control measurement of zero° or zero mm. This control represents the ideal measurement (i.e. no error). Inter-observer and Intra-observer concordance was tested using Kundall coefficient of concordance. Correlation between the results of the study observers was done using Pearson moment correlation test (r). A probability value (p value) less than 0.05 was considered significant.

Results

All TKA procedures were successfully completed using the templates without resorting to conventional instrumentation systems. The PST technique was found to be less invasive, compared with CI, because of the elimination of intra-medullary (IM) rods. There were 84 pieces of jigs and fixtures in the CI set, compared with only two for the PST technique. Unlike the PST technique, the conventional technique required setting up, assembling and dismantling of numerous pieces of instruments. It also required spatial arrangements to provide an adequate space for the surgeon and the assistant and an easy access to the knee joint and instruments. CI systems also involved several steps of sizing, alignment measurements, and bone cutting. The mean time for bone cutting was 9 min with a surgical assistant and 11 min without an assistant as compared to 15 and 30 min for conventional technique, respectively. The smoothness of bone cutting, as measured by steel shims was better than that of CI as only two out of six cases (four for conventional technique) had gaps of 1 mm or more between bones and implants.

The computer-assisted analysis of six random CT scans showed mean errors for alignment and bone resection within 1.7° and 0.8 mm (maximum 2.3° and 1.2 mm). The reliability test showed that the positioning of the templates and the alignment of the subsequent femoral and tibial bone cuts had a mean error of 0.67°. The maximum error was 2.5°, which was recorded for the posterior sloping of one of the tibial cuts for one observer. The mean error in positioning the templates for the level of bone cutting was 0.32 mm (maximum 1 mm). For qualitative analysis, it was apparent (without even using Kappa statistics) that all measured values were within 3° indicating complete inter-observer and intra-observer agreement. For quantitative analysis using Friedman test and Kendall concordance coefficient, there was an overall significant agreement between the observers (p<0.05). The concordance coefficient was high indicating a considerable inter-observer agreement for all measured parameters except femoral cutting level that had a relatively low concordance coefficient. Comparison between **different recorded measurements for the same observer** (intra-observer variation test) showed significant agreement (p value <0.003) and the concordance coefficient was very high. This means that there was no difference after repeating the same test by the same observer and there was a considerable intra-observer agreement. Femoral rotation was measured from only 3 (out of 5) observers, as the navigation monitor suddenly signed off, and it was not possible to operate the system further at the time of this experiment. Based on the available data, the mean error of rotation was 1.86° (St D 0.02° and the maximum error was 2.84° of excessive external rotation), as compared to the pre-operative planning of 3° external rotation. The observers were able to do the experiment without surgical assistants. They found the templates to be user-friendly and could be uniquely positioned, and held with one or 2 hands.

Discussion

Navigation and robotic techniques have recently been introduced into clinical practice and they have proved to be more accurate than conventional instrumentation systems [3, 9, 16, 28, 30, 31, 35, 36]. They have eliminated the use of alignment guides. However, navigation techniques still require the use of conventional instruments for making the various bone cuts and they even require additional instruments and technical steps such as registration and tracking. This adds to the complexity of the procedure and leads to prolonged operative time. The overwhelming intra-operative information can ultimately take senior surgeons away from their comfort zone and interrupt their learning curve. All the above drawbacks have limited the broad clinical application of robotics and navigation techniques.

Unlike navigation and robotics, PST did not require computer equipments in the operating room nor did it require registration process. Also, PST needed no tracking, pin insertion or continuous line of sight. The main the advantages of the PST technique were the ease of use (two-piece instrumentation system), the significant reduction of bone cutting time (up to 9 min) and the elimination of medullary canal perforation. The PST technique required only CT images and a personal computer with the specific software. The services of RP machine and template production were performed off campus, obviating the need to purchase such equipment. Designing the templates could be transferred to the RP machine using electronic mail. Patient-specific templating can be applied to any TKA prosthesis provided that manufactures are willing to provide the CAD files of their prostheses for preoperative planning. The patient's initials, hospital number, and side of the knee can be engraved on the templates.

The cost of PST technique is less than robotics, navigation and CI systems. Information from manufacturers indicated that the actual cost of manufacturing a set of CI system is about $ 30,000. The instruments must be discarded after 5 years and the estimated average use is around 150 operations. Based on this information, the cost of manufacturing is around $ 200 for each operation. In this study, the cost of two templates ($ 200) was equal to the estimated cost of manufacturing the CI per one TKA procedure. The cost of a single CT scan in this study ($ 100) was less than the cost of sterilizing one set of CI ($ 180). Currently, there are hidden costs for the use of CI systems such as storage, transportation and training for nurses and surgeons and more importantly, the cost of the operating room time that is wasted during the setting up, assembling, dismantling, and washing of the numerous pieces of instruments. The use of PST does not have any of the above hidden costs. On the other hand, current navigation systems still require CI and this double instrumentation system raise the cost of TKA procedure significantly. The cost of a navigation system is around $ 150,000 with a life span of roughly 5 years. Based on average use, the estimated cost per one TKA procedure would be more than $ 1000.

The majority of clinical application of rapid prototyping comes from dentistry and maxillofacial surgery [13]. Rapid prototyping machines work as 3-D printers to produce physical models from CAD data. Orthopaedic applications were confined to the production of models and guides rather than tools or instruments. Brown et al. [2] reported successful and cost effective use of rapid prototyping in the surgical treatment of fractures in 117 patients, suggesting that rapid prototyping is the future of trauma surgery. Radermacher [33] and Portheine [32] reported their pioneering work of using rapid prototyping in spinal, hip, and knee surgery. Their work on TKA was to produce templates that can guide conventional cutting blocks. Although they dispensed of the medullary alignment guides, the templates did not replace the conventional instrumentations. The main criticism to this approach was the drawbacks of the additional preoperative preparation and the use of CT scans that involve cost and radiation. Literature review did not reveal any study that developed patient-specific instruments (cutting blocks) that completely replace conventional instrumentation.

There are drawbacks of the PST technique. The radiation exposure from CT scans is a concern, but it may be justified by the benefits. Intra-operative measurement and adjustment is limited. However, surgeons rely on conventional four in one femoral cutting blocks. Robotic techniques also have limited intra-operative adjustments and rely on the accuracy of preoperative planning that is well documented [3, 21, 31]. The template design can be modified for controversial conditions. In our study, there was a cadaveric specimen that had a fixed flexion defor-

mity that required developing two femoral templates with different options for the level of resection of the distal femur. Another drawback is the lack of support for soft tissue balancing. In conventional techniques, surgeons use their own judgment to perform soft-tissue balancing. In the PST technique, the accurate preoperative sizing and alignment should lead to precise bone cutting that will diminish the need for soft tissue release. The ease and speed of performing bone cuts using the PST technique may allow the surgeon to focus his efforts on soft tissue balancing if needed. Another drawback is changes in the routine practice of TKA by shifting certain surgical steps from the intra-operative to the preoperative stage. Although this may save on precious operative time, some surgeons may not tolerate such a change.

It appears that the PST technique has several advantages over conventional instrumentation systems. The PST technique is also a practical alternative to navigation and robotics. It confines the computational work to the pre-operative stage and provides the surgeon with only two patient-specific instruments (cutting blocks) that are easy to use, less invasive, and time saving. The technique has the potential to be used as a training tool. Although this laboratory study proved the concept of PST and validated its accuracy, further clinical validation is required to confirm the results of this study.

Acknowledgement. Authors thank Keyworth Institute, University of Leeds, UK; the Radiology Department, St. Luke Hospital Bradford, UK; DePuy International Ltd, Leeds, UK; Materialise, Belgium; The Engineering and Physical Sciences Research Council (EPSRC), UK; The Arthritis Research Council (ARC), UK; and The Institute for Computer Assisted Orthopaedic Surgery, Pittsburgh, USA.

References

1. Brouwer RW, Jakma TS, Bierma-Zeinstra SM, Ginai AZ, Verhaar JA (2003) The whole leg radiograph: standing versus supine for determining axial alignment. Acta Orthrop Scand 74: 565–568
2. Brown GA, Firoozbakhsh K, DeCoster TA, Reyna JR Jr, Moneim M (2003) Rapid prototyping: The future of trauma surgery? J Bone Joint Surg Am 85(Suppl 4): 49–55
3. Chauhan SK, Scott RG, Breidahl W, Beaver RJ (2004) Computer-assisted knee arthroplasty versus a conventional jig-based technique. A randomised, prospective trial. J Bone Joint Surg Br 86: 372–377
4. Delp SL, Stulberg SD, Davies B, Picard F, Leitner F (1998) Computer-assisted knee replacement. Clin Orthop Relat Res 354: 49–56

5. Dennis DA, Channer M, Susman MH, Stringer EA (1993) Intramedullary versus extramedullary tibial alignment systems in total knee arthroplasty. J Arthroplasty 8: 43–47

6. DiGioia AM III, Jaramaz B, Colgan BD (1998) Computer assisted orthopaedic surgery; image guided and robotic assistive technologies. Clin Orthop Relat Res 354: 8–16

7. Ecker ML, Lotke PA, Sindsor RE, Cella JP (1987) Long-term results after total condylar knee arthroplasty. Significance of radiolucent lines. Clin Orthop Relat Res 216: 151–158

8. Fehring TK, Odum S, Griffin WL, Mason JB, Nadaud M (2001) Early failure in total knee arthroplasty. Clin Orthop Relat Res 392: 315–318

9. Haaker, RG, Stockheim M, Kamp M, et al. (2005) »Computer-assisted navigation increases precision of component placement in total knee arthroplasty.« Clin Orthop Relat Res 433: 152–159.

10. Hafez MA (2006) Computer-assisted total knee arthroplasty using patient-specific templates. MD thesis, Medical School, The University of Leeds

11. Hafez MA, Chelule K, Seedhom BB, Sherman KP (2006) Computer-assisted total knee arthroplasty using patient-specific templating. Clin Orthop Relat Res 444: 184–192

12. Hafez MA, Chelule K, Seedhom BB, Sherman KP, Jaramaz B, DiGioia AM III (2005) Patient-specific instrumentation for TKA: Testing the reliability using a navigation system. In: Symposium on Less and Minimally Invasive Surgery for Joint Arthroplasty: Fact and Fiction (MIS Meets CAOS). San Diego, CA, USA, pp 585–590

13. Harris J, Rimell J (2002) Can rapid prototyping ever become a routine feature in general dental practice? Dent Update 29: 482–486

14. Ilahi OA, Kadakia NR, Huo MH (2001) Inter- and intraobserver variability of radiographic measurements of knee alignment. Am J Knee Surg 14: 238–242

15. Incavo SJ, Coughlin KM, Beynnon BD (2004) Femoral component sizing in total knee arthroplasty: size matched resection versus flexion space balancing. J Arthroplasty 19: 493–497

16. Jakopec M, Harris SJ et al. (2001) The first clinical application of a »hands-on« robotic knee surgery system. Comp Aided Surg 6: 329–339

17. Jazrawi LM, Birdzell L, Kummer FJ, Di Cesare PE (2000) The accuracy of computed tomography for determining femoral and tibial total knee arthroplasty component rotation. J Arthroplasty 15: 761–766

18. Jenny JY, Boeri C (2004) Low reproducibility of the intra-operative measurement of the transepicondylar axis during total knee replacement. Acta Orthrop Scand 75: 74–77

19. Kalairajah Y, Simpson D, Cossey AJ, Verral GM, Spriggins AJ (2005) Blood loss after total knee replacement: Effects of computer-assisted surgery. J Bone Joint Surg Br 87: 1480–1482

20. Kim YH (2001) Incidence of fat embolism syndrome after cemented or cementless bilateral simultaneous and unilateral total knee arthroplasty. J Arthroplasty 16: 730–739

21. Kinzel V, Scaddan M, Bradley B et al. (2004) Varus/valgus alignmen of the femur in total knee arthroplasty. Can accuracy be improved by pre-operative CT scanning? Knee 11: 197–201

22. Koshino T, Takeyama M, Jiang LS, Yoshida T, Saito T (2002) Underestimation of varus angulation in knees with flexion deformity. Knee 9: 275–279

23. Laskin RS (2003) Instrumentation pitfalls: you just can't go on autopilot! J Arthroplasty 18 (Suppl 1): 18–22

24. Liow RYL, Murray DW (1997) Which primary total knee replacement? A review of currently available TKR in the United Kingdom. Ann R Coll Surg Engl 79: 335–340

25. Lonner JH, Laird MT, Stuchin SA (1996) Effect of rotation and knee flexion on radiographic alignment in total knee arthroplasties. Clin Orthop Relat Res 331: 102–106

26. McPherson E, Roidis N, Song M et al. (2002) Location of positive culture in treatment of infected TKA. SICOT/SIROT XXII World Congress, San Diego, CA, p 407

27. McPherson EJ, Patzakis MJ, Gross JE, Holtom PD, Song M, Dorr LD (1997) Two-stage reimplantation with a gastrocnemius rotational flap. Clin Orthop Relat Res 341: 73–81

28. MDA (2002) Evaluation of image guided surgery systems. Official report of the »Medicines and Healthcare Products Regulatory Agency« MDA 01025. Department of Health, UK

29. Moreland JR, Bassett LW, Hanker GJ (1987) Radiographic analysis of the axial alignment of the lower extremity. J Bone Joint Surg Am 69: 745–749

30. Nabeyama R, Matsuda S, Miura H, Mawatari T, Kawano T, Iwamoto Y (2003) The accuracy of image guided knee replacement based on computed tomography. J Bone Joint Surg Br 86: 366–371

31. Perlick L, Bathis H, Tingart M et al. (2004) Navigation in total-knee arthroplasty: CT-based implantation compared with the conventional technique. Acta Orthrop Scand 75: 464–470

32. Portheine F, Ohnsorge JA, Schkommodau E et al. (2004) CT-Based planning and individual template navigation in TKA. In: Stiehl JB, Konermann WH, Haaker RG (eds) Navigation and robotics in total joint and spine surgery. Springer, Berlin Heidelberg New York Tokyo, pp 336–342

33. Radermacher K, Portheine F, Anton M, Zimolong A, Kaspers G, Rau G, Staudte H-W (1998) Computer assisted orthopaedic surgery with image-based individual templates. Clin Orthop 354: 28–38

34. Sharkey PF, Hozack WJ, Rothman RH, Shastri S, Jacoby SM (2002) Insall Award paper. Why are knee replacements failing today? Clin Orthop Relat Res 404: 7–13

35. Siebert W, Mai S, Kober R, Heeckt PF (2002) Technique and first clinical results of robot-assisted total knee replacement. Knee 9: 173–180

36. Stulberg SD (2003) How accurate is current TKR instrumentation? Clin Orthop Relat Res 416: 177–184

37. Teter KE, Bergman D, Colwell CW (1995) Accuracy of intramedullary versus extramedullary tibial alignment cutting systems in total knee arthroplasty. Clin Orthop Relat Res 321: 106–110

Part II B Minimally Invasive Surgery: Total Knee Arthroplasty

Principles of MIS in Total Knee Arthroplasty

F. Benazzo, S. Stroppa, S. Cazzamali, L. Piovani, M. Mosconi

Introduction

In the past few years a growing interest has arisen on minimal invasive surgical (MIS™) techniques. In orthopedic surgery, in particular, minimally invasive total knee arthroplasty (TKA) has gained special attention. Minimally invasive techniques in joint arthroplasty had, however, a premature birth. In other terms, surgeons have been implanting prosthetic components, already in use and designed without any constraints deriving from the surgical exposure, through reduced skin and soft tissue incisions. Those are either analogous to the traditional ones but smaller or newer and obtained using more innovative approaches and »ad hoc« instruments.

MIS is, therefore, still evolutionary and this is giving rise to several innovative trends in arthroplasty. Defining MIS only based on the incision size is inappropriate: smaller scars should not be the final goal, but only the consequence of a procedure that aims at an increased preservation of the existing and still functional tissues. In total knee arthroplasty, minimally invasive surgery basically means preserving the extensor mechanism. The surgical exposure of the knee joint for bone resection and prosthetic components implantation needs to be performed with the least possible damage to:

- The vastus medialis and quadriceps tendon. Von Langebeck's approach, conventionally the most used, involves an incision between tendon and VMO that, after scaring, hinders active contraction and active and passive flexion-extension for a long time. Allowing a patient to undergo a faster rehabilitation and functional recovering is considered one of the most important pillars in MIS TKA;
- The patella and patellar tendon and their blood perfusion. Eversion of the patella stretches the patellar tendon, altering blood perfusion. This induces tendon shortening which can result in a *patella baja* that is not correlated to unintentional alterations of the joint line.

Three key topics need to be addressed as an overview to MIS TKA:

- The diverse surgical approaches and the instruments enabling them;
- New prosthetic components designed »ad hoc« for MIS (a field that offers unlimited development opportunities);
- The possibility to combine MIS and computer assisted navigation, as a method to control implant alignment and ligament balancing when the surgical approach does not allow a complete and continuous visualization of the joint.

Surgical Techniques

Surgical techniques can be classified into 2 categories: »traditional-mini« (frontal) and »fully innovative« techniques (medial and lateral; ◻ Fig 25.1).

The »mini midvastus snip« and »mini-subvastus« techniques belong to the first category, whereas the

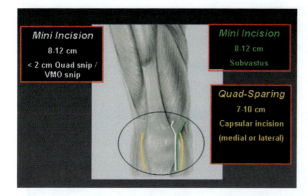

Fig. 25.1. Mininvasive approaches to the knee

»Quad-Sparing™« technique, in the medial and lateral versions, belongs to the second one.

In frontal, midvastus and subvastus, *MIS* techniques, philosophy and surgical steps are substantially equivalent to those of more traditional approaches [1–3].

Minimal invasiveness is reached through surgical approaches designed to preserve tissue and dedicated instruments designed to work in smaller spaces than those available in the past.

The quad-sparing™ technique, instead, brought in true innovation: this new surgical approach avoids any disruption of the vastus medialis obliquus (VMO) – in the medial variant – [4–6] and the vastus lateralis obliquus (VLO) – in the lateral variant – [7] throughout the surgical procedure.

All the surgical steps included in the traditional medial and lateral approaches have been modified and the instrument design changes have not only been determined by the reduced incision size but also by the different, i.e. non-frontal, approach.

Patients and Methods

Between June 2003 and December 2005, we performed 52 TKAs with the *MIS* Quad-Sparing™ technique using a medial approach and 114 TKAs with the *MIS* mini-midvastus technique.

The patients suffered from osteoarthritis unresponsive to conservative treatments. TKAs performed in patients with rheumatoid arthritis and revision TKAs are not included in this study.

An important parameter considered in the study was the patient weight, specifically as related to the amount of subcutaneous fat in the distal part of the thigh.

In both patient groups the same posterior cruciate retaining knee implant model was used.

In the patients operated with the Quad-Sparing™ technique the traditionally stemmed plate was substituted with a »pegged« plate during the first year and with a modular MIS plate during the past year.

In the post-operative follow-up, the following parameters have been monitored and evaluated:
- Blood loss in terms of crude loss through the drain in the first 4 hours after surgery, as well as hemoglobin count immediately post-surgery, and in the 1st and in the 3rd day after surgery;
- range of motion (ROM);
- implant alignment accuracy, as evaluated by measuring α and β angles on frontal X-ray projections, and γ and σ angles on lateral projections [8].

Results

The patients who underwent knee replacement with a *MIS* Quad-Sparing™ (QS) technique had an average blood loss of 370 cc in the first 4 hours after surgery, whereas for those operated with a *MIS* mini-midvastus technique the average blood loss was 360 cc.

Average hemoglobin loss for the two groups of patients was compared to that of a reference sample (patients operated with a traditional approach). Average hemoglobin loss for the patients operated with a QS approach was 1.4 points lower in the immediate post-op, 1.3 points lower on day 1 after surgery, and 1.9 points lower on day 3 after surgery. Patients operated with a mini midvastus technique had an average hemoglobin loss 1.3 points lower post-operatively, 1.5 points lower on day 1 and 1.7 points lower on day 3 after surgery. All differences were statistically significant.

Patients operated with *MIS* Quad-Sparing™ left the hospital 5 (±3) days after surgery. This group had an average ROM of 100.1±4.7° at hospital discharge, 112.3±4.9° one month, 120.1±5.3° three months, 125.7±6.2° six months, 128.8±5.7° one year and 129±4.7° two years after surgery.

Figure 25.2 shows a comparison between these findings and those obtained with a traditional technique.

Patients operated with *MIS* mini midvastus left the hospital 6 (±3) days after surgery; this group had average ROM

25

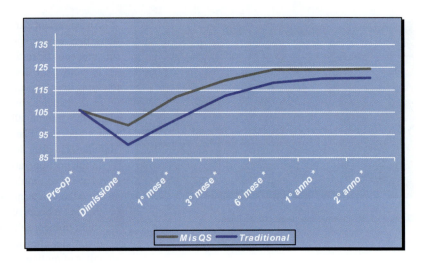

☐ **Fig. 25.2.** Comparison between two
groups of patients: QS and traditional
approaches

of 99.9±4.1° at hospital discharge, 111.7±5.1° one month,
119.7±4.7° three months, 126.1±5.3° six months, 129.1±6.1°
one year and 128.7±4.1° two years after surgery.

Implant alignment accuracy evaluation yielded
α=94.7° (sd 2.2), β=89.1° (sd 1.6), γ=4.6° (sd 1.0) and
σ=86.6° (sd 2.0) with *MIS* Quad-Sparing™ and α=94.4°
(sd 2.0), β=89.3° (sd 1.0), γ=4.4° (sd 1.2) and σ=86.3°
(sd 2.5) with *MIS* mini midvastus.

Discussion

The objectives to pursue in *MIS* TKA are the following:
- Eliminate or reduce possible damage to the quadri-
  ceps.
- Avoid eversion of the patella in order to prevent dam-
  age to the quadriceps and patellar tendons.
- Avoid overstressing the medial and lateral ligaments
  by trying to reduce too much the incision length.
- Achieve faster and better functional recovery as com-
  pared to standards with traditional techniques.
- Reduce blood loss.
- Achieve implant alignment accuracy comparable to
  that obtainable with traditional techniques.

We believe that the above listed goals can be met addressing three different factors:
- new surgical approaches;
- new surgical instruments;
- new prosthetic implants.

We have now innovative instruments which facilitate new
surgical approaches. Tibial plates with shorter stems and
new modular tibial plates -in which the stem extension
can be inserted after implanting the plate or which can
be assembled onto the stem after the latter has been im-
planted- are now available.

As previously mentioned, the new surgical approaches
are based on two different principles:
- the anterior approaches employ surgical instruments
  of reduced size, but substantially follow the traditional
  technique philosophy;
- the medial and lateral approaches implement innovative surgical procedures.

In both cases, the objectives are achievable only by using
new dedicated surgical equipment. However, while in the
first case the traditional instruments were basically only
reduced in size, in the second case they needed to be
completely re-designed.

The extent to which invasiveness can be minimized,
depends exclusively on the quality of the instruments
available to the surgeon. It is important to understand,
however, that it is not possible to reduce the incision below a threshold which depends on implant size.

In order to obtain the best possible results from these
new techniques, the choice must be based on clinical
evidence.

Exclusion criteria for both groups were:
- Deformity >15° (in either varus or valgus);
- flexion contracture >10°-15°;

- pre-operative ROM <90°;
- severe osteoporosis (which excludes most RA patients);
- *Patella baja*, and/or low VMO insertion;
- revision TKA.

With the anterior mini approaches, some of these exclusion criteria can be disregarded (in particular the height of the patella and the height of the VMO insertion) also based on surgeon's experience. Besides clinical evidence, the choice between a frontal or Quad-Sparing™ approach should be based on how familiar the surgeon is with those two techniques and instruments.

Although some authors have described the lateral approach and used it as a routine technique, we believe that it should only be used in knees with valgus deformities above 10°. The proven increased risks for the subcutaneous vascularity associated with a lateral approach do not justify such a choice in less severe valgus deformities, even if it makes ligament balance in the external compartment easier.

Lastly, navigation also needs to be considered as an option in *MIS* TKA. It can add value to the procedure if, and only if, the surgeon is in an advanced phase of his MIS learning curve, i.e. when the surgeon's experience can compensate for the incomplete and discontinuous visualization of the joint.

References

1. Laskin RS (2003) New techniques and concepts in total knee replacement. Clin Orthop 416: 151–153
2. Laskin RS, Beksac B, Phongjunakorn A, Pittors K, Davis J, Shim JC, Pavlov H, Petersen M (2004) Minimally invasive total knee replacement through a mini-midvastus incision: an outcome study Clin Orthop 428: 74–81
3. Scuderi GR, Tenholder M, Capeci C (2004) Surgical approaches in mini-incision total knee arthroplasty Clin Orthop 428: 61–67
4. Tria AJ Jr, Coon TM (2003) Minimal incision total knee arthroplasty. Clin Orthop 416: 185–190
5. Tria AJ Jr (2004) Minimally invasive total knee arthroplasty: the importance of instrumentation. Orthop Clin N Am 35: 227–234
6. Tria AJ Jr (2003) Advancements in minimally invasive total knee arthroplasty. Orthopedics 26 (8): s859–863
7. Goble ME, Justin DF (2004) Minimally invasive total knee replacement: principles and technique. Orthop Clin N Am 35: 235–245
8. Ewald FC (1989) The knee society total knee arthroplasty roentgenographic evaluation and scoring system. Clin Orthop 248: 9–12

MIS Total Knee Arthroplasty with the Limited Quadriceps Splitting Approach

J.L. Cook, G.R. Scuderi

Introduction

In 1974, the first total knee arthroplasty (TKA) was introduced [6, 7]. An extensile approach was utilized with a 20–25 cm midline skin incision. Most commonly, a long medial parapatellar arthrotomy was made [8], although some surgeons preferred a subvastus [5] or midvastus [4] approach. This was followed by extensive soft tissue dissection, as well as eversion and lateral dislocation of the patella. This exposure helped to facilitate appropriate placement of both cutting instruments as well as the components themselves. Over the past 30 years, the techniques of attaining symmetric flexion and extension gaps, ligament balancing, and recreating anatomic alignment have been improved upon so that excellent long term results have been obtained in follow up studies approaching 20 years in length [3, 9, 10, 12, 14, 16].

In the late 1990's, minimally invasive surgery (MIS) for knee arthroplasty was introduced. The theoretical advantages of less invasive surgery included: diminished post-operative morbidity, a reduction in post-operative pain, a decrease in blood loss, and a quicker recovery. While several approaches were initially described, none replaced the standard extensile technique. However, Repicci's work with unicondylar knee replacement encouraged further interest in a limited surgical approach [11, 13]. His successful techniques provided the foundation for MIS total knee replacement.

Several limited approaches have evolved from the traditional extensile approach including: the limited quadriceps splitting approach, also known as the limited medial parapatellar arthrotomy, the limited midvastus approach, the limited subvastus approach, and the quadriceps sparing approach. While limiting surgical dissection is the goal of MIS TKA, the integrity of the procedure must not be compromised. Therefore, it is important to note that each of these approaches can be easily converted to the traditional extensile approach if greater exposure is necessary. Not all patients are candidates for minimally invasive surgery. In general, knees with large deformities often require more soft tissue dissection and may even need releases to correct a deformity. Therefore, deformity should be limited to less than 15 degrees of varus and less than 20 degrees of valgus [15]. Larger deformities require greater exposure and cannot be safely performed with a minimally invasive technique. Additionally, the patient should have a minimum pre-operative range of motion of 90 degrees [15]. If a flexion contracture is present, it must be less than 10 degrees [15]. Larger contractures again require more extensive releases and thus cannot be easily accomplished with a minimally invasive approach. Furthermore, patients with complicating medical problems such as rheumatoid or inflammatory arthritis, diabetes, and those patients whom have had prior surgery should be considered for the more traditional extensile exposure [15]. Those patients whom have had previous surgery often have extensive scar tissue which may need to be released to provide adequate exposure of the knee, thus prohibiting a minimally invasive approach. Clinically, we have also noted that muscular males, obese patients, large femurs, or a short patella tendon typically require greater exposure with the traditional techniques [1].

Methods

The Limited Quadriceps Splitting Approach

The surgical preparation is no different then our standard approach. After preoperative antibiotics are administered, the leg is routinely prepped and draped, and the tourniquet is inflated. The limited quadriceps splitting approach is the most versatile of the minimally invasive approaches because it has evolved from a traditional medial parapatellar arthrotomy performed by most surgeons. The learning curve for this technique is short as surgeons gradually reduce the length of the skin incision and the arthrotomy into the quadriceps tendon in order to gain exposure of the knee joint. With lateral subluxation of the patella, instead of eversion, both the femur and tibia can be visualized without extending the arthrotomy high into the quadriceps tendon. Exposure and placement of the instrumentation does require placing the knee in various positions of knee flexion throughout the procedure, as well as careful placement of the retractors by the surgical assistant. There are several key points that are detailed below.

A straight anterior midline skin incision is made from the superior border of the patella to the superior aspect of the tibial tubercle (Fig. 26.1). This is accomplished with the knee in extension. The incision is usually 10–14 cm in length. The skin incision is made as small as possible in every patient, but is extended as needed during the procedure to allow for adequate visualization and to avoid excess skin tension. There is a direct correlation with the height of the patient, the BMI, and the length of the skin incision. All patients are informed pre-operatively that the smallest incision will be used, but that it may be extended as necessary to safely perform the procedure. We also observed that as the knee is brought from extension to flexion, the skin will stretch do to its elasticity and the exposure gains approximately 3 cm in length. However, during the procedure, the skin incision is watched very carefully, especially at the superior and inferior apices. When the apex forms a V (V sign) (Fig. 26.2a), the skin is not under any undo tension. However if the V flattens out and begins to form a U (U sign) (Fig. 26.2b), or worse, becomes transverse, the skin incision should be lengthened to avoid unnecessary injury or tearing of the skin. Small full-thickness medial and lateral flaps are created over the extensor mechanism. Release of the deep fascia proximally beneath the skin, superficial to the quadriceps tendon, facilitates mobilization of the skin and enhances exposure. The elasticity of

the skin allows for broader exposure as the knee is brought into a flexed position.

Prior to the arthrotomy, the quadriceps tendon, along the path of the arthrotomy and the medial retinaculum, is injected with 1% lidocaine and epinephrine. This injection has dramatically reduced the post-operative bleeding and has also contributed to a reduction in the post-operative hemoglobin drop. The limited medial parapatellar arthrotomy extends only 2–4 cm into the quadriceps tendon. With this limited arthrotomy the patella can then be subluxed laterally, allowing adequate exposure of the joint. In contrast to the traditional approach, the patella is not everted. If there is difficulty displacing the patella laterally, or if the patella tendon is at risk of injury, the arthrotomy can easily be extended proximally into the quadriceps tendon until adequate exposure can be achieved.

As the knee is flexed to 90 degrees, retractors can be placed both medially and laterally to help aid in exposure, avoid undue skin tension, and to protect the supporting soft tissue structures. In order to aid visualization and

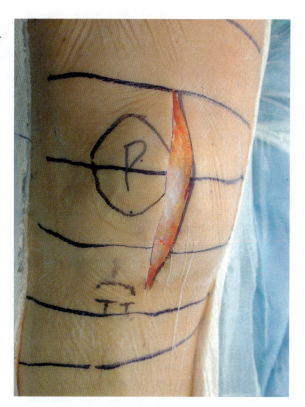

 Fig. 26.1. The skin incision

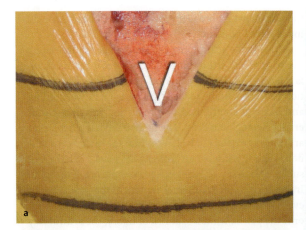

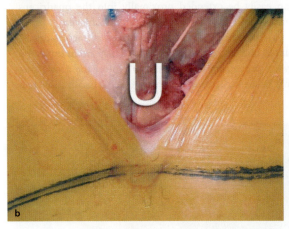

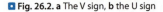

Fig. 26.2. a The V sign, **b** the U sign

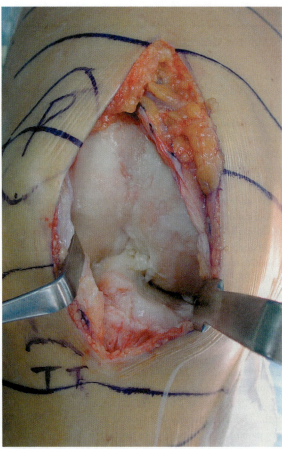

Fig. 26.3. The mobile window

avoid undue tension to the skin, the surgical assistants should be instructed in appropriate placement of retractors and positioning of the knee. Although we use Homan retractors, which have been bent to 90 degrees, specialized retractors are not required. By using differential force, the arthrotomy can be moved as a »mobile window« from medial to lateral and from superior to inferior as necessary (■ Fig. 26.3). With experience, it will become obvious that the bone preparation and resection is performed at different angles of knee flexion. That is why the patient should have at least a 90 degree arc of motion preoperatively. In addition, as the bone is resected from the proximal tibia and distal femur, there is more flexibility to the soft tissue envelope and greater exposure is achieved.

For the limited quadriceps splitting approach, standard instrumentation is too cumbersome and difficult to place appropriately. Modified 4 in 1 multi-referencing instruments (Zimmer, Warsaw, IN) are useful in performing MIS TKA. Alignment guides and cutting blocks, for both tibia and femur, are designed similar to standard instrumentation, but have been reduced in size and geometrically changed to facilitate placement within a smaller soft tissue envelope. This is of particular importance because the patella is no longer everted and there is limited access to the lateral compartment. Although the instrumentation has been modified to fit in a smaller space, there is no difference in the surgical technique. Since the instruments are reduced in size, care must be taken to make sure they are securely fixed to the bone. Screw fixation, in contrast to smooth nails, is more secure and is used routinely. In addition, the saw blades are narrower in order to avoid impingement of the modified instruments.

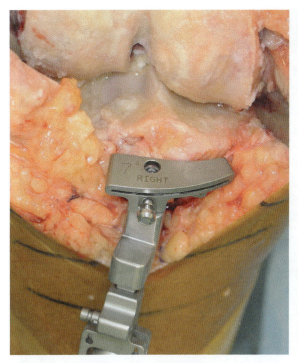

Fig. 26.4. Extra-medullary guide for the tibia

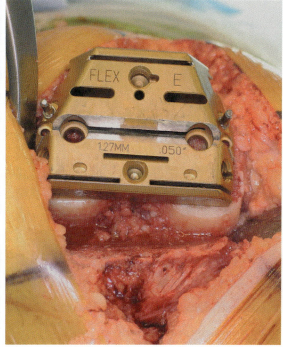

Fig. 26.5. The femoral AP cutting guide

The order of bone resection is dependent upon the surgeon's preference, but we recommend cutting the tibia first. The removal of bone from the proximal tibia will impact both the flexion and extension gap, thereby facilitating preparation of the femur. Tibial resection is accomplished with the assistance of an extramedullary guide that is side specific and medially biased. (◘ Fig. 26.4) The tibial guide is centered on the tibial tubercle and set at the appropriate depth, approximately 10 mm from the uninvolved side, and slope, approximately 7 degrees of posterior slope. The tibia is resected perpendicular to the mechanical axis, while the knee is positioned in 90 degrees of flexion.

Once the proximal tibial bone has been removed, there is laxity of the joint in both flexion and extension, facilitating the placement of femoral instrumentation. An intra-medullary femoral cutting guide, which references the most prominent condyle, is inserted into the distal femur. The distal femur is resected with the appropriate degree of valgus, as determined during the pre-operative planning. Following resection of the distal femur, either the anteroposterior (AP) axis or the epicondylar axis is determined. The femur is sized and the

AP cutting block is secured in the appropriate degree of external rotation (◘ Fig. 26.5). Once the cutting block is securely in place the bone is resected.

Following resection of the femoral bone, laminar spreaders are used to distract the knee joint at 90 degrees of flexion. At this point the medial and lateral menisci are removed, along with the residual fibers of the anterior cruciate ligament and posterior femoral osteophytes (◘ Fig. 26.6). Since we prefer a posterior stabilized knee, the posterior cruciate ligament (PCL) is resected at this time as well. However, for surgeons who prefer a posterior cruciate retaining design, the mini-incision approach provides appropriate exposure. At this point the soft-tissue balance is checked with a space block and alignment rod. The collateral ligaments should be balanced. If there is any inequality, the proper soft-tissue releases should be performed. The release for a residual varus deformity has been well described and includes sub-periosteal elevation of the deep and superficial medial collateral ligament. This release can be performed with the mini-incision approach without excessive subcutaneous dissection along the proximal medial tibia by sub-periosteal release of

26

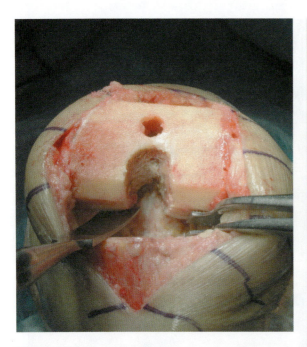

Fig. 26.6. Preparing the posterior femur

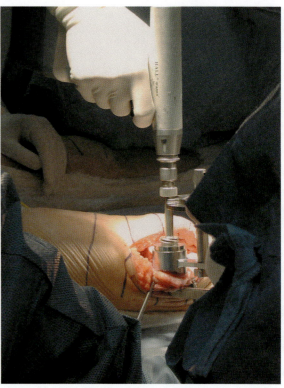

Fig. 26.7. Patella preparation

the MCL. A lateral release for a valgus deformity can be performed through the medial arthrotomy. The »pie crust« technique selectively releases the arcuate ligament, the iliotibial band and the lateral collateral ligament with preservation of the popliteus tendon.

Once it is determined that the knee is appropriately balanced, the finishing cuts are performed on both the femur and tibia to allow trialing with the provisional components. The knee is flexed to 90 degrees and the bone is resected from the femoral intercondylar notch to accommodate the posterior stabilized femoral component. To gain exposure to the proximal tibial surface, the knee is hyperflexed and externally rotated. In this position the femur falls beneath the extensor mechanism and does not interfere with visualization of the proximal tibia. The appropriately sized tibial template is positioned in the correct rotation and the tibia is prepared for the final component.

It is our preference to prepare the patella after femoral and tibial resection. Following removal of the bone from the proximal tibia and distal femur, there is about a 20 mm gap, resulting in laxity of the soft-tissue envelope, which allows easier manipulation of the patella during preparation. With the knee in either full extension or

slight flexion the patella is tilted. However, the entire extensor mechanism does not have to be twisted or everted. Following measurement of the patella thickness, the appropriate sized reamer is used to resect the patella to the appropriate depth (Fig. 26.7). The three holes for the patellar prosthesis can be made at this time and a trial button placed. The final thickness of the resurfaced patella is measured and compared to the original thickness.

At this point, all the provisional components are inserted. It is usually easier to insert the tibia tray first. In order to do this, the knee is hyper-flexed and externally rotated so that the tibia is sub-luxed forward through the arthrotomy. The tibial tray is then seated in place. The knee is then brought back to 90° of flexion, and with distraction of the joint, the flexion space opens and the trial femoral component is impacted in place. The provisional tibial articular surface is then inserted. If there is difficulty gaining exposure and inserting the tibial articular surface, the knee is placed in mid-flexion, about 45 – 60 degrees, and the articular surface is guided into place. Finally, the trial patellar button is placed. After the provisional components are trialed and felt to be appropriate with excellent range of motion, stability, and patellar tracking, they are removed and the bone is prepared for cementation of the final components. The knee is copiously irrigated with pulsatile lavage and dried thoroughly. Once the cement is of the appropriate viscosity, the knee is hyper-flexed and externally rotated so that the tibia is again brought forward. Cement is placed on the proximal tibia and into the stem hole, and the tibial tray is impacted into place, being sure that it is fully seated on the proximal tibial bone and set at the appropriate rotation. Any excess cement is removed with forceps. The knee is brought back to 90 degrees of flexion. Cement is placed along the anterior and distal femur as well as on the posterior condyles of the implant. The femoral component is then impacted in place. Any excess cement is removed with forceps. A careful inspection of the posterior recess and along the margins of the implant should confirm that there is no cement debris. A reduction is performed with a provisional tibial articular surface. The patella is cemented in place and held with the patellar clamp until the cement hardens. The knee is assessed for appropriate balance range of motion, and patellar tracking. If results are satisfactory, the provisional tibial articular surface is removed and the final tibial polyethylene insert is locked in place. If there is difficulty inserting the final tibial polyethylene component, the knee can be placed in mid-flexion and with a front loading tibial tray the polyethylene insert can be guided into place.

With the final components in place (■ Fig. 26.8), the tourniquet is released and any bleeding is addressed with electrocautery. The tourniquet is then re-inflated for closure and the knee is copiously irrigated with an antibiotic solution. The arthrotomy is closed over a suction drain in an interrupted fashion using absorbable suture. The deep tissues and the subcutaneous layer are closed with absorbable suture and the skin is closed with staples. A sterile dressing is applied. The drain is hooked up to a re-infusion Ortho PAT system (Hemonetics). The drain remains in situ for 24 hours.

While we have just described the technique with modified standard instruments, computer navigated surgery with smaller and precise instrumentation has recently been introduced and aids in the placement and verification of the cutting guides (■ Fig. 26.9). The addition of

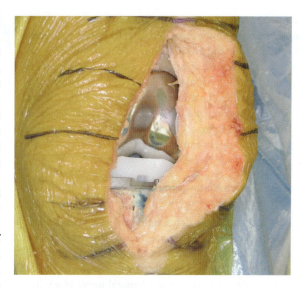

■ **Fig. 26.8.** The final components

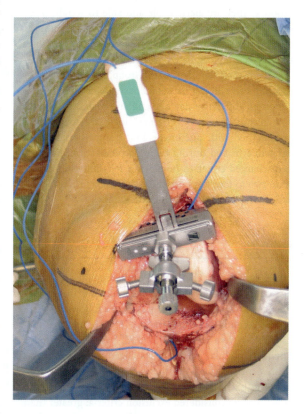

■ **Fig. 26.9.** Computer-navigated resection of the distal femur

computer navigation is still evolving but it appears to be another means of optimizing minimally invasive surgery. It can enhance and restore surgeon confidence in a reduced visibility field. Computer navigation can provide dynamic tracking of instruments, real time feedback on the angle and depth of bone resection (■ Fig. 26.10), and with some instrumentation, such as the AxiEM system (Medtronics, Denver, CO), determination of soft tissue balance and range of motion (■ Fig. 26.11).

Postoperative Management

All patients receive the same regimen of pain management as conducted through our anesthesia department, with patients placed on a patient controlled analgesia pump and either maintaining an epidural catheter overnight (for bilateral patients) or receiving a femoral nerve block (for unilateral patients). Continuous passive motion is started in the recovery room. The patients begin full weight bearing ambulation and active range of motion exercises as soon as they are alert, stable and able to weight bear. Twice daily physical therapy for range of motion, ambulation, and strengthening begins on postoperative day one. Patients are anticoagulated with Lovenox® (enoxaparin sodium injection, Sanofi-Aventis Group, Bridgewater, NJ). Patients receive 30 mg subcutaneously twice daily beginning on postoperative day one and are treated for a total of 12 days after surgery. Pharmacologic anticoagulation is augmented with pneumatic foot pumps, which they wear while in bed during their hospitalization. Patients are discharged either to home or a rehabilitation center within two to four days depending on their progress with physiotherapy and their social situation.

Results

Minimally invasive TKA with a limited quadriceps splitting arthrotomy is an alternative technique with satisfactory results when the above key steps are followed.

In a recently published report, 118 consecutive primary TKA's were reviewed [17]. All patients received a cemented, modular, posterior-stabilized prosthesis (Nex-Gen LPS or LPS Flex Prosthesis, Zimmer, Warsaw, IN). Realizing that this procedure is not for all patients, the following were considered exclusion criteria: greater than 20° of deformity (anatomic axis alignment greater than

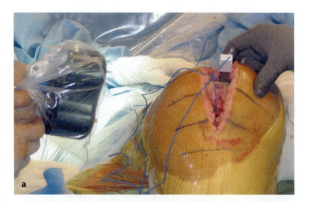

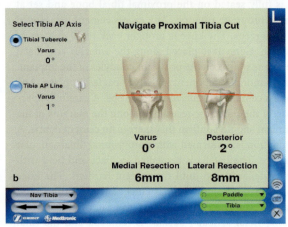

■ Fig. 26.10a,b. Computer probe on the resected tibia (**a**); computer screen with data (**b**)

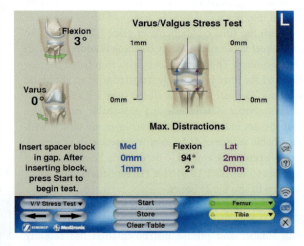

■ Fig. 26.11. Computer navigation provides dynamic feedback on soft tissue balance and intra-operative range of motion

25° of valgus, or greater than 15° of varus as measured on the preoperative AP standing radiograph), previous open procedures to the knee, any previous knee incisions other than arthroscopy portals, any compromise of the soft tissue envelope, or patients whose knees required a complex reconstruction with bone graft and/or prosthetic augmentation.

The surgery was performed through as small of an incision and arthrotomy as possible. Data was collected on multiple variables as outlined below. Comparisons of these variables were made between two groups based on the length of the incision in extension and the extent of the arthrotomy. A clinical decision was made to set the cutoff point at 14 cm. Those patients with incisions measuring less than 14 cm were considered mini-incisions and were labeled Group 1. Group 2 patients had standard incisions measuring greater than or equal to 14 cm.

The following pre-operative information was recorded from the patients' office records and radiographic files: diagnosis, gender, age, weight, height, and body mass index (BMI), preoperative motion, radiographic alignment, Insall-Salvati ratio, and hemoglobin and/or hematocrit levels. Body mass index was determined by a simple formula based on the height and weight of the patient: BMI = weight in kg/(height in m). A standard set of radiographs including standing AP view, a lateral view with the knee flexed 45°, and a Merchant patella view were reviewed for all patients. Deformity in the AP plane was determined by measuring the anatomic axis. The Insall-Salvati ratio was calculated from the pre-operative lateral radiograph. Post-operative component and limb alignment were all measured.

Intra-operative data was collected including the length of the incision and arthrotomy, femoral trans-epicondylar width, implant size and tourniquet time. Post-operative information included: changes in hemoglobin and hematocrit in the recovery room, post-operative day one and post-operative day three; blood loss from the re-infusion drain; transfusion requirements; progress with physiotherapy including range of motion, ambulatory distance, and stair climbing; length of stay; discharge disposition; and complications.

As mentioned above, the cohort was divided into two groups. Group 1 had 69 patients (58%) who had an incision smaller than 14 cm and a limited quadriceps splitting arthrotomy. The average incision length in full knee extension for Group 1 was 11.84 cm (range, 9.5–13.9 cm). The average length of the incision with the knee flexed to

90° was 15.67 cm (range 12.7–19.0 cm). Group 2 had 49 patients (42%) who had an incision in extension greater than or equal to 14 cm and a standard medial parapatellar arthrotomy. The average incision length in full knee extension for Group 2 was 15.92 cm (range, 14.0–21.0 cm). The average length at 90° of knee flexion was 20.14 cm (range, 16.5–25.5 cm).

The average age of the entire cohort was 65.4 years (range 45–84 years) and there was no difference between the two groups. When looking at the pre-operative diagnosis, Group 1 had 67 patients (97%) with osteoarthritis and 2 patients (3%) with osteonecrosis. There were no patients with rheumatoid arthritis. Group 2 had 44 patients (90%) with osteoarthritis, 4 patients (8%) with rheumatoid arthritis and 1 patient (2%) with osteonecrosis. The mini-incision patients had better preoperative knee flexion (117° versus 109°, p=0.01) and an overall arc of motion (116° versus 107°, p=0.03), were shorter (3.8 cm difference, p=0.02), and lighter (10.0 kg difference, p=0.01). Age, pre-operative alignment, pre-operative flexion contracture, Insall-Salvati ratios, and body mass index did not differ between the two groups. There were roughly twice as many women as men in the study (79 women versus 39 men). Of the 39 men in the study, 13 (33%) were able to have the mini-incision procedure. Twenty-six men (67%) had the standard-incision procedure. Of the 79 women, 56 (71%) had a mini-incision procedure, compared with 23 women (29%) who had a standard-approach procedure. These gender differences were significant (p=0.0001). If only the women are analyzed, the average body mass index was significantly smaller in the MIS group (BMI 29.5 kg/m versus 34.2 kg/m, p<0.05)

Patients in Group 1 had narrower femoral transepicondylar widths by 6.7 mm (p<0.0001). Differences in epicondylar width remained significant when broken down by gender. Among the male patients only, those patients in the mini-incision group still had narrower femurs than patients who had standard procedures (89.5 mm versus 93.2 mm, p=0.03). Female patients showed a similar difference (80.2 mm versus 83.6, p=0.001). There was also a difference in component sizing with patients in group 1 averaging one size smaller in the femoral and tibial components (p<0.0001). In Group 1, the average LPS femoral component was a size E, with a mediolateral (ML) dimension of 68 mm and an AP dimension of 61.5 mm. In Group 2, the average LPS femoral component size was F (ML dimension 72 mm, AP dimension 65.5 mm). The average tibial component was a size 4 in the patients who had a mini-incision procedure (ML: 66 mm, AP: 46 mm), and size 5 in the patients who had a standard procedure (ML: 74 mm, AP: 46 mm). Average polyethylene (PE) thickness was the same in each group. There was no difference between the tourniquet time or the operative time in the groups.

The amount of blood re-infused from the postoperative drain was less in the mini-incision group, analyzed as the mean (292 versus 683 cc, p<0.0001) and the median (238 versus 600 cc, p<0.0001). Postoperative day 3 hemoglobin measurements were similar between the groups. However, Group 1 had reduced transfusion requirements, requiring 0.1 units per patient on average, compared with 0.6 units per patient in Group 2 (p=0.03). In Group 1, seven patients required transfusion, each receiving one unit. Five of these patients had autologous transfusions whereas two received allogeneic blood. In Group 2, 12 transfusions were given at an average of 1.5 units per transfusion. Seven patients received autologous blood only, four received allogeneic blood only, and one had a combination of autologous and allogeneic units.

The average length of hospital stay was similar in the two groups: 3.9 days for patients in Group 1, and 4.2 days for patients in Group 2. The similarity in the length of stay is probably multi-factorial considering the implementation of a multidisciplinary approach to patient discharge. The clinical pathways integrate the orthopedic service with anesthesia, nursing, physiotherapy, social service, and home care. There is also an initiative to reduce the length of stay, which impacts patient discharge planning. Thirty-eight percent of the patients in Group 1 were discharged directly to their homes compared with 24% of patients in Group 2. By post-operative day 3, the patients who had mini-incision procedures were walking an average 5.8 meters further and climbing 1.2 more stair-steps than patients who had standard procedures, but these differences were not significant. On postoperative day 3, the patients who had mini-incision procedures had better flexion than patients who had the standard procedures (p=0.014), with an average 4° of difference. The average post-operative flexion for Group 1 on day 3 was 92 degrees (range 48–120 degrees), compared to an average of 88 degrees in Group 2 (range 69–105).

While one of the major concerns with the use of minimally invasive TKA is that it will compromise the positioning of components, this is not the case. Radiographic review in this study population revealed that the average alignment of the prosthesis and the overall limb alignment were consistent with previously published reports [2, 7].

Summarizing our initial experience, 58% of patients could be performed with a limited quadriceps splitting approach [17]. The average incision length in extension was 11.7 cm (range 9.5 to 13.3 cm). It was readily apparent that the MIS approach was more applicable to women since 71% of females had a mini-incision compared to only 33% of males. The mini-incision knees also had better pre-operative knee flexion (117° vs. 109°) and an overall better arc of motion (116° vs. 107°). The mini-incision patients were also shorter in stature, lighter in weight, had a lower body mass index, and smaller femurs. While one of the major concerns with the use of smaller exposures for TKA is that it decreases visualization of landmarks and therefore compromises the positioning of the components, this is not the case. With careful attention to intra-operative details, component position and limb alignment can be achieved that is comparable to a standard approach. The same can be said for intra-operative complications. Additionally, in experienced hands, shortening the incision does not increase the operative time [15].

Discussion

Minimally invasive total knee arthroplasty has gained popularity over the last several years. The limited quadriceps splitting incision is part of the continuum of these modified approaches with limited access and visibility. The learning curve for this technique is short since the arthroplasty is performed with the same surgical technique using modified and smaller instruments that are more adaptable to the limited operative field. With a gradual shortening of the skin incision and medial parapatellar arthrotomy, a smaller and comfortable operative field will be obtained.

Our clinical experience has been observed by others. Coon and co-workers recently reported on their experience with minimally invasive TKA using both the MIS mini-incision and the MIS quadriceps sparing techniques [18]. They found a significantly shorter length of stay of 3.4 days versus 5.9 days for the traditional approach. Minimally invasive patients had a lower transfusion requirement of 4% versus 34%. Looking at the early functional outcome, minimally invasive patients walked three times farther on the third post-operative day (176 feet versus 58 feet) and had a better range of motion. This study also reported a potential cost reduction to the healthcare system as surgeons performing minimally invasive surgery improve their operative efficiency and further reduce the hospital length of stay.

The definition of success with minimally invasive TKA is dependent upon the expectations of the surgeon, patient, and family. Patients have overwhelmingly become interested in the concept of minimally invasive surgery because of the anticipation of lower morbidity and a more rapid recovery. However, they need to realize that the clinical outcome is not solely dependent on the length of the incision. We recommend that during pre-operative counseling, patients are informed that they will receive the smallest incision possible to allow for proper placement of the prosthesis rather than guaranteed an incision of a specific length. Success is also multi-factorial and depends on the appropriate blood loss management, effective pain control, a comprehensive physiotherapy program and a supportive social services network.

Optimizing patient selection and paying specific attention to the operative details will insure clinical success. Experience has demonstrated that there are certain patient characteristics that are better suited for minimally invasive TKA. A shorter, thinner female patient with a lower body mass index, a narrower femur, and better pre-operative range of motion is better suited for minimally invasive surgery. Caution needs to be taken with patients who have rheumatoid arthritis or inflammatory arthritis, limited range of motion with severe fixed angular deformity or prior surgery. Regarding the surgical technique, it is important to pay attention to the intra-operative details. The surgical procedure has not essentially changed from the standard techniques. The real difference is that the procedure is performed in an operative field with limited visibility. The addition of modified and smaller instruments has made it easier to access the joint with little or no damage to the extensor mechanism. Training of the surgical assistants to position the knee and retractors for specific surgical steps will greatly facilitate the operation. Finally, minimally invasive TKA can easily be converted to a more extensile approach if there is any difficulty with exposure, positioning the instrumentation or the implants during the arthroplasty. It is important to remember that TKA is historically a successful operation and the minimally invasive surgical technique should not compromise the outcome.

References

1. Bonutti PM, Neal DJ, Kester MA (2003) Minimal incision total knee arthroplasty using the suspended leg technique. Orthopedics 26(9): 899–903
2. Brassard MF, Insall JN, Scuderi GR, Colizza W (2001) Does modularity affect clinical success? A comparison with a minimum 10-year follow up. Clin Orthop 388: 26–32
3. Colizza W, Insall J, Scuderi G (1995) The posterior stabilized total knee prosthesis: assessment of polyethylene damage and osteolysis after a ten year minimum follow-up. JBJS 77: 1716–1720
4. Engh GA, Holt BT, Parks NL (1997) A midvastus muscle-splitting approach for total knee arthroplasty. J Arthroplasty 12: 322–331
5. Hofmann AA, Plaster RL, Murdock LE (1991) Subvastus (southern) approach for primary total knee arthroplasty. Clin Orthop 269: 70–77
6. Insall J, Ranawat C, Scott WN, Walker P (1976) Total condylar knee replacement. Preliminary report. Clin Orthop 120: 149–154
7. Insall J, Tria A, Scott W (1979) The total condylar knee prosthesis. The first five years. Clin Orthop 145: 68–77
8. Insall JN: A midline approach to the knee. J Bone Joint Surg 53A: 1584–1586
9. Malkani A, Rand J, Bryan R, Wallrich S (1995) Total knee arthroplasty with the kinematic condylar prosthesis. A ten year follow-up study. JBJS 77: 423–431
10. Ranawat C, Flynn W, Saddler S, Hansraj K, Maynard M (1993) Long-term results of the total condylar knee arthroplasty. A 15-year survivorship study. Clin Orthop 286: 96–102
11. Repicci JA, Eberle RW (1999) Minimally invasive surgical technique for unicondylar knee arthroplasty. J South Orthop Assoc 8: 20–27
12. Ritter MA, Herbst SA, Keating EM, Faris PM, Meding JB (1994) Long term survivorship analysis of a posterior cruciate retaining total condylar total knee arthroplasty. Clin Orthop 309: 136–145
13. Romanowski MR, Repicci JA (2002) Minimally invasive unicondylar arthroplasty: Eight-year follow-up. J Knee Surg 15: 17–22
14. Scott RD, Volatile TB (1986) 12 years experience with posterior cruciate retaining total knee arthroplasty. Clin Orthop 205: 100–107
15. Scuderi GR, Tria AJ (2005) Minimally invasive total knee arthroplasty. Insall and Scott Surgery of the Knee, 4th edn. Elsevier, Amsterdam
16. Stern S, Insall J (1992) Posterior stabilized prosthesis. Results after follow-up of nine to twelve years. JBJS 74: 980–986
17. Tenholder M, Clarke HD, Scuderi GR (2005) Minimal incision total knee arthroplasty: the early clinical results. Clin Orthop Rel Res 440: 67–76
18. Coon TM, Tria AJ, Lavernia C, Randall L (2005) The economics of minimally invasive total knee surgery. Semin Arthro 16: 235–238

Total Knee Replacement through a Mini-Mid-Vastus Approach

R.S. Laskin

Introduction

The results of total knee replacement over the past 30 years have been excellent. The operation has been shown to relieve pain and increase the ability of patients to function and participate in activities of daily living. Over and above this these results have been shown to be long-lasting, with many ten and fifteen year follow up studies in the peer reviewed literature [1–3] using a variety of implant designs.

Traditionally, these primary total knee replacements have been performed through a median parapatellar incision. The incision extended proximally for several inches into the junction between the rectus tendon and the vastus medialis muscle. The suprapatellar bursa was extensively opened, the knee was hyper-flexed and the patella was everted. All of this was done through a skin incision that normally measured somewhere between 15 and 18 cm in length.

Despite our excellent long-term results using this type of surgical exposure we did note, however, that the recuperation was prolonged. Patients often had difficulty regaining flexion. Physical therapy requirements were often intensive with patient's not able to normally resume their activities of daily living for about three or more months after surgery.

Over the past 10 to 15 years, minimally invasive approaches have been used to treat a variety of other surgical conditions including chronic gallbladder disease, torn anterior cruciate ligaments, ruptured ovarian cysts, and median nerve compression in the carpal tunnel. The premise in all of those surgeries had been that by limiting the amount of disruption of the deep tissues during the surgery the recuperative time could be sped up, blood loss could be diminished, and postoperative pain could be decreased. Orthopaedic surgeons conjectured whether similar type outcomes could be obtained if we could perform primary knee replacements to more limited exposures. Could we perform the surgery by not extensively disrupting the quadriceps musculature and suprapatellar pouch and still obtain adequate exposure for proper component position and ligament balancing? Would the results of doing this be less pain at the surgery, a faster recuperation, and possibly less blood loss? Bearing all of this in mind, however, had to still perform the surgery in a manner which enabled us to properly expose the important anatomic features so as to minimize the chance of inadvertent damage to bony capsular, vascular or neurological structures.

What Is a Minimally Invasive Knee Replacement?

Although it is well ingrained in the lay literature, using the word minimal to describe these procedures is incorrect. Webster's dictionary defines minimal as the least possible or barely adequate [4]. The least possible incision might be one resulting from the insertion of arthroscope, but at the present time no one is suggesting performing primary total knee replacements arthroscopically. Furthermore no surgeon attempts to do an operation through an exposure that is »barely adequate.« A more appropriate term might be »lesser invasion totally replacement« or »lesser soft tissue dissection total knee replacement«. Having said that, and although we all agree that minimally invasive is the incorrect appellation, its widespread use will lead me to use a MIS as an acronym for this type of surgery throughout this chapter.

There have been several MIS approaches described over the last few years. Among these are the limited rectus incision [5], the sub vastus incision [6], the »quad sparing« [5] approach, and the mini-mid vastus. It is this last approach, a modification of the standard mid vastus approach originally described by Engh [7] that we have used for the past four years, and the one that I will describe in this chapter.

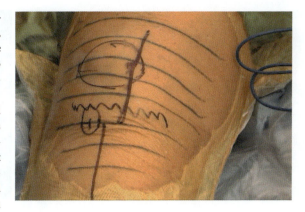

☐ Fig. 27.1. The skin incision begins approximately 2 cm proximal to the superior border of the patella and then crosses the medial third of the patella and extends distally to the level of the tibial tubercle

The Mini-Mid-Vastus MIS Approach to the Knee

The skin incision for a mini-mid-vastus approach is longitudinal and centered over the medial one third of the patella. It begins approximately 1 or 2 cm proximal to the patella and then extends down to the level of the tibial tubercle (☐ Fig. 27.1). Making the skin and capsular incision is facilitated if the knee is kept in a 45° partially flexed position. This can be achieved by placing several rolled towels or sheets under the knee during the exposure or placing the foot on a sandbag placed under the surgical drapes.

The exact length of the skin varies, dependent upon many factors. Scuderi [5] has noted a direct correlation between the width of the femoral condyles and the required skin incision, when used a mid quad split MIS approach. We have shown that the length of the incision depends upon a height of the patient. In our series it could be as long as 13 to 14 cm for the tall obese patient, down to 8–10 cm for the shorter thin patient. Since the length of the incision depends on the size of the patient's leg and the patient's height giving any absolute value for the average skin incision land has no meaning. Furthermore, the skin incision may (and should) be further lengthened if the surgeon notices any undue tension on the skin, especially distally.

The deep capsular incision extends around the medial border of the patella and down along the proximal tibia adjacent to the patella tendon to the level of the tibial tubercle. Proximally the incision extends about 1–2 cm above the patella and then is turned medially for about 2 cm as a muscle splitting incision of the vastus medialis obliquus (☐ Fig. 27.2).

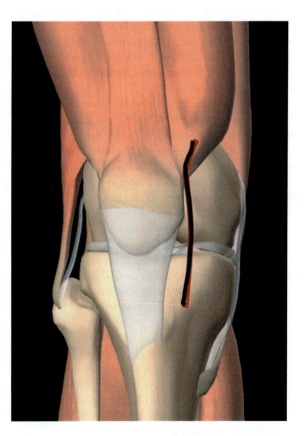

☐ Fig. 27.2. The capsular incision begins around the patella and extends distally to the level of the tibial tubercle. Proximally it extends for about 2 cm proximal to the superior pole of the patella and then turns medially for 2 cm as a muscle splitting incision into the VMO

27

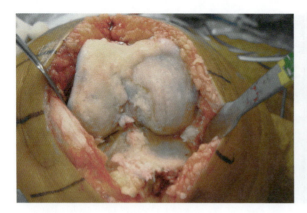

■ **Fig. 27.3.** The distal femur is easily visualized through the mini-mid-vastus approach

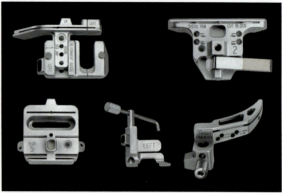

■ **Fig. 27.4.** Instrumentation designed and validated for use in the smaller capsular incision (Genesis II, Smith and Nephew, Tn USA)

The knee is then extended and the patella is then displaced laterally but not everted. A PCL retractor is used laterally to hold the patella and its displaced position. The lateral patello-femoral ligament can usually be identified then and tenotomized from within outwards. The knee is now flexed again to about 45°.

A medial capsular flap is elevated from the tibia to the level of the mid coronal plane, and approximately 50% of the fat pad is removed. Finally the tibial spines are resected. This last step opens the knee several millimeters and allows more easily placement of the resection instruments. Both condyles are now under direct vision (■ Fig. 27.3), allowing their subsequent resection from above downward without inadvertent soft-tissue damage or bone fracture.

To facilitate performing the surgery smaller instruments that will fit within the surgical wound without tension on the skin edges have been used (■ Fig. 27.4). These have been validated to be equally accurate as the standard instruments we had previously been using for the prior nine years.

Exposing the knee through a mini-mid vastus incision requires changing the flexion angle at various points during the procedure. For example, to visualize the anterior femur the knee has to be extended to allow the soft tissue window to move proximally. Likewise, to visualize the tibial plateau surfaces the knee has to be flexed to move the soft tissue window distally.

The author's personal preference is to first resect the distal femur using anterior referencing instruments. (Genesis II, Smith and Nephew, Memphis Tn). Rotational

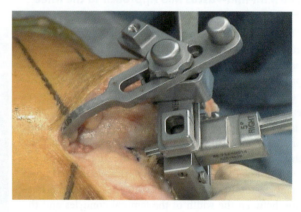

■ **Fig. 27.5.** Anterior referencing instrumentation rotationally oriented from the mid trochlear (Whiteside) line

alignment of the cutting guide is referenced off the mid trochlear line of Whiteside (■ Fig. 27.5). The femur is then sized after which the anterior, posterior and chamfer surfaces are resected using the appropriately sized cutting block.

After making the posterior femoral resection the tibia can easily be subluxed forward 1–2 cm. Either an intra-medullary or extra-medullary guide is then used to position the tibial cutting block. The medial half of the tibia is resected first after which the resected medial surface serves as a cutting platform for cutting the lateral half of the tibia. If a posterior stabilized prosthesis is to be used, the posterior cruciate ligament is resected at this stage.

Any remaining peripheral osteophytes are removed and the flexion and extension spaces are assessed for rectangularity. If necessary, the appropriate soft-tissue release can then be performed. For example, an elevation of the medial capsular flap can easily be performed for the fixed varus knee, and a release of the postero-lateral capsule and iliotibial band made for the fixed valgus knee. It is difficult, however, to release those structures that insert on the lateral epicondyle. If this type of lateral release is proposed pre-operatively, a standard median parapatellar should probably be used.

With the knee distracted by a laminar spread while at 90° of flexion, any posterior femoral osteophytes are removed with a curved osteotome and curette (■ Fig. 27.5). The flexion and extension spaces are compared for equality of size. If necessary at this stage, a further resection of the distal femur or proximal tibia is performed.

The patella is then lifted upward. It is resected from above downward (that is from medial to lateral) if an on-set implant is to be used, or reamed from the medial side of the knee if an inset implant is chosen.

To cement the tibial component, the tibia is flexed maximally and acutely subluxed forward using a PCL retractor posteriorly to allow full visualization of the resected tibial plateau surface (■ Fig. 27.6). This is the only time during the operation where such full flexion and anterior translation of the tibia is required. The surgeon should use cement during its high viscous phase to avoid running of the acrylic posteriorly. The author routinely uses Palacos (Biomet, Warsaw, Ind) since it remains viscous throughout almost its curing phase. Any remaining peripheral cement is removed, after which the femoral component is cemented in place. A trial bearing surface is inserted, the knee extended and the cement allowed to cure. After tourniquet deflation and securing of hemostasis, the permanent bearing is inserted.

If a posterior stabilized implant is chosen, it may be difficult to insert the permanent bearing with the knee flexed. The technique used by the author is to start insertion of the bearing with the knee flexed and then to extend the knee to about 30° of flexion. At this point the bearing may be fully seated using an impactor (■ Fig. 27.7). The knee is closed in a routine manner over close suction drains.

Post-operatively, the patient is placed in a compression bandage with a supplemental cold packs or a continuous cooling pad. The patient is begun on passive range of motion in a CPM machine within a few hours

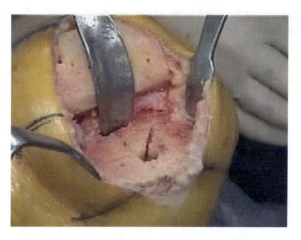

■ **Fig. 27.6.** The tibia is subluxed forward only for cementation of the tibial component

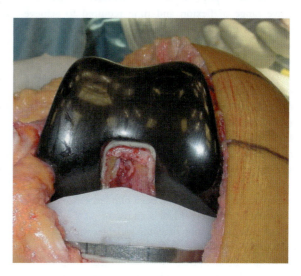

■ **Fig. 27.7.** The Genesis II Oxinium tri-compartmental total knee cemented in place trough a mini-mid vastus incision

after surgery, beginning at about 70° degrees of flexion. The CPM machine is advanced daily and this is combined with active and passive knee flexion exercises with the physical therapist. Since the routine in the author's hospital to use a femoral nerve block and continuous epidural catheter for analgesia after surgery, the patient walks with a soft knee splint on the leg for 1–2 days, after which this is discontinued.

Results of Total Knee Replcement Performed Through a Mini-Mid-Vastus Approach

In 2004 we reported on a prospective series of patients with osteoarthritis to whom it was proposed that their primary knee replacement surgery be performed through a mini-mid-vastus approach [8]. We excluded patients who had previously undergone an open surgical procedure on their knee, but did not exclude patients because of body mass index, gender or deformity. Thirty two patients were enrolled in this group. They were compared with a group of patients who had undergone a primary knee replacement through a standard medial parapatellar approach during the previous year.

We evaluated the patients both before and after surgery using the Knee Society rating system clinically and radiographically, entering the findings into a computerized database. A physical therapist measured the patient's passive range of flexion and time required to achieve specific rehabilitation milestones. The amount of pain medication that was used both in the epidural catheter and thereafter orally during the hospitalization was recorded by the anesthesia pain management team. They likewise measured pain level using a visual analog scale (VAS) multiple times during the day while the patients were awake. Closed suction blood drainage during the 24 hours after surgery was measured. The patients were evaluated at the first and second post-operative visits which normally occurred at 4–6 weeks, and 8–10 weeks, respectively). The radiographs were evaluated by an independent radiologist who had been blinded as to the type of surgical approach that had been used.

The data distribution of all the variables was examined and the relationship of each demographic and clinical variable to the outcome variables was examined. Nonparametric tests, such as the Man-Whitney test were used for non parametric data, and contingency table analysis was used to evaluate categorical data. T-tests were used for group comparisons of normally distributed continuous data.

General linear models were used to test variables that showed statistically significant relationships to the outcomes n vicariate models, with an alpha level being set at 0.05. The study was approved by the Institutional Review Board of the Hospital for Special Surgery.

The average patient age for the MIS group was 70 years (range = 62–78 years), while in the standard group it was 68 years (range = 58–75 years; p=0.4). There was no statistical difference in the height, weight, age, and BMI pre-operative alignment, pre-operative Lahey Clinic Score, or Function Score between the two groups. The patients in the MIS group had slightly better flexion pre-operatively (112° vs. 107°) and a slightly higher Knee Score than did the patients in the standard incision group, and the difference in both were statistically significant (p=0.03 and p=0.02, respectively).

The average tourniquet time for the MIS group was 58 min, while it was 51 min in the median parapatellar group. The difference was due to the requirement in the MIS group to reposition the knee to move the surgical window and replace the retractors at several stages during the operation. There were no lateral retinacular releases required in either group.

The patient's perception of pain as well as the amount of analgesics required by the patient were statistically less in the MIS group. The VAS in patients with the MIS incision was statistically less on every day in the hospital. The total PCA volume used by the patients in the MIS group was statistically lower than that in the standard incision group. The salutary effect on relief of pain was carried forth even after the epidural catheter was removed. We were able to convert the amount of analgesics used orally after removal of the epidural catheter into morphine sulfate equivalents. The MIS group used statistically lower amounts of morphine sulfate equivalents than did the standard group (p=0.008). We feel that this diminished pain is a major salutary effect of this surgical approach.

A second beneficial effect of this surgical approach was related to the rate of regaining flexion after the operation. By the second post-op day over 70% of the patients in the MIS group had achieved more than 80° of flexion, whereas in the standard group this degree of flexion was usually not obtainable until the 4th day after surgery. Since the MIS group had a slightly greater passive flexion pre-operatively, an ANOVA evaluation with pre-operative passive flexion as the covariate and post operative flexion as the dependent variable was performed. Even with this analysis, the MIS patients continued to have a more rapid return of flexion. What this meant was that patients in the MIS group reached their functional milestones which permitted discharge from the hospital, approximately 20% faster than the cohort of the patients in the standard incision group.

This increase of flexion was seen at the 6 weeks follow up examination as well. By three months the groups results in both groups were starting to approach each other and by one year they were essentially similar with no statistical difference.

There was no statistical difference in the amount of blood loss between the two groups. This could have been predicted, since blood loss after knee replacement is more likely from the cut bone surfaces and pin-hole tracts than from the soft tissues, and the bone cuts in both groups of patients were the same.

These benefits in pain relief and more rapid return of motion and function would be of no value if the implants were not properly inserted nor the knee properly balanced. We found, however that the position and alignment of the individual implants, the post operative stability, and the Knee Scores as evaluated after surgery were equal and excellent for both groups.

We had one patient with a skin complication in this entire series. This was a patient in the MIS group who developed a small skin slough at the most distal aspect of the wound. This healed with local skin care without any evidence of infection. We learned that the skin incision must be made long enough to prevent undue tension, especially distally, and that the surgeon's threshold for lengthening the skin incision in this area should be very low.

We subsequently performed a feasibility study of one hundred consecutive patients who were scheduled for a primary knee replacement to see what factors made the surgery through a mini-mid-vastus approach possible and which factors made the surgery extremely difficult to perform [9].

We found that the ideal patient was less than 71 inches in height and weighed less than 175 lbs. Having said that however, we were able to perform this surgical approach on patients as tall as 76 inches, and as heavy as 250 lbs. Calculating a BMI in these patients is of little value. There are some obese patients with a high BMI in whom the obesity is mainly truncal, with resultant thin legs. Those patients do as well as patients with a lesser BMI but with equally thin legs. To the contrary there are obese patients with a high BMI in whom the obesity is both truncal and peripheral. It is extremely difficult to perform an MIS approach in these patients.

The »optimal« patients should have at least 80°–90° of pre-operative flexion, less than a 15° flexion contracture, and a varus deformity or valgus deformity less than 20°. Finally the patient should not have had any open surgical procedures on the knee; although a prior arthroscopic procedure was not a contraindication.

The morbidly obese or highly muscular patient initially presented as a contraindication to this type of approach. Most recently we have been able to use this approach in some of these patients by extending the quad tendon split 1–2 cm more proximal before turning medially into the VMO.

Again in this study of 100 patients we found excellent position of the femoral and tibia components in both the sagittal and coronal planes and excellent stability in both planes. There were no infections, and no skin healing problems.

The standard midvastus incision may, or may not, result in electromyographic changes in that muscle after surgery. Dalury [10, 11] has shown that it does not, while Parentis [12] has shown that it does. Their studies, however were all made on 6–8 cm mid-vastus splitting incisions. Our regimen involves only a 2 cm split in the muscle, placing the split far distal to the neurological innervation of the muscle. Likewise a 2 cm split is distal to the descending genicular artery on the medial side of the knee.

This surgical approach is extensile and allows excellent visualization of both femoral condyles allowing a standard resection from above downward under direct vision. Furthermore, since it is a modification of already familiar surgical incision it is easy to teach and easy for surgeons to understand.

It has been alleged that a minimally invasive approach will somehow jeopardize the long term results of the arthroplasty. The major causes of total knee replacement failure are mal-positioning of the implants, knee imbalance, infection, and polyethylene failure [13]. In our two studies the implants were not mal-positioned, the knees were balanced and there were no infections. Furthermore, the implants that we used (Genesis II, Smith and Nephew, Tn) were ones that we had previously used for over 8 years in standard incision knee replacements with good longevity of the polyethylene.

What we did find, however, was that the salutary effects of this type of limited exposure were mainly related to the first 6–12 months after surgery. By one year after surgery patients' findings were similar to those who had undergone a standard larger surgical approach. However, the limited exposure patients arrived at that point with less pain and a more rapid return of their function. There must be a reality check, however between surgeons and their patients. This is a major surgical procedure, and there still is some pain after surgery and during the recuperative period. Patients must still participate in a vigorous physical therapy program if they are to expect the best outcomes.

References

1. Buechel F Sr, Buechel F Jr, Pappas MJ, D'Alesio J (2001) Twenty year evaluation of meniscal bearing and rotating platform knee replacements. Clin Orthop 388: 41–50
2. Ritter MA, Berend ME, Meding JB, Keating EM, Faris PM, Crites BM (2001) Long term follow-up of anatomic graduated components posterior cruciate retaining total knee replacement. Clin Orthop 388: 51–57
3. Hofmann AA, Evanich JD, Ferguson RP, Camargo MP (2001) Ten to 154 year clinical follow-up of the cementless natural knee system. Clin Orthop 388: 85–94
4. Webster's Ninth New Collegiate Dictionary (2002) Merriam-Webster INC, Springfield, Ma, p 756
5. Scuderi GR, Tenholder M, Capeci C (2004) Surgical approaches in mini incision total knee arthroplasty. Clin Orthop 428: 61–67
6. Pagnano M (2005) The anatomy of the extensor mechanism with particular reference to quadriceps sparing minimally invasive total knee arthroplasty: clinical, cadaveric, and high resolution MRI analysis of 200 knees. Clin Orthop 440: 62–68
7. Engh GA, Hold BT, Parks NL (1997) A midvastus muscle splitting approach for total knee arthroplasty. J Arthroplasty 12:322–331
8. Laskin RS, Beksac B, Phongjunakorn A, Pittors K, Davis J, Shim J, Pavlov H, Petersen M (2004) Minimally invasive total knee replacement through a mini-midvastus incision. Clin Orthop 428: 74–81
9. Laskin RS (2005) Minimally invasive total knee arthroplasty. The results justify its use. Clin Orthop 440: 54–59
10. Dalury DF, Jiranek WA (1999) A comparison of the midvastus and paramedical approaches for total knee arthroplasty. J Arthroplasty 14: 33–37
11. Dalury DF (2004) Does the midvastus approach compromise the vastus medialis obliquus? Arch Am Acad Orthop Surg 5: 454–459
12. Parentis MA, Rumi MN, Deol GS (1999) A comparison of the vastus splitting and median parapatellar approaches in total knee arthroplasty. Clin Orthop 367: 107–116
13. Sharkey PF, Hozack JW, Rothman R (2002) Why are total knee arthroplasties failing today? Clin Orthop 404: 7–13

Quadriceps Sparing Total Knee Arthroplasty in Association with Electromagnetic Navigation

R.K. Alan, A.J. Tria

Introduction

Since the introduction of the total condylar knee replacement in 1974, improvements and modifications have changed total knee arthroplasty (TKA) in many aspects [1–3] The result of these modifications has led to excellent long-term outcomes [4]. Other adjustments have been made to facilitate component insertion and surgical technique. Some of the changes have contributed significant advancements and have withstood the test of time and the rigors of objective testing, while others have fallen out of favor. Caspari, Whipple, and Goble attempted to perform a TKA with arthroscopic assistance and were unable to complete the procedure. Unfortunately, they did not publish any details concerning their work; however, this was one of the earliest attempts to perform a TKA with a less invasive approach.

Repicci developed the minimally invasive unicondylar knee arthroplasty (UKA) during the early 1990's. He and others have shown that the surgical approach reduced the morbidity, blood loss, hospital stay and recovery time [5–8]. The latest innovation in joint arthroplasty has been to extend the techniques and principles of minimally invasive surgery to TKAs. These changes have been made with the overall goal of improving outcomes for the patient. Ideally, minimally invasive surgery for TKA should maintain or improve upon the longevity of standard TKA, maintain the quality and safety of traditional TKAs, and decrease the morbidity and recovery time.

»Mini« TKA has contributed a decreased surgical incision length and decreased soft tissue disruption. The minimized approaches typically incise the quadriceps tendon, the vastus medialis, or the subvastus interval [9–15]. The quadriceps sparing TKA uses a capsular incision that extends from the superior pole of the patella to 2 cm below the tibial joint line. The benefit of the quadriceps sparing minimally invasive technique is aligned with the mini principles but aims to maintain the complete integrity of the extensor mechanism. The surgical approach of quadriceps sparing TKA does not extend the arthrotomy proximally into the quadriceps tendon, the vastus medialis, or the subvastus interval. The early results are promising and have shown earlier increased range of motion (ROM), shorter hospital stay, decreased blood loss, decreased pain, and earlier return to function without compromising alignment, knee scores, and patient safety [16, 17].

During the time period when the minimally invasive TKA techniques were being developed, there were many investigators working on navigational systems to assist the clinical surgery [18–21]. The senior author (AJT) was initially opposed to the use of these devices in conjunction with the minimally invasive TKA because of the additional time necessary to devote to the technique and the associated learning curve. Now the imageless systems are improved. Percutaneous arrays are no longer required; direct line of site with a camera is no longer necessary; and the time requirements are reduced to reasonable values. Navigation is more user friendly and has become a routine part of the minimally invasive TKA at our medical center.

Indications

The indications for the surgery are more restrictive than the standard TKA. The patient should have symptomatic, radiographically confirmed osteoarthritis that has failed medical management. Patella baja is a relative contraindication because it is more difficult to sublux the patella laterally. Rheumatoid patients are not the best candidates because the bone is often osteoporotic and can be injured during the course of the surgery with the smaller approach. The patient should be in good overall medical health and should not have significant co-morbidities that would preclude an operation that can be 50% longer than a standard TKA. The knee alignment should be no greater than 10 degrees of varus, 15 degrees of valgus, or 10 degrees of flexion contracture. Obesity also represents a problem for the surgery and an overall weight of 225 pounds is used as a cutoff. The BMI has not proven to be helpful at all. The *distribution* of the weight and the relationship between the thigh length and knee circumference is more important and it may be possible to establish a ratio of these two measurements that will be more clinically relevant. The knee should have at least 105 degrees of motion.

The anatomy of the vastus medialis has some effect upon the degree of difficulty of the exposure. There are three types of insertions for the vastus medialis: a high insertion into the quadriceps tendon above the level of the patella, a standard insertion into the superomedial aspect of the patella, and a low insertion at the mid portion of the patella. The lower the insertion, the more difficult the exposure becomes. The vastus insertion into the midlevel of the patella makes the procedure extremely difficult and is an indication for extension of the exposure and for the use a mini approach.

Over the past four years, the senior author has seen a gradual increase in the number of quadriceps sparing surgeries that have been performed. The percentage has increased from 28% to 39% of the entire number of arthroplasties per year. This increase is more related to the referral patterns of the practice than to any change in the indications. The mini approaches now represent 33% of the cases. Thus, smaller incisions now affect roughly three quarters of the TKAs that are performed annually.

Surgical Technique

The patient is positioned supine on the operating-room table and a tourniquet is applied to the upper thigh. The leg is sterilely prepped and draped in the traditional fashion and a leg holder (Innovative Medical Products, Plainville, Connecticut, USA) is used for positioning of the limb throughout the entire procedure (◘ Fig. 28.1). The leg holder is valuable in this type of surgery because the knee is typically in the flexed position from 30 to 60 degrees for most of the operation and holding this by hand is cumbersome and time consuming. Most of the surgeries are performed under tourniquet control. A curvilinear skin incision is made from the superior pole of the patella to the tibial joint line just medial to the patella and patella tendon (◘ Fig. 28.2). This is essentially the same incision

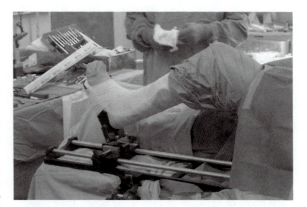

◘ **Fig. 28.1.** The leg holder allows both flexion-extension and internal-external rotation

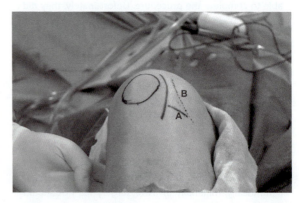

◘ **Fig. 28.2.** The medial incision extends from the superior margin of the patella to 2 cm below the joint line. »A« is the tibiofemoral joint line and »B« is the medial femoral condyle margin

used for the minimally invasive medial compartment UKA. An arthrotomy is made in line with the skin incision from the superomedial border of the patella approximately two centimeters below the tibial joint line. Both the varus and valgus knee can be replaced through the medial arthrotomy, however, a lateral arthrotomy similar to one for a lateral UKA can be used for the valgus knee. With either approach, care is taken to avoid extension of the arthrotomy into the quadriceps tendon, the vastus medialis, or the subvastus interval.

The knee is then brought into full extension and the patellar fat pad is excised. Without fully everting the patella, the articular surface is removed using a free hand technique with an oscillating saw. A patellar clamp is currently under development to eliminate the need for free hand resurfacing. The patellar cut is carried out early in the procedure in order to provide more working room in the knee joint. Resurfacing of the patella is not mandatory but facilitates the exposure. A metal protector is placed over the patellar surface to shield it from the retractors that are used throughout the remainder of the procedure if the bone is soft (◘ Fig. 28.3).

While the knee remains in full extension, the anterior surface of the femur is cleared to visualize the femoral sulcus for later femoral sizing and positioning. The femoral dynamic reference frame (DRF) is attached to the medial aspect of the femoral metaphysis about 2 cm above the joint line and medial to the femoral sulcus area to avoid interference with the femoral cuts (◘ Fig. 28.4). The DRF is the equivalent of the arrays that are used with the line of sight systems. The tibial DRF is attached to the medial tibial metaphyseal area 2 cm distal to the joint line and just above the insertion of the pes anserinus. The emitter (the equivalent of the camera in the line of sight systems) is covered with a sterile bag and is kept in the field for the duration of the operative procedure (◘ Fig. 28.5). The hip center of rotation is established with rotation of the lower limb and the land marking is completed with the pointer probe (◘ Fig. 28.6).

The knee is then flexed to 45 degrees and the anterior and posterior cruciate ligaments are resected from the intercondylar notch. Following resection of the cruciates and visualization of the notch, the antero-posterior (AP) axis line of Whiteside is established (◘ Fig. 28.7). The paddle probe is placed on the end of the uncut femur and the distal femoral varus or valgus versus the mechanical axis of the knee is recorded (◘ Fig. 28.8). An intra-medullary rod is introduced into the femoral canal (◘ Fig. 28.9).

A cutting guide is then attached to the intra-medullary reference and the distal femur is resected from medial to lateral. The angle of this cut is adjusted to correct the distal femoral surface to neutral versus the mechanical axis. During the distal femoral cutting, the intra-medullary reference must be removed and the cut must be completed by using the partially cut condyles to guide the saw blade for the remainder of the resection. The paddle probe is then placed on the end of the cut surface to verify that the cut is neutral. The flexion of the cut is kept the same as the original flexion of the natural distal femur (◘ Fig. 28.10).

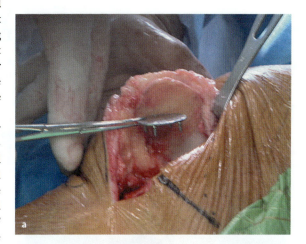

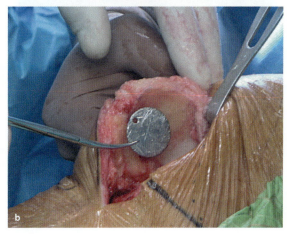

◘ **Fig. 28.3a,b.** The metal protector is placed on the patellar cut surface to protect it from the retractors during the remainder of the procedure

28

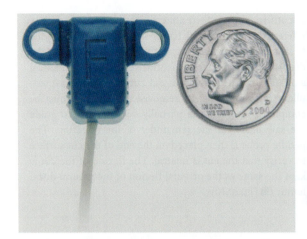

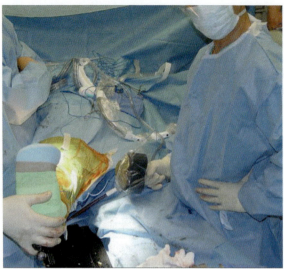

Fig. 28.5. The emitter is wrapped with a sterile cover and kept in the surgical field

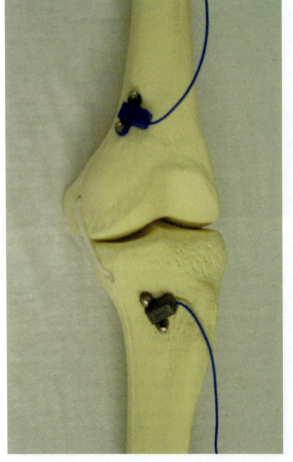

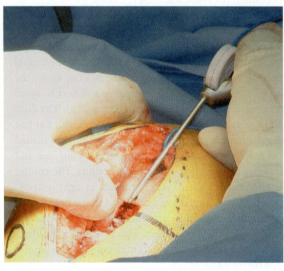

Fig. 28.6. The pointer probe is used to identify specific sites on the femoral and tibial side of the knee

Fig. 28.4a. The DRF is the size of an American dime. **b** The DRFs are attached with two screws to the medial aspect of the femur and the tibia

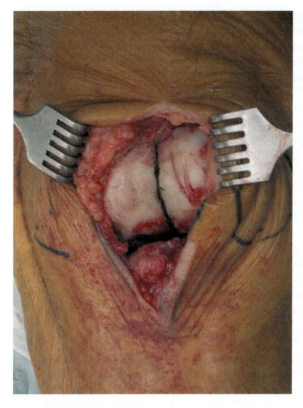

Fig. 28.7. Whiteside's antero-posterior axis line is drawn on the surface of the femur

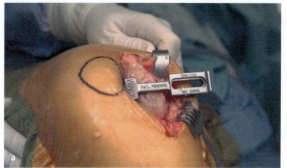

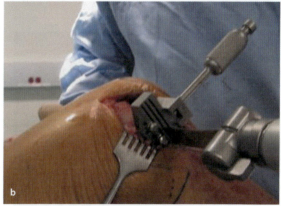

Fig. 28.9. a The intra-medullary guide is inserted into the femoral canal with a plate that references the medial femoral condyle. **b** The side cutting guide is attached to the intra-medullary plate on the medial side of the femur

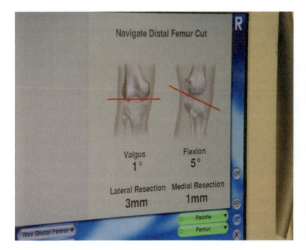

Fig. 28.8. The EM screen shows the mechanical varus or valgus of the actual distal femur before the cut is made

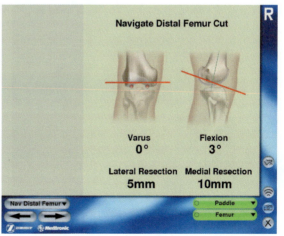

Fig. 28.10. The EM screen with the paddle placed on the distal femoral cut surface to check that the cut is neutral versus the mechanical axis

The tibial surface is resected next using an extra-medullary guide. The alignment guide for the quadriceps sparing system is very similar to that for a standard total knee but it directs the saw blade from the medial aspect of the tibia (❑ Fig. 28.11). The varus-valgus, flexion-extension, and depth of the resection are all controlled in a similar fashion to a standard cutting guide but with the EM paddle probe in the cutting slot to again verify the cut (❑ Fig. 28.12).

After alignment of the tibial guide is completed, the cut is initiated with the knee in 70 degrees of flexion. Sometimes, the tibial surface can be resected as a single piece, similar to the standard technique. However, if the soft tissues are particularly stiff, or the knee is a larger size, it may be necessary to cut the tibial proximal fragment into two or three pieces to facilitate the removal and to protect the posterior neurovascular structures. The three piece approach removes the medial one half of the tibia as a single piece similar to the resection for a medial UKA. The lateral one half is then cut into two pieces, anterior and posterior and removed in sequence (❑ Fig. 28.13). After the tibial resection is completed, the paddle is placed on the cut surface to confirm that the cut is perpendicular to the long axis of the tibia and that the slope is in the range of 5 to 7 degrees posteriorly angulated (❑ Fig. 28.14).

With both the distal femoral and proximal tibial resections completed, the extension space is checked with a spacer block and extra-medullary rods (❑ Fig. 28.15). Ligament balancing is conducted in the normal fashion with the standard soft tissue releases. With the 20 mm of bone resected from the surfaces, it is not difficult to release either the medial collateral ligament complex or the ilio-tibial band and the lateral ligament complex. The EM system can check the degree of laxity in millimeters on both the medial and lateral side of the knee in full extension when stress is applied with the spacer block in place. If the laxity is 1–2 mm on each side, the balance is acceptable. Once alignment and balance in extension are confirmed, the knee is flexed to 70 degrees and the femoral sizing guide (tower) is used to set the external

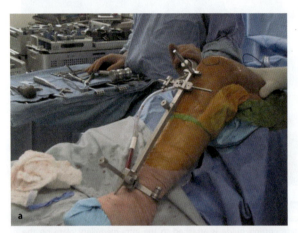

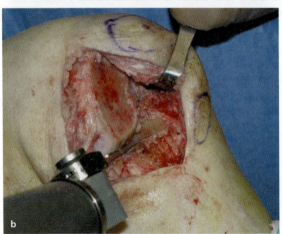

❑ **Fig. 28.11. a** The extra-medullary tibial cutting guide directs the saw blade from the medial aspect of the knee. **b** The medial one half of the proximal tibial resection can be removed using a technique similar to the unicondylar resection. Then, the saw blade can be inserted into the slot cut to complete the lateral resection

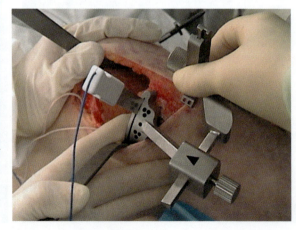

❑ **Fig. 28.12.** The EM paddle is placed into the tibial cutting slot to check the cut before it is completed

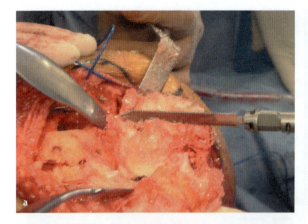

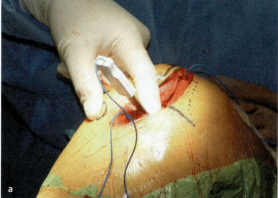

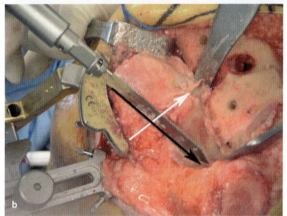

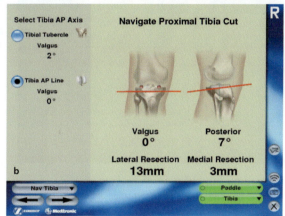

Fig. 28.13. a The proximal tibial resected bone can be removed using a three piece technique if the knee is tight or the fragment is of a larger size. This figure shows the antero-posterior cut with a reciprocating saw in an open knee procedure. **b** The white arrows shows the previous antero-posterior cut and the black arrow traces the oblique cut from medial to lateral to remove the antero-lateral fragment

Fig. 28.14. a The paddle is placed on the tibial cut surface. **b** The EM screen shows the tibial cut as recorded with the paddle probe

rotation and to determine the size of the femoral component (**Fig. 28.16). The EM land marking has already indicated a femoral size at the start of the surgery and the clinical measurement should be confirmed. The tower references the posterior condyles of the femur but must also be adjusted so that it is parallel to the antero-posterior axis line if either condyle is deficient posteriorly.

A probe is attached to the tower and used to reference the anterior femur for sizing (**Fig. 28.17). A preliminary cut is made across the anterior surface of the femur, setting the rotation and avoiding cortical notching.

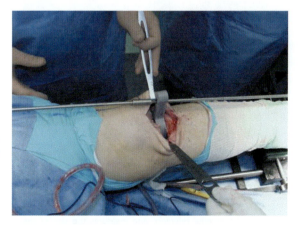

Fig. 28.15. The extension space is checked using a standard spacer block and extramedullary rods

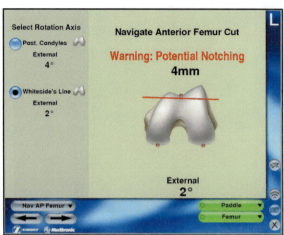

Fig. 28.18. The EM screen shows the anterior femoral cut. The cut is 4 mm below the anterior cortex and should be adjusted. It is 4 degrees externally rotated versus the posterior condylar axis and 2 degrees externally rotated versus Whiteside's line

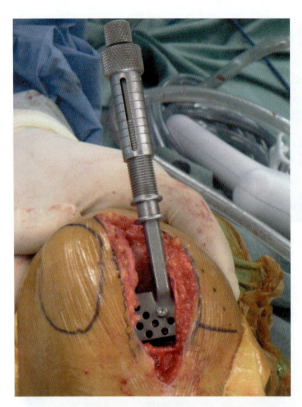

Fig. 28.16. The tower is an instrument that references the posterior femoral condyles and sets the external rotation of the femoral cuts

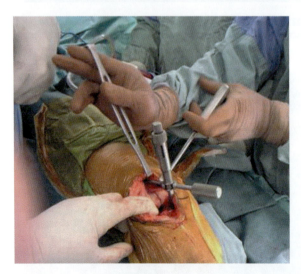

Fig. 28.17. The anterior reference arm measures the size of the femoral component and sets the location of the preliminary external rotation cut

The EM paddle probe can be set into the anterior cutting slot of the femoral guide before the cut is initiated and can confirm the external rotation versus the posterior condylar axis and the anteroposterior axis. It can also confirm that the anterior cut will not notch the femoral cortical surface (Fig. 28.18). The finishing block is positioned medial to lateral in full extension while resting on the previously made external rotation cut (Fig. 28.19). The femoral finishing cuts are completed with the knee in 70 degrees of flexion (Fig. 28.20).

After completion of the femoral and tibial cuts, the working space in the knee is dramatically increased. The final checks of the flexion and extension gaps are completed and alignment and balance are adjusted in the standard fashion. The gaps in flexion and extension can be evaluated with the EM to check that the laxity on the medial and lateral sides is 1 to 2 mm in each position (Fig. 28.21).

The tibial sizing plate is attached to a curved handle that avoids internal rotation. The guide has two deployable hooks that reference the posterior cortex of the proximal tibia (Fig. 28.22). The plate is centered medial to lateral and externally rotated using the tibial tubercle, the femoral box cut, and the malleoli of the ankle as reference points. The drilling and broaching are completed in the standard fashion.

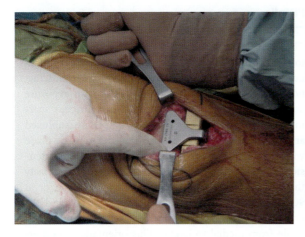

◨ **Fig. 28.19.** A plate is attached to the femoral finishing block and rests on the anterior cut surface. The block is centered medial to lateral and pinned in place

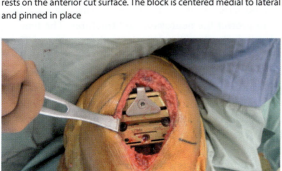

◨ **Fig. 28.20.** The knee is flexed to 70 degrees and the finishing cuts are completed

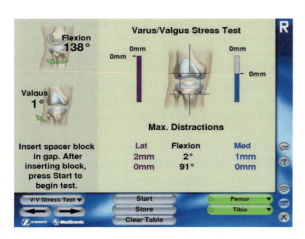

◨ **Fig. 28.21.** The EM screen records the laxity of the knee at 2 and 91 degrees of flexion

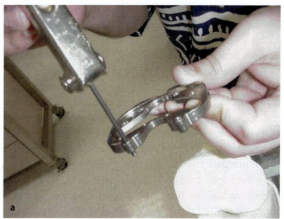

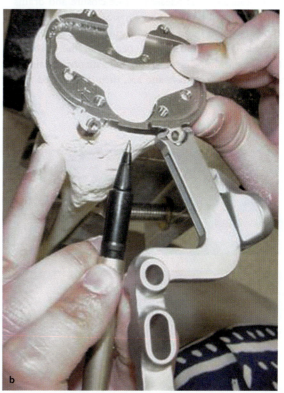

◨ **Fig. 28.22. a** The tibial sizing plate has two posterior hooks that can be deployed to reference the posterior cortex of the tibia on either the medial or lateral side, or both. **b** The handle for the tibial plate angles around the patellar tendon to avoid internally rotating the component while positioning the plate

28

The trial components are inserted in the following order: tibia, femur, polyethylene tray, and patella. Patellar tracking, ligament balance, range of motion, and overall alignment are checked for the final time before cementing. The EM is again used to confirm that the knee is in proper overall alignment, that the gaps are balanced, and that the knee does come to full extension. The bone surfaces are prepared and the components are cemented in the same order as the trial components. The tibial component is now two pieces with a stem that is inserted through the plate and torqued into position. The shorter keel on the implant makes it much easier to insert in full extension and allows improved visualization for the cementing (Fig. 28.23).

The tourniquet is released before closure and drains are placed for cell saver suction. Physical therapy is started on the afternoon of surgery with full weight bearing as tolerated. DVT prophylaxis is begun on the first day after surgery with enoxaparin. The patients remain in the hospital for two days and are, then, transferred to a rehabilitation center.

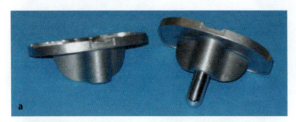

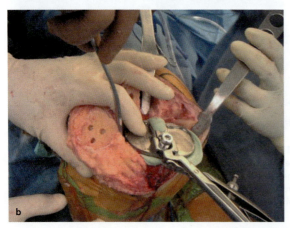

 Fig. 28.23. a The MIS tibial component has a shorter keel for ease of insertion. **b** A drop down screw can be inserted through the tray

Pitfalls

The most important way to avoid many of the pitfalls is to choose the appropriate knee for the surgical procedure. Expanding the indications is sometimes enticing; however, it will often lead to difficulties with exposure and lead to early failures. During the quadriceps sparing surgery, the tibia is seldom completely subluxed anterior to the femur. Therefore, the cuts must be made with the knee in different degrees of flexion and extension as opposed to the standard open knee arthroplasty that references the knee either in full extension or at 90 degrees of flexion. The distal femoral cut and the proximal tibial cut are performed with a captured saw blade from medial to lateral. This orientation is different than the standard approach and with less visibility of the posterior aspect of the knee, the surgeon must be sure to protect the neurovascular structures. The femoral cut does become much easier with experience. The tibial cut can deviate from the perpendicular because the lateral aspect is not fully visualized. This is a step that is significantly improved with the EM navigation because the alignment can be checked both before and after the cut is completed. With greater experience it is also possible to see the entire lateral aspect of the tibia in full extension.

Cement removal is a bit more tedious with the minimally invasive surgery technique. Palacos cement is much easier to use because of its prolonged doughy phase and the components should be cemented with separate mixes. The tibial component is cemented first. The MIS tibia is much easier to position in full extension and the lateral side of the knee is much easier to see with the new prosthesis. It is important to fully visualize the lateral aspect of the tibia during the cementing. The tibia should be kept under compression with a spacer block while waiting to cement the femoral component. There have been three tibial loosenings and these seem to have occurred because of liftoff of the tray while the cement is setting up.

Male knees with extremely large femoral components are difficult to complete and the surgeon should not hesitate to extend the incision if necessary.

The EM navigation does not perform the operation and should be used as another tool but not as the final, and only confirming instrument. It does, however, add another checking system that improves the accuracy of the overall surgical procedure.

Results

The senior author has now completed over 400 of the minimally invasive quadriceps sparing surgeries since February of 2002. Some 75 of the operations have been done under EM control. The procedure now requires about 50 percent more time (total tourniquet time of 70 min) than the standard TKA (total tourniquet time of 45 min). The EM navigation adds 12 minutes to the procedure. The blood loss is 20% less as measured by intra-operative and post-operative cell saver collections and transfusions. The average length of stay has decreased by two days from the standard TKA. Pain scores, pain medicine requirements, and physical therapy participation have all improved in the quadriceps sparing TKA population when compared to the standard TKA. Greater ROM in the range of 20 to 30 degrees has been measured for quadriceps sparing TKA and this difference persists for at least three months. Post operative alignment as determined radiographically has shown no statistically significant difference from matched controls undergoing standard TKA over the same time period and Knee Society Scores are the same in both populations.

There are three tibial component loosenings, one early infection, two late infections, and 2 tibial components are in 7 degrees of varus. Two of the tibial loosenings have been revised using a standard tibial tray with a stem. The early infected knee was removed and re-implanted with success. The two varus tibias have not required surgical correction. One of the late infections has been removed and reinserted and the other is pending further surgery. The EM cases have no outliers. There have been two cases using the EM system that have produced grossly misleading measurements that were ignored (incidence of 2.6%). The post-operative x-rays showed that the clinical decision was correct. On one occasion, the EM system failed in the middle of the procedure and had to be abandoned.

Conclusions

Minimally invasive TKAs are in the early stages of development and are improving in a step-wise fashion. The quadriceps sparing minimally invasive surgery TKA does not violate the extensor mechanism or the supra-patellar pouch. The early results have shown decreased blood loss, hospital stay, pain scores, pain medication requirements, and time till participation in physical therapy while con-

currently increasing early ROM [16, 17]. Combining the procedure with EM navigation control adds a degree of increased accuracy and confirms each step of the procedure. However, the EM is not correct 100% of the time and should be used as an additional surgical tool rather the primary reference. The surgeon must still control the entire operative procedure and make the final decisions. The findings have also shown Knee Society Scores and radiographic alignment outcomes that are comparable to standard TKAs without significantly increasing complications or compromising patient safety. The short term results appear to be promising. Long term results and clinical trials comparing the different minimally invasive surgery techniques will certainly need to be completed; however, there is little doubt that smaller exposures with limited arthrotomies controlled with navigational tools will become more common in the next few years.

References

1. Insall J, Ranawat CS, Scott WN, Walker P (1976) Total condylar knee replacement: preliminary report. Clin Orthop Relat Res 120: 149–54
2. Insall J, Tria AJ, Scott WN (1979) The total condylar knee prosthesis: the first 5 years. Clin Orthop Relat Res 145: 68–77
3. Insall JN, Hood RW, Flawn LB, Sullivan DJ (1983) The total condylar knee prosthesis in gonarthrosis. A five to nine-year follow-up of the first one hundred consecutive replacements. J Bone Joint Surg 65: 619–628
4. NIH Consensus Statement on Total Knee Replacement December 8–10 (2004) J Bone Joint Surg Am 86A: 1328–1335
5. Repicci JA, Eberle RW (1999) Minimally invasive surgical technique for unicondylar knee arthroplasty. J South Orthop Assoc Spring 8: 20–27
6. Argenson JN, Flecher X (2004) Minimally invasive uni-compartmental knee arthroplasty. Knee 11: 341–347
7. Price AJ, Webb J, Topf H, Dodd CA, Goodfellow JW, Murray DW, Oxford Hip and Knee Group (2001) Rapid recovery after oxford unicompartmental arthroplasty through a short incision. J Arthroplasty 16: 970–976
8. Gesell MW, Tria AJ Jr (2004) MIS unicondylar knee arthroplasty: surgical approach and early results. Clin Orthop Relat Res 428: 53–60
9. Scuderi GR, Tenholder M, Capeci C (2004) Surgical approaches in mini-incision total knee arthroplasty. Clin Orthop Relat Res 428: 61–67
10. Bonutti PM, Mont MA, McMahon M, Ragland PS, Kester M (2004) Minimally invasive total knee arthroplasty. J Bone Joint Surg Am 86A (Suppl 2): 26–32
11. Haas SB, Cook S, Beksac B (2004) Minimally invasive total knee replacement through a mini midvastus approach: a comparative study. Clin Orthop Relat Res 428: 68–73

12. Laskin RS (2004) Minimally invasive total knee replacement using a mini-mid vastus incision technique and results. Surg Technol Int 13: 231–238

13. Laskin RS, Beksac B, Phongjunakorn A, Pittors K, Davis J, Shim JC, Pavlov H, Petersen M (2004) Minimally invasive total knee replacement through a mini-midvastus incision: an outcome study. Clin Orthop Relat Res 428: 74–81

14. Laskin RS (2005) Minimally invasive total knee arthroplasty: the results justify its use. Clin Orthop Relat Res 440: 54–59

15. Boerger TO, Aglietti P, Mondanelli N, Sensi L (2005) Mini-subvastus versus medial parapatellar approach in total knee arthroplasty. Clin Orthop Relat Res 440: 82–87

16. Tria AJ, Coon TM (2003) Minimal incision total knee arthroplasty: early experience. Clin Orthop Relat Res 416: 185–190

17. Berger RA, Sanders S, Gerlinger T, Della Valle C, Jacobs JJ, Rosenberg AG (2005) Outpatient total knee arthroplasty with a minimally invasive technique. J Arthroplasty 20 (Suppl 3): 33–38

18. Stulberg SD, Loan P, Sarin V. Computer assisted navigation in total knee replacement: results of an initial experience in thirty-five patients. J Bone Joint Surg Am 84(Suppl) 90–98, 2002.

19. Sparmann M, Wolke B, Czupalla H, Banzer D, Zink A (2003) Positioning of total knee arthroplasty with and without navigation support. J Bone Joint Surg (Br) 85: 830–835

20. Jenny JY, Boeri C, Picard F, Leitner F (2004) Reproducibility of intraoperative measurement of the mechanical axes of the lower limb during total knee replacement with a non-image based navigation system. Comput Aided Surg 9: 161–165

21. Schicho K, Figl M, Donat M, Birkfellner W, Seemann R, Wagner A, Bergmann H, Ewers R (2005) Stability of miniature electromagnetic tracking systems. Phys Med Biol 50: 2089–2098

MIS Total Knee Arthroplasty with a Subvastus Approach

M.W. Pagnano

Introduction

Performing minimally invasive total knee arthroplasty through a subvastus approach makes sense on an anatomic basis, on a scientific basis and on a practical basis. Anatomically, the subvastus approach is the only approach that saves the entire quadriceps tendon insertion on the patella [1–5] (Fig. 29.1). Scientifically, the subvastus approach has been shown, in prospective randomized clinical trials, to be superior to the standard medial parapatellar arthrotomy and to the so-called quad-sparing arthrotomy [3, 6, 7] (Table 29.1). Practically, MIS TKA with a subvastus approach is reliable, reproducible and efficient and allows the MIS technique to be applied to a broad group of patients not just a highly selected subgroup [8] (Table 29.2).

It is now accepted widely that the tenets of minimally invasive (MIS) total knee arthroplasty (TKA) include: a smaller skin incision, no eversion of the patella, minimal disruption of the suprapatellar pouch, and minimal disruption of the quadriceps tendon. To what degree any one of those factors contribute to improvements in post-operative function remains unclear. Our initial attempts at MIS TKA using the short medial arthrotomy (sometimes referred to as the quad-sparing approach) and the mini-midvastus splitting approaches were frustrated by some substantial technical difficulties. We then modified the subvastus approach to the knee to meet the tenets of MIS TKA and found that it markedly facilitated MIS surgery and allowed it to be applied to a broader group of patients. When coupled with instruments designed specifically for small incision surgery the modified subvastus approach is reliable, reproducible and safe. Using a simple set of retractors this procedure can be done without making any blind cuts or free-hand cuts and that enhances surgical accuracy and patient safety.

Surgical Technique

The incision starts at the superior pole of the patella, ends at the top of the tibial tubercle and measures 3.5 inches (8.8 cm) in extension. Surgeons should start with a traditional 6- to 8-inch incision and then shorten the incision length over time. The medial skin flap is elevated to clearly delineate the inferior border of the vastus medialis obliquus muscle. The fascia overlying the VMO is left intact as this helps maintain the integrity of the muscle belly itself throughout the case. The anatomy is very consistent. The inferior edge of the VMO is always found more inferior and more medial than most surgeons anticipate. The muscle fibers of the VMO are oriented at a 50-degree angle and the VMO tendon always attaches to the mid-pole of the patella. It is very important to save this edge of tendon down to the mid-pole. That is where the retractor will rest so that the VMO muscle itself is protected throughout the case. The arthrotomy is made along the inferior edge of the VMO down to the mid-pole of the patella (do not be tempted to cheat this superiorly as that will hinder, not help, the ultimate exposure; Fig. 29.2).

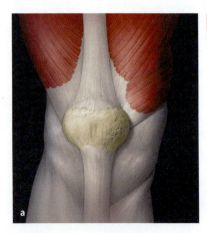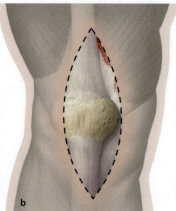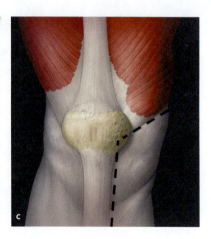

Fig. 29.1a–c. Anatomy of the extensor mechanism. a The vastus medialis obliquus (VMO) tendon consistently inserts at the mid-pole of the patella at a 50-degree angle relative to the long axis of the femur. **b** When looking through a surgical incision one could easily mis-identify the most prominent part of the VMO (the point closest to the patella, akin to the bow of the ship) as the most inferior part of the VMO. Because that most prominent portion often lies close to the superior pole of the patella some surgeons might then mis-takenly presume that the VMO inserts at the superior pole of the patella. Additional medial dissection will delineate the inferior bor-der of the VMO which is more inferior and more medial than most surgeons anticipate. **c** The arthrotomy for the subvastus exposure parallels the inferior border of the VMO, intersects the patella at the mid-pole and then is turned straight distally to parallel the medial margin of the patellar tendon (Copyright Mayo Foundation used with permission)

Table 29.1. Prospective randomized trials of the subvastus approach in total knee arthroplasty

Authors	Patients Randomized [n]	Study Variable	Key Findings
Roysam and Oakley [7]	89	Subvastus versus medial parapatellar approach	1. Subvastus had earlier straight leg raising p<0.001 2. Subvastus used fewer narcotics week one p<0.001 3. Subvastus had greater knee flexion at 1 week p<0.001
Aglietti et al. [6]	60	Subvastus versus Zimmer Quad-Sparing approach	1. Subvastus had earlier straight leg raising p=0.004 2. Subvastus had better flexion at 10 days p=0.01 3. Subvastus had better flexion at 30 days p=0.03
Faure et al. [3]	20	Subvastus versus Medial parapatellar approach	1. Subvastus had greater strength at 1 week and 1 month 2. Subvastus had fewer lateral releases done 3. Subvastus was preferred by patients 4:1

Table 29.2. Clinical results with the minimally invasive subvastus approach in 103 consecutive patients with osteoarthritis [8]

Gender	Age [years]	Weight [pounds]	Operative time [minutes]	Functional outcomes mean (in days)
61 female 42 male	66 (40–90)	198 pounds (137–305)	58 minutes (35–115)	1. Hospital stay 2.8 days 2. Normal daily activities 7 days 3. No walker: 14 days 4. No cane: 21 days 5. Drive 28 days 6. Walk ½ mile 42 days 7. Flexion at 8 weeks 116 degrees

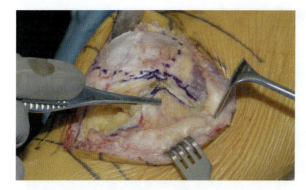

◻ **Fig. 29.2.** The arthrotomy starts medially along the inferior border of the VMO and extends to the mid-pole of the patella at the same 50-degree angle as the muscle fibers of the VMO

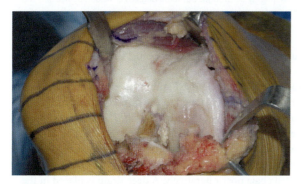

◻ **Fig. 29.3.** With surprisingly little force the patella is retracted completely into the lateral gutter. The knee is then flexed to 90 degrees providing exposure of both condyles of the distal femur

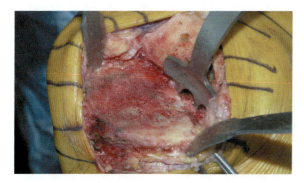

◻ **Fig. 29.4.** The tibia is prepared next and that is done in order to provide more working room for subsequently sizing and rotating the femoral component (the most difficult part of any MIS TKA). Good exposure of the entire surface of the tibia is accomplished with 3 retractors placed precisely: a pickle-fork retractor posteriorly to provide an anterior drawer; and bent-Homan retractors medially and laterally to protect the collaterals and define the perimeter of the tibial bone

This proximal limb of the arthrotomy parallels the inferior edge of the VMO and is made at the same 50 degree angle relative to the long axis of the femur. At the mid-pole of the patella the arthrotomy is directed straight distally along the medial border of the patellar tendon. A 90 degree bent-Homan retractor is placed in the lateral gutter and rests against the robust edge of VMO tendon that was preserved during the exposure. Surprisingly little force is needed to completely retract the patella into the lateral gutter. The knee is then flexed to 90 degrees providing good exposure of both distal femoral condyles. (◻ Fig. 29.3) If the patella does not slide easily into the lateral gutter, typically it is because a portion of the medial patello-femoral ligament remains attached to the patella. That occurs if the proximal limb of the arthrotomy is made in too horizontal a fashion rather than at the 50 degree angle that parallels the VMO. By releasing that tight band of tissue the patella will translate laterally without substantial difficulty.

The distal femur is cut with a modified intra-medullary resection guide. Bringing the knee out to 60 degrees of flexion better exposes the anterior portion of the distal femur. When a very small skin incision is used the distal femur is cut one condyle at a time with the intra-medullary portion of the cutting guide left in place for added stability. If a slightly longer skin incision is used the distal cutting guide can be pinned in place and both condyles cut in a standard fashion.

The proximal tibia is cut next and by doing that more room is made for subsequently sizing and rotating the femoral component (the most difficult part of any MIS TKA). Three retractors are placed precisely to get good exposure of the entire surface of the tibia: a pickle-fork retractor posteriorly provides an anterior drawer and protects the neurovascular structures; and bent-Homan retractors medially and laterally protect the collaterals and define the perimeter of the tibial bone (◻ Fig. 29.4). The tibial resection is carried out with an extra-medullary guide optimized for small incision surgery. The tibia is cut in one piece using a narrow but thick saw blade that fits the captured guide. The narrow blade is more maneuverable in the smaller guide and provides better tactile feedback for the surgeon to detect when the posterior and lateral tibial cortices have been cut.

The femoral sizing and rotation guide is thin enough that it can be pinned to the distal femur and the knee can still be brought out to 60 degrees of flexion to visualize the anterior femur for accurate sizing (◻ Fig. 29.5).

At 60 degrees of flexion a retractor is placed anteriorly and the surgeon can see under direct vision that the femoral cortex will not be notched. Clearing some of the synovium overlying the anterior femoral cortex helps ensure that femoral sizing is accurate. The femoral finishing guide is adjusted medially or laterally. Femoral rotation is confirmed by referencing the surgeon's choice of the posterior condyles, Whiteside's line or the transepicondylar axis each of which can be defined with this subvastus approach. After the femoral and tibial cuts are made the surgeon can carry out final ligament releases and check flexion and extension gap balance in whatever fashion is desired.

Patellar preparation with this surgical approach is left until the end. Cutting the patella is not required for exposure and preparing the patella last the risk of inadvertent damage to the cut surface of the patella is minimized. The patella cut is done free-hand or with the surgeon's choice of cutting or reaming guides. When a patellar cutting guide is used, the trial components are removed as then the entire limb can shorten, taking tension off the extensor mechanism and allowing easier access to the patella for preparation.

The modular tibial tray is cemented first, then the femur and finally the patella. The tibia is subluxed forward with the aid of the pickle-fork retractor and the medial and lateral margins of the tibia are exposed well with 90 degree bent-homan retractors. Care is taken to remove excess cement from around the tibial base plate, particularly postero-laterally. The femur is exposed for cementing by placing bent human retractors on the medial and lateral sides above the collateral ligament insertions on the femur. A third retractor is placed under the VMO where it overlies the anterior femur. Cement is applied to the entire undersurface of femoral implant prior to impaction. Special attention is paid to removing excess cement from the distal lateral surface of the femur as this area is difficult to see after the patella is cemented in place. At this point, the real tibial insert can be placed or a trial insert can be used at the surgeon's discretion. The patella is cemented last. After the cement has hardened, the knee is put through a range of motion and final balancing and patellar tracking are assessed.

The tourniquet is deflated so that any small bleeders in the subvastus space can be identified and coagulated. The closure of the arthrotomy starts by re-approximating the corner of capsule to the extensor mechanism at the mid-pole of the patella. Then 3 interrupted zero-vicryl su-

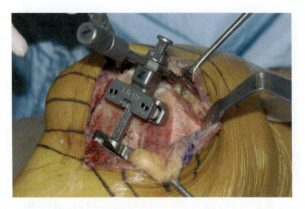

■ **Fig. 29.5.** The femoral sizing and rotation guide is designed to be pinned to the distal femur and is thin enough that the knee can subsequently be brought out to 60 degrees of flexion to visualize the anterior femur for accurate sizing

tures are placed along the proximal limb of the arthrotomy. (■ Fig. 29.6) These sutures can usually be placed deep to the VMO muscle itself and grasp either fibrous tissue or the synovium attached to the distal or undersurface of the VMO instead of the muscle itself. These first 4 sutures are most easily placed with the knee in extension but are then tied with the knee at 90 degrees of flexion to avoid over-tightening the medial side and creating an iatrogenic patella baja post-operatively. A deep drain is placed in the knee joint and the distal/vertical limb of the arthrotomy is closed with multiple interrupted zero-vicryl sutures placed with the knee in 90 degrees of flexion. The skin is closed in layers. Staples are used, not a subcuticular suture. More tension is routinely placed on the skin during MIS TKA surgery than in standard open surgery and our experience suggests the potential for wound healing problems is magnified if the skin is handled multiple times as is the case with a running subcuticular closure.

Discussion

Minimally invasive total knee arthroplasty with a subvastus approach has proved reliable, reproducible and efficient in our experience. The technique is amenable to step-wise surgeon learning and can be applied to a substantial range of patients who require total knee arthroplasty not just a selected subgroup. There are patients who are not good candidates for any MIS TKA procedure including those with marked knee stiffness, fragile skin,

management program, a rapid rehabilitation protocol and appropriate patient expectations. How much each of those contribute versus how much the surgical technique contributes to early functional improvement has not been determined scientifically.

References

1. Pagnano MW, Meneghini RM, Trousdale RT (2006) Anatomy of the knee with special reference to quadriceps sparing TKA. Clin Orthop, in press
2. Chang CH, Chen KH, Yang RS, Liu TK (2002) Muscle torques in total knee arthroplasty with subvastus and parapatellar approaches. Clin Orthop 398: 189–195
3. Faure BT, Benjamin JB, Lindsey B, Volz RG, Schutte D (1993) Comparison of the subvastus and paramedian surgical approaches in bilateral knee arthroplasty. J Arthroplasty. 8: 511–516
4. Gore DR, Sellinger DS, Gassner KJ, Glaeser ST (2003) Subvastus approach for total knee arthroplasty. Orthopedics 26: 33–35
5. Hoffman AA, Plaster RL, Murdock LE (1991) Subvastus (Southern) approach for primary total knee arthroplasty. Clin Orthop 269: 70–77
6. Aglietti P; Baldini A (2005) A prospective, randomized study of the mini subvastus versus quad-sparing approaches for TKA. Presented at the Interim Meeting of the Knee Society. New York, NY September 8, 2005
7. Roysam GS, Oakley MJ (2001) Subvastus approach for total knee arthroplasty: a prospective, randomized, and observer-blinded trial. J Arthroplasty 16: 454–457
8. Pagnano MW, Leone JM, Hanssen AD, Lewallen DG (2005) Minimally invasive total knee arthroplasty with an optimized subvastus approach: a consecutive series of 103 patients. Presented at American Academy of Orthopaedic Surgeons Annual Meeting 2005, Washington DC

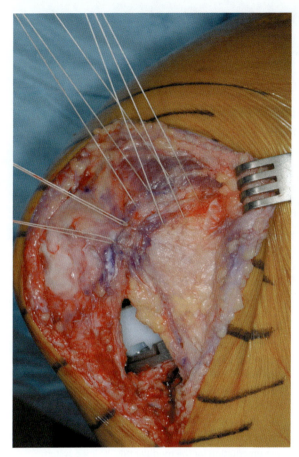

◾ **Fig. 29.6.** The tourniquet should be let down and any small bleeders in the subvastus space should be cauterized. The closure is then done by first re-approximating the corner of capsule at the mid-pole of the patella. Then 3 interrupted sutures are placed through the deep layer of synovium to close the knee joint itself. Those 4 sutures are tied with the knee at 90 degrees of flexion to avoid creating iatrogenic patella baja

or marked obesity. Similarly, any knee with patella baja will be markedly difficult with an MIS approach because subluxing the patella laterally is often not possible. In those cases a traditional skin incision and more extensile exposure are in the interest of patient and surgeon alike.

Surgeons should be aware that changes in surgical technique alone are unlikely to provide the dramatic early improvements in postoperative function that some surgeons have described after MIS TKA. Maximizing the early gains after surgery (minimal pain, early ambulation, rapid hospital discharge) typically requires a combination of advanced anesthetic techniques, a multimodal pain

Minimally Invasive Total Knee Replacement in Tibia First Technique with the INNEX® Knee System

A.M. Halder, S. Köhler, G. Pap, W. Neumann

Introduction

Since excellent long term results have been reported [8, 12, 14, 20, 22, 31, 32, 35, 39, 40, 42] a growing number of younger patients are receiving total knee replacement. These active patients expect fast recovery with early mobilization and short rehabilitation to reassume work and sports as soon as possible. Additionally, decreasing financial resources in public health systems force surgeons to minimize surgical trauma to be able to shorten hospital stay and thereby costs. The main reason for prolonged rehabilitation still is extensive soft tissue trauma with eventual wound healing problems and extensor mechanism disturbance. Therefore, after minimally invasive unicompartimental knee replacement had been established [34], minimally invasive techniques for total knee replacement have been developed [5–7, 15, 17, 33, 43, 45–47].

Unfortunately, minimally invasive total knee replacement is not well defined yet. Various clinical parameters could be taken into consideration, such as skin incision length, extent of transection of the retinaculum, the tendons and muscles of the extensor apparatus and the joint capsule as well as the amount of bone resection and patella manipulation [7]. Although important for patient's satisfaction skin incision length should not be the only determinant [7] and it varies considerably with knee position. If the goal of minimally invasive total knee replacement is less pain and rapid recovery, trauma to the extensor mechanism is probably the decisive factor and should be minimized.

Therefore, we have chosen the subvastus approach for minimally invasive total knee replacement as the integrity of the vastus medialis muscle and its tendon is preserved [37]. The patella is lateralized but not everted and patella surface resection is not mandatory for adequate exposure. At the same time, the approach allows direct anterior access to the knee and thereby soft-tissue balancing. In contrary to other existing procedures, in our operative technique the tibia is cut first and all subsequent bone cuts are soft-tissue tension referenced. In cooperation with the ZIMMER company we have developed a minimal invasive instrumentation for the modular INNEX® knee system

Indication

Especially in the beginning, patients for minimally invasive total knee replacement should be carefully selected and indication for the minimally invasive procedure should be restrictive not to compromise patient care and run into intra-operative problems.

The medial side is easy to access and mild to moderate varus knees with less than 10° varus angle are an ideal indication. Severe varus knees need releases beyond the extent of minimal incisions. As access to the lateral side is more difficult and therefore lateral ligament releases are hard to carry out we limit the indication to mild and passively correctable valgus knees with less than 15° valgus angle. A flexion contracture should not exceed 15° as extensive posterior releases are hard to perform through minimal incisions. Flexion should be possible to about 90°

to be able to lateralize the patella. Additionally, access to the anterior soft tissues is limited.

A high body mass index makes a patient less suitable for minimally invasive total knee replacement as a thick subcutaneous tissue layer additionally obstructs sight. On the other hand, an extremely thin subcutaneous tissue layer is hard to retract and tends to develop wound healing problems. Finally, a narrow femur is easier to handle minimal invasively as soft-tissue traction is mainly on the lateral side. In summary, »the ideal patient for a minimal incision total knee arthroplasty … seems to be a thin woman with a low body mass index, a narrow femur, and good pre-operative range of motion« [44].

Pre-Operative Diagnostics

Preoperative diagnostics include a single leg-stance X-ray of the knee joint in the a-p plane to indicate the operation and to estimate the size of the components. A lateral X-ray in 90° flexion shows the posterior slope of the tibia plateau and the height of the patella. An axial view of the patella in 30° flexion reveals patella tilt or subluxation. A long leg X-ray with the load on both legs is used to determine the mechanical and anatomical axes of the leg. The femoral angle alpha, representing the difference between the two, in necessary to choose the appropriate femoral angle bushing for the distal femoral cut. Furthermore the amount of tibia resection perpendicular to its longitudinal axis can be estimated.

Operative Technique

Tourniquet

The operation is carried out in general or spinal anesthesia. We do not routinely use a tourniquet as post-operative pain is significantly reduced without it [1, 28, 49]. Furthermore, it clamps the quadriceps muscle and thus interferes with its tension. For the described minimal invasive subvastus approach optimal muscle relaxation is needed. Finally, it is safer to control bleeding throughout the procedure than only at the end as one might miss perforating vessels on the posterior surface of the vastus medialis muscle. If it becomes necessary to apply the tourniquet it should be placed as far superiorly as possible and be inflated at most 100 mmHg above systolic blood pressure [28, 50].

Positioning

The patient is in the supine position. The knee is flexed to 90°. We routinely use a supporting roll on the table as well as a lateral support to position the leg in extension as well as high flexion easily and reliably. Of course, a knee positioner could be used alternatively as the flexion position of the knee has to be changed frequently throughout the procedure to optimize access to the tibia and femur through the incision and make best use of the soft-tissue window. Access to the tibia is easier from the top in high flexion while pulling on the tibial head in the anterior direction leaving the femur posteriorly. Access to the femur is easier from the front in 90° of flexion leaving the tibia inferiorly.

Approach

The procedure is initiated with a midline skin incision starting from the superior pole of the patella down to about 2 cm inferior to the joint line level. While the superior part of the skin incision is needed to insert the femoral component, the inferior part is needed for the tibial cut. The subcutaneous tissue is cut down to the level of the fascia in line with the skin incision. Then it is bluntly separated from the fascia on top of the vastus medialis muscle and the medial retinaculum. The dissection is advanced in superior direction underneath the skin on the medial side on top of the vastus medialis muscle (◘ Fig. 30.1). The medial retinaculum is incised just medially of the patella and the patella tendon. Two Langenbeck retractors elevate subcutaneous tissue and skin and sharp dissection is advanced superiorly along the inferior border of the vastus medialis muscle down medially to the inter-muscular

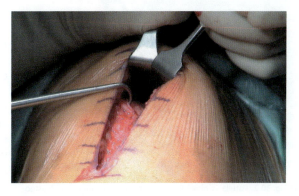

◘ **Fig. 30.1.** Subcutaneous subvastus approach with patella lateralised

septum. Then dissection is continued bluntly with a swab to lift the vastus medialis from the septum as far superiorly as possible. This should be performed up to the adductor hiatus. Care must be taken not to harm the femoral artery and vein [38]. Finally, the joint capsule is incised underneath the vastus medialis muscle in superior direction up to the superior pouch.

Inside the joint, the anterior part of the medial meniscus, the anterior cruciate ligament, the anterior part of the lateral meniscus and the inferior part of the Hoffa fat pad are resected. Partial resection of the Hoffa fat pad prevents painful impingement post-operatively [23]. The patella is now lateralized stretching the vastus medialis muscle across the anterior inferior femur. A 90° angulated Homann retractor is inserted on the lateral side to expose the lateral tibial plateau and keep the patella lateralized. Two 90° angled Homann retractors are inserted on the medial side and posteriorly in the intercondylar notch.

Patella

The patella is tilted 90° upward with the leg extended (◘ Fig. 30.2). If the patella is preserved, we perform a circumferential denervation and remove peripheral osteophytes. For patella replacement the patella is clamped with the patella forceps to ensure the correct resection height and cut through its slot with an oscillating saw. The central anchoring hole is drilled as far superior and medially as possible and the trial patella is inserted to check its fit.

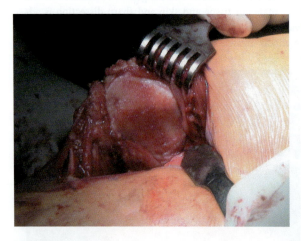

◘ **Fig. 30.2.** Patella is tilted 90° upward for denervation and osteophyte removal

Tibia Resection

We routinely use the modular INNEX® knee system for unconstrained or semi-constrained, mobile or fixed primary and revision total knee replacements. For extramedullary aiming the tibial alignment guide is fixed with a pin proximally in the center of the tibial plateau and distally around the ankle joint in 90° knee flexion. Rotation is adjusted with reference superiorly to the medial aspect of the tibial tuberosity and inferiorly to the centre of the ankle joint or the second metatarsal bone. Then the guide is aligned parallel to the axis of the tibia resulting in perpendicular tibia resection with a fixed slope of 6°. For intra-medullary aiming – preferred by us – the tibial canal is opened with a drill through the footprint of the anterior cruciate ligament. An intra-medullary rod is inserted, the tibial alignment guide is slid onto it and the rotation position is fixed with a pin.

With a stylus tibia resection height is determined (◘ Fig. 30.3). To restore the joint line tibia resection is usually performed 10 mm inferior to the level of the healthier compartment corresponding to 10 mm minimum implant thickness. The tibia cutting block is fixed medially with pins and the alignment guide is removed (◘ Fig. 30.4). Tibia resection is carried out with an oscillating saw. Care must be taken not to damage the patella tendon. Both Homann retractors should be placed between the tibia plateau and the collateral ligaments to protect them especially as the lateral compartment is not entirely visible. If the posterior cruciate ligament should be preserved an osteotome is used to protect its tibial insertion. The saw cut should be entirely completed to be able to remove the resected bone in one piece as later resection of the posterior residues is difficult. The tibia cutting block is removed.

Femoral Resection

Osteophytes from the femur and tibia are now resected and a preliminary medio-lateral ligament balancing is done. In minimally invasive technique it is easier to access the medial compartment but releases on the lateral side are still possible with the Homann retractor between tibia or femur and the lateral collateral ligament. The intra-medullary canal of the femur is opened with a drill usually slightly medial and anterior to the roof of the intercondylar notch and an intra-medullary rod is inserted.

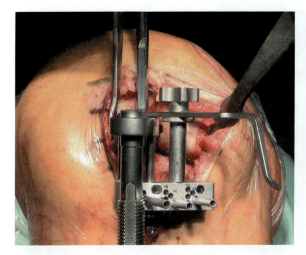

Fig. 30.3. Tibia resection height is determined with a stylus

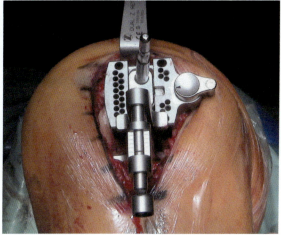

Fig. 30.5. Tensioner turns ap cutting block into 3°-5° external rotation

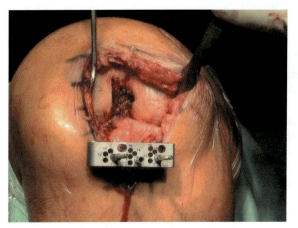

Fig. 30.4. Tibia cutting block is fixed medially with pins

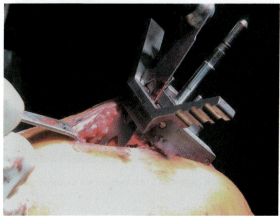

Fig. 30.6. Anterior femur resection

Anterior femoral resection is facilitated and muscle violation prevented with a modified Z-retractor elevating the vastus medialis muscle from the distal femur. The size of the femoral component is determined with a gauge referring to the distance from the anterior femoral cortex to the posterior femoral condyles. The femoral angle bushing is chosen as preoperatively planned. The respective a-p cutting block is slid onto the intra-medullary rod and its anterior surface is adjusted in line with the anterior femoral cortex with the help of a stylus.

The tensioner is inserted turning the a-p cutting block into an external rotation of about 3–5° resulting from equal tension on the medial and lateral side (Fig. 30.5). If the rotation alignment guide cannot be inserted, ligament tension is too high and the tibia should be resected again, if tension is too low, additional spacers should be inserted with the rotation alignment guide. Then the a-p cutting block is fixed with two pins and the rotation alignment guide is removed. The anterior and posterior femoral resections are performed with an oscillating saw (Fig. 30.6).

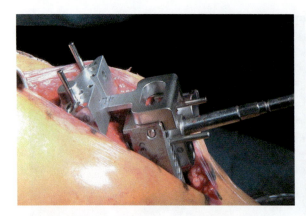

Fig. 30.7. Alignment of distal femur cutting block

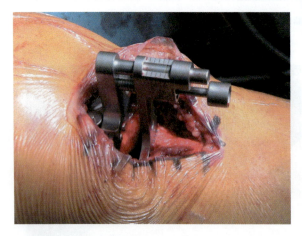

Fig. 30.8. Extension gap height is checked with the tensioner

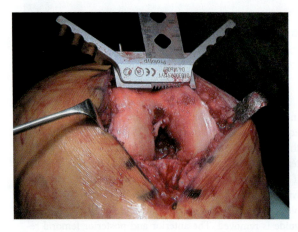

Fig. 30.9. Distal femur resection

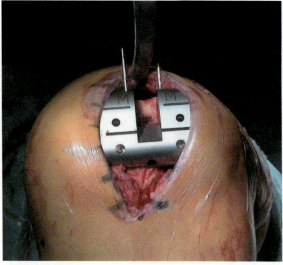

Fig. 30.10. Facet cutting guide is aligned with reference to the patella groove

The flexion gap should be rectangular and the tibial surface should be parallel to the epicondylar axis. The resulting stability in flexion is tested with the spacer.

In flexion contracture posterior osteophytes should now be removed and the posterior capsule released. The distal femoral cutting block is slid on top of the a-p cutting block and fixed with two pins (■ Fig. 30.7). The a-p cutting block and the intra-medullary rod are removed. Prior to the distal femoral resection the resulting tension is now checked with the tensioner (■ Fig. 30.8). If necessary, the resection level is adjusted so that the extension gap exactly matches the flexion gap. Then distal femoral resection is performed and the distal femoral cutting block is removed (■ Fig. 30.9). Finally both flexion and extension gaps are checked with the spacer for equality and stability.

Now the respective chamfer resection guide is inserted (■ Fig. 30.10). Care must be taken not to trap soft tissues medially or laterally. Medio-lateral positioning of the guide is done with reference to the width of the femoral condyles and the position of the patella groove. The chamfer resection guide is fixed with two pins and the anterior and posterior chamfer resections are carried out. The trochlea recess for the femoral component is cut out with an osteotome and the chamfer resection guide is removed.

30

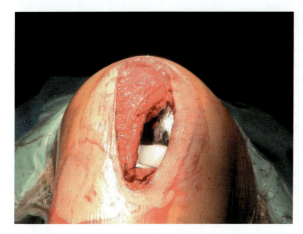

Fig. 30.11. Range of motion, stability and patella tracking is checked

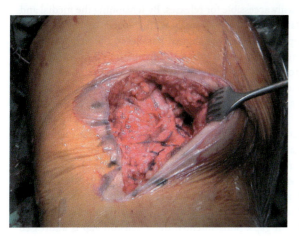

Fig. 30.12. Retinaculum suture

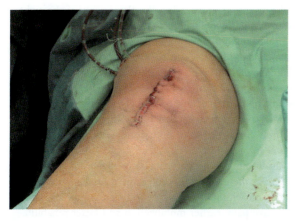

Fig. 30.13. Skin suture

Trial Reduction

The trial femoral component is inserted and the posterior femoral condyles are adapted. The size of the trial tibial component is chosen depending on the size of the tibial plateau. The height of the onlay is determined according to the height of the flexion and extension gaps and attached to the trial tibial component. Both are inserted and rotated into the ideal position with the patella reduced by repeated flexion and extension while maintaining optimum tibia coverage. In extension the tibial trial component is fixed in place with two pins and the knee is flexed. The peg holes are drilled as well as the central stem hole and the instruments are removed.

The bony surfaces are cleaned thoroughly. We always cement the tibial and if required the patella component. Then the tibial onlay is inserted. In minimally invasive knee replacement we implant a cementless femoral component as access to its sides is limited and therefore removal of excess cement is difficult. Finally, the knee joint is moved with the patella reduced to check range of motion, stability and patella tracking [11]. For wound closure the medial retinaculum, subcutaneous tissue and skin are sutured in flexion. Suturing of the vastus medialis muscle or tendon is not necessary as it is not transected at all [12, 13].

Discussion

Approach

In less invasive techniques for total knee replacement the standard median parapatellar approach is shortened as well as the necessary skin incision [36]. The patella is still everted or at least completely lateralized. As in standard total knee replacement techniques this approach allows good visualization and surgery on both tibial and femoral condyles from the front. However, it violates the vastus medialis tendon as well as the quadriceps tendon and therefore with regard to our above mentioned definition should not be regarded as minimal invasive.

In the so called quad-sparing approach the incision ranges »from the superior pole of the patella to the tibial joint line« [47] transecting the medial retinaculum as well as the inferior part of the vastus medialis tendon as its insertion sometimes inferiorly reaches the middle third of the patella [2]. Although this approach violates the vastus medialis tendon it allows no patella eversion and only limited patella lateralization. Therefore, access to and visualization of the lateral compartment is limited and surgery is solely done from the medial side. Consequently, releases and resections on the lateral side are difficult and the risk of lateral prosthetic overhang is increased. Moreover, the important distal femoral cut is at risk to be imprecise as the oscillating saw is guided by the cutting block fixed to the soft medial side wall of the medial condyle. To perform the subsequent resections it is advantageous to further reduce tension and resect the patellar surface even if this is clinically not indicated.

Another way to reduce tension in the soft tissues is to advance the incision directly into the vastus medialis muscle as midvastus approach [24–27] or as VMO snip [5–7]. Even though many minimally invasive techniques for total knee replacement use this approach it violates the vastus medialis muscle by splitting its distal fibers and endangers its innervation [30] and the politeal vascular bundle [10].

For these reasons we use a minimally invasive technique for total knee replacement using a subcutaneous subvastus approach. The subvastus approach has proven to be less harmful for the extensor apparatus than the parapatellar approach [13, 16, 21]. It preserves the integrity of the vastus medialis muscle [41] and its tendon elevating it bluntly from the inter-muscular septum to be able to completely lateralize the patella. Nor an incision of the vastus medialis tendon neither a separation of its muscle fibers is necessary. Patella blood supply and stability are preserved [29] and the risk of patella dislocation is minimized. The patella is not everted what could cause post-operative extensor weakness [6]. Therefore, the approach results in less blood loss, less post-operative pain, earlier mobilization and faster rehabilitation [4, 9, 37]. However, compared to the standard parapatellar approach, the operative procedure is more demanding and operation time is prolonged [4]. Furthermore, the surgeon has to rely on sufficient relaxation of the vastus medialis muscle for adequate exposure. In our approach, skin incision length is reduced by subcutaneous preparation superior to the patella.

Soft Tissue Balancing

In most existing techniques for minimally invasive total knee replacement, soft-tissue tension referenced bone cuts are difficult or even impossible if access is limited to the medial side. Soft-tissue referenced bone cuts require access from the front to insert a ligament tensioner or spacer to determine tension on the medial and lateral side separately in flexion and extension. In these techniques the femur is cut first and the subsequent resections are bone referenced. The femoral epicondyles could serve as bony landmarks. However, if access is limited to the medial side the lateral epicondyle is hidden.

The subcutaneous subvastus approach allows access from the front for soft tissue tension referenced bone cuts with a tensioner or spacer. In our technique, we perform the tibial cut first: All subsequent resections on the femur are based on the perpendicular tibial cut and are soft tissue tension referenced. The tibial cut reduces overall tension and the soft tissues on the medial and lateral side are easily accessible for releases. By tensioning the medial and lateral soft tissues equally with a spacer or tensioner the epicondylar axis is aligned parallel to the tibial cut. This maneuver usually turns the femur into 3–5° of external rotation. Corresponding to the size of the femoral component, the level of the posterior femoral condyle resection is determined and thereby the flexion gap.

If the flexion gap is imbalanced, ligament releases are carried out as necessary. In flexion the medial and lateral soft tissues as well as the posterior joint capsule are easily accessible for releases. As the flexion gap is wider, the releases usually are less extensive than in extension. Releasing soft tissues in flexion starts balancing the extension gap, too, as most ligaments constrain both gaps. Subsequently, the extension gap is addressed second and usually only needs fine tuned releases. This procedure minimizes the need for releases in extension and prevents over-releasing the flexion gap if the tight extension gap would be addressed first. This especially is important if a mobile bearing is used. Furthermore, balancing the flexion gap first allows releasing the medial collateral ligament from anterior to posterior as the anterior bundle tightens in flexion whereas the posterior bundle tightens in extension. Finally, the important distal femoral resection is carried out with the cutting block securely fixed on top of both condyles ensuring a high degree of precision.

In summary, the subcutaneous subvastus approach preserves the integrity of the vastus medialis muscle and its tendon without patella eversion resulting in less post-operative pain, earlier mobilization and faster rehabilitation. At the same time it allows access from the front for soft tissue tension referenced bone cuts with a tensioner or spacer to obtain balanced flexion and extension gaps of identical size.

However, compared to the standard parapatellar approach, the operative procedure is more demanding and depends on adequate muscle relaxation. Therefore, we recommend to gradually adopt the minimally invasive technique. First, one should switch from standard to minimal invasive instrumentation and get used to it. Then skin and tendon incision could be shortened without patella eversion. Finally, the whole vastus medialis muscle could be left intact and pulled across the distal femur to lateralize the patella. Thereby, the increased risk of component mal-positioning immanent to all minimal invasive total knee replacement techniques is minimized.

Results

Since minimal invasive techniques for unicondylar knee replacement have been introduced by Repicci [34] similar techniques for total joint replacement have been developed. Consequently, minimally invasive total knee replacement is a new evolving technique lacking long term results. Therefore, most authors solely describe their new technique [48] and – at most – early results. As the benefit of minimal invasive total knee replacement is expected to be evident within the first weeks or months after the operation these early results are meaningful and most of them are encouraging:

Some authors use the quad-sparing approach. Tria [47] has followed 70 minimal invasive total knee replacements for 9 months and noticed less intra-operative blood loss, shorter length of stay and increased range of motion by 20° with similar implant accuracy to standard total knee replacements. He reported no infections or wound complications, but the operative procedure took twice as long. Berger [3] reported that 48 of 50 consecutive patients with minimal invasive total knee replacement chose to go home the day of surgery but he had three readmissions. He described no intra-operative complications.

More authors use a modified midvastus approach. Bonutti reported 210 [97%] good to excellent results of a total of 216 minimally invasive total knee replacements according to the Knee Society Score two to four years post-operatively. Six underwent manipulation and five re-operation because of deep infection or component misplacement. In a matched pairs study all 32 minimal invasive total knee replacements had excellent results while only 29 of 32 standard total knee replacements rated excellent. Laskin [27] compared 32 minimally invasive total knee replacements with 26 standard open replacements six weeks post-operatively. In the minimally invasive knee replacements the increase in the Knee Society Score was higher and the average pain score was lower. The alignment and position of the components was normal in both groups. Haas [18] followed 40 minimally invasive knee replacements for one year and reported faster regain of motion and greater range of motion one year post-operatively. He reported no difference in leg alignment, no infections, extensor mechanism or neurovascular complications.

To summarize, most authors report less pain, faster regain of motion with accelerated rehabilitation and good to excellent short term results. Our own early results indicate less pain post-operatively with faster regain of motion and accelerated rehabilitation, but the procedure was more demanding and the operative time was prolonged. However, in changing existing successful total knee replacement techniques the main goal must be not to compromise the long term result for the patient. Therefore, as long-term results are not available yet, the main concern is correct component positioning and leg alignment. Dalury [11] compared 30 minimally invasive knee replacements with 20 standard knee replacements. He reported early advantages of minimal invasive total knee replacement like less pain, faster regain of motion but points out three cases of varus mal-alignment to conclude that minimal incisions impede surgeon's vision and thereby influence component alignment and the long-term result negatively. Consequently, to start with minimal invasive total knee replacement we recommend:

- to carefully select the patient for minimal invasive total knee replacement,
- to schedule twice the time as for standard total knee replacement,
- to gradually adopt the minimal invasive technique [5],
- to check component alignment intra-operatively with fluoroscopy,
- to convert to a standard approach if component alignment is in doubt and
- to measure skin incision length in extension as the result will be more satisfying for the surgeon.

References

1. Abdel-Salam A, Eyres KS (1995) Effects of tourniquet during total knee arthroplasty A prospective randomised study. J Bone Joint Surg Br 77: 250–3

2. Andrikoula S, Tokis A, Vasiliadis HS, Georgoulis A (2006) The extensor mechanism of the knee joint: an anatomical study. Knee Surg Sports Traumatol Arthrosc 14(3):214–220

3. Berger RA, Sanders S, Gerlinger T, Della Valle C, Jacobs JJ, Rosenberg AG (2005) Outpatient total knee arthroplasty with a minimally invasive technique. J Arthroplasty 20: 33–38

4. Boerger TO, Aglietti P, Mondanelli N, Sensi L (2005) Mini-subvastus versus medial parapatellar approach in total knee arthroplasty. Clin Orthop Relat Res 440: 82–87

5. Bonutti PM, Mont MA, Kester MA (2004) Minimally invasive total knee arthroplasty: a 10-feature evolutionary approach. Orthop Clin North Am 35: 217–226

6. Bonutti PM, Mont MA, McMahon M, Ragland PS, Kester M (2004) Minimally invasive total knee arthroplasty. J Bone Joint Surg 86: 26–32

7. Bonutti PM, Neal DJ, Kester (2003) MA Minimal incision total knee arthroplasty using the suspended leg technique. Orthopedics 26: 899–903

8. Buechel FF Sr (2002) Long-term followup after mobile-bearing total knee replacement. Clin Orthop Relat Res 404: 40–50

9. Chang CH, Chen KH, Yang RS, Liu TK (2002) Muscle torques in total knee arthroplasty with subvastus and parapatellar approaches. Clin Orthop Relat Res. 398:189–195

10. Cooper RE Jr, Trinidad G, Buck WR (1999) Midvastus approach in total knee arthroplasty: a description and a cadaveric study determining the distance of the popliteal artery from the patellar margin of the incision. J Arthroplasty 14: 505–508

11. Dalury DF, Dennis DA (2005) Mini-incision total knee arthroplasty can increase risk of component malalignment. Clin Orthop Relat Res. 440: 77–81

12. Elkus M, Ranawat CS, Rasquinha VJ, Babhulkar S, Rossi R, Ranawat AS (2004) Total knee arthroplasty for severe valgus deformity. Five to fourteen-year follow-up. J Bone Joint Surg 86: 2671–2676

13. Faure BT, Benjamin JB, Lindsey B, Volz RG, Schutte D (1993) Comparison of the subvastus and paramedian surgical approaches in bilateral knee arthroplasty. J Arthroplasty 8: 511–516

14. Gill GS, Joshi AB, Mills DM (1999) Total condylar knee arthroplasty. 16- to 21-year results. Clin Orthop Relat Res 367: 210–215

15. Goble EM, Justin DF (2004) Minimally invasive total knee replacement: principles and technique. Orthop Clin North Am. 35: 235–245

16. Gore DR, Sellinger DS, Gassner KJ, Glaeser ST (2003) Subvastus approach for total knee arthroplasty. Orthopedics 26: 33–35

17. Gregori A (2005) Minimally invasive navigated knee surgery: a European perspective. Orthopedics 28: 1235–1239

18. Haas SB, Cook S, Beksac B (2004) Minimally invasive total knee replacement through a mini midvastus approach: a comparative study. Clin Orthop Relat Res 428: 68–73

19. Hofmann AA, Plaster RL, Murdock LE (1991) Subvastus (Southern) approach for primary total knee arthroplasty. Clin Orthop Relat Res 269: 70–77

20. Ito J, Koshino T, Okamoto R, Saito T (2003) 15-year follow-up study of total knee arthroplasty in patients with rheumatoid arthritis. J Arthroplasty 18: 984–992

21. Keblish PA (2002) Alternate surgical approaches in mobile-bearing total knee arthroplasty. Orthopedics 25: 257–264

22. Kelly MA, Clarke HD (2002) Long-term results of posterior cruciate-substituting total knee arthroplasty. Clin Orthop Relat Res 404: 51–57

23. Kramers-de Quervain IA, Engel-Bicik I, Miehlke W, Drobny T, Munzinger U (2005) Fat-pad impingement after total knee arthroplasty with the LCS A/P-Glide system. Knee Surg Sports Traumatol Arthrosc 13: 174–178

24. Laskin RS (2003) New techniques and concepts in total knee replacement. Clin Orthop Relat Res 416: 151–153

25. Laskin RS (2004) Minimally invasive total knee replacement using a mini-mid vastus incision technique and results. Surg Technol Int 13: 231–238

26. Laskin RS (2005) Minimally invasive total knee arthroplasty: the results justify its use. Clin Orthop Relat Res 440: 54–59

27. Laskin RS, Beksac B, Phongjunakorn A, Pittors K, Davis J, Shim JC, Pavlov H, Petersen M (2004) Minimally invasive total knee replacement through a mini-midvastus incision: an outcome study. Clin Orthop Relat Res 428: 74–81

28. Manen Berga F, Novellas Canosa M, Angles Crespo F, Bernal Dzekonski J (2002) Effect of ischemic tourniquet pressure on the intensity of postoperative pain. Rev Esp Anestesiol Reanim 49: 131–135

29. Matsueda M, Gustilo RB (2000) Subvastus and medial parapatellar approaches in total knee arthroplasty. Clin Orthop Relat Res 371: 161–168

30. Parentis MA, Rumi MN, Deol GS, Kothari M, Parrish WM, Pellegrini VD Jr (1999) A comparison of the vastus splitting and median parapatellar approaches in total knee arthroplasty. Clin Orthop Relat Res 367: 107–116

31. Pavone V, Boettner F, Fickert S, Sculco TP (2001) Total condylar knee arthroplasty: a long-term followup. Clin Orthop Relat Res 388: 18–25

32. Ranawat AS, Ranawat CS, Elkus M, Rasquinha VJ, Rossi R, Babhulkar S (2005) Total knee arthroplasty for severe valgus deformity. J Bone Joint Surg Am 87: 271–284

33. Reid JB, Guttmann D, Ayala M, Lubowitz JH (2004) Minimally invasive surgery-total knee arthroplasty. Arthroscopy 20: 884–889

34. Repicci JA, Eberle RW (1999) Minimally invasive surgical technique for unicondylar knee arthroplasty. J South Orthop Assoc Spring 8: 20–27

35. Ritter MA, Berend ME, Meding JB, Keating EM, Faris PM, Crites BM (2001) Long-term followup of anatomic graduated components posterior cruciate-retaining total knee replacement. Clin Orthop Relat Res 388: 51–57

36. Rittmeister M, Konig DP, Eysel P, Kerschbaumer F (2004) Minimally invasive approaches to hip and knee joints for total joint replacement. Orthopade 33: 1229–1235

37. Roysam GS, Oakley MJ (2001) Subvastus approach for total knee arthroplasty: a prospective, randomized, and observer-blinded trial. J Arthroplasty 16: 454–457

38. Scheibel MT, Schmidt W, Thomas M, von Salis-Soglio G (2002) A detailed anatomical description of the subvastus region and its

30

clinical relevance for the subvastus approach in total knee arthroplasty. Surg Radiol Anat 24: 6–12

39. Schroder HM, Berthelsen A, Hassani G, Hansen EB, Solgaard S (2001) Cementless porous-coated total knee arthroplasty: 10-year results in a consecutive series. J Arthroplasty 16: 559–567

40. Schwitalle M, Salzmann G, Eckardt A, Heine J (2001) Late outcome after implantation of the PFC modular knee system. Z Orthop Ihre Grenzgeb 139: 102–108

41. Scuderi GR, Tenholder M, Capeci C (2004) Surgical approaches in mini-incision total knee arthroplasty. Clin Orthop Relat Res. 428: 61–7

42. Sharma S, Nicol F, Hullin MG, McCreath SW (2005) Long-term results of the uncemented low contact stress total knee replacement in patients with rheumatoid arthritis. J Bone Joint Surg Br 87: 1077–1080

43. Stulberg SD (2005) Minimally invasive navigated knee surgery: an American perspective. Orthopedics 28: 1241–1246.

44. Tenholder M, Clarke HD, Scuderi GR (2005) Minimal-incision total knee arthroplasty: the early clinical experience. Clin Orthop Relat Res 440: 67–76

45. Tria AJ Jr (2003) Advancements in minimally invasive total knee arthroplasty. Orthopedics 26: 859–863

46. Tria AJ Jr (2004) Minimally invasive total knee arthroplasty: the importance of instrumentation. Orthop Clin North Am 35: 227–234

47. Tria AJ Jr, Coon TM (2003) Minimal incision total knee arthroplasty early experience. Clin Orthop Relat Res 416: 185–190

48. Vail TP (2004) Minimally invasive knee arthroplasty. Clin Orthop Relat Res 428: 51–52

49. Vandenbussche E, Duranthon LD, Couturier M, Pidhorz L, Augereau B (2002) The effect of tourniquet use in total knee arthroplasty. Int Orthop 26: 306–309

50. Worland RL, Arredondo J, Angles F, Lopez-Jimenez F, Jessup DE (1997) Thigh pain following tourniquet application in simultaneous bilateral total knee replacement arthroplasty. J Arthroplasty 12: 848–852

Part II C Minimally Invasive Surgery and Navigation: Total Knee Arthroplasty

Valgus Approach to Total Knee Arthroplasty

T.M. Seyler, M.A. Mont, J.F. Plate, P.M. Bonutti

Introduction

Since the first total condylar knee replacement in 1974 [1], standard total knee arthroplasty has been in development. With recent advances in surgical techniques, prosthetic designs, and evolution of instrumentation, standard total knee arthroplasties have demonstrated excellent long-term results with survival rates of 95% [1–5]. However, short-term results have often showed less favorable results. Standard total knee arthroplasty is a procedure that is frequently associated with a tremendous amount of pain and functional limits. Patients often require an intensive rehabilitation program with multiple hours of physical therapy per day for the first six weeks after these procedures.

The functional outcomes and patient satisfaction after standard total knee arthroplasty may not be as optimal as what has been reported in the literature. Most studies have assessed the outcome after standard total knee arthroplasty utilizing objective criteria, such as the Knee Society clinical rating system and the Knee Society roentgenographic evaluation system. However, there is little information published considering subjective, patient-reported functional status or patient satisfaction after these procedures. The patient's judgment about the outcome of the procedure is equally important since the ultimate goal of this treatment option is pain relief and long-term satisfaction. Various studies have described a discrepancy between how surgeons perceive total knee arthroplasty and how patients assess their outcome. Bullens and col-

leagues [6] used a visual analog scale to assess satisfaction after total knee arthroplasty in a group of 108 patients (126 total knee arthroplasties) with short-term to medium-term follow-up. A comparison between subjective visual analog scale results and objective outcome measurement systems such as the Knee Society clinical rating system and Western Ontario and McMasters universities osteoarthritis index revealed only poor correlations. This comparison suggested that the criteria for satisfactory outcomes after total knee arthroplasty for patients and surgeons differ, and it appeared that surgeons are more satisfied than patients after the procedure. Dickstein et al. [7] studied the dissatisfaction rate of 79 patients by interviews and physical examinations after total knee arthroplasty 6 and 12 months postoperatively. They found that one third of the respondents expressed dissatisfaction from the operation. Robertsson and coworkers [8] reported on patient satisfaction after total knee arthroplasty in 27,372 knees registered in the Swedish joint registry. Stratified by underlying disease such as osteoarthritis or rheumatoid arthritis, there were 18% of the female patients (n=14,609) and 16% of male patients (n=6,556) with osteoarthritis unsatisfied or uncertain with the outcome of total knee arthroplasty, whereas, in the rheumatoid arthritis group the corresponding fractions were 14% (n=2,568) and 15% (n=635), respectively. The overall percentage of dissatisfied patients was 8%. Trousdale et al. [9] assessed patients concerns before undergoing total hip or total knee arthroplasty. The two greatest concerns were postoperative pain and length of recovery. Patient concerns and expectations must be addressed and balanced with the known risks associated with current techniques for total knee arthroplasty.

Standard total knee arthroplasty is usually a highly invasive open procedure with large incisions up to 30 centimeters and that does not spare muscles. Operative steps such as eversion of the patella, section of the quadriceps tendon, and tibio-femoral dislocation, may lead to permanent muscular dysfunction and weakness. As a consequence, extensive physical therapy is frequently required to obtain optimal function of the replaced joint. Minimally invasive total knee arthroplasty may be able to address these concerns.

The driving focus that directs the development of minimally invasive knee arthroplasty includes patient concerns with postoperative pain, prolonged rehabilitation, and less than optimal functional outcomes after standard total knee arthroplasty. From a surgeons' perspective, patient demand, rapid recovery process, and potential health care savings are the most important driving forces. The introduction of unicondylar knee arthroplasty in the 1990's was a milestone in knee arthroplasty surgery. Repicci's work [10] with these smaller components further stimulated interest in minimally invasive surgery. Soon surgeons began applying the limited approach utilized for unicondylar knee arthroplasty to total knee arthroplasty with encouraging short-term results.

The authors believe that the advantages of minimally invasive total knee arthroplasty are multifold [11]. With all these factors in mind, the present valgus approach to total knee arthroplasty is an attempt to minimize soft tissue damage, reduce postoperative pain and recovery time, and achieve better functional outcomes. Various key features of the valgus approach technique have been developed and successfully applied to date.

Key Features

The following section reviews the key features and discusses the rationale for the use in the valgus approach to total knee arthroplasty:

- *Small incision approach:* The incision is about twice the length of the patella (between 6 and 11 cm) (◘ Fig. 31.1). Minimizing the incision length has been a gradual process in this surgical technique. As surgeons become comfortable with this procedure the incision should be gradually decreased. This small incision approach utilizes a mobile skin window. As

the knee is brought into flexion or extension, the skin incision exposes different portion of the joint. By flexing the knee, posterior structures become visible, while when extended anterior joint structures are exposed. The principles of technique are somewhat similar to shoulder rotator cuff surgery, in which it has been successfully used for years. Using a symbiotic stress-relaxation technique for the retractors, the mobile skin window is an important factor in gaining selective exposure of the knee joint.

- *The position of the incision and postoperative pain*: This may be a cosmetic feature but the limited length and the lateral position of the incision is certainly appreciated by patients requesting this minimal invasive procedure. In addition, there are less nerve plexi on the lateral side than on the anterior side of the knee, which appears to significantly decrease pain postoperatively. Related to this, is the fact that in standard total knee arthroplasty it is extremely painful to bend the knee from the front of an incision, which is necessarily for rehabilitation. With the valgus approach technique, bending in the front of the knee is not effected and allows for a faster rehabilitation by decreasing pain.

- *The procedure is muscle-sparing:* A key element of the valgus approach is the sparing of the quadriceps muscle (◘ Fig. 31.2). The current method shares many similarities with the mid-vastus approach, where only small amounts of the vastus medialis obliquus are split. However, the valgus approach goes through the iliotibial band only and does not necessitate any invasion of the quadriceps muscle. The muscle-sparing nature of the valgus approach may contribute to earlier recovery and less pain for the patient as described in various studies.

- *The patella is not everted:* The patellar capsule is released superiorly and inferiorly. This provides exposure of the entire knee joint and the patellar can be easily mobilized for patellar preparation that just involves cutting the patella *in situ* on top of the femoral trial component (◘ Fig. 31.3). It has been reported that full eversion of the patella may cause more of the damage found in standard total knee arthroplasty. Mahoney et al. [12] assessed quadriceps function after standard total knee arthroplasty. Patients were asked to rise from a 16-inch chair without using their arms. At three months postoperatively, only 40% of patients that underwent standard total knee arthroplasty were able to arise from the chair without arm support. The same test was performed six months postoperatively, with only 64% of patients showing the ability to arise unassisted, suggesting weakness of the quadriceps muscles after these procedures. In contrast, Bonutti and coworkers [13] performed the described test on 420 patients who underwent minimally invasive total knee arthroplasty using a technique that does not require patella eversion. At 3.5 weeks after surgery, 90% of the patients could rise from a 16-inch chair without arm support. These findings suggest that quadriceps function is more rapidly restored when the patella is not everted.

— *Downsized instrumentation and navigation:* Downsized instrumentation is essential for optimizing outcomes of minimally invasive total knee arthroplasty. A major goal of less invasive approaches is to reduce soft tissue invasion. With less bulky instrumentation, downsized 40% from traditional instrumentation for standard total knee arthroplasty, soft-tissue invasion is limited. The use of cut bone surfaces, after the initial bone cuts are made, can serve as a guide without utilizing additional instruments to complete bone cuts. The excision of bone may be accomplished in a piecemeal manner.

— *Computer-Aided Navigation:* Accuracy and positioning of components is of great importance in total knee arthroplasty. The use of modern navigation systems avoids intra-medullary instrumentation and increases accuracy. Each component must be correctly positioned in all six degrees of freedom to guarantee optimal axial alignment. Intra-medullary rods can lead to embolic showering of the lungs [14–16] and the use of navigation may be advantageous to avoid intra-medullary instrumentation and subsequent complications. In addition, extra-medullary positioning of cutting guides allows bone to be resected and removed with substantially less traction applied to the quadriceps muscle and other soft tissue structures.

— *The knee joint is not dislocated or subluxed:* The valgus approach allows for the cuts to be made on the femur and the tibia in situ. The tibia does not have to be dislocated in front of the femur as for most standard total knee arthroplasty procedures (▫ Fig. 31.4). This is facilitated by the method and the order of bone cuts as well as the small keel on the tibial component. In addition, this may minimize capsular damage and reduces post-operative pain.

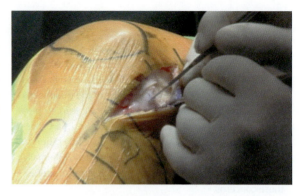

▫ **Fig. 31.1.** Small incision approach with an incision about twice the length of the patella (between 6 and 11 cm)

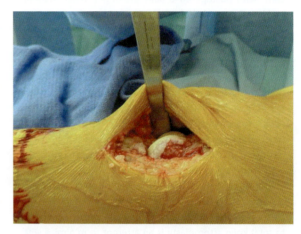

▫ **Fig. 31.2.** In the valgus approach, small parts of the vastus medialis obliquus are split, whereas the quadriceps muscle is spared

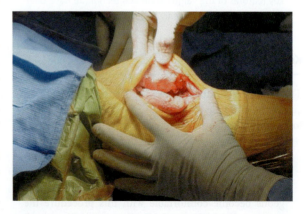

▫ **Fig. 31.3.** Complete eversion of the patella is avoided, thus sparing potential quadriceps and patella tendon damage

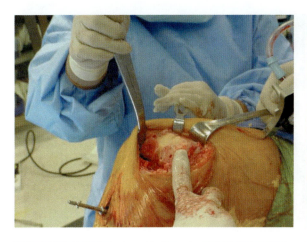

Fig. 31.4. In the valgus approach, femoral and tibial cuts are *in situ* without dislocation of the knee joint to minimize capsular damage

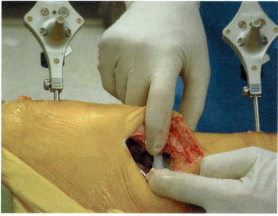

Fig. 31.5. In comparison to intra-medullary rods, percutaneous navigation pins are utilized in this novel surgical technique

In summary, the authors believe that all of these features are important for the valgus approach and distinguish it from standard approaches to total knee arthroplasty. This is certainly an evolutionary approach and needs further refinements, but it will change the way patients perceive the results of total knee arthroplasty.

Surgical Technique

The patient is placed in a supine position on the operating table. In a standard manner, skin preparation and draping, as well as a tourniquet are applied. The authors usually keep the medial and lateral malleoli, as well as the medial side of the knee free, so that navigational mapping can be done. Two different methods of holding the leg have been explored, one with a traditional leg holder, which is a convenient way to achieve variable flexion and extension, versus a suspended leg technique [17], which is similar to arthroscopic knee procedures, where the leg is hung over a padded bolster, allowing the surgeon to progressively flex and extend the knee. This suspension increases gravity forces and enhances posterior soft tissue exposure and joint distraction.

A lateral incision twice the size of the patella is then made (◻ Fig. 31.1). The typical lateral incision is made from slightly below the Gerdy's tubercle to the lateral epicondyle of the femur. The skin and underlying subcutaneous tissue is then incised revealing the iliotibial band.

With the incision of the iliotibial band, the surgeon can easily expose the proximal tibia as well as the distal femur from the lateral side. Through the lateral arthrotomy, the fat pad is excised together with the anterior horn of the lateral meniscus. Next, a release of the capsule from the anterior tibia to mobilize the patella laterally is undertaken. Dissection is continued by utilizing soft-tissue retractors underneath the patellar tendon and across to the medial side of the tibia, releasing any soft tissue that is necessary. Attention should then be directed to the proximal soft tissue. Symbiotic use of retractors with the knee in extension allows visualization of the suprapatellar pouch. The fat and synovial tissue from the anterior surface of the distal femur can be removed, including any plica bands.

At this point, the navigation system is set up. The use of navigation in minimally invasive total knee arthroplasty avoids intra-medullary instrumentation and with this particular approach applies considerably less strain to the quadriceps muscle mechanism and soft tissue (◻ Fig. 31.5). A tracker is set up ten to twelve centimeters proximal to the distal femur angled at 45 degrees placed from lateral to medial. Likewise, a similar tracker is placed at ten to twelve centimeters below the tibial joint line. Once the femoral and tibial anchors are in place, the navigation software is used to map the center of the hip, various landmarks of the femur (both epicondyles, center of the knee, and antero-posterior axis [Whiteside's line]), the tibial landmarks (condylar surfaces, tibial spine cen-

31

ter, and anterior tibia), as well as the ankle landmarks (center of the ankle, medial and lateral malleoli).

The distal femoral cut (◘ Fig. 31.6a) is made by positioning the resection guide in relation to three axes of freedom: (1) varus/valgus; (2) flexion/extension; and (3) distal resection depth. The tibia is then cut *in situ* (◘ Fig. 31.6b), without dislocating the tibia on the femur using a similar resection guide, again, considering the three axes of freedom. At this point, it is certainly possible to resect only three-quarters of the anticipated cut to avoid the risk of cutting the medial collateral ligament. However, the surgeon may have to get used to taking out cut bone in a piece-meal fashion rather than the full bone piece as known in standard (large-incision) total knee arthroplasty.

Next, attention is re-directed to the femur where a T-bar device is used to re-map the femoral rotation landmarks. With the distal femur and the proximal tibia cut, it is straightforward to use the epicondylar rotation guide, which is based on the 90 degree relationship between Whiteside's antero-posterior axis and the surgical transepicondylar axis. One arm of the epicondylar rotation guide is placed along the Whiteside's antero-posterior axis and the other arm is aligned with the lateral epicondyle. These points are marked to guarantee accurate assessment of rotation for the next step. The final preparation of the femur is done by using templates from radiographs and a femoral sizing guide, which is linked to the navigation unit to ensure the appropriate rotation.

After the tibial and femoral cuts are completed, the patella is retracted and cut with the knee in full extension. This cut can be made either in situ on top of the femoral trial component or with minimal subluxation medially. However, the patella is always cut without everting the patella in this surgical approach. Patella preparation can be performed earlier if there is difficulty with exposing the femur.

The surfaces can be checked with the navigation devices to ensure appropriate alignment. Next, the trial components are placed and the process of balancing is accomplished by ranging the knee while checking patella tracking and collateral ligament balance. After satisfactory tracking and balancing, the components are cemented. Typically in the valgus approach, the tibia is implanted first. An additional step is made to ensure careful removal of any excess cement, especially medially. Then the femur and the patella are cemented in place. Finally, range of motion, balancing, and patella tracking

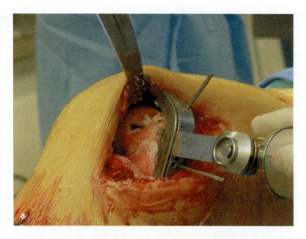

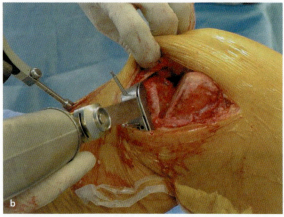

◘ **Fig. 31.6a,b.** The femoral (**a**) and tibial (**b**) cut is made *in situ* with down-sized instrumentation to facilitate the lateral approach

is assessed again. The joint is thoroughly irrigated and then closed (◘ Fig. 31.7).

Results

While there is a significant learning curve with this approach, preliminary results are encouraging. Seyler and colleagues [18] reported the results of a pilot study comparing this valgus approach (26 patient, 26 knees) to a standard medial parapatellar approach (53 patients, 53 knees) to total knee arthroplasty. At a mean follow-up of two years, patients in the lateral approach group had minimal anterior knee pain and reduced analgesic use.

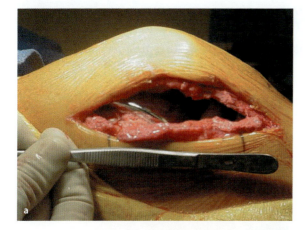

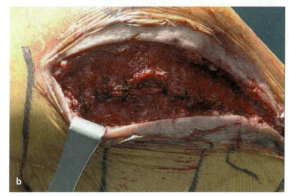

Fig. 31.7a,b. Small lateral incision after installation and thorough irrigation of all components (**a**) and capsular closure (**b**)

A radiographic evaluation demonstrated no difference in various radiographic indices between both groups. In particular, the three-month data revealed that the lateral approach has been superior to the standard medial parapatellar approach to total knee arthroplasties, with Knee Society Objective scores having a higher mean (97 points) when compared to the standard approach (91 points). Furthermore, most of these patients were able to perform straight-leg raises immediately after surgery and had a reduction in length of hospitalization. Gait studies demonstrated kinematics more closely mimicking normal knee kinematics compared with the standard approach in which the gait pattern rarely stimulated normal knee kinematics at the same time point.

Discussion

Several studies have demonstrated excellent long-term results of standard total knee arthroplasty [2–5]. Despite these excellent results, returning to activities of daily living and persistent post-operative pain remains a challenge for some patients. These patients continue to be unsatisfied with the results of the surgery. This finding was highlighted by various authors [6, 7], who reported that up to one-third of the patients who underwent total knee arthroplasty were unhappy with the outcome post-operatively. Minimally invasive approaches to total knee arthroplasty such as the present valgus approach may be able to enable patient to return to normal function more quickly and decreases postoperative pain and rehabilitation needs [18].

Patients undergoing total knee arthroplasty have not only concerns such as postoperative pain relief, length of recovery, but also specific functional goals such as the ability to walk, climbing stairs, kneeling, as well as returning to low-impact sports [9]. While these are reasonable expectations, media exposure is often misleading, which sometimes may increase these expectations to an unreasonable level for minimally invasive techniques. However, our clinical investigations and our experience with minimally invasive total knee arthroplasty demonstrated that some of these goals may be obtainable in the future.

The valgus approach to total knee arthroplasty offers tremendous advantages over standard total knee arthroplasty approaches. It is done through a small laterally-located incision, which reduces pain and functional limitations post-operatively. Many patients have also been quite happy with the cosmetic nature of placing the incision laterally, although the authors suggest that this approach should not be considered to be a cosmetic procedure but rather an opportunity to address patient concerns such as postoperative pain and a long rehabilitation process. The muscle-sparing nature of this procedure further reduces recovery time, improves functional outcome and gait pattern. In addition, features such as lack of patella eversion and avoiding dislocation of the tibio-femoral joint may offer more advantages. Computer navigation allows for accurate component implantation and may diminish the risk of side effects such as embolic events may. However, as every new technique this approach has a significant learning curve and further refinements are needed to allow its general use for any orthopaedic surgeon. Although the present technique can be difficult and time-consuming, the short-term results are promising, which should outweigh the extra effort required to learn this technique.

References

1. Insall J, Ranawat CS, Scott WN, Walker P (1976) Total condylar knee replacement: preliminary report. Clin Orthop Relat Res 120: 149–154

2. Stern SH, Insall JN (1992) Posterior stabilized prosthesis. Results after follow-up of nine to twelve years. J Bone Joint Surg Am 74: 980–986

3. Buechel FF Sr (2002) Long-term follow-up after mobile-bearing total knee replacement. Clin Orthop Relat Res 404: 40–50

4. Keating EM, Meding JB, Faris PM, Ritter MA (2002) Long-term follow-up of nonmodular total knee replacements. Clin Orthop Relat Res 404: 34–39

5. Font-Rodriguez DE, Scuderi GR, Insall JN (1997) Survivorship of cemented total knee arthroplasty. Clin Orthop Relat Res 345: 79–86

6. Bullens PH, van Loon CJ, de Waal Malefijt MC, Laan RF, Veth RP (2001) Patient satisfaction after total knee arthroplasty: a comparison between subjective and objective outcome assessments. J Arthroplasty 16: 740–747

7. Dickstein R, Heffes Y, Shabtai El, Markowitz E (1998) Total knee arthroplasty in the elderly: patients' self-appraisal 6 and 12 months postoperatively. Gerontology 44: 204–210

8. Robertsson O, Dunbar M, Pehrsson T, Knutson K, Lidgren L (2000) Patient satisfaction after knee arthroplasty: a report on 27,372 knees operated on between 1981 and 1995 in Sweden. Acta Orthop Scand 71: 262–267

9. Trousdale RT, McGrory BJ, Berry DJ, Becker MW, Harmsen WS (1999) Patients' concerns prior to undergoing total hip and total knee arthroplasty. Mayo Clin Proc 74: 978–982

10. Repicci JA, Eberle RW (1999) Minimally invasive surgical technique for unicondylar knee arthroplasty. J South Orthop Assoc 8: 20–27; discussion 27

11. Bonutti PM, Mont MA, McMahon M, Ragland PS, Kester M (2004) Minimally invasive total knee arthroplasty. J Bone Joint Surg Am 86-A (Suppl 2): 26–32

12. Mahoney OM, McClung CD, dela Rosa MA, Schmalzried TP (2002) The effect of total knee arthroplasty design on extensor mechanism function. J Arthroplasty 17: 416–421

13. Bonutti PM, Mont MA, Kester MA (2004) Minimally invasive total knee arthroplasty: a 10-feature evolutionary approach. Orthop Clin North Am 35: 217–226

14. Barre J, Lepouse C, Segal P (1997) Embolism and intramedullary femoral surgery. Rev Chir Orthop Reparatrice Appar Mot 83: 9–21

15. Ries MD, Rauscher LA, Hoskins S, Lott D, Richman JA, Lynch F Jr (1998) Intramedullary pressure and pulmonary function during total knee arthroplasty. Clin Orthop Relat Res 356: 154–160

16. Mont MA, Jones LC, Rajadhyaksha AD et al. (2004) Risk factors for pulmonary emboli after total hip or knee arthroplasty. Clin Orthop Relat Res 422: 154–163

17. Bonutti PM, Neal DJ, Kester MA (2003) Minimal incision total knee arthroplasty using the suspended leg technique. Orthopedics 26: 899–903

18. Mont MA, Seyler TM, Ragland PS (2005) Gait analysis of total hip resurfacing arthroplasty: a comparison study to hip osteoarthritis and standard total hip arthroplasty patients. J Arthroplasty (submitted)

31

Implications of Minimally Invasive Surgery and CAOS to TKR Design

P.S. Walker, G. Yildirim, J. Sussman-Fort

Introduction

Based on the long-term follow-up data of some of the earlier designs, and the gradual evolution in design since then, the evidence is that today's knee replacements can provide satisfactory function for one to two decades or even longer. This applies whether posterior cruciate retaining or substituting, whether fixed bearing or mobile bearing. However all of the long-term data was obtained for standard incisions giving full exposure, and mechanical instrumentation using intra-medullary or extra-medullary guides for overall alignment. The relatively small percentages of failures were due mainly to misalignment and instability and, in some circumstances, to polyethylene wear. With the recent introduction of MIS and CAOS, an important question is the impact that these new surgical modalities will have on total knee design, and on the short and long-term results. Early experience with smaller incisions with less invasion of muscle tissue has shown advantages in the recovery period, but disadvantages at the time of surgery due to the more limited exposure. In fact, the required space for placing the jigs and fixtures and accessing the saw blades, and the size of present total knee components, places a lower limit on the size of the incision.

Technique

The technique problems can be addressed in a number of ways. Jigs and fixtures can be streamlined and designed to fit the contours of the bones on the medial sides of the femur and tibia. Saw blades can be made narrower with less oscillation displacement, or side-cutting blades or drills could be applied. Using navigation techniques, the direct placement of pins for attaching the slotted cutting guides can eliminate the need for more invasive fixturing and the use of intra-medullary rods. Cutting tools themselves can be navigated, side-stepping the requirement for cutting guides altogether [22]. However as indicated, the size and shape of the total knee components is not compatible with very small incisions, and often tissue is unduly stretched for access. The possibility is then raised of modifying existing components, or even redesigning completely, to allow for the smallest incisions possible.

Modularizing total knee components is one possibility. For example, the femoral component can be divided either in the sagittal or the frontal planes (◘ Fig. 32.1). The former might be equivalent to a »double uni« with each uni having a hemi patella flange. The latter might be equivalent to a non-flanged component, with a patella flange added separately. Such schemes can involve »split lines« over one or more of the bearing surfaces. A sagittal plane split down the center of the patella flange could be acceptable if this area was recessed so that there was no contact with the patella. On the other hand, a transverse split just above the femoro-tibial contact areas, might compromise the patello-femoral bearing in high flexion. If there was a close mechanical join between the modular parts, the problem of fretting would have to be dealt with. Modular components could also be prone to relative movements over time due to differential bone remodel-

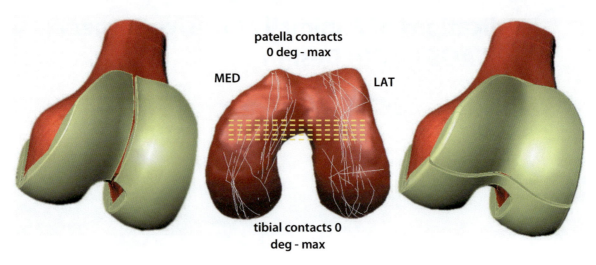

◘ Fig. 32.1. Possibilities for modularizing a femoral component for ease of insertion. The central figure shows the paths of the centers of the patello-femoral and femoro-tibial contacts of 6 knee specimens, in the full range of flexion. The yellow dashed area shows the contact region of the patella in the range 120–135 degrees. The sagittally divided femoral component (*left*) would have not discontinuity of contacts so long as the center of the patella did not contact the bottom of the groove. The frontally divided femoral component (*right*) would result in a discontinuity of patella tracking in high flexion

ing. In addition, there are stringent alignment requirements at surgery.

Modularization of tibial components may be easier and more sound mechanically. The simplest solutions merely involve a reduction in the depth of the fixation posts rather than modularization. For example, four small posts have shown long-term durability in cemented application for PC-retaining designs [1] (◘ Fig. 32.2). »Mini-keels« consisting of a shortened central post, with lateral and medial projecting keels of large surface area are already being applied. Although long-term clinical data is not available at this time, theoretical (FEA) and experimental studies have supported their validity [7]. It is relatively easy to design a modular central post, introduced after the tibial platform has been positioned on the upper tibia. This scheme has the advantage of more closely replicating components which have a long history of successful fixation, but the disadvantages of requiring close tolerances if a taper fit is used, and the requirement of correctly assembling the parts at surgery.

Reducing the size of total knee components to the point of »double unis« with a separate patella flange comprising a set of modular components which can be used selectively for each case, has been advanced by Aubaniac and others. The amount of bone removal is relatively small

using such an approach while the existing bone surfaces can be more easily used as 'templates' in order to more accurately restore the original sagittal profiles of the joint, which would especially be beneficial in the sagittal plane from a kinematic point of view. In fixing components to the femur, the use of keels cemented (or uncemented) into slots has proved to be durable. Curved femoral components can even be »wrapped around« the posterior femur, an advantage for accommodating high flexion. If components for the femur and tibia were housed completely in slots, along the lines of the original polycentric design, surgical preparation of the bone could be greatly simplified. At this time, such a modular component approach may be most appropriate for limited deformity and when both cruciates are preserved. However, it does offer the prospect of achieving more normal function, and it is compatible with small incisions.

Avoiding the use of cement has advantages for small incision surgery. The use of uncemented femoral components has shown similar long-term success as cemented, but there is a requirement for accurate bone preparation and component costs have been higher. On the tibial side, uncemented components have had mixed results, although the use of hydroxyapatite on metal trays has shown promising results [8]. More recently, composite

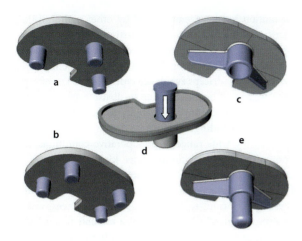

Fig. 32.2a–e. Tibial trays designed for easier access through small incisions. **a** Three medium length posts. **b** Four short length posts. **c** Mini-keel. **d,e** Mini-keel with central post introduced after placement of the tray on the tibia

tool or milling cutter rather than a saw, in which case the volume of bone to be removed should be minimized favoring the curved cuts mentioned above rather than the more traditional 'square cuts' which require much more bone removed. Another way in which bone removal can be reduced for the femoral component is a reduction in the extent of the intercondylar region for the posterior cruciate substituting cam and post. On the tibial side, the bone removal could be reduced by removing primarily those areas beneath the femoral-tibial contact areas, which may also be an advantage to fixation.

Notwithstanding the various possibilities for reducing the size of the components, a parallel reduction in the size of the incisions needs to take into consideration the access necessary to various regions of the joint, for the removal of excess cement for example. A further limitation on the size of the incision relates to soft tissue procedures including removal of unwanted tissue and ligament balancing. To some degree the use of arthroscopic techniques, possibly augmented by computer-assisted navigation could be envisioned, but only if the benefits of yet smaller incisions would justify the greater difficulty of the surgery.

tibial components have been fabricated, consisting of plastic fused into a trabecular metal backing. Not only has this provided excellent fixation to date, but backside wear is prevented. Notwithstanding the extra costs, enhancements in the surgical precision of bone preparation using CAOS could well lead to a renewal of interest in uncemented components, which could reduce operating time and even extend the duration of the fixation beyond that of cement.

However, a present drawback to using uncemented components is the limited accuracy of using saw blades. It would be an advantage to both improve the accuracy of the bone preparation and the amount of bone removed. This would require a change in the design of the components. On the femoral side, contoured cuts could be made which removed only a few millimeters from the distal femur. To achieve such cuts accurately, several approaches are possible. The first is to use a robotically controlled milling cutter or burring tool, although this would require the acceptance of an active robot. A second approach is a passive robot where the surgeon controls the progress of the cutting tool but where the boundaries are controlled by the robotic arm. The boundaries match the geometry of the implant itself. A third approach, a variant of the passive robot arm, is a cutting tool where the power to the tool is cut off when the tool reaches the prescribed boundaries [26]. Such approaches preferably utilize a burring

Criteria for Design and Improvements

Returning to conventional total knee components, computer-assisted surgery offers the benefits of more accurate placement and alignment, while smaller incisions can improve recovery [4]. These factors alone may improve the function of the knee in the short and long term. However to take full advantage of the capabilities of CAOS and MIS, it is useful to re-examine the fundamentals of total knee design itself, with the goal of achieving the optimal performance for each patient. It has been found that with the most commonly used types of total knee, patients were unable to perform many of the functions they would like to, unlike their age-matched controls [25]. The particular activities were those requiring both high flexion and high muscle force. Hence, one of the deficiencies may be the inability of the muscles to generate the necessary forces and torques, probably due to many years of diminished use [18], as well as capsular fibrosis. Prolonged quadriceps weakness may be due to the repeated shifting of the load to the opposite unaffected limb [14]. It is self-evident that an inadequate maximum flexion angle will limit many activities. The functional ranges after TKR were found to be even less than the passive ranges [10] which again may be related to muscle strength.

Diminished proprioception is another factor which might reduce function. It has been well documented that loss of the ACL with resulting instability reduces proprioception, even after rehabilitation or reconstruction [11]. Nevertheless, after TKR with the anterior cruciate resected, it was found that proprioception could be restored if attention was given to correct collateral ligament balancing [3]. In any case, the absence of one or both cruciates does not necessarily result in an inferior result. In a large series of bilateral cases with a different type of knee on each side, knees which retained both cruciates were preferred by the patients to either PCL sacrificing or substituting types. However, equal to the cruciate preserving knees were medial (or lateral) pivot knees, where the medial side provided almost complete stability in the A-P direction [17].

Another mechanical factor in total knees is the movement of the femoral-tibial contact points as a function of flexion, during different activities. Based on fluoroscopic motion studies of 811 total knees of different types it was stated that »… normal knee kinematics are difficult to obtain after TKR. Multiple kinematic abnormalities, including reduced posterior femoral rollback, paradoxical anterior femoral translation, reverse axial rotation patterns, and femoral condylar lift-off commonly are present« [9]. These authors did, however, find that ACL and PCL preservation implants were closest to normal. PS types of implant did show less variation in A-P translation due to their more dished tibial surfaces but this would inhibit both posterior displacement with flexion (until the cam became active) and reduced internal-external rotation. Abnormal kinematics in the sagittal plane was also determined by measuring the angle of the patella ligament to the long axis of the tibia, when the patient performed different exercises, up to a maximum of 90 degrees flexion [16]. Compared with normal intact knees, the TKRs all showed an almost constant ligament angle of about 10 degrees compared with normal where the angle steadily reduced from about +20 degrees to minus 5 degrees during flexion. This implied that there was too much anterior tibial displacement in extension, and too little in flexion. Such sagittal plane abnormalities described above would have major effects on the lever arms of the muscles, the torque generated by the quadriceps, on the ligament and capsular lengths, and even on proprioception. The importance of the role of both cruciates in obtaining normal motion has been emphasized by other authors [5]. »Sacrifice of the ACL removes a constraint to the anterior displacement of the tibia produced by quadriceps contraction near full extension. Patients with ACL deficiency developed a quadriceps avoidance type of gait.« The effect of the weakened quadriceps due to disuse even prior to the TKR, would diminish the ability to perform biomechanically demanding functions.

Given the wide range of pre-operative conditions, it is not surprising that »normal knee kinematics are difficult to obtain after TKR« and that there is a wide range of motion patterns postoperatively. Nevertheless it is still necessary to formulate design goals for total knees, with the ultimate aim of achieving the best possible functional results in each case. Even for the less able patients, femoral-tibial geometry which maximized the extension moment for a given quadriceps force, would be an advantage. It has been suggested previously that »after implantation of the knee replacement, the motion of the knee in any activity is indistinguishable from the motion of the knee in its healthy intact state« [22]. This is an ideal which is not possible to achieve generally due to the status of the muscles and soft tissues. Hence the design criterion can be modified to something which is testable in the laboratory using cadaveric specimens or even a computer model: »after implantation of the TKR, the neutral path of motion and the constraint throughout the flexion range is indistinguishable from that of the knee in its intact state.« The neutral path of motion can be described by the successive positions of a defined transverse axis in the distal femur, projected on to the upper tibia, as the knee is flexed from zero to maximum. In one model, synchronous rotations were found to occur about a transverse axis through the epicondyles, and a vertical axis in the tibia emerging on the medial inner slope [6, 13]. This model has recently been refined to emphasize the »surgical epicondylar axis« [2]. Such motion is due to relative stability on the medial side, together with a lateral femoral condyle which moves progressively posteriorly with flexion, and anteriorly with extension, driven by the cruciate ligaments. The center of the femur also moves posteriorly with flexion, (approximately half the amount of the lateral side) which is often termed »femoral rollback«. The external femoral rotation with flexion can hence be thought of as a consequence of the stable medial side, lax lateral side, and the guiding action of the cruciate ligaments. It is possible that this scheme provides substantial A-P stability yet allows for freedom of internal-external rotation at the same time.

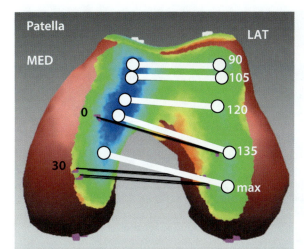

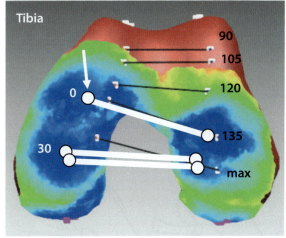

Fig. 32.3. Typical paths of the centers of contacts for the patello-femoral and femoro-tibial joints, on the distal end of the femur. When the knee is brought into extension, the contact on the medial side moves anteriorly on the femur and tibia (white arrow). This is due in part to the upsweep on the anterior tibia (see *white arrow* on Fig. 32.4). This anterior contact may stabilize the knee in extension and inhibit further extension

It is also an important characteristic of the normal knee that there is both A-P and rotational laxity about the normal path of motion. It is suggested that these major ingredients of knee motion, medial stability, lateral posterior displacement with flexion, and some laxity about the neutral position, should be the major design criteria for a total knee replacement regarding kinemat-

ics [12]. An important phenomenon in this connection is produced by a combination of the cruciates and the shape of the condyles on the medial side. As the knee is brought into extension, the medial contact area shifts substantially anteriorly, onto the upsweep of the anterior medial tibial plateau (◘ Fig. 32.3). This may produce an important braking action to further extension and may also impart a feeling of stability. To achieve the above goals with a TKR which retained both cruciates, the medial femoral-tibial conformity should provide the maximum A-P stability throughout flexion, consistent with the surgical requirement of being able to position the tibial component to be compatible with the cruciates in the full range of flexion. However the cruciates will provide the required »rollback with flexion« and »rollforward with extension«, mainly on the lateral side. At the other extreme, for a knee without cruciates, the medial conformity should again be maximized, but now the rollback and rollforward would need to be provided by some other means such as an intercondylar cam [23, 24] or by the geometry of the condylar surfaces [21, 22]. The cams of the PS type of designs today are usually designed to provide posterior femoral displacement after mid-flexion [15]. For the first half of flexion, the femur will preferentially locate at the bottom of the tibial dish, with relatively little AP sliding or rotation. For a posterior cruciate retaining (CR) type of design, the cruciate produces the posterior displacement, but there is usually less constraint in the tibial surfaces allowing more AP and rotational laxity. However such cams or retention of the PCL, do not automatically provide rollforward with extension. This has to be accomplished either by the femur relocating into the bottom of the tibial dish, or by some other cam or surface guided mechanism.

Included in the above goals for kinematics should be the ability to achieve high flexion [19]. In the anatomic knee this is achieved by posterior displacement on the lateral side, and not surprisingly, the impingement between the femur and the tibia at maximum flexion occurs on the medial side (◘ Fig. 32.4). The main object for a TKR is that the posterior bone of the femur does not impact on the posterior edge of the plastic which could limit flexion as well as damage the plastic and cause loosening. Experiments have been performed in the laboratory to determine the factors which influence the angle of flexion at which impingement occurred (◘ Fig. 32.5). The most influential factor limiting flexion was exposed cancellous bone on the posterior cut surfaces of the femur.

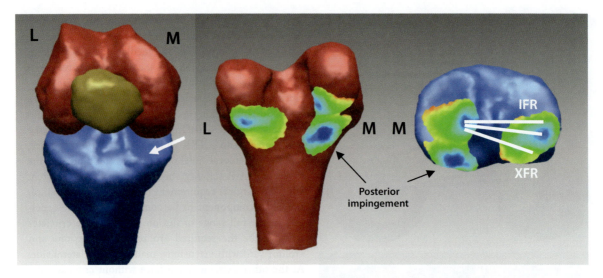

◼ **Fig. 32.4.** Reconstructions of the relative positions of the femur, tibia and patella in a test machine which simulated rising from a low squatting position at 135–155 degrees flexion. The medial posterior femoral cortex contacted the posterior edge of the tibia. When the tibia was rotated the pivot point occurred on the medial side and the lateral contact extended to the extreme posterior

32

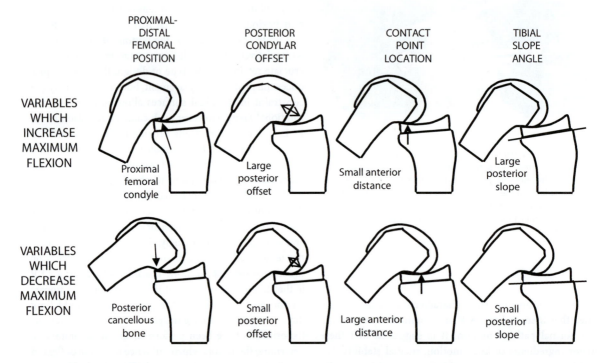

◼ **Fig. 32.5.** Surgical and design factors affecting the maximum flexion angle of a total knee before impingement occurred on the posterior edge of the plastic. The largest effects were due to the placement (and size) of the femoral component on the femur. These findings were obtained from laboratory experiments where the femoral component position and the contact location of the femur on the tibia were controlled

This could be caused by a femoral component placed too distally (an inadequate distal cut) or too anteriorly (an excessive posterior cut). The choice of too small a component would also have the same effects. Another factor in such placement is an inadequate posterior condylar offset which has been shown to correlate with reduced flexion clinically [20]. In addition, in the above laboratory experiments, inadequate posterior femoral displacement, and inadequate posterior tibial slope also led to early impingement. Hence to achieve high flexion, appropriate design factors in parallel with accurate surgical technique are required. The latter can be achieved more easily using computer assisted surgery. A crucial factor in obtaining optimal kinematics throughout the flexion range is the restoration of correct ligament balancing. CAOS can play a major role here in achieving this [27].

Summary and Conclusions

The possible advantages of MIS in regard to recovery and function have led to a streamlining of the jigs and fixtures and design changes to TKR components to improve access. One approach has been to reduce the post sizes of the tibial baseplates or to use a central modular post. Another approach has been to use a set of modular compartmental components including a patella flange. The use of CAOS has improved the accuracy of the bone cuts and has facilitated ligament balancing. However, the combination of MIS and CAOS can go even further in optimizing the performance of TKR for each patient. By defining the kinematic goals to include medial side stability, lateral rollback and rollforward, and AP and optimal laxity throughout flexion; a TKR may perform more like the normal knee. Motion guidance can be by retention of both cruciates, or by cams, or by guide surfaces. CAOS can provide for less bone resection, more accurate cuts to facilitate cementless fixation, and improved soft tissue balancing.

Acknowledgements. The studies illustrated in Figs. 32.1, 32.3, 32.4 and 32.5 were carried out at the Laboratory for Minimally-Invasive Surgery, New York University – Hospital for Joint Diseases Orthopaedic Program, by the following: Gaurav Aggarwal (City College, New York), Daniel Hennessy. Gregg Klein, MD, Jon Sussman-Fort (Columbia University), Peter S. Walker, PhD, Brian White, MD, and Gokce Yildirim (Columbia University).

References

1. Archibeck MJ, Berger RA, Barden RM, Jacobs JJ, Sheinkop MB, Rosenberg AG, Galante JO (2001) Posterior cruciate ligament-retaining total knee arthroplasty in patients with rheumatoid arthritis. J Bone Joint Surg 83A(8): 1231–1236
2. Asano T, Akagi M, Nakamura T (2005) The functional flexion-extension axis of the knee corresponds to the surgical epicondylar axis. J Arthroplasty 20(8): 1060–1067
3. Attfield SF, Wilton TJ, Pratt DJ, Sambatakakis A (1996) Soft-tissue balance and recovery of proprioception after total knee replacement. J Bone Joint Surg (Br) 78-B(4): 540–545
4. Berger RA, Sanders S, Gerlinger T, DellaValle C, Jacobs JJ, Rosenberg AG (2005) Outpatient total knee arthroplasty with a minimally invasive technique. J Arthroplasty 20(7) (Suppl 3): 33–38
5. Chaudhari AM, Dyrby CO, Andriacchi TP (2005) The importance of the ACL for the function of the knee: relevance to future developments in total knee arthroplasty. In: Bellemans J, Ries MD, Victor J (eds) Total knee arthroplasty. Springer, Berlin Heidelberg New York Tokyo, pp 121–125
6. Churchill DL, Incavo SJ, Johnson CC, Beynnon BD (1998) The transepicondylar axis approximates the optimal flexion axis of the knee. Clin Orthop Relat Res 356: 111–118
7. Coleman JC, Pendleton JE, Johnson TS (2006) Effect of stem geometry on fixation of cemented tibial baseplates under posterior stabilized loading conditions, vol. 31. Trans Orthopaedic Research Society, Chicago
8. Cross MJ, Parish EN (2005) A hydroxyapatite-coated tibial total knee replacement: prospective analysis of 1000 patients. J Bone Joint Surg (Br) 87-B: 1073–1076
9. Dennis DA, Komistek RD, Mahfouz MR, Haas BD, Stiehl JB (2003) Multicenter determination of in vivo kinematics after total knee arthroplasty. Clin Orthop Relat Res 418: 37–57
10. Dennis DA, Komistek RD, Stiehl JB, Walker SA, Dennis KN (1998) Range of motion after total knee arthroplasty. J Arthroplasty 13(7): 748–752
11. Fremerey RW, Lobenhoffer P, Zeichen J, Skutek M, Bosch U, Tscherne H (2000) Proprioception After rehabilitation and reconstruction in knees with deficiency of the anterior cruciate ligament. J Bone Joint Surg (Br) 82-B(6): 801–806
12. Haider H, Walker PS (2005) Measurements of constraint of total knee replacement. J Biomech 38: 341–348
13. Hollister AM, Jatana S, Singh AK, Sullivan WW, Lupichuk AG (1993) The axes of rotation of the knee. Clin Orthop Relat Res 290: 259–268
14. Mizner RL, Snyder-Mackler L (2005) Altered loading during walking and sit-to-stand is affected by quadriceps weakness after total knee arthroplasty. J Orthop Res 23: 1083–1090
15. Nakayama K, Matsuda S, Miura H, Higaki H, Otsuka K, Iwamoto Y (2005) Contact stress at the post-cam mechanism in posterior-stabilized total knee arthroplasty. J Bone Joint Surg (Br) 87-B: 483–488
16. Pandit H, Ward T, Hollinghurst D, Beard DJ, Gill HS, Thomas NP, Murray DW (2005) Influence of surface geometry and the cam-post mechanism on the kinematics of total knee replacement. J Bone Joint Surg (Br) 87-B: 940–945

17. Pritchett JW (2004) Patient preferences in knee prostheses. J Bone Joint Surg (Br) 86-B(7): 979–982
18. Silva M, Shepherd EF, Jackson WO, Pratt JA, McClung CD, Schmatzried TP (2003) Knee strength after total knee arthroplasty. J Arthroplasty 18(5): 605–611
19. Sultan PG, Most E, Schule S, Li G, Rubash HE (2003) Optimizing flexion after total knee arthroplasty. Clin Orthop Relat Res 416: 167–173
20. Victor J, Banks S, Bellemans J (2005) Kinematics of posterior cruciate ligament-retaining and –substituting total knee arthroplasty. J Bone Joint Surg (Br) 87-B: 646–655
21. Walker PS (2001) A new concept in guided motion total knee arthroplasty. J Arthroplasty 16 (Suppl): 157–163
22. Walker PS (2005) Bearing surfaces for motion control in total knee arthroplasty. In: Bellemans J, Ries MD, Victor J (eds) Total knee arthroplasty. Springer, Berlin Heidelberg New York Tokyo, pp 295–302
23. Walker PS, Sathasivam S (1999) The design of guide surfaces for fixed-bearing and mobile-bearing knee replacements. J Biomech 32: 27–34
24. Walker PS, Sathasivam S (2000) Controlling the motion of total knee replacements using intercondylar guide surfaces. J Orthop Res 18(1): 48–55
25. Weiss JM, Noble PC, Conditt MA, Kohl HW, Roberts S, Cook KF, Gordon MJ, Mathis KB (2002) What functional activities are important to patients with knee replacements? Clin Orthop Relat Res 404: 172–188
26. Wolf A, Mor AB, Jaramaz B, DiGioia III AM (2004) How can CAOS support MIS TKR and THR? – Background and significance. In: Hozak WJ, Krismer M, Nogler M, Bonutti PM, Rachbauer F, Schaeffer JL, Donnelly WJ (eds) Minimally invasive total joint arthroplasty. Springer, Berlin Heidelberg New York Tokyo, pp 182–185
27. Zalzal P, Papini M, Petrucelli D, deBeer J, Winemaker MJ (2004) An in vivo biomechanical analysis of the soft-tissue envelope of osteoarthritic knees. J Arthroplasty 19(2): 217–223

Fluoroscopy-Based Navigation in Genesis II Total Knee Arthroplasty with the *Medtronic »Viking« System*

F.-W. Hagena, M. Kettrukat, R.M. Christ, M. Hackbart

Introduction

Mal-alignment reduces the survival of total knee replacements. The imbalance of the soft-tissue results in instability of the replaced knee joint. This leads to functional deficits and increased wear.

Computer-assisted technology has been introduced into orthopaedic surgery based on the knowledge that it can improve the precision of surgical procedures. Computerized three-dimensional imaging has been the prerequisite to adapt these techniques. In total knee replacement an optimized alignment to the mechanical axes of the lower limb in comparison to the traditional instrumentation is required. The additional aim is to achieve a correct soft-tissue balancing.

Computer-assisted surgical procedures are based on CT-scan analysis and kinematic evaluation of the anatomy of the lower limb. The acquisition of fluoroscopic imaging for navigation has been described in traumatological procedures [3] Fluoroscopic navigation with the Medtronic system has been widely used in spine surgery [2]. The advantages are a minimum of radiation exposure and the exact and reproducible fixation of pedicle screws. Fluoroscopic-assisted navigation offers a high level of precision and surgical safety [3].

These advantages of minimal radiation and of reproducible accuracy are adapted for the development of a stable software and new instruments for fluoroscopic-assisted navigation in total knee arthroplasty.

The goal is to plan preoperatively and to adjust intra-operatively to the individual anatomy, and to navigate the surgical tools and cutting guides to reduce the human errors. After evaluation of medical images (CT, MRI, fluoroscopy) and correlation to anatomical landmarks, determined by sensors mounted on surgical instruments the physician can be guided during performance [2, 3]. At any time the surgeon is able to simulate and to control the precision of each single step of the procedure. This technology leads to a new approach to documenting the individual procedure and performing follow-up studies in the future.

Requirements

Data related to the individual patient's anatomy are required for computer-assisted surgery. Function of the extremity is a prerequisite for the kinematic acquisition of these data. In case of an ankylosis of the adjacent joints (i.e. the hip or ankle joints) the necessary mobility can not be expected. The ankylosing osteoarthritis of the knee also may be an exclusion for kinematic evaluation of the extremity.

For the CT-based navigation preoperative imaging and evaluation has to be performed. This technique needs very sophisticly logistic planning. Even more the radiation exposition for the patients is critical in the routine of total knee replacement. Additionally, the amount of costs have to be considered in relation to the achieved improvement of accuracy on a regular base.

Navigation is »only« a supplementary instrument for the implantation of the knee arthroplasty. For optimal use a learning curve is necessary. Failures may be expected if navigation is only used in »special« cases. Navigation integrated in the routine surgical procedure has to follow these principles: availability, reproducibility, cost-effectiveness and safety. To correspond with these criteria the effort and the costs have to correlate with efficacy. The equipment has to be appropriate to the integration into the routine. Under these postulations the CT-based navigation is at least controversial for the routine of total knee arthroplasty.

In fluoroscopy-assisted navigation of TKA the individual lower limb is evaluated radiographically including all joints: the hip, the knee and the ankle joint. After acquisition of these images in two planes the mechanical axis of the limb is calculated in 3 dimensions.

The availability of these data is not restricted in any way. This information is stored and is available for controls and quality management. The time for fluoroscopic investigation and image acquisition is 8 min and less than 1 min of fluoroscopic radiation.

The surgeon estimates the individual quality of the images and is able to include this information into the further decisive steps of the surgical procedure. The additional time of data acquisition in the operation theatre does not increase the overall time considerably.

Having registered the axes of the limb the surgeon outlines the anatomic landmarks of the femoral condyles and of the tibia plateau with a mobile diode which is mounted to a probe. After complete data evaluation a 3D model of the extremity is calculated. The discrimination of the data is of less than 2 mm and smaller than 2° within the acceptable limits.

Surgical Procedure

The patient is in supine position. A tourniquet is put on the thigh. It may be inflated at any time during the procedure.

A pre-patellar longitudinal skin incision is carried out. To mount the femoral navigation frame this incision is proximally extended about 4 cm longer. Mediopatellar opening of the joint. Proximal and distal of the joint line the navigation frames are mounted to transosseous fixed pins.

Two fluoroscopic images are taken of the joints: the femoral head in 45° angle and in a.p. and lateral view of the knee and ankle joint. The center of the femoral head is identified on the monitor. After registration of the mechanical axes the intra-articular landmarks of the femoral condyles and of the proximal tibia are determined with a free diode. The mechanical femoral axis is defined by the relation of the intercondylar center, the epicondylar axis and the »Whiteside line« at the distal femur to the center of the femoral head. The tibial axis is determined by the a.p. alignment perpendicular to the center of the tibial head and to the center of the distal tibia. The rotational alignment is depending on the midtransversal axis at the tibial head diverging 10° of the posterior corticalis axis and at the center of the joint surface of the distal tibia.

The resection guides are registered and the osteotomies of the joint surfaces are performed with the navigated instruments. During each step it is possible to adjust the cutting guides within the limits of less than 2 degrees of deviation to the navigated axes.

At any time an intraoperative clinical control and revision is possible. The program and the controls have to be coordinated.

The system offers the control of the alignment of the trial implants. Dynamic testing during continuous motion and at 0°, 30° and 90° flexion enables the test of the soft tissue balancing. All these tests are documented automatically.

Experience with Fluoroscopic Navigation

Experimental data of fluoroscopic navigation had been presented after cadaver surgery [1]. After further clinical testing the technology of fluoroscopy-assisted navigation had been introduced for clinical studies. At each stage of development a very sophisticated documentation of all data had been collected. The documentation of each step of the surgical procedure is an excellent contribution to quality control and quality improvement. This is a very important advantage of navigation.

During the phase of development of fluoroscopy-assisted navigation an integration of the system into the routine program was not possible. The testing of new instruments has been time consuming. With up to 4 total knee replacements the same day it is not possible to use the navigation system at each procedure because there has been only one set of instruments for navigation available. After some experience and the development of adequate equipment, we are now able to state that the application of the system is now stable, safe and reproducible.

Results

We had the opportunity to start with the clinical application of the fluoroscopic navigation »Viking« in our clinic in May 2001. Out of a total of 240 TKA within the last year, we were able to use the fluoroscopic-assisted navigation system in 50 of the Genesis II TKA. During the early phase of this study we were not able to increase the frequency of application considerably. It is our goal to use the navigation system in each case to achieve optimal results for all patients.

To evaluate the accuracy of the new fluoroscopic navigation system all these patients are introduced into a prospective study design in comparison to traditional implantation techniques. The results of this study is not yet available.

Alignment

The advantage of this system is a control of accuracy at any time of the procedure and it allows an online documentation. Surgical time is slightly increased by the acquisition of the fluoroscopic images (■ Fig. 33.1). We have to admit that it is still a more time-consuming procedure in comparison to the traditional instrumentation with alignment rods.

We check the alignment of the resection planes regularly during the surgical procedure. The real presentation of the fluoroscopic images on the touch-screen facilitates the imagination of the surgeon during the procedure. A virtual line representing the anatomical structures and the position of the limb may have a negative influence on the surgeons' compliance. The intraoperative control shows a very high accuracy of less than 2° degrees deviation (■ Fig. 33.2).

It is essential that there are no contraindications for the application of the fluoroscopic-assisted navigation. In contrast, kinematic-based navigation may be limited in case of ankylosing disease of the hip and of the knee which is going to be operated.

Control of the Results Intraoperatively

It is possible to control the results of alignment. The control studies did not show any failure that was related to the navigation system. Even in cases of very severe deformities of the femur or of the tibia (i.e. posttraumatic deformities) the intraoperative control with alignment rods did confirm the exact alignment and the correct implantation of the arthroplasty (■ Fig. 33.3).

Testing of Soft-Tissue Balancing

Fluoroscopic-assisted navigation with the »Viking« system (Medtronic) offers a great advantage after implantation of the trial implants. It is now possible to check the soft-tissue balancing dynamically and in various degrees of flexion. The tests are documented in neutral 0° and in 90° of flexion. The tests are performed for the following parameters:
- a.p. translation (anterior drawer sign),
- varus- and valgus stress,
- rotational stability.

After these dynamic tests it is still possible to improve soft-tissue balancing by adequate procedures. It is interesting to note that using the »Viking« navigation system we can see that there is hardly any correction of the resection necessary because of the accuracy of implantation of the TKA.

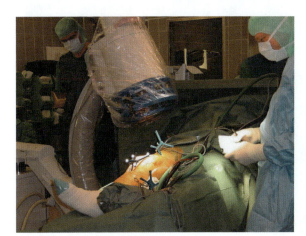

■ **Fig. 33.1.** Acquisition of the center of the femoral head with mounted navigation frames at the knee

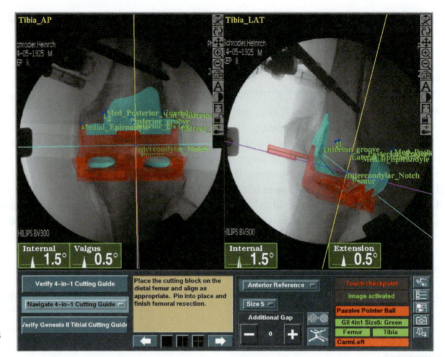

■ **Fig. 33.2.** The real fluoroscopic image of the knee in combination with the virtual image of the implant on the screen and the results after resection

33

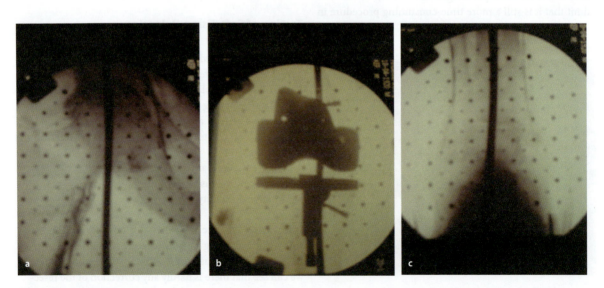

■ **Fig. 33.3a-c.** Intraoperative fluoroscopic control after insertion of the trial-implants with the alignment rod. **a** Center of the femoral head, **b** the knee, **c** center of the ankle

The mean values show excellent results. The tests before the closure of the capsule cause an increased laxity at 90° flexion. The rotating platform of the Genesis II TKA provides a high degree of rotational capacity (◻ Fig. 33.4). After finishing the knee replacement the manual controls did not give any sign of pathologic laxities (◻ Table 33.1).

◻ **Table 33.1.** Fluoroscopic-assisted navigation: Genesis II/ rotating platform (n=50)		
Level of evaluation	**Results (median)**	**Standard deviations**
V/V lateral 0°	2,3 mm	0,1 – 5,8 mm
V/V lateral 90°	2,9 mm	–2,7 – 14,3 mm
a.p. lateral 0°	1,9 mm	–5,4 – 6 mm
a.p. lateral 90°	2,9 mm	–8,0 – 6,4 mm
I/E rotation 0°	3,6°	0 – 7,0°
I/E rotation 90°	9°	2,0 – 16,9°

V/V Varus/Valgus, *a.p.* Translation, *I/E* internal/external rotation.

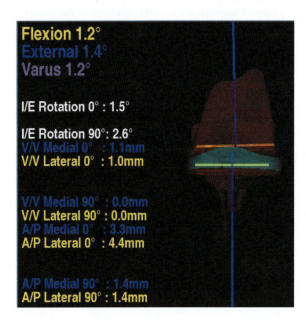

Flexion 1.2°
External 1.4°
Varus 1.2°

I/E Rotation 0° : 1.5°

I/E Rotation 90°: 2.6°
V/V Medial 0° : 1.1mm
V/V Lateral 0° : 1.0mm

V/V Medial 90° : 0.0mm
V/V Lateral 90° : 0.0mm
A/P Medial 0° : 3.3mm
A/P Lateral 0° : 4.4mm

A/P Medial 90° : 1.4mm
A/P Lateral 90° : 1.4mm

◻ **Fig. 33.4.** Visualization and documentation of the soft-tissue balancing at 0° and 90° of flexion

Limitations of Alignment

The improvements of the designs of knee arthroplasties include the development of better instrumentation techniques to achieve a reproducible alignment to the mechanical axis of the lower limb.

There are still some controversial publications in terms of the navigation-guided instruments. Some of the critical cuts and positions of the implants are depending on the visual analysis by the surgeon.

Variables for alignment in TKA
▬ Intercondylar femoral center
▬ Transepicondylar axis of the femur
▬ Rotation of the tibia
▬ Center of the distal tibia
▬ Position of the patella implant

It is well accepted that it is not possible to define the epicondyles as a point at the distal femur. Using the fluoroscopic-assisted navigation system it is possible to exactly define the center of the femoral head and of the distal tibial joint surface. But still it is difficult to accurately describe the rotation of the tibia.

Time of Surgical Procedures

A continuous reduction of the total time of the surgical procedures have been registered for the fluoroscopic-assisted navigation during the experience of more than 12 months. With a total time of 90 min cut to finish of surgery a reasonable time has been achieved. This is not only true for the senior author but also for 3 senior surgeons at our hospital. This could be demonstrated during various visits of other colleagues. We are now going to include the online documentation of the timing into our software program.

The testing of soft-tissue balancing is a new part of the surgical procedure which justifies additional time. The graph demonstrates the »learning curve« during the first applications of the navigation system (◻ Fig. 33.5). The black line »trial alignment« of this graph shows the time of laxity tests that are about 10 minutes unchanged. It is expected that this time will be reduced in the future also.

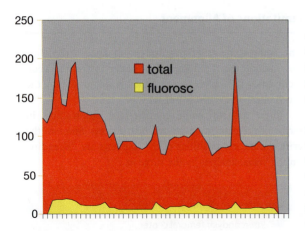

Fig. 33.5. Additional time for navigation

Additional Efforts for Navigation

Navigation in total knee arthroplasty is in a stage of development. At the phase of application it is not only time-consuming. During the first 20 navigated TKA one more nurse has been needed to adjust the camera during the navigation. The use of fluoroscopic investigation and registration took more time during the first cases than it was necessary later. The exact positioning and the stable fixation of the navigation frames has been established after our experience. The development of special instruments for navigated total knee arthroplasty will help to reduce the time of surgery even more.

Discussion

Various systems to navigate the total knee arthroplasties are already available. Kinematic-based navigation shows the advantage that it is applied independently of any imaging. The disadvantage seems to be the limitation in case of severe joint contracture and ankylosis of the knee and of the adjacent hip joint. Also patients with greater masses of soft tissues surrounding the knee are excluded of this method. The results do not confirm a higher degree of reproducibility. As limiting factors for kinematic based-navigation
- the variability of the surgeons,
- the value of surface registrations and
- movements of the navigation frames
had been identified as problems [4].

The CT-based navigation may give the highest degree of accuracy. The fact that this method is depending on CT scan preoperatively is restricting its application. This technology is not available in all hospitals and it needs more time and more radiation exposure for the image acquisition and it is very expensive in the routine.

Fluoroscopic navigation seems to give the best solution. It offers a very high degree of accuracy and the best way of reproducibility. The reduction of radiation using the fluoroscopy is an advantage for the surgeon [5]. At any time the update of the imaging is available. It is less time-consuming than the CT-based navigation. The online imaging on the screen offers an excellent compliance for the surgeon. The time for surgery used for documentation and laxity tests seems in good relation to the improved quality.

Prospective studies are planned to verify the significance of this system.

References

1. Carson C, Lyons C, Salehi A (2002) Accuracy validation of an image guided surgical system for total knee arthroplasty. Orthopedic Research Society, 48th Annual Meeting, Dallas, Abstract
2. Foley KT, Simon DA, Rampersaud YR (2000) Virtual fluoroscopy. Oper Tech Orthop 10: 77–81
3. Hofstetter R, Slomczykowski M, Sati M, Nolte L-P (1999) Fluoroscopy as an imaging means for computer-assisted surgical navigation. Computer Aided Surg 4: 65–79
4. Stulberg D, Loan P, Sarin V (2001) Computer-assisted total knee replacement surgery: an analysis of an initial experience with Orthopilot system. Computer Aided Surg 6: 124
5. Suhm N, Jacob Al, Nolte L-P, Regazzoni P, Messmer P (2000) Surgical Navigation based on fluoroscopy – clinical application for computer-assisted distal locking of intramedullary implants. Computer Aided Surgery 5: 391–400

33

Minimally Invasive-Navigated Extra-Medullary Preparation in Total Knee Arthroplasty with the »Stryker« System

R.L. Wixson, M. MacDonald

Introduction

Recent advances in total knee replacement have involved the use of computer assisted navigation (CAN) and minimally invasive surgical (MIS) approaches. The goal of using CAN has been to increase the accuracy and reproducibility of implant placement and limb alignment. The goal of limiting the surgical exposure with MIS techniques has been to reduce the pain associated with the procedure and to achieve a more rapid recovery. The combination of CAN with a minimally invasive approach in total knee replacement has the potential to achieve improved alignment and implant placement while doing the surgery through a smaller incision with reduced exposure.

Failure to achieve restoration of appropriate neutral mechanical alignment has been associated with an increased late failure rate, particularly in knees with 3° of varus mal-alignment or greater [1–4]. A number of authors have demonstrated a series of inaccuracies due to variations in the saw cut and mechanical instruments [5,6]. In comparative studies of navigation and conventional techniques, CAN has been shown to result in significantly less mal-alignment based primarily on analysis of long-standing radiographs [7–9]. In a series of studies the range of cases with less than 3° of varus varied from 67–84% with conventional techniques compared to 89–98% of navigated cases [10–15].

Minimally invasive surgical techniques in total knee replacement have less disruption of the extensor mechanism and do not require eversion of the patella. The goal of MIS is to reduce the amount of pain and scarring associated with the procedure and to improve the patient experience, through a more rapid recovery as well as improved function and range of motion [16–18]. With the reduced exposure in MIS surgery, it is more difficult to place the instruments and make the bone cuts accurately. Concern over an increase in cases of mal-alignment has been documented by several authors [5, 19, 20]. However, navigation, due to its inherent ability to verify the bone cuts and adjust it at each step of the process, has the advantage of being able to be used with minimally invasive techniques by providing maintenance of accurate, reproducible alignment.

From previous experience the author had found that the use of navigation resulted in more reproducible establishment of appropriate neutral mechanical alignment than with conventional intra-medullary instruments [13]. With the development of minimally invasive methods for total knee replacement, the author modified the technique to use it with navigation under the assumption that, with navigation, the surgical procedure could be done with the same degree of accuracy and reliability as had been done with the larger incision. The goal of this chapter is to describe the surgical technique for minimally invasive total knee replacement with the Stryker[1] imageless navigation system along with preliminary results.

---

[1] Stryker Corporation, Kalamazoo, Michigan, USA

Methods

The computer-assisted system used in this series of knee replacements was the Stryker Navigation unit. With this system, navigation trackers are rigidly fixed to the tibia and femur with percutaneous pins to which are attached a locking mechanism with an attachment arm for the trackers. The trackers are wireless »active« devices, powered by a small sterile battery. On each tracker are a series of light emitting diodes (LED) that transmit a series of infrared light signals. A free-standing navigation unit consisting of three infrared cameras connected to a computer monitors the position of each tracker and the spatial relationship of each LED on each tracker. With the establishment of a coordinate system, changes in position of each tracker are transformed into changes in position of any anatomic point identified on the femur and tibia with a wireless LED »pointer« device. The knee navigation software can then determine the positions of the femur and tibia, the instruments used to make the bone cuts as well as the angle, orientation and depth of each of the cuts.

With limited space inside the incision with an MIS approach, the pins for fixation of the trackers are placed outside the incision with a percutaneous technique. For both the tibia and femur, two self-tapping bicortical external fixator type pins are placed from lateral to medial. An external locking mechanism[2] is placed over the pins and tightened, creating a rigid attachment for the navigation tracker which is positioned to face the cameras on the navigation unit. Following placement of rigidly fixed trackers on the tibia and femur, the trackers are activated to establish communication channels with the computer navigation system. The hip center is identified by moving the hip gently through a range of motion. An algorithm in the software adjusts for any pelvic motion.

In this series, the knee incision was a limited midvastus exposure. The skin incision begins just above the superior border of the patella, is carried slightly medially over the edge of the patella and ends just medial to the mid-point of the tubercle. At the top of the incision, at the level of the superior pole of the patella, a small cut is made through the tendon into the muscle of the vastus medius in line with the fiber orientation followed by releasing the capsule superiorly. The periosteum and capsule can then be elevated off of the medial tibia just below the joint line.

The patella can then be subluxed laterally, exposing the intercondylar area and a portion of the lateral femoral condyle to remove the anterior lateral meniscus and anterior cruciate ligament. With the trochlear groove visualized, an electro-cautery knife is used to mark the trochlear groove or Whiteside's line [21].

Once the exposure is complete the bony landmarks of the distal femur and tibia are identified through a registration process. The medial epicondyle is identified and the pointed tracker used to mark the sulcus below the medial epicondyle [22]. The lateral epicondyle is registered by flexing the knee to 20°, retracting the patella and palpating the tip of the pointer and the prominence of the epicondyle. The knee is then flexed to 80° and the center of the distal femur registered. The pointer is then placed parallel to the electro-cautery mark made earlier in the trochlear groove to register Whiteside's line [21]. The computer software identifies the AP axis of the femur as the average of the measurements made for the epicondylar axis and Whiteside's line with the degrees of difference between the two displayed.

The surfaces of the distal anterior femoral cortex, medial and lateral distal condyles and medial and lateral posterior condyes are then mapped and registered with multiple points. With the tibia retracted forward, the tibial center and AP axis are identified. This is followed by the mapping of the medial and lateral condylar surfaces. The center of the ankle is determined by registering the tips of the medial and lateral malleoli and using the pointer to identify a point that is 55% lateral and 45% medial to the bi-malleolar points. With both trackers in place, the initial alignment, range of motion and range of varus-valgus stability are determined and recorded.

One of the premises behind using an MIS approach for a TKR is that by removing the bone needed for the surgery, the operative space is opened up, which facilitates the reduced exposure surgery [16, 18]. In this series the bone cut order was distal femur followed by proximal tibia. This allowed adequate space for making the remaining femoral cuts and setting rotation. The current version of the software recognizes which cut is being made by the position of the tracker attached to each cutting block. The computer automatically moves to the screen displaying the cut to be made, eliminating the need for the surgeon to manually move from screen to screen during the bone resection process.

With the navigated MIS approach, the distal femoral cutting block with a navigation tracker attached, can be

---

[2] Ortholock – Stryker Corporation, Kalamazoo, Michigan, USA

placed in any position with the appropriate plane and depth of cut with guidance from the navigation system by watching the computer monitor. The author uses both an open solid block that fits into this space as well as an adjustable slotted block (◘ Fig. 34.1). The desired plane of the distal femoral cut of 0° varus-valgus and 3° flexion makes the cut approximately perpendicular to the axis of the distal half of the femur identified by a standard intra-medullary rod. Once the correct plane is established, the software displays the planned cut orientation and the amount of bone that would be resected from each distal femoral condyle (◘ Fig. 34.2). The surgeon needs to base the decision for depth of cut on the type of deformity, the amount of wear on each condyle and the thickness of the implant to be placed. For a knee with an intact distal medial femoral condyle and an implant that was 8 mm thick, the author would resect 8 mm from the distal femur.

The cut is made with an oscillating saw from the medial or antero-medial side, removing the medial distal femoral condyle first. Once completed, a small flat metal plate can be placed over the entire surface of the distal femur, the cut verified and any further small adjustments made. Once the femoral cut has been completed, the same cutting block used on the femur is placed against the antero-medial aspect of the tibia and pinned into place using the monitor display to adjust the positioning for 0° of varus-valgus, the appropriate amount of posterior tilt and depth of bone resection. Rather than resect the full proximal tibia as one piece, as is done frequently with a standard approach, the author has found it easier to make multiple cuts and take it out in pieces.

Once the distal femoral and proximal tibia cuts have been made, the space opens up as the soft tissues relax allowing a double pronged retractor to be placed around the

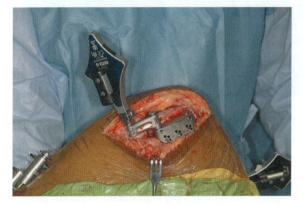

◘ **Fig. 34.1.** Navigated distal femoral cutting block pinned to the medial femoral condyle with a limited incision

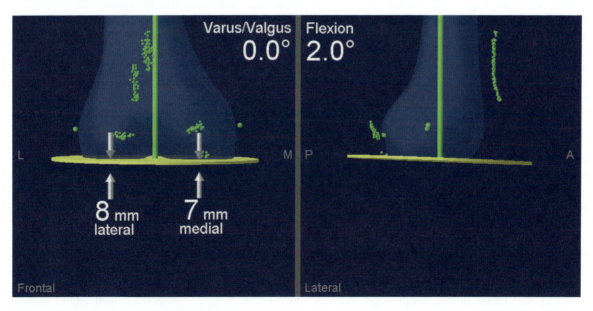

◘ **Fig. 34.2.** Computer monitor display for distal femoral cut

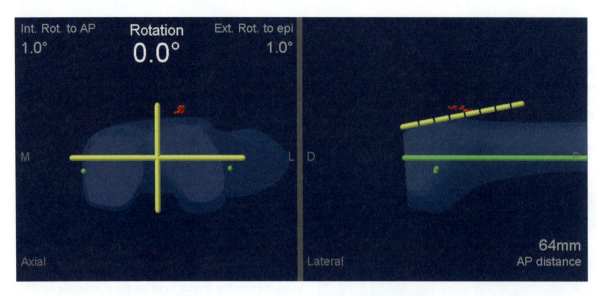

Fig. 34.3. Monitor display of femoral rotation and planned anterior resection line

lateral femoral condyle to retract the patella and expose the face of the distal femoral cut with the knee flexed. The feet of a navigated rotational and anterior-posterior sizing instrument are placed beneath the femoral condyles and the device rotated until 0° of rotation is achieved. In this system, the monitor displays the rotation relative to the palpated epicondyles, Whiteside's line and the average of those two values, which is what the author most frequently relies on. The device is fixed with 3.2 mm pins placed into each condyle through holes in the guide. At this point, the knee is flexed with limited access to the supracondylar area. A navigation tracker is then placed onto the guide with calibrated marks for each size of implant with the monitor displaying the plane of the cut line as it intersects with the mapped points on the distal anterior cortex of the femur (Fig. 34.3). Once the size of the implant has been chosen, the rotation guide and pins are removed and the four-in-one cutting block is used to resect the remaining femoral condyles and chamfer.

Once all of the bone cuts have been made, the joint can be distracted with spreaders with mobile discs on the ends that fit between the posterior condyles and the cut tibial surface with the knee in flexion for debridement of meniscal remnants, loose bodies and osteophytes. If a posterior cruciate substituting design is indicated, the PCL can be removed at this time. The tibial surface can

now be completely exposed for verification using the navigation software and any adjustments in the cut made to bring it to 0° of varus-valgus.

With the bone cuts made and verified, both the tibial and distal femoral cut surfaces should be in 0° ± 0.5° of varus-valgus alignment. With placement of the trial components, the overall limb alignment can be assessed with the navigation software throughout the range of motion and any necessary soft-tissue balancing performed. The patella is most easily cut with the knee in extension where it can be everted without stress on the tissues. Once all the cuts have been made, the bone surfaces are cleaned with pulsatile lavage and drying in preparation for cementing the implants into place.

During the preparation of the knee, with each bone cut and resection, the exposure becomes easier as the soft tissues relax as the space is opened up. As the implants are cemented into place, the opposite is true and the soft tissues become tighter, again limiting the exposure. The author prefers to cement all three components with a single mix of bone cement. To facilitate this, the tibia is cemented first using the cement in a low viscosity state where it flows easily, usually within two minutes of initial mixing. The patella is cemented next by extending the knee and everting the patella the cement applied to the cut surface and compressed with a patellar clamp which

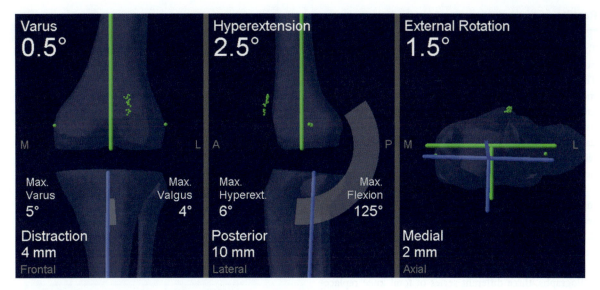

□ Fig. 34.4. Display of final alignment and range of motion

is then removed. The author has found that with the knee flexed and the patella subluxed laterally, the pressure of the patella against the lateral condyle and a lateral retractor are adequate to hold the patella in place during the rest of the cementing procedure. With the small incision, there is not enough exposure to leave a patellar clamp in place while cementing the femur.

After completing the patella, cement is applied to the femoral bone surfaces and the inside of the femoral component. To avoid scratching the femoral component, the author uses flat 3 mm thick plastic inserts that fit into the tibial base plate and provide a protective and gliding surface for the femoral component as the implant is impacted into place. With the femoral component in place, the knee is extended to about 20° of flexion, the tibial base plate protector removed and a trial tibial component inserted. With all the components in place and the cement still in a dough stage, the knee can be extended, the trackers placed back on their attachments and the software on the monitor used to be sure the cement sets up with the knee in complete extension and neutral alignment. Following hardening and debridement of the cement, the tourniquet is released and hemostasis obtained. Following placement of modular insert, the final ROM, alignment and soft tissue laxity are recorded after which the knee is closed in a routine manner (□ Fig. 34.4).

Long standing radiographs, taken at intervals postoperatively, were used to assess the final alignment. For patients whose hips were not visible on the long film, the pelvic radiograph, taken at the same time, was overlaid on the long film to create a single image of the entire lower extremity for analysis. An image analysis software program[3] was then used to mark the center of the femoral heads, center of the knee, center of the talar dome, the femoral joint line and the tibial tray on the radiographs to determine the radiographic alignment. Reliability of repeated measures with this technique was assessed with a Cronbach's Alpha value of 0.990. Cases with rotated views of the components were excluded from the analysis due to the effect of any persistent flexion contracture and rotation on the apparent alignment of the limb.

Study and evaluation of the patients and their clinical results has been approved by the Northwestern University Institutional Review Board (IRB). The patients in the study were informed and consented about the nature of the study and the use of the information. Data collection and analysis were done using Microsoft Access[4] and SPSS.[5]

[3] Sigma Pro – SPSS Software, Chicago, Illinois, USA
[4] Microsoft Corporation, Redmond, Washington, USA
[5] SPSS, Inc., Chicago, Illinois, USA

Results

To evaluate the outcome of using an MIS Navigated approach, the results were compared to two earlier series. The first is a conventional total knee where a standard median parapatellar incision with patellar eversion and intra-medullary instruments with mechanical blocks was used. The second is a series of total knees using the standard median approach but with navigated cutting blocks without an intra-medullary device. ◻ Table 34.1 shows the demographics and characteristics of the three groups.

◻ Table 34.2 shows the navigational values achieved in surgery in the MIS navigated cases and an earlier series using navigation with a standard incision with no difference in values for the key bone cuts and alignment between the two approaches.

Using the alignment derived from the long standing radiographs, three different series of total knee replacements were compared (◻ Fig. 34.5). These are a group of cases done by the senior author using standard intra-medullary instruments with a goal of 6° of anatomic alignment, a group of navigated cases using a long standard medial parapatellar incision with eversion of the patella and a goal of 0° of mechanical alignment, and the current group of navigated cases using an MIS mid-vastus incision with subluxation of the patella and a goal of 0° of

alignment. The values are in ◻ Table 34.3 and demonstrate a significant reduction in the range of post-operative radiographic alignment along with a significant decrease in the percentage of cases outside of a 3° range of mechanical alignment from neutral between the navigated groups and the manual group (p=0.00). There was not a significant difference between the two navigated groups with standard and MIS incisions (p=0.12).

◻ **Table 34.1.** Characteristics of the groups of patients compared to total knees done with MIS and navigation

	Standard Incision Intra-medullary	Standard Incision Navigation	MIS Incision Navigation
Osteoarthritis	94.6%	94.9%	98.8%
Age	67.3	69.0	69.3
Gender % M:F	42:58	35:65	31:69

◻ **Table 34.2.** Intra-operative navigation values (degrees) at surgery comparing a standard medial incision with patellar eversion and an MIS mid-vastus incision with patellar subluxation

Measure	Standard	MIS
Initial Alignment		
– Varus (%)	67.6	64.5
– Valgus (%)	29.7	29.0
– Neutral (%)	2.7	6.5
Distal femoral cut varus/valgus	0.0° ± 0.3°	0.2° ± 0.4°
Distal femoral flexion	1.1° ± 1.3°	2.8° ± 0.7°
Distal femoral rotation	0.1° ±0.3°	0.2° ± 0.8°
Proximal tibial varus/valgus	0.0° ± 0.3°	0.1° ± 0.4°
Final alignment	0.0° ± 0.7°	0.0° ± 0.6°

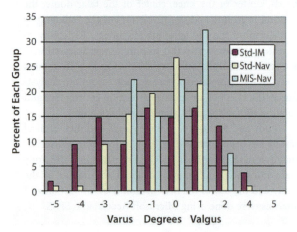

◻ **Fig. 34.5.** Percentage distribution in one degree increments of mechanical alignment, on the basis of long standing radiographs, for each of the three groups: standard incision intra-medullary (IM); standard incision navigation; and MIS navigation.

◻ **Table 34.3.** Comparison of the radiographic alignment on long standing films between total knees done with either: standard long incision intra-medullary, standard long incision navigation and MIS navigation mid-vastus incision

Method	Mean	Std. Dev.	Range
Standard incision intra-medullary	0.3° Varus	2.3°	8.7°
Standard incision navigation	0.5° Varus	1.4°	6.1°
MIS mid-vastus navigation	0.2° Varus	1.3°	4.1°

Discussion

The primary goal of navigation is to achieve reproducible mechanical alignment to minimize the likelihood of late mechanical failure due to mal-alignment [1–4]. Achievement of complete extension and ligament balancing throughout the range of motion are also facilitated by having navigation for guidance. The primary goal of reducing the incision size is to reduce the pain and morbidity associated with a total knee replacement to achieve a quicker and more comfortable recovery for the patient. By reducing the incision, limiting the disruption of the extensor mechanism and not everting the patella, the use of MIS offers the possibility of improved range of motion and functional outcomes for the patients [16–18]. In total knee replacement, computer-assisted navigation is used as an alternative to traditional intra-medullary and mechanical block-based instruments with improved reproducibility of mechanical alignment [10–15]. Its use in minimally invasive surgery can allow the surgeon to achieve the same intra-operative accuracy as with larger, more traditional incisions.

In this series of MIS navigated total knees, on the basis of long standing radiographs, the results with navigation, using either a standard or MIS approach are equivalent and superior to the previous experience using standard intra-medullary instruments. This suggests that the combination of navigation and MIS techniques may be a preferred approach for total knee replacement.

References

1. Berend M, Ritter M, Meding J et al. (2004) Tibial component failure mechanisms in total knee arthroplasty. Clin Orthop 428: 26
2. Jeffery R, Morris R, Denham R (1991) Coronal alignment after total knee replacement. J Bone Joint Surg 73B: 709
3. Lotke P, Ecker M (1977) Influence of positioning of prosthesis in total knee replacement. J Bone Joint Surg 59A: 77
4. Moreland J (1988) Mechanisms of failure in total knee arthroplasty. Clin Orthop 226: 49
5. Bathis H, Perlick L, Tingart M, Perlick C, Luring C, Grifka J (2005) Intraoperative cutting errors in total knee arthroplasty. Arch Orthop Trauma Surg 125(1): 16–20
6. Plaskos C, Hodgson AJ, Inkpen K, McGraw RW (2002) Bone cutting errors in total knee arthroplasty. J Arthroplasty 17: 698–705
7. Chauhan SK, Scott RG, Breidahl W, Beaver RJ (2004) Computer-assisted knee arthroplasty versus a conventional jig-based technique. A randomised, prospective trial. J Bone Joint Surg 86B(3): 372–377
8. Decking R, Markmann Y, Fuchs J, Puhl W, Scharf HP (2005) Leg axis after computer-navigated total knee arthroplasty: a prospective randomized trial comparing computer-navigated and manual implantation. J Arthroplasty 20(3): 282–288
9. Haaker RG, Stockheim M, Kamp M, Proff G, Breitenfelder J, Ottersbach A (2005) Computer-assisted navigation increases precision of component placement in total knee arthroplasty. Clin Orthop Relat Res 433: 152–159
10. Anderson KC, Buehler KC, Markel DC (2005) Computer assisted navigation in total knee arthroplasty. J Arthroplasty 20(7): 132–138
11. Bathis H, Perlick L, Tingart M, Luring C, Zurakowski D, Grifka J (2004) Alignment in total knee arthroplasty. A comparison of computer-assisted surgery with the conventional technique. J Bone Joint Surg 86B(5): 682–687
12. Jenny JY, Boeri C (2001) Computer-assisted implantation of total knee prostheses: a case-control comparative study with classical instrumentation. Comp Aided Surg 6(4): 217–220
13. Kim SJ, MacDonald M, Hernandez J, Wixson RL (2005) Computer Assisted navigation in total knee arthroplasty: improved coronal alignment. J Arthroplasty 20(7): 123–131
14. Matsumoto T, Tsumura N, Kurosaka M, Muratsu H, Kuroda R, Ishimoto K, Tsujimoto K, Shiba R, Yoshiya S (2004) Prosthetic alignment and sizing in computer-assisted total knee arthroplasty. Intern Orthop 28(5): 282–285
15. Sparmann M, Wolke B, Czupalla H et al. (2003) Positioning of total knee arthroplasty with and without navigation support. J Bone Joint Surg 85B: 830
16. Bonutti PM, Mont MA, McMahon M, Ragland PS, Kester M (2004) Minimally invasive total knee arthroplasty. J Bone Joint Surg 86A(S2): 26–32
17. Laskin RS, Beksac B, Phongjunakorn A, Pittors K, Davis J, Shim JC, Pavlov H, Petersen M (2004) Minimally invasive total knee replacement through a mini-midvastus incision: an outcome study. Clin Orthop Relat Res 428: 74–81
18. Tria AJ Jr, Coon TM (2003) Minimal incision total knee arthroplasty: early experience. Clin Orthop Relat Res 416: 185–190
19. Dalury DF, Dennis DA (2005) Mini-incision total knee arthroplasty can increase risk of component malalignment. Clin Orthop Relat Res 440: 77–81
20. Fisher DA, Watts M, Davis KE (2003) Implant position in knee surgery: a comparison of minimally invasive, open unicompartmental, and total knee arthroplasty. J Arthroplasty 18(7): 2–8
21. Whiteside L, Arima J (1995) The anteroposterior axis for femoral rotational alignment in valgus total knee arthroplasty. Clin Orthop 321: 168
22. Berger RA, Rubash HE, Seel MJ, Thompson WH, Crossett LS (1993) Determining the rotational alignment of the femoral component in total knee arthroplasty using the epicondylar axis. Clin Orthop 286: 40–47

Part II D   Navigation and Minimally Invasive Surgery in Unicompartmental Knee Arthroplasty (UKA)

Navigated Minimally Invasive Surgery Unicompartmental Knee Replacement

J.-Y. Jenny

Introduction

The accuracy of implantation is an accepted prognostic factor for the long-term survival of unicompartmental knee replacement (UKR) [1–3]. However, most UKR systems offer a limited and potentially inaccurate instrumentation that relies on substantial surgeon judgment for prosthesis placement. Rates of inaccurate implantation as high as 30 per cent have been reported with conventional, free hand instrumentation [4]. Intra-medullary femoral guiding device can improve these results [5, 6], but does not allow reproducible optimal implantation.

Computer-assisted systems have been developed for to-tal knee replacement (TKR), and have proved allowing a higher precision of implantation for such implants in comparison to conventional instruments [7–9]. The OrthoPilot® system (Aesculap, Tuttlingen, Germany) has also been validated in clinical use by a prospective, randomized study [10]. This system is considered as non-image based, because it only relies on an intra-operative cinematic analysis of the lower limb.

In a first stage, we developed an adaptation of this technique for implantation of a conventional, fixed bearing UKP (☐ Fig. 35.1a), without any extra-medullary or intra-medullary guiding device, suitable for either conventional or mini-invasive approach. We hypothesized that the navigation system will allow placing the prosthesis in a better position than the conventional technique, and that the radiological results will be different based on the type of instruments used. In a second stage, we devel-

oped a new implant dedicated to a navigated technique (☐ Fig. 35.1b), using the concept of extra-articular fixation of the resection guides to further decrease the invasiveness of the procedure. The present study reports the early radiological results of two groups of patients in whom a UKP was implanted with a navigated instrumentation and MIS approach, with a comparison with a historical group operated on with a conventional, open navigated technique and a concurrent group operated on with the same navigation technique for a TKR, used as the gold standard for navigated implantation of a knee prosthesis.

Operative Techniques

Conventional Navigated Technique

The used navigation system is an intra-operative non-image based one (OrthoPilot®, AESCULAP, Tuttlingen, FRG; ☐ Fig. 35.2) [11]. After a medial parapatellar approach, typically 18 cm of length, three infrared localizers were implanted on screws in the distal femur and in the proximal tibia, and strapped on the dorsal part of the foot. The relative motion of two adjacent localizers was tracked by an infrared camera (Polaris®, Northern Digital, Toronto, Canada). The dedicated software calculated the center of rotation of this movement, and so defined the respective centers of rotation of the hip, knee and ankle joints. With these centers were calculated the mechanical axes of both femur and tibia on both coronal and sagittal planes. A localizer was then fixed on tibial or femoral resection

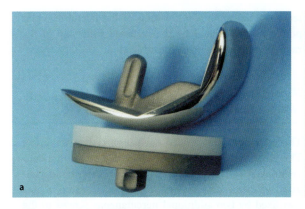

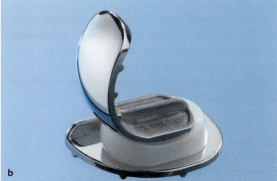

Fig. 35.1a,b. The implants: conventional UKR (**a**), dedicated UKR (**b**)

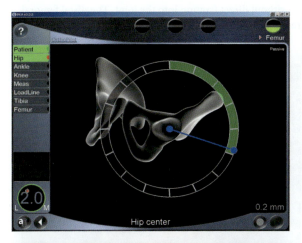

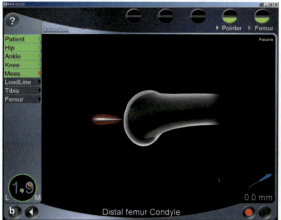

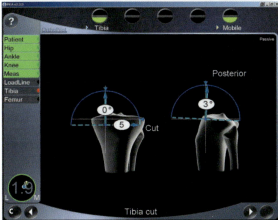

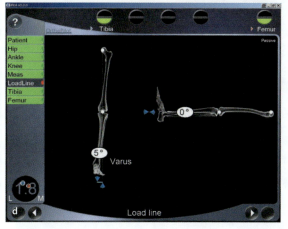

Fig. 35.2a–d. Conventional navigated operative technique: registrations of joint center of motion (example: hip) (**a**), registration of bony landmarks (example: distal femoral condyle) (**b**), orientation of the resection blocks (example: proximal tibial resection) (**c**), control with the trial implants (**d**)

blocks, and the software displayed on line the orientation of this block in comparison to the mechanical axes of the bone. The surgeon could fix the block with the desired orientation before performing the bony resection with a classical motorized saw blade. The trial implants were tested, and the definitive prosthesis was cemented if the test was satisfactory.

Mini-invasive Navigated Technique with Conventional Implants

The same non-image based navigation system was used, but the instruments were modified to allow their placement through a 8 cm skin incision (◘ Fig. 35.3). However the software had to be modified, as the minimal invasive approach did not allow the direct palpation of the lateral

femoro-tibial joint. The position of the lateral articular points was calculated by the software with help of the radiographic pre-operative planification.

Mini-invasive Navigated Technique with Dedicated Implants

The same non-image based navigation system was used. The proximal tibial resection was performed with a conventional motorized saw blade guided by a free hand navigated orienting device. For the femoral resection, a bow was fixed by two additional percutaneous screws to the distal femur. The bow was navigated to be oriented along the knee flexion axis, and the femoral guide was fixed on it, without direct fixation into the joint. The distal femoral resection was performed with a burr (◘ Fig. 35.4).

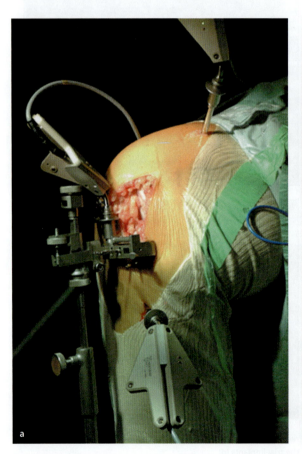
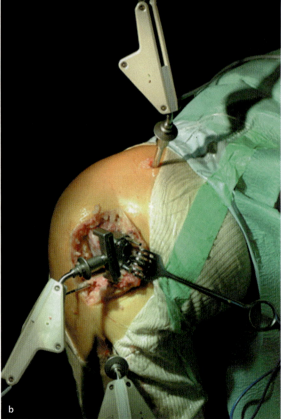

a

b

◘ **Fig. 35.3a,b.** Mini-invasive navigated technique with conventional implants: tibial resection (**a**), femoral resection (**b**)

35

Navigated TKR Technique

This technique has been described more extensively elsewhere [12]. It is basically the same technique as for UKR implantation with the conventional navigated technique.

Material and Methods

90 patients have been operated on for a medial osteoarthritis at the authors' institution from January 2001 to September 2002 with implantation of a UKR with the conventional navigated instrumentation. From October 2002 to December 2004, the mini-invasive navigated technique with conventional implants was used in 108 cases. The conventional, fixed bearing prosthesis (Search® UKR, AESCULAP, Tuttlingen, FRG – see Fig. 35.4a) was designed to

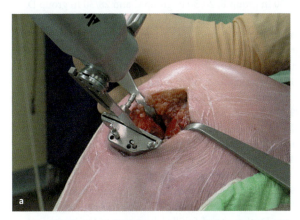

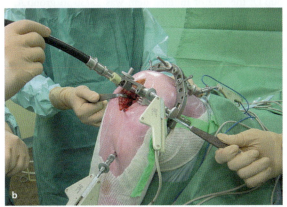

◻ Fig. 35.4a,b. Mini-invasive navigated technique with dedicated implants: tibial resection (**a**), femoral resection (**b**)

be implanted as follows: coronal femoro-tibial mechanical angle of 0 to 5 degrees of remaining varus deformation, coronal orientation of the femoral component of 90±2 degrees in comparison to the coronal femoral mechanical axis, sagittal orientation of the femoral component of 90±2 degrees in comparison to the distal anterior femoral cortex, coronal orientation of the tibial component of 90±2 degrees in comparison to the coronal tibial mechanical axis, sagittal orientation of the tibial component of 88±2 degrees in comparison to the proximal posterior tibial cortex.

From September 2004 to December 2005, the mini-invasive navigated technique with dedicated implants was used in 50 cases. The dedicated, mobile bearing prosthesis (Univation® UKR, AESCULAP, Tuttlingen, FRG – see Fig. 35.4b) was designed to be implanted as follows: coronal femoro-tibial mechanical angle of 0 to 5 degrees of remaining varus deformation, coronal orientation of the femoral component of 90±5 degrees in comparison to the coronal femoral mechanical axis, sagittal orientation of the femoral component of 80±5 degrees in comparison to the distal anterior femoral cortex, coronal orientation of the tibial component of 85 to 90 degrees in comparison to the coronal tibial mechanical axis, sagittal orientation of the tibial component of 85 to 90 degrees in comparison to the proximal posterior tibial cortex. Tolerances were greater than for the conventional, fixed bearing prosthesis because of the complete congruence between femoral and tibial implants.

From October 2002 to December 2004, 205 patients have been operated on for a global varus osteoarthritis at the authors' institution by means of a TKR. The used prosthesis (E-motion® TKR, AESCULAP, Tuttlingen, FRG) was designed to be implanted as follows: coronal femoro-tibial mechanical angle of 0±3 degrees, coronal orientation of the femoral component of 90±2 degrees in comparison to the coronal femoral mechanical axis, sagittal orientation of the femoral component of 90±2 degrees in comparison to the distal anterior femoral cortex, coronal orientation of the tibial component of 90±2 degrees in comparison to the coronal tibial mechanical axis, sagittal orientation of the tibial component of 90±2 degrees in comparison to the proximal posterior tibial cortex.

All patients had a complete radiological examination in the first three months after the index procedure, with AP and lateral plain knee X-rays and AP and lateral long leg X-rays.

30 conventional UKR implanted with the conventional navigated technique (group A), 30 conventional UKR

implanted with the mini-invasive navigated technique (group B), 30 dedicated UKR implanted with the mini-invasive navigated technique (group C) and 30 TKR implanted with the conventional navigated technique (group D) were randomly selected and compared. By the selected patients, the following angles were measured on long leg X-rays by a unique observer (JYJ):

- mechanical femoro-tibial angle (normal = 0°, varus deformation was measured with a positive angle);
- coronal orientation of the femoral component in comparison to the mechanical femoral axis (normal = 90°, varus deformation was measured with an angle <90°);
- sagittal orientation of the femoral component in comparison to the distal anterior femoral cortex (normal = 90°, flexion deformation was measured with an angle <90°);
- coronal orientation of the tibial component in comparison to the mechanical tibial axis (normal = 90°, varus deformation was measured with an angle <90°);
- sagittal orientation of the tibial component in comparison to the proximal posterior tibial cortex (normal = 90°, flexion deformation was measured with angle <90°).

Individual analysis was performed as follows: one point was given for each fulfilled item, giving a maximal accuracy note of 5 points; the accuracy note was compared between all groups with an ANOVA test with post-hoc Bonferrini-Dunn correction. Prosthesis implantation was considered as satisfactory when the accuracy note was 5 (all fulfilled items); the rate of satisfactory implanted prostheses was compared in all groups with a Chi-square test. Mean angular values in all groups were compared for each criterion with an ANOVA test with post-hoc Bonferrini-Dunn correction; the rate of prostheses implanted within the desired range for each criterion was also compared in all groups with a Chi-square test. All statistical tests were performed with a 0.05 limit of significance.

Results

120 patients were selected: 55 men and 65 women, with a mean age of 66 years (range, 51 to 82 years). Mean body mass index was 29.5 (range, 20.6 to 44.3). Mean preoperative coronal femoro-tibial mechanical angle was 8 degrees (range, 2 to 15 degrees). There were 51 grade 2, 56 grade

3 and 13 grade 4 degenerative changes according to Ahlback [13].

Radiographic results at the early follow-up are reported in the ◘ Tables 35.1 and 35.2.

Global accuracy note was 4.5 ± 0.6 degrees in group A, 3.3±1.2 degrees in group B, 3.6±1.0 degrees in group C and 4.2±0.8 degrees in group D; the rate of perfect implantation was 18/30 in group A, 13/30 in group B, 12/30 in group C and 17/30 in group D.

Mean femoro-tibial angle was 1.5 ± 2.2 degrees in group A, 0.5±3.1 degrees in group B, 2.9±2.8 degrees in group C and 0.2±2.7 degrees in group D; the rate of fulfilled item was 25/30 in group A, 22/30 in group B, 22/30 in group C and 27/30 in group D.

Mean coronal orientation of the femoral component was 89.1±1.4 degrees in group A, 91.1±5.0 degrees in group B, 86.0±3.9 degrees in group C and 90.3±1.4 degrees in group D; the rate of fulfilled item was 26/30 in group A, 23/30 in group B, 20/30 in group C and 28/30 in group D.

Mean sagittal orientation of the femoral component was 89.6±1.6 degrees in group A, 87.6±3.5 degrees in group B, 90.1±4.6 degrees in group C and 88.6±2.7 degrees in group D; the rate of fulfilled item was 27/30 in group A, 21/30 in group B, 21/30 in group C and 24/30 in group D.

Mean coronal orientation of the tibial component was 89.1±1.4 degrees in group A, 91.1±5.0 degrees in group B, 87.6±4.2 degrees in group C and 90.1±1.7 degrees in group D; the rate of fulfilled item was 28/30 in group A, 24/30 in group B, 24/30 in group C and 27/30 in group D.

Mean sagittal orientation of the tibial component was 89.6±1.3 degrees in group A, 87.6±3.5 degrees in group B, 88.3±2.5 degrees in group C and 89.8±3.1 degrees in group D; the rate of fulfilled item was 28/30 in group A, 24/30 in group B, 24/30 in group C and 26/30 in group D.

For all items, there was a significant difference between all groups as a whole; there was no significant difference between groups A and D; there was a significant decrease of the quality of results in groups B and C in comparison to groups A and D.

Discussion

Navigation systems have proved to improve the accuracy of implantation of a TKR [7–10, 14], and can be considered as the golden standard for knee-replacement surgery. The precision of the used system was experimentally calculated to be of 1° for angle measurement and of 1 mm

Table 35.1. Radiographic results in degrees (mean, maximum, minimum, standard deviation)

	Group A (n=30)	Group B (n=30)	Group C (n=30)	Group D (n=30)
Coronal femoro-tibial mechanical angle	1.5 5 -4 2.2	0.5 8 -8 3.1	2.9 8 -3 2.8	0.2 6 6 2.7
Coronal orientation of the femoral component	89.1 92 85 1.4	91.1 100 76 5.0	86.0 94 79 3.9	90.3 93 86 1.4
Sagittal orientation of the femoral component	89.6 92 86 1.6	87.6 96 78 3.5	90.1 105 80 4.6	88.6 97 80 2.7
Coronal orientation of the tibial component	89.1 92 86 1.4	91.1 94 83 5.0	87.6 93 70 4.2	90.1 94 85 1.7
Sagittal orientation of the tibial component	89.6 93 86 1.3	87.6 92 84 3.5	88.3 94 82 2.5	89.8 92 84 3.1

Table 35.2. Radiographic results: number of prostheses in the desired angular range

	Group A (n=30)	Group B (n=30)	Group C (n=30)	Group D (n=30)
Coronal femoro-tibial mechanical angle	25	22	22	27
Coronal orientation of the femoral component	26	23	20	28
Sagittal orientation of the femoral component	27	21	21	24
Coronal orientation of the tibial component	28	24	24	27
Sagittal orientation of the tibial component	28	24	24	26
Optimally implanted prosthesis	18	13	12	17

for distance measurement [15]. However, outliers still can occur. There are several possible additional reasons for the observed errors: lack of precision of the radiological measurement technique, lack of rigid fixation of the resection block on the bone, lack of precise guiding of the saw blade by the resection blocks bending of the saw blade [16]. These causes of errors are a part of all systems. But a modification of the reference software should not bring other causes of errors.

UKR is a valuable alternative to high tibial osteotomy [17] or TKR for the treatment of isolated medial osteoarthritis [4, 18–21]. However, the exact indications are still controversial, as some authors have reported a low survival rate of such implants [22]. Inaccurate implantation is an accepted factor for early failure [1, 3]. There is no general agreement on the ideal positioning of a UKR, and the positioning we wanted to achieve can only be seen as a personal opinion. However the goal of an instrumentation is to allow the surgeon to place the prosthesis in the position he decided himself. It is then valuable to compare the positioning of the three groups of UKR implantation techniques, which were expected to implant the prosthesis in the same position, whatever this position should be. Most instrumentation offer unprecise guiding systems, which mainly rely on the surgeon's skill [5]. Even intra-medullary guiding systems do not offer reproducible optimal implantation technique [6]. The conventional navigated instrumentation used in this study is similar to that used for TKR implantation. It allowed getting a significant higher rate of implantation into the desired angular range on post-operative X-rays for all criteria in comparison to the manual technique. It also allowed a significant higher rate of global satisfactory implantation, with all measured angles within the desired range by one given patient. These rates were similar to that obtained with the reference TKR software.

The conventional navigation technique involves conventional skin incision and approach, with splitting of the vastus medialis muscle and lateral subluxation of the patella. We developed a navigated minimal invasive technique, which allows performing the whole procedure through a shorter skin incision. Our first experience is interesting. All procedures succeeded with a 7 to 10 cm long skin incision. However, we observed a decrease in the quality of implantation of the prosthesis with the minimal-invasive navigated technique for both conventional and dedicated implants. The calculation of the location of the anatomic point was less precise than the direct palpation, and this point has to be addressed in the future development. However, we observed no clinical influence on the short-term functional results. We hope that the use of the dedicated implant with full congruency will allow compensating for this decreased accuracy of implantation.

We did not yet study the influence of the minimally invasive approach on the rehabilitation time. This point has already been investigated, and minimal invasive procedures might allow an earlier discharge and faster rehabilitation [23].

The follow-up of the navigated prostheses is currently too short to know if clinical outcome or survival rates will be improved. Longer follow-up is required to determine the respective advantages and disadvantages of this techniques and the potential benefit of a mini-invasive implantation.

Conclusion

Navigated implantation of a UKP with the used, non-image-based system allowed to improve the accuracy of the radiological implantation without any significant inconvenient and with little change in the conventional operative technique. Mini-invasive implantation was effective, but the accuracy did not reach that of the conventional navigated technique. Minimally invasive techniques have to be validated, because a loss of accuracy will negatively influence long term outcomes.

References

1. Cartier P, Sanouillier JL, Grelsamer RP (1996) Unicompartmental knee arthroplasty surgery. 10-year minimum follow-up period. J Arthroplasty 11: 782–788
2. Hernigou P, Deschamps G (1996) Prothèses unicompartimentales du genou. Rev Chir Orthop 82 (Suppl 1): 23
3. Lootvoet L, Burton P, Himmer O, Piot L, Ghosez JP (1997) Prothèses unicompartimentales de genou: influence du positionnement du plateau tibial sur les résultats fonctionnels. Acta Orthop Belg 63: 94–101
4. Tabor OB Jr, Tabor OB (1998) Unicompartmental arthroplasty: a long-term follow-up study. J Arthroplasty 13: 373–379
5. Argenson JN, Chevrol-Benkeddache Y, Aubaniac JM (2002) Modern cemented metalbacked unicompartmental knee arthroplasty: a 3 to 10 year follow-up study. J Bone Joint Surg 84A: 2235–2239
6. Jenny JY, Boeri C (2002) Accuracy of implantation of a unicompartmental total knee arthroplasty with 2 different instrumentations: a case-controlled comparative study. J Arthroplasty 17: 1016–1020
7. Decking R, Markmann Y, Fuchs J, Puhl W, Scharf HP (2005) Leg axis after computer-navigated total knee arthroplasty: a prospective randomized trial comparing computer-navigated and manual implantation. J Arthroplasty 20: 282–288
8. Stockl B, Nogler M, Rosiek R, Fischer M, Krismer M, Kessler O (2004) Navigation improves accuracy of rotational alignment in total knee arthroplasty. Clin Orthop 426: 180–186
9. Victor J, Hoste D (1998) Image-based computer-assisted total knee arthroplasty leads to lower variability in coronal alignment. Clin Orthop 428: 131–139
10. Saragaglia D, Picard F, Chaussard C, Montbarbon E, Leitner F, Cinquin P (2001) Mise en place des prothèses totales du genou assistée par ordinateur: comparaison avec la technique conventionelle. Rev Chir Orthop 87: 18–28
11. Jenny JY, Boeri C (2003) Unicompartmental knee prosthesis implantation with a non-image-based navigation system: rationale, technique, case-control comparative study with a conventional instrumented implantation. Knee Surg Sports Traumatol Arthrosc 11: 40–45
12. Jenny JY, Boeri C (2001) Computer-assisted implantation of total knee prostheses: a case-control comparative study with classical instrumentation. Comput Aided Surg 6: 217–220
13. Ahlback S (1968) Osteoarthrosis of the knee. A radiographic investigation. Acta Radiol Diagn 277 (Suppl): 1–72
14. Jenny JY, Boeri C (2001) Implantation d'une prothèse totale de genou assistée par ordinateur. Etude comparative cas-témoin avec une instrumentation traditionnelle. Rev Chir Orthop 87: 645–652
15. Delp SL, Stulberg SD, Davies B, Picard F, Leitner F (1998) Computer assisted knee replacement. Clin Orthop 354: 49–56
16. Plaskos C, Hodgson AJ, Inkpen K, MacGraw RW (2002) Bone cutting errors in total knee arthroplasty. J Arthroplasty 17: 698–705
17. Schai PA, Suh JT, Thornhill TS, Scott RD (1998) Unicompartmental knee arthroplasty in middle-aged patients: a 2- to 6-year follow-up evaluation. J Arthroplasty 13: 365–372
18. Newman JH, Ackroyd CE, Shah NA (1998) Unicompartmental or total knee replacement? Five-year results of a prospective, randomized trial of 102 osteoarthritic knees with unicompartmental arthritis. J Bone Joint Surg 80B: 862–865
19. Robertsson O, Borgquist L, Knuston K, Lewold S, Lidgren L (1999) Use of unicompartmental instead of tricompartmental prostheses for unicompartmental arthrosis in the knee is a cost-effective alternative. 14,437 primary tricompartmental prostheses were compared with 10,624 primary medial or lateral unicompartmental prostheses. Acta Orthop Scand 70: 170–175
20. Robertsson O, Dunbar M, Pehrsson T, Knutson K, Lidgren L (2000) Patient satisfaction after knee arthroplasty: a report on 27,372 knees operated on between 1981 and 1995 in Sweden. Acta Orthop Scand 71: 262–267
21. Squire MV, Callaghan JJ, Goetz DD, Sullivan PM, Johnston RC (1999) Unicompartmental knee replacement. A minimum 15-year follow-up study. Clin Orthop 367: 61–72
22. Bert JM (1998) 10-year survivorship of metal-backed, unicompartmental arthroplasty. J Arthroplasty 13: 901–905
23. Price AJ, Webb J, Topf H, Dodd CA, Goodfellow JW, Murray DW (2001) Rapid recovery after oxford unicompartmental arthroplasty through a short incision. J Arthroplasty 16: 970–976

Minimal Invasive Navigated Unicondylar Knee Replacement with the DePuy Ci-System

H. Bäthis, L. Perlick, C. Lüring, M. Tingart, J. Grifka

Introduction

The results of unicondylar knee arthroplasties have improved steadily since their introduction over 30 years ago [3]. This might be contributed to the development of better implants, appropriate patient selection, the use of thicker and better polyethylene, and better surgical technique [20].

The endeavor to preserve the anatomy and kinematics of the normal knee to enable better function and faster recovery, led to the development of the minimally invasive technique [8, 15]. Despite the favor of preserving undamaged soft tissue the surgeon has a reduced overview and is in risk of component mal-position [7]. Furthermore, most unicompartmental knee arthroplasty systems offer limited and potentially inaccurate instrumentation, which causes a surgeon's judgment to play a large role in prosthesis placement.

This might explain why Tabor et al. found an inaccurate implantation with conventional freehand instrumentation in 30% of the patients [19]. This problem is enhanced when using a limited view as mentioned above [7].

Due to correlation between accuracy of implantation and long-term results, navigation systems have been developed to improve the accuracy of component alignment. Using a conventional incision length, Jenny et al. reported superior results when using the computer-assisted technique [10].

The aim of this study was to analyze the accuracy of post-operative leg alignment and component orientation in minimally invasive computer-assisted UKR, when using a non-image-based navigation system with a specific instrument set. We hypothesized that the computer-assisted procedure will prevent overcorrection and lead to a more precise component orientation and thereby might improve patient long term outcome.

Surgical Technique Navigated Unikondylar Knee Replacement

The image-free Ci-Navigation-System® (DePuy I-Orthopaedics, Munich, Germany) has an optical tracking unit, which detects passive reflecting marker spheres by an infrared camera. The Ci-System is built as a very small computer system which can be placed independently from the position of the camera system near to the surgeon's position. It is controlled by either a draped touch-screen monitor or footswitch (◘ Fig. 36.1).

A 7–9 cm skin incision is made from the superior medial edge of the patella and extended distally and the joint was exposed in the technique described by Repicci et al. [15]. Two reference arrays with passive marker spheres are rigidly attached to both, the femoral and the tibial bone through stitch incisions. The center of the hip is determined by a pivoting algorithm. Specific anatomic landmarks (e.g. the anterior cruciate ligament insertion, the borders of the medial plateau, the medial and lateral malleolus) are digitized at the beginning of the operation with a navigation pointer. Bone-surface information is gained by sliding the pointer on top of the medial tibial plateau and the medial femoral condyle (◘ Fig. 36.2). Based

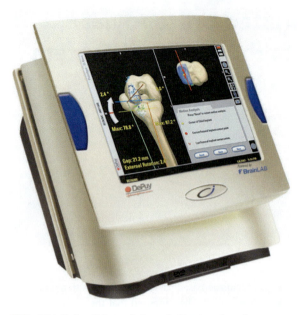

Fig. 36.1. DePuy Ci-System®. Controlled by draped touch-screen or footswitch

on these data, the system creates an adapted bone model of the specific patient's anatomy. With additional information about the desired leg alignment, a planning proposal for the component orientation is generated and can be adjusted to the surgeon's preferences (■ Fig. 36.3). The system provides a kinematical analysis, in which the implant contact areas between the femoral and tibial component are visualized throughout the range of motion (■ Fig. 36.4).

A set of specialized instruments are provided for the navigation based technique of the Preservation® Uni-System such as fine-adjustable resection guides and a universal navigated instrument handle (■ Fig. 36.5).

Comparable to the conventional technique, the resection of the proximal tibia is performed first. The tibial slope is adapted to the individual patient's anatomy. The orientation of the resection guide is controlled by the navigation system. Each resection is verified with the system to identify cutting errors. Using spacer blocks, the knee is balanced both in flexion and extension. The surgeon has the opportunity at every step of the procedure to check for the leg alignment and joint stability, especially

36

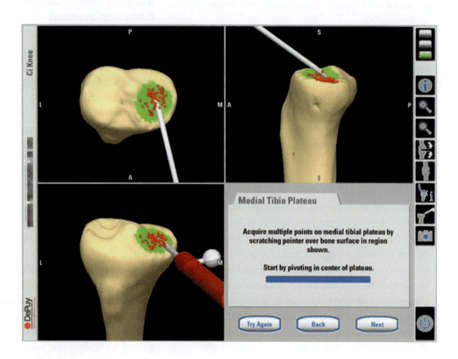

Fig. 36.2. Digitization of the bone-surface on the medial tibial plateau.

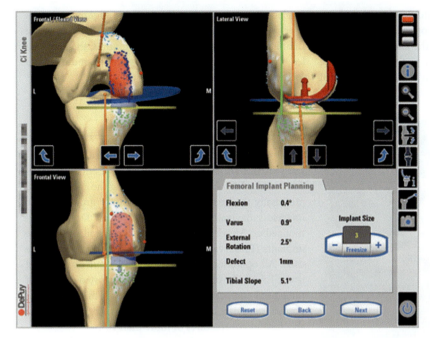

Fig. 36.3. Proposal for the component orientation based on the desired leg alignment. Prosthesis position and size can be modified to the surgeons preference

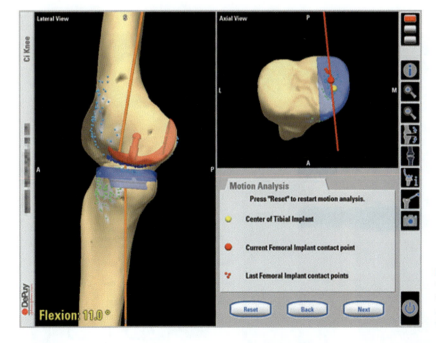

Fig. 36.4. Motion analysis. Simulation of the contact areas between femoral and tibial component of according to the planned position before any bone cut is performed

to prevent from overcorrection into a valgus leg-alignment (■ Fig. 36.6). According to an optimized component orientation, the distal femoral and the additional femoral resections are performed using a multi-cutting guide with the control of the navigation system. Using trial implants, the range of motion and leg alignment can be checked again. After cementing of the components, the final implant position, the range of motion, the achieved leg axis and the joint stability are examined and digitized for case-records.

Study Design and Patients

Forty patients scheduled for UKR were enrolled prospectively in this single-centre study. The patients were randomized by lot to a control group using the conventional minimally invasive technique or a study group using a imageless navigation system (Ci®-System, DePuy I-Orthopaedics, Munich, Germany). In both groups the same implants (Preservation®, DePuy Inc., Warsaw, USA) were used. All operations were performed by one experienced team. Exclusion criteria were advanced osteoarthritis of the lateral compartment, insufficiency of the anterior or posterior cruciate ligament, severe varus/valgus instability and flexion contractures of more than 10°.

The patients in both groups were comparable regarding age, gender and preoperative leg deformity. In the computer-assisted group (study group), 14 female and 6 male patients were included. The mean age was 65 years

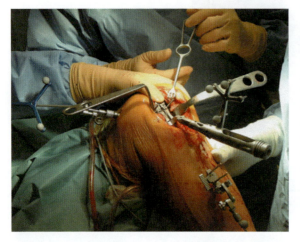

■ **Fig. 36.5.** Specialized instruments for minimal invasive technique. Example: Navigation controlled universal instrument handle with femoral all in one cutting guide

36

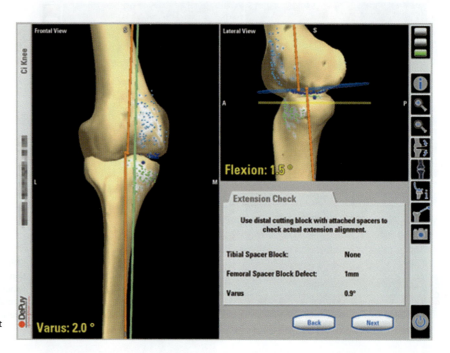

■ **Fig. 36.6.** Alignment check. The surgeon is in control of the leg alignment and stability throughout the whole procedure

(range: 49–73 yrs.) and the mean pre-operative deformity was 4.7 degrees varus. In the conventional surgical technique (control group), 12 female and 8 male patients were included with a mean age of 67 years (range: 45 to 74 yrs.) and a mean pre-operative deformity of 5.6 degrees.

The leg alignment and the component orientation were evaluated on standardized pre- and post-operative full length weight-bearing radiographs by two independent observers. Data of both groups was compared using unpaired t-tests. Level of statistical significance was determined for $p < 0.05$.

Results

Mechanical Leg Axis

In both groups we aimed on a post-operative alignment of 2 degrees of varus from the mechanical axis. The mean pre-operative mechanical axis femoro-tibial angle was corrected from 4.7 degrees varus to 1.6 degree varus (SD 1.2°) in the navigated group. In the conventional group, a mean pre-operative deformity of 5.6 degrees was corrected to 1.4 degrees (SD 2.4°). In the navigated group, one case with a slight overcorrection (1° valgus) was

found, while there were 4 patients (maximum 3° valgus) in the conventional group (■ Fig. 36.7). The results were statistically significant (p=0.008).

Frontal Plane Alignment

For the coronal orientation of the tibial component, we found a mean angle of 89 degrees (SD 0.9°, range 88° to 91°) in the navigated group, while the mean angle in the conventional group 88.7 degrees (SD1.8°, range 85° to 92°) (p=0.04)

The mean deviation from the neutral axis was 0.7 degree (SD 1.5°, range 2° valgus to 3° varus) in the computer assisted group and 1.1 degrees (SD 1.9° range: 2° valgus to 5° varus) in the conventional group (p=0.12).

Sagital Plane Alignment

In the computer-assisted group, the mean flexion-extension alignment was 0.9 degrees (SD 2.5° range: 4° flexion to 5° extension), while in the conventional group it was 1.7 degrees (SD 4.4° range: 6° flexion to 10° extension) (p=0.028).

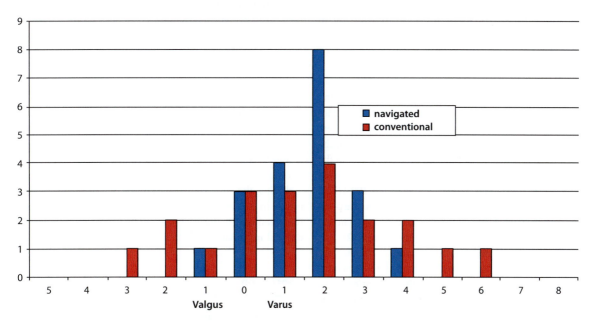

■ **Fig. 36.7.** Results of leg alignment. Navigation group compared to conventional technique

The tibial slope was adjusted to the natural slope. In the study group, the posterior slope of the tibial component was 4.7 degrees (SD 1.4°), in the conventional group it was 5.8 degrees (SD 1.6)

Surgical Data

No conversion from computer assisted surgery to the conventional technique was required in this study. The mean time for surgery (skin to skin) was 77 min (SD 14 min) in the computer-assisted group and 58 min (SD 11 min) in the conventional group. There were no complications (e.g. infections, fractures) due to the fixation of the reference bases.

Discussion

In recent years there has been a resurgence of interest in doing unicompartmental knee replacement [13]. This method appears to be a valuable alternative to high tibial osteotomy or TKA for treating patients with isolated medial osteoarthritis.

Unicompartmental replacement has distinct advantages. It has been reported to be much less invasive than total knee replacement, preserving the undamaged soft-tissue and articular structures and restoring the joint to more normal function [1]. The time needed for recovery is considerably lower, particularly when a reduced or minimally invasive approach is used [13].

Unfortunately, there is no consensus on the amount of ideal correction of the pre-operative deformity. Many experienced surgeons advocate under-correction of the mechanical axis by 2 to 3 degrees [2, 4, 6, 9, 18] because over-correction might result in medio-lateral subluxation of the femoro-tibial articulation or produce excessive force on the unresurfaced compartment with early secondary degeneration [5, 7]. Kennedy and White who analyzed 100 UKRs reported that superior results were obtained when the post-operative mechanical axis of the operated limb fell in the center of the knee or slightly medial to the center [12].

Inaccurate implantation is a well-accepted factor for early failure [4, 14, 16]. Rates of inaccurate implantation of 30% have been reported with conventional instrumentation [21]. Minimally invasive unicondylar knee arthroplasty is a technically demanding procedure [17] because the limited view may further alter the accuracy

and reproducibility when accessing implant positioning and post-operative limb alignment.

Fisher et al. [7] compared the minimally invasive with the standard open UKR. They found a higher variance of post-operative limb alignment when using the minimally invasive technique (mean 3.5° varus, SD 2, range 3° valgus to 8° varus) compared with the standard approach (mean 4.3° varus, SD 1.2, range 2° varus to 8° varus). Further, significant mal-alignment was seen for the tibial implant position in the frontal plane, and for the femoral implant position in the lateral plane. However, in their study, the precision of the post-operative determination of component alignment was limited by the size of the radiographs (18-inch size).

Recently, Keene et al. compared the accuracy of leg alignment in a bilateral unicondylar replacement using navigated technique on one side and conventional technique on the other. In their study the same navigation system (Ci-System) was used. They found a significant better alignment in the navigated group [11]. Using the Orthopilot® system, Jenny and Boeri [10] reported a significantly higher rate of correct component implantation in all planes. 60% of the computer-assisted prosthesis had a satisfactory alignment compared with 20% of cases in the conventional group [10]. For the femoro-tibial mechanical angle they reported a range of 5 degrees varus to 4 degrees valgus in the computer-assisted group compared with 10 degrees varus to 10 degrees valgus in the conventional group. These findings are comparable to our results. Aiming on a post-operative leg axis of 2 degrees varus, 95% of patients in the navigated group and 70% in the conventional group were within a range of 0 degree to 4 degrees varus leg axis.

Additional operating time is needed when using navigation systems in unicondylar knee arthroplasty. However, after an initial learning curve, the computer-assisted surgical procedure was increased by 29 minutes. The work flow is user friendly and does not afford any special computer knowledge. Particularly, the spezialized instrument set including the fine adjustable cutting guide seems to be useful in achieving an exact plane adjustment. Further, the kinematics analysis appears to be useful providing additional information before performing the first resection.

Conclusion

Navigated minimally invasive unicondylar replacement with specific instruments leads to a superior accuracy in reconstruction of limb alignment. Additional and valuable information is provided to the surgeon intra-operatvely in order to achieve the planned leg- and component alignment.

References

1. Ackroyd CE, Whitehouse SL, Newman JH, Joslin CC (2002) A comparative study of the medial St Georg sled and kinematic total knee arthroplasties. Ten-year survivorship. J Bone Joint Surg Br 84: 667–672

2. Ansari S, Newman JH, Ackroyd CE (1997) St. Georg sledge for medial compartment knee replacement. 461 arthroplasties followed for 4 (1-17) years. Acta Orthop Scand 68: 430–434

3. Banks SA, Fregly BJ, Boniforti F, Reinschmidt C, Romagnoli S (2005) Comparing in vivo kinematics of unicondylar and bi-unicondylar knee replacements. Knee Surg Sports Traumatol Arthrosc 13: 551–556

4. Cartier P, Sanouiller JL, Grelsamer RP (1996) Unicompartmental knee arthroplasty surgery. 10-year minimum follow-up period. J Arthroplasty 11: 782–788

5. Deshmukh RV, Scott RD (2001) Unicompartmental knee arthroplasty: long-term results. Clin Orthop 392 272–278

6. Engh GA, McAuley JP (1999) Unicondylar arthroplasty: an option for high-demand patients with gonarthrosis. Instr Course Lect 48: 143–148

7. Fisher DA, Watts M, Davis KE (2003) Implant position in knee surgery: a comparison of minimally invasive, open unicompartmental, and total knee arthroplasty. J Arthroplasty 18: 2–8

8. Fuchs S, Rolauffs B, Plaumann T, Tibesku CO, Rosenbaum D (2005) Clinical and functional results after the rehabilitation period in minimally-invasive unicondylar knee arthroplasty patients. Knee Surg Sports Traumatol Arthrosc 13: 179–186

9. Heck DA, Marmor L, Gibson A, Rougraff BT (1993) Unicompartmental knee arthroplasty. A multicenter investigation with long-term follow-up evaluation. Clin Orthop 286: 154-159

10. Jenny JY, Boeri C (2003) Unicompartmental knee prosthesis implantation with a non-image-based navigation system: rationale, technique, case-control comparative study with a conventional instrumented implantation. Knee Surg Sports Traumatol Arthrosc 11: 40–45

11. Keene G, Simpson D, Kalairajah Y (2006) Limb alignment in computer-assisted minimally-invasive unicompartmental knee replacement. J Bone Joint Surg Br 88: 44–48

12. Kennedy WR, White RP (1987) Unicompartmental arthroplasty of the knee. Postoperative alignment and its influence on overall results. Clin Orthop 221: 278–285

13. Laskin RS (2001) Unicompartmental knee replacement: some unanswered questions. Clin Orthop 392: 267–271

14. Lootvoet L, Burton P, Himmer O, Pilot L, Ghosez JP (1997) A unicompartment knee prosthesis: the effect of the positioning of the tibial plate on the functional results. Acta Orthop Belg 63: 94–101

15. Repicci JA, Eberle RW (1999) Minimally invasive surgical technique for unicondylar knee arthroplasty. J South Orthop Assoc 8: 20–27

16. Riebel GD, Werner FW, Ayers DC, Bromka J, Murray DG (1995) Early failure of the femoral component in unicompartmental knee arthroplasty. J Arthroplasty 10: 615–621

17. Romanowski MR, Repicci JA (2002) Minimally invasive unicondylar arthroplasty: eight-year follow-up. J Knee Surg 15: 17–22

18. Stockelman RE, Pohl KP (1991) The long-term efficacy of unicompartmental arthroplasty of the knee. Clin Orthop 271: 88–95

19. Tabor OB, Jr., Tabor OB (1998) Unicompartmental arthroplasty: a long-term follow-up study. J Arthroplasty 13: 373–379

20. Tanavalee A, Choi YJ, Tria AJ (2005) Unicondylar knee arthroplasty: past and present. Orthopedics 28:1423–1425

21. Voss F, Sheinkop MB, Galante JO, Barden RM, Rosenberg AG (1995) Miller-Galante unicompartmental knee arthroplasty at 2- to 5-year follow-up evaluations. J Arthroplasty 10: 764–771

Hands-on Robotic Unicompartmental Knee Replacement

A Prospective Randomized Controlled Clinical Investigation of the Acrobot® System

J. Cobb

Introduction

A variety of different technologies have been exploited to improve reliability in orthopaedic surgery. Entirely passive guidance using camera based tracking alone has been extensively developed at one extreme [1, 2], while fully active robots have been developed at the other [3, 4]. Surgical camera-based navigation has been shown to reduce the number of outliers as defined by radiographic criteria, but improvement in outcome has been hard to document [5–8]. The fully active robots have also had problems [9, 10] preventing their acceptance in the wider community. In the Mechatronics in Medicine Laboratory, my colleague Professor Brian Davies has been leading a team developing robots for medical use for over 15 years. His 'Probot' was the first robotic device to operate upon a human being, performing semi-automated prostatectomy in 1991, before the clinical trials of robodoc in total hip replacement started. We developed the concept of an active constraint device from a notion of 'hands on robotics' to a fully fledged system in the course of the 1990s. We were sure that robotics were the only way to achieve serious accuracy, yet equally certain that an entirely active robot, that cut the surgeon out of the loop, was going to be hard to accept for most orthopaedic surgeons. Professor Davies' concept was that the surgeon should remain in control at all times, with the device merely 'holding the surgeons hand'. To achieve this aim, the device had to be fully back-drivable, yet be stiff enough to resist a surgeon's attempt to do the wrong thing. To achieve this aim needed two devices in series: a gross positioning device that was active, and could

be locked off, and a back-drivable device mounted on the end. Once the area of interest was approached, the gross positioner was locked off, and the active constraint device activated. The surgeon then held a force control handle. With a digitizing probe end, he was able to register using fiducial markers in early work, and anatomic registration in all human trials. After co-registration of the pre-operative plan with the patient's anatomy, the probe was exchanged for a series of cylinder and spherical cutters which were pushed by the surgeon but actively constrained by the device, within software constraints.

The initial devices were very large in order to obtain the stiffness needed, while a later version, that underwent clinical trials in total knee arthroplasty, was more maneuverable, but the gross positioning device was not really stiff enough to withstand holding an active constraint head on the end of it, and the forces that were applied to the head. The most recent evolution was a better compromise, with a very stiff gross positioning device, and a lighter 5 axis active constraint head.

While developing technology is a fairly full time activity, finding the right avenue for its exploitation is another. There is no point in developing a technology for an operation that is widely held to be very successful already, with a large and skilled workforce performing the procedure without assistance and little reported error. We therefore concentrated upon the knee rather than the hip. Despite wanting to go straight for unicompartmental knee arthroplasty, it was felt that any device should be pluri-potential, able to perform a total knee arthroplasty too, and so the early devices had to be able to remove large volumes of bone in several planes, to enable the bone ends to be machined precisely. The penalty of the time it takes a milling tool to remove large quantities of bone was a major barrier to further development, so the next device was developed with the specific aim of performing unicompartmental arthroplasties. While there is a significant revision rate for total knee replacement, there is a rather higher one for unicompartmental knee arthroplasty (UKA) [11]. This area of unicompartmental knee arthroplasty had some significant attractions, as the high failure rate was attributed to surgeon skill, while as a minimally invasive procedure, that only needed to resect very small amounts of bone, meant that it was well suited to a semi-robotic application [11–15]. We therefore hoped to be able to show that surgeons could be helped in a demanding technical field.

Another of the problems for computer-assistance devices has been the reporting of their impact: a sufficiently sensitive measure of implant position is required to detect how accurately the implant has been positioned. Plane radiographs have been used to evaluate the position of components, but the use of computerized tomography greatly enhances the ability of the investigator to measure this [16]. The risk of a type-II error, of failing to detect a difference in accuracy by using an insufficiently accurate metric can be overcome by the use of pre- and post-operative CT. The dose of radiation, and the cost of the scans are both issues that have prevented this technology from being adopted widely thus far. The comparison of angles between radiographs and CT scanograms has been made [17], and there is no systematic error between the two technologies, simply less accuracy is obtainable by plain radiography, if position in three dimensional space is being sought.

The primary variable used in any clinical trial is still contentious. In the knee, clinical scores, while extensively validated, are confounded by the variability between patients, and do not directly measure surgical accuracy. A knee replacement may be inserted inaccurately in a number of ways, each of which will influence function adversely, yet the ability of the patient to recover from surgery is hugely variable, and in the short term may confound any measurements which may simply report how resilient a patient is.

The hard end point of varus valgus alignment is the variable that is reported most extensively as both measurable and significant. Knees that are left in too much varus, or thrust into too much valgus will be more likely to fail early [18, 19]. This angle can be measured with plain X-rays, so has been fairly extensively validated. There have not been many other series reported where any other variables have been reliably measured and found significant. This is most probably because it is excessively difficult to measure accurately angles in the other 3 axes, and translation in any of the 3 axes are also hard to quantify with plane radiographs.

We therefore undertook a prospective, randomized, double blind (patient and evaluator), controlled trial of minimally invasive unicompartmental knee arthroplasty using a novel hands-on robotic assistant, the Acrobot® System.

Patients, Materials and Methods

Recruitment

After satisfactory piloting of the device in a small number of cases, 31 patients already on the waiting list for medial Unicompartmental Knee Replacement (UKA), and who fulfilled the entry criteria (inclusion and exclusion), were invited to participate in the study.

All accepted the invitation to participate and were blinded as to the type of treatment. In 3 subjects, surgery was planned for both knees, in separate sessions, so the total number of knees studied was 34.

Patients continued to benefit from the standard medical care, during and after the study, in accordance with the usual practice. Randomization and post-operative assessment were performed blind by independent parties. The clinical investigation was approved by the Ethics Committee and the Medicines and Healthcare products Regulatory Agency (MHRA).

Inclusion and Exclusion Criteria

Male and female subjects, aged over 18 years, requiring UKA on and radiographic grounds, able to understand the study requirements, willing to participate in the study and to sign an informed consent form fulfilled the general inclusion criteria. Knee specific inclusion criteria were that the disease was limited to the medial compartment, that the acl was intact, that the varus deformity could correct fully in 10 degrees of flexion, and that there was at most a minor fixed flexion contracture. Stressed radiographs were not taken preoperatively by any of the contributing surgeons, in routine practice, so were not used in the study.

Patients were excluded from this trial principally if they had any factors that would jeopardize their completion of the trial. Two CT scans were needed, and an operation that was predicted to be significantly longer than normal. In addition, clamps were used that were still prototypes, and would be difficult in fat legs. Patients with a body mass index of 31 or more, conditions leading to osteoporosis or serious neurological conditions, women of childbearing age, and those with increased risk of DVT were therefore excluded from the trial.

Four subjects (total of 6 knees) were withdrawn from the study. In the first withdrawn subject, an intra-operative decision was made to switch from UKA to TKR (Total Knee Replacement). A second subject, already operated on one knee, perforated a duodenal ulcer in the post-operative period; whilst the patient was reviewed at six weeks as per protocol, he was not fit for the planned second operation. In three further subjects, the reason for withdrawal was the unavailability of the Acrobot® System. The system is large and complex having been developed for the purpose at Imperial College. A technical problem with some internal cabling meant that it was not available for a short period when 3 cases were booked. Postponing operations for any reason had considerable political implications at the time, so the 3 subjects despite being randomized to the robotic arm had to be re-allocated into the conventional surgery arm. As the 3 subjects were not treated per randomization scheme, this was considered a protocol violation, and the subjects were not included in the final analysis. All patients recruited are included, however, in the analysis of the safety data.

Data from all the 27 remaining subjects (corresponding to 28 knees, as one subject had UKA on both knees) were analyzed. Recruitment started in December 2003. The last patient was assessed in July 04. All 27 subjects performed the 6 and 18 weeks post-operative assessment.

Preoperative Planning

All patients had a pre-operative CT scan, lying supine. The affected leg was placed in a splint, with the foot pointing upwards. A bag of saline was placed lateral to the knee to correct some of the varus and avoid bone touching bone on the medial side which causes difficulty with segmentation. Slices were taken through the hips, knees and ankles. The scans were saved as DICOM files from which the bones were extracted using a semi-automated segmentation al-

gorithm [20]. The bone surfaces were then used to plan every case, with the surgeon choosing exactly where he wanted to position the components and which size fitted best for every case, whether robotic or conventional. The tibia was sized and positioned by the surgeon to recreate a joint line in keeping with the lateral compartment with a 4 mm bearing at least. All patients had a varus deformity that corrected fully clinically in 10 degrees of flexion, but in each case, the surgeon chose the orientation of the tibial cut, and the height of the joint line based on a match with the lateral compartment, and proximal tibia. This sometimes left the joint line in slight varus (◘ Fig. 37.1a). Each case was planned individually, by each surgeon, who chose to plan each case on its merits. Rotation of the component in relation to the shape of the proximal tibia, the position relative to the tibial tubercle and the ankle joint was selected by the surgeon at his discretion. The femoral component was positioned using the flexion facet of the condyle, which is relatively preserved in anteromedial arthritis [12]. The component was fitted to this curve in the sagittal plane by eye, having been aligned to the axis of the femur, and translated and rotated from that at the discretion of the surgeon to the most appropriate position on the condyle (◘ Fig. 37.1a). This is at variance with the designers instructions, where the soft tissue tension in both flexion and extension determines how much distal femur is resected. Our experience with the ct based planning in total knee arthroplasty led us to believe that leaving the centre of rotation of the femoral component where it was pre-operatively was safe in knees with fully correctable varus. Additional increments of 0.5 mm could be taken from the extension gap if needed at operation. The plans were then printed and brought to theatre on the day, for the surgeon to use as a visual aid.

Operative Procedure

The Acrobot® System is a novel hands-on robotic device for orthopaedic surgery. It is the latest prototype in a series that have been developed at Imperial College in the Mechatronics in Medicine Laboratory, and more recently by The Acrobot Company [20 a spin out from the Laboratory. It consists of a high speed cutter that is mounted on a robotic device. The robotic device actively prevents the surgeon from cutting bone away outside the area defined in the pre-operative plan, but servo-assists the surgeon when the drill is within the area of bone to be milled away (■ Fig. 37.2). One surgeon carried out the 13 robotic cases; 4 other surgeons joined him in carrying out the 15 conventional cases. After asking advice, the potential conflicts of interest of the author posed an issue that would have been difficult to overcome had he performed all the control operations too. All surgeons whose patients were entered into the trial were performing unicompartmental knee replacements regularly.

Study Hypothesis

The primary hypothesis was that the Acrobot® System would achieve more reliable angular alignment prostheses. and corresponding tibio-femoral alignment in the coronal plane than would conventional instrumentation. From our review of the literature, tibio-femoral angles measured and reported for conventional UKA use different cut-off points, with authors using 2°, 3°,5° and 10° as being the cut-off point between accurate and inaccurate, with the proportion achieving the degree of accuracy varying with the width of the margin of error, between 48% and 92% [19, 21–25].

We were confident that the system could be very accurate, but from our experience with previous devices and understanding of the limitations of the system and the ability to measure small differences we knew that we could reliably detect a change in alignment of 1°. We should thus be able to measure within 2° of the angle planned in >99.9% of UKA patients, versus a predicted percentage of 48% of cases achieving this close an alignment with conventional surgery from the studies reported above.

Method of Measurement

For the purpose of the study, we defined the angle of tibio-femoral alignment as the angle between the femoral axis and the tibial axis in the coronal plane. The angles (mechanical angle, tibial component angle, femoral component angle) and mechanical axes (of the femur and the tibia) were measured from CT scans.

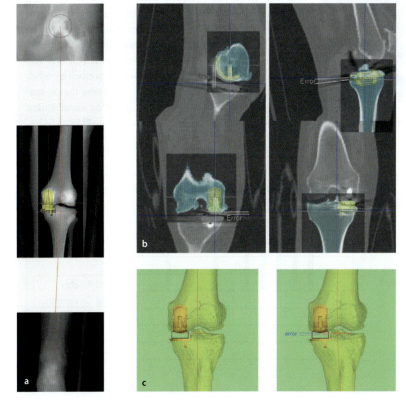

■ **Fig. 37.1. a** Planned positions of the components on CT; **b** co-registration of the planned and achieved positions for both components; **c** two close-up views of the joint illustrating the tibio-femoral angular error

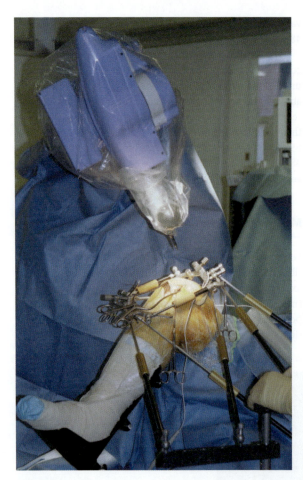

■ **Fig. 37.2.** Acrobot system in the operating theatre

Numbers were calculated for significance level α of 0.05 and a power of 80% (β=0.20), based on a two-sample test of proportions and a 2-sided test hypothesis using SPSS*. Yate's correction for continuity was applied. 26 completed subjects (13 per group) would be sufficient to detect a difference, in support of the hypothesis.

The primary outcome measure was the change in tibio-femoral angle, defined as the difference between the planned and achieved angles in the coronal plane. The measured values were transformed into dichotomous data (*i.e.* an angle of less than ±2° into 0; a difference greater than ± 2° into 1). These two groups were compared by Fisher's exact test.

To test this hypothesis, involving the confident measurement of angles and translations to less than a degree, a method had to be devised that was accurate enough. The post-operative CT scan, was co-registered with the pre-operative plan (■ Fig. 37.3) by a medical physicist who was blinded as to from which group the patient came. The resulting change in varus-valgus alignment was calculated from the proximal/distal translation error (achieved vs. planned), obtained in millimeters, for both the femoral and the tibial components. These measurements were transformed into angular values using the inverse tangent generated by the width of the joint and the translation error. This measurement was reproducible, based upon a software analysis of position. Every other variable was also measured but, since they have not been described by other authors, comparison is not possible. Following the co-registration, the bone was subtracted, allowing visualization of the two positions, planned and achieved (■ Fig. 37.4).

■ **Fig. 37.3.** Primary outcome measurement: difference in tibio-femoral alignment between planned and achieved in the coronal plane. Note that one of the Acrobot cases has a value of 0 degrees

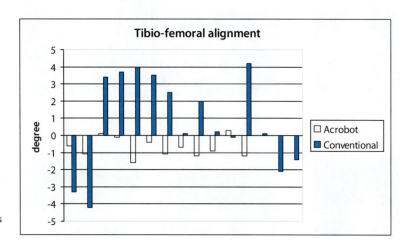

37

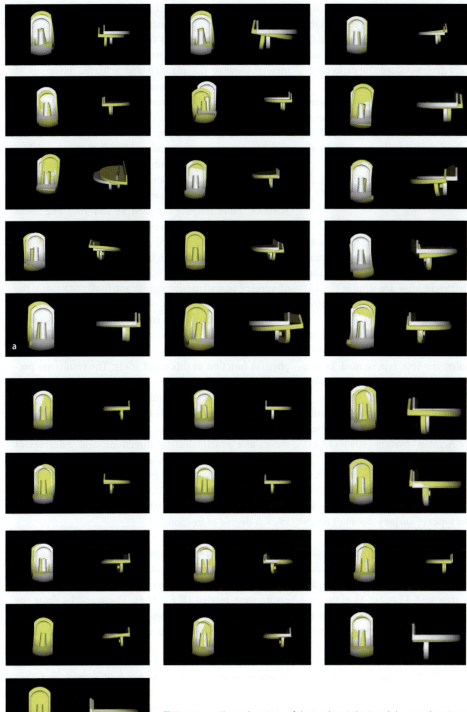

■ **Fig. 37.4. a** Planned position of the implant (*white*) and the actual position achieved (*yellow*) in the control group. **b** Planned position of the implant(*white*) and the actual position achieved (*yellow*) in the acrobot group

Secondary outcome parameters studied included the American Knee Society (AKS) Score [26] and Western Ontario and McMaster Universities Osteoarthritis (WOMAC) [27] index, pre-operatively and at 6 and 18 weeks, all adverse events and specifically device-related and procedure-related complications, and the operating times.

Differences in pre- and post-surgery AKS scores were compared by Mann-Whitney U test. WOMAC Scores were also analyzed by Mann-Whitney U test. Means are followed by the standard deviation in brackets in all cases.

Results

The two groups of patients (Acrobot® System vs. conventional surgery) are homogeneous for baseline characteristics. Male subjects are more common than female ones (15/12), frequencies of left/right knee are similar (13/15) and the mean age is 70.1 (5.6) years. The pre-operative AKS score is 101.4 (13.93).

With respect to the type of surgery, the conventional and Acrobot® groups have a mean age of 70.4 and 69.8 years, respectively, females are less represented in the Acrobot® System group (5/7) and left knees are more frequent in the conventional group (8/5).

Pre-operative Knee Society scores were higher in subjects who underwent conventional surgery with respect to those treated with the Acrobot® System [104.9 (13.43) vs 97.3 (13.90)].

Operating time (skin to skin) has a mean of 95 (18.1) minutes and it is higher in Acrobot® treated subjects (104 (16.6) vs. 88 (16.3) min). The difference in mean operating time between the two types of surgery does not reach significance.

The difference between the tibio-femoral angles planned and achieved were transformed into dichotomous data (angles ≤ ±2° or > ±2°) and a cross tabulation, angles vs. type of surgery, was performed. 13 out of 13 of the Acrobot® cases were implanted with tibio-femoral alignment in the coronal plane within 2° of the planned position [ranging between -1.6 and 0.3°, mean of −0.65°(0.59)], while of the conventionally performed cases, only 6 out of 15 [ranging between -4.2 and 4.2°, mean of -0.84°(2.75)] achieved this level of accuracy. Both Pearson chi-square and Fisher's exact test, (the latter more reliable than the former for this data distribution), were calculated and results are statistically significant (p=0.001). The primary

hypothesis (that the use of an active constraint robotic assistant improves prosthesis positioning in the coronal plane) is thus supported by this data.

This difference in accuracy is further illustrated by images showing the planned and achieved positions of the implants after the bones were superimposed upon one another and then subtracted (Fig. 37.4) by a blind assessor.

Differences between pre- and post-surgery AKS scores in the two groups were calculated for all 28 knees and data analyzed by the Mann-Whitney U test at 6 and 18 weeks. Values within subjects treated with conventional surgery show a wider dispersion, ranging from 3 to 83, with the Acrobot® cases ranging between 38 and 107; The mean increase in AKS score was twice as large in the Acrobot® System group [65.2 (18.36) versus 32.5(27.46)]; median values are more than three times higher in the Acrobot® System group (62 versus 19). The difference between type of surgery is statistically significant (p=0.004) using the non parametric test.

During the study, each subject's WOMAC scores were measured. There was no significant difference between the two groups in the three score for pain, stiffness and physical function in this small study. The results are presented in Table 37.1.

The deviations of alignment from the pre-operative plan were measured in all 6 degrees of freedom (3 degrees of translation, in the medial/lateral, anterior/posterior, and proximal/distal directions; and 3 degrees of rotation, in the varus/valgus, flexion/extension, and axial directions). The variations from the planned position are shown graphically (Fig. 37.5) They show that the acrobot assisted group have consistently more accurate results in each degree of freedom.

The translational and rotational errors have been combined to form measures of compound translational and rotational errors, for both femur and tibia [28]. Plots of improvements in AKS scores at 18 weeks versus these errors were plotted (Fig. 37.6). These graphs show the difference between the two groups with the Acrobot® group having higher scores and lower errors, with closer clustering of results.

During the course of the study, 4 'non serious' adverse events were registered: 3 in Acrobot® System and 1 in conventionally treated subjects. In no case did the adverse event lead to the subject's withdrawal. Details are reported in Table 37.2. Three serious adverse events occurred in 3 subjects: 1 in the Acrobot® subjects and 2 in conventionally

Table 37.1. WOMAC scores

	Change in Pain Score	Change in Stiffness Score	Change in Physical Function Score
Control			
Average	6	2	17
Median	7	3	18
Standard deviation	2	2	11
Acrobot			
Average	8	3	24
Median	8	3	23
Standard deviation	3	2	10

Table 37.2. Non serious adverse events

Type of surgery	Days after surgery	Event	Severity	Causality
Acrobot System	21	Swollen leg	Mild	Probably related to surgical procedure.
Acrobot System	4	Skin blister in peri-scar area	Mild	Certainly related to surgical procedure.
Acrobot System	21	Swollen ankle	Mild	Possibly related to surgical procedure and conditions of the patient.
Conventional	2	Bilateral swollen legs	Intermediate	Unlikely related to the condition of the patient (OA).

Table 37.3. Serious adverse events

Type of surgery	Days after surgery	Event	Severity	Relationship	Outcome
Acrobot System	1	Acute urinary retention	Intermediate	Possibly related to the conditions of the patient	Resolved with TURP
Conventional	1	Perforated peptic ulcer	Severe	Probably related to the conditions of the patient and the surgical procedure	Laparotomy
Conventional	9	Myocardial infarction	Intermediate	Possibly related to the conditions of the patient	Recovered well

treated subjects. Details are reported in Table 37.3. While all adverse events are likely to be procedure related, none was considered to be directly related to the study itself.

Discussion

In this prospective randomized controlled trial we confirmed that the risk of inaccuracy in arthroplasty can be reduced using an active constraint device. All (13 out of 13) of the Acrobot® cases achieved angles of tibio-femoral alignment on the coronal plane within the target zone of ±2°, while only 6 out of 15 cases performed conventionally were within this zone(p=0.001). The patients did have longer operations, but clinical outcome at this early stage does not show that they have suffered as a result.

Functional scores were used to measure clinical outcomes at six and 18 weeks post-operatively. There was a real concern before the trial that the extra 4 stab wounds in the skin, and the bone clamps introduced through them, together with the longer operating time would result in poorer function in the short term. Differences

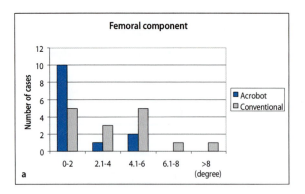

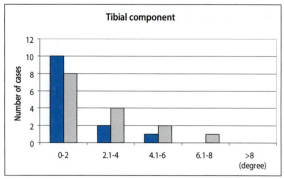

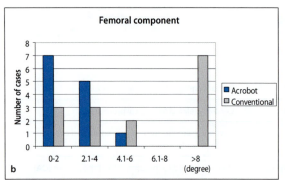

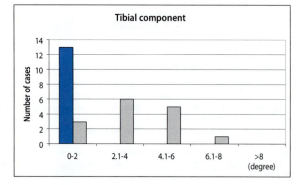

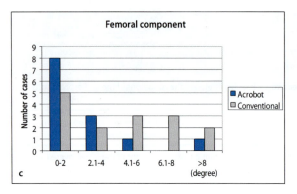

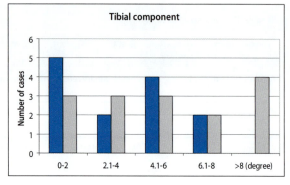

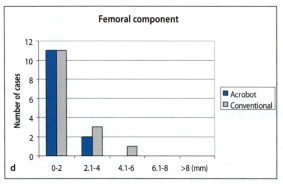

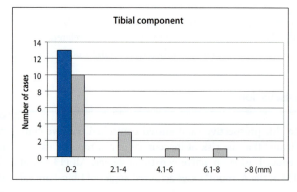

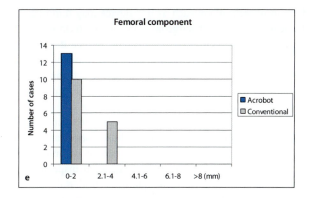

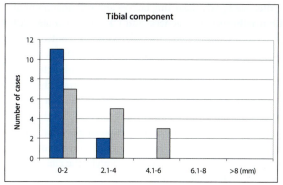

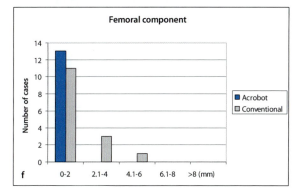

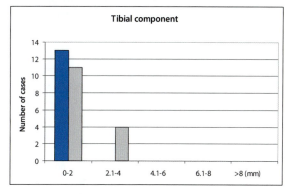

Fig. 37.5. a Absolute value of alignment error in the varus/valgus direction. Acrobot® cases range between 0.2 and 4.8° with a mean of 1.5 (1.4) versus 0.1, 9.8, and 3.4 (2.4). **b** Absolute value of alignment error in the flexion/extension direction. Acrobot® cases range between 0 and 4.1° with a mean of 1.39 (1.1) versus 0, 14, and 4.9 (3.4). **c** Absolute value of alignment error in the axial direction. Acrobot® cases range between 0.1 and 8.4° with a mean of 2.8 (2.5) versus 0.7, 13.1, and 5.1 (3.7). **d** Ab- solute value of alignment error in the medial/lateral direction. Acrobot® cases range between 0.1 and 2.3 mm with a mean of 0.8 (0.6) versus 0.1, 7, and 1.9 (1.7). **e** Absolute value of alignment error in the anterior/poste- rior direction. Acrobot® cases range between 0 and 2.8 mm with a mean of 0.9 (0.8) versus 0, 4.8, and 1.9 (1.5). **f** Absolute value of alignment error in the proximal/distal direction. Acrobot® cases range between 0 and 1.1 mm with a mean of 0.5 (0.3) versus 0, 4.3, and 1.2 (1.1)

between pre and post-surgery Knee Society scores were calculated for each subject and data analyzed by the Mann-Whitney U test. At 6 weeks post-op, while patients were still blinded as to which group they were in, the Acrobot® System patients had improved more than the control group; this difference is statistically significant (p=0.004). The WOMAC scores in this small study did not show a significant difference (p=0.06).

Operating time (skin to skin) was higher in Acrobot® treated subjects (104 (16.6) vs. 88 (16.3) minutes), but the difference between the two types of surgery fails to reach significance.

This study has a number of shortcomings. It uses a six and 18 week score from the American Knee Society as a clinical end point which, while repeatable, and blinded, has been shown to have inter and intra-observer errors that are substantial [29]. No long-term follow up is yet presented. The patients are being followed prospectively, although the assessment can no longer be blinded. The series is small, principally because the power calculation performed suggested that we could achieve significance quickly. For ethical and regulatory reasons, it was agreed that no more Acrobot® procedures than those strictly nec- essary would be performed until the device had met regu- latory approval. All of the Acrobot® cases were performed by the first author, while the control group were performed by four colleagues who were regularly performing UKAs. It was felt that this would minimize potential bias from an interested party. Learning curves are well documented within arthroplasty in general and UKA in particular. All the surgeons performing the UKAs in the control arm had undertaken more than 10 similar procedures previously, while the Acrobot® had been proven with extensive laboratory tests before the study to demonstrate that the system worked satisfactorily. The variations in short term clinical outcomes may be due to surgeon bias, but the correlation between accuracy and function implies that there is a real relationship here: if the joint line and orientation can be planned and reproduced accurately, the chances of a good clinical result are higher.

Joint replacement today remains an expensive process, in which experience remains at a premium. The intro-

duction of technology such as this device may diminish the learning curve of surgeons who are in training or acquiring a new technique. This should reduce the cost of arthroplasty, by increasing access, and reducing risk of error. The drive towards minimal access arthroplasty continues, fuelled by patient demand, and the pressure to reduce costs. Technology such as an active constraint robot may enable this process without the unacceptable risks of inaccuracy and its attendant clinical sequelae.

The use of CT scans in the assessment of implant accuracy has enabled a much more detailed inspection of the impact of surgical technique to be undertaken. It has also shown that each degree of freedom can now be measured.

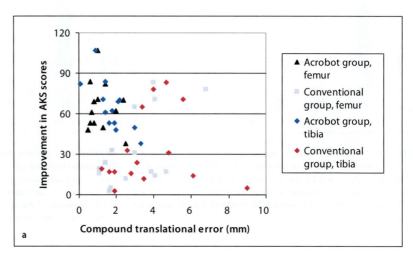

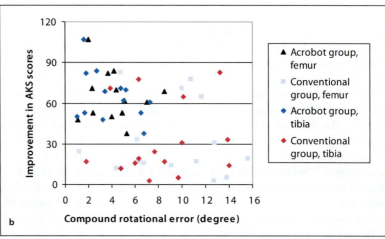

Fig. 37.6a, b. Difference between pre-operative and post-operative AKS scores against Compound rotational error

How Accurate Is Good Enough?

We still do not know how accurate the surgeon needs to be to obtain reliably good results: we simply set about trying to be as accurate as we could be. While the relationship between accuracy and outcome in arthroplasty has been suspected, it has been difficult to prove radiographically [29, 30]. Without a way of ensuring accuracy, there has been a reluctance on behalf of surgeons to address the issue: measuring the inaccuracy of an implantation is pointless unless there is something which can be done to prevent it. The post-operative CT scan protocol we have developed allows the precise position of any implant to be determined. It is our suggestion that this precision of post-operative measurement provides a more sensitive method of investigation of the joint following arthroplasty. A joint that is functioning poorly will frequently be shown to have some significant technical error, whether in angular positioning, translation, or sizing of component, or a combination of these.

The Future

The use of detailed pre-operative planning and an active constraint device will reduce the chances of a patient being exposed to the risk of poor function, and early joint failure. This prototype system has been shown to be both accurate and reliable. The widespread adoption of such technology however is far from certain, as it is costly, and time-consuming. The challenge facing all such technologies is to provide improved outcomes in the long term without huge costs in the short term. In the area of minimally invasive joint replacement there may be the opportunity for such exploitation. By permitting the creation of bone surfaces that can be sculpted into complex shapes, and by liberating the joint designers from the simple shapes made by an oscillating saw, materials that are not currently easily used may come into play. Robotic systems like the 'acrobot' thus pave the way for novel implant designs to be developed that may facilitate more truly bone conserving arthroplasty.

Acknowledgements. We would like to thank Messrs J. Patel, J. Youngman, A. Fazal, and N. Ashwood who planned and performed surgery in the conventional arm, and Sister Linda Stringer and the theatre staff in The Middlesex Hospital; Dr. Robin Richards in the Department of Medical Physics in UCL for help in the blinded post-operative assessment. We are grateful to Dr. Lucio Fumi, Wyfold Consultancy Ltd, for the guidance, monitoring and statistical analysis of the study.

The investigation was funded by The Acrobot Co Ltd, with support from the Sackler Institute for Musculoskeletal Research, UCL.

References

1. Stulberg SD, Loan P, Sarin V (2002) Computer-assisted navigation in total knee replacement: results of an initial experience in thirty-five patients. J Bone Joint Surg Am 84-A (Suppl 2): 90–88
2. Bathis H et al. (2004) Alignment in total knee arthroplasty. A comparison of computer-assisted surgery with the conventional technique. J Bone Joint Surg Br 86(5): 682–687
3. Siebert W et al. (2002) Technique and first clinical results of robot-assisted total knee replacement. Knee 9(3): 173–180
4. Bargar WL, Bauer A, Borner M (1998) Primary and revision total hip replacement using the Robodoc system. Clin Orthop 354: 82–91
5. Mielke RK et al. (2001) Navigation in knee endoprosthesis implantation--preliminary experiences and prospective comparative study with conventional implantation technique. Z Orthop Ihre Grenzgeb 139(2): 109–116
6. Jenny JY, Boeri C (2001) Computer-assisted implantation of total knee prostheses: a case-control comparative study with classical instrumentation. Comput Aided Surg 6(4): 217–220
7. Hart R et al. (2003) Total knee arthroplasty implanted with and without kinematic navigation. Int Orthop 27(6): 366–369
8. Clemens U, Miehlke RK (2003) Experience using the latest OrthoPilot TKA software: a comparative study. Surg Technol Int 11: 265–273
9. Nogler M et al. (2001) Contamination risk of the surgical team through ROBODOC's high-speed cutter. Clin Orthop 387: 225–231
10. Nogler M et al. (2001) Excessive heat generation during cutting of cement in the Robodoc hip-revision procedure. Acta Orthop Scand 72(6): 595–599
11. Knutson K et al. (1994) The Swedish knee arthroplasty register. A nation-wide study of 30,003 knees 1976–1992. Acta Orthop Scand 65(4): 375–386
12. Goodfellow JW et al. (1988) The Oxford Knee for unicompartmental osteoarthritis. The first 103 cases. J Bone Joint Surg Br 70(5): 692–701
13. Argenson JN, Chevrol-Benkeddache Y, Aubaniac JM (2002) Modern unicompartmental knee arthroplasty with cement: a three to ten-year follow-up study. J Bone Joint Surg Am 84-A(12): 2235–2239
14. Svard UC, Price AJ (2001) Oxford medial unicompartmental knee arthroplasty. A survival analysis of an independent series. J Bone Joint Surg Br 83(2): 191–194
15. Murray DW, Goodfellow JW, O'Connor JJ (1998) The Oxford medial unicompartmental arthroplasty: a ten-year survival study. J Bone Joint Surg Br 80(6): 983–989

16. Stockl B et al. (2004) Navigation improves accuracy of rotational alignment in total knee arthroplasty. Clin Orthop 426: 180–186

17. Jeffcote B, Shakespeare D (2003) Varus/valgus alignment of the tibial component in total knee arthroplasty. Knee 10(3): 243–247

18. Kennedy WR, White RP (1987) Unicompartmental arthroplasty of the knee. Postoperative alignment and its influence on overall results. Clin Orthop 221: 278–285

19. Hernigou P, Deschamps G (2004) Alignment influences wear in the knee after medial unicompartmental arthroplasty. Clin Orthop Relat Res 423: 161–165

20. Jakopec M et al. (2001) The first clinical application of a »hands-on« robotic knee surgery system. Comput Aided Surg 6(6): 329–339

21. Voss F et al. (1995) Miller-Galante unicompartmental knee arthroplasty at 2- to 5-year follow-up evaluations. J Arthroplasty 10(6): 764–771

22. Emerson RH Jr et al. (2002) Comparison of a mobile with a fixed-bearing unicompartmental knee implant. Clin Orthop 404: 62–70

23. Jenny JY, Boeri C (2003) Unicompartmental knee prosthesis implantation with a non-image-based navigation system: rationale, technique, case-control comparative study with a conventional instrumented implantation. Knee Surg Sports Traumatol Arthrosc 11(1): 40–45

24. Jenny JY, Boeri C (2002) Accuracy of implantation of a unicompartmental total knee arthroplasty with 2 different instrumentations: a case-controlled comparative study. J Arthroplasty 17(8): 1016–1020

25. Cartier P, Sanouiller JL, Grelsamer RP (1996) Unicompartmental knee arthroplasty surgery. 10-year minimum follow-up period. J Arthroplasty 11(7): 782–788

26. Insall JN et al. (2002) Correlation between condylar lift-off and femoral component alignment. Clin Orthop 403: 143–152

27. Babis GC et al. (2002) Double level osteotomy of the knee: a method to retain joint-line obliquity. Clinical results. J Bone Joint Surg Am 84-A(8): 1380–1388

28. Reuben JD et al. (1998) Cost comparison between bilateral simultaneous, staged, and unilateral total joint arthroplasty. J Arthroplasty 13(2): 172–179

29. Liow RY et al. (2000) The reliability of the American Knee Society Score. Acta Orthop Scand 71(6): 603–608

30. Lotke PA, Ecker ML (1977) Influence of positioning of prosthesis in total knee replacement. J Bone Joint Surg Am 59(1): 77–79

Navigated Unicompartmental Knee-Replacement – Genesis-Accuris-System

K. Buckup, L.-Chr. Linke

Introduction

Many studies have shown excellent long-term results for unicompartmental knee replacement [1, 2, 4, 17]. Survival times for both, unicompartmental and total knee replacements are similar. By preserving the cruciate ligaments in unicompartmental replacements, better proprioception and physiological kinematic outcome are shown compared to total knee replacements. The rate of postoperative infections and the total costs are also less [11, 25].

Various authors have shown that clinical results for unicompartmental knee replacements can be improved by using minimally invasive techniques. Price et al and Müller et al. have shown that there is no difference in technical implantation quality between the minimally invasive and the standard procedure [16, 20, 22, 23]. Müller reports equal quality of implant position in both groups, but also points out that in a great number of cases the implant position was not within the ideal range. In the meantime a number of publications reporting on navigation systems for knee replacements came out. The reporting of good postoperative results for total knee replacements implanted with computer-assisted navigation systems had encouraging effected on their use for minimally invasive implanted unicompartmental systems [15, 19, 27]. Jenny et al. reported better technical results for the implantation of unicompartmental knee replacements when using computer assisted navigation in comparison to conventional techniques [10]. In a prospective study on minimally invasive implanted unicompartmental knee replacements, Perlick et al. could show improved position of the axis for those protheses implanted with computer assisted navigation [19].

Patients and Methods

A population of 38 patients was divided into two groups. The 23 patients allocated to group 1 underwent a minimally invasive procedure. The remaining 15 patients of group 2 also had minimally invasive treatment plus computer-assisted navigation during the procedure. Patients of group one had surgery between June 2003 and July 2004, patients of group two between February 2005 and November 2005.

Details of all patients are listed in ▣ Table 38.1.

▣ **Table 38.1.** Details of the two groups of patients

	Gr. 1 Conventional	Gr. 2 Navigated
Male/female	15/8	7/8
Mean age in years Range	69,6 (54–85)	72,1 (52–86)
Primary osteoarthritis	21	14
asept. Osteonecrosis – Ahlbäck's disease	2	1
Tibial implant full polyethylene/metal backed	16/7	11/4

Indications for Surgery

21 patients of group 1 had primary osteoarthrosis and in 2 Ahlbäcks disease was diagnosed. In group 2 14 patients presented with primary osteoarthritis and 1 patient had osteonecrosis of the medial femoral condyle.

Pre-operative Management

Anamnesis including assessment potential relevant systemic diseases. (I.e. PAVK, diabetes, neurological condition). Assessment of joint mobility and stability.

Radiological Investigations

Anterior/posterior and lateral views of the knee joint with the patient standing and fully weight-bearing (pre-operative – standing, post-operative – lying down).

Anterior/posterior views of the knee joint in 25° flexion with the patient standing and fully weight-bearing. These views show »true« defects of the cartilage reflected by the degree of reduction of joint space. Despite Rosenberg et al. who were asking for a flexion of 45°, an angle of 25°–30° seems to be sufficient in order to assess the degree of arthrosis [26]. For many elderly people, higher degrees of flexion are not acceptable due to pain and instability.

Tangential views of the femuro-patellar joint in 30° and 60° of flexion in order to assess possible femuro-patellar arthrosis and alignment of the kneecap. Anterior/posterior leg views with the patient standing to assess to the leg axis and possible varus-deformity.

Pre- and post-operative frontal and sagittal of the knee and whole leg views to assess the leg axis were performed [6].

Methods

We operated with the specific set of instruments for minimal invasive implantation for Accuris unicompartmental knee replacement in onlay technique (Smith & Nephew GmbH, Osterbroogksweg 71, 22869 Schenefeld, Germany).

This was combined with the Brain LAB Vector-vision uni-knee system by Brain LAB (Brain LAB AG, Ammerthalstr. 8, 85551 Heimstetten, Germany).

The Vector-Vision uni-knee uses a 3D statistical model of the knee joint based on arthritic knee joints of several patients worldwide, which are integrated into a CT database. A 7–9 cm skin incision was made from the superior medial edge of the patella and extended distally. After arthrotomy marginal osteophytes were resected from the medial femoral condyle and the medial femoral trochlear groove. The medial meniscus was resected and large tibial osteophytes were removed. This allowed passive correction of the knee joint's varus deformity preserving normal tension of the medial collateral ligament. Two reference arrays with passive marker spheres are rigidly attached to both the femoral and tibial bone through skin incisions (◘ Fig. 38.1). Specific anatomic landmarks (i.e. insertion point of the anterior cruciate ligament, borders of the medial plateau and the medial and lateral malleolus) were determined at the beginning of the operation. The center of the hip joint was determined by a pivoting algorithm. Additional surface information was gained by sliding a pointer across the medial tibial plateau and the medial femoral condyle.

Based on the obtained data, the system created an adapted bone model of the patient's anatomy specific and offered a planning proposal for component orientation (◘ Fig. 38.2). The images were shown in two-dimensional axial, coronal and sagittal views. Prior to the first bone resection, the surgeon was informed about the expected leg axis (◘ Fig. 38.3). The laxity of ligament could be monitored throughout the entire range of motion. Furthermore, the system provided a kinematics analysis.

After successful registration of the patient with the pointer tool, a 2 mm shim was introduced into the joint gap to tighten the ligaments. The Accuris minimally invasive unicompartmental knee system is unique in the respect of achieving ligamentous balancing before osteotomies are made. Once the joint had been balanced with the joint balancing shims, all osteotomies were then referenced off the shim. This allowed accurate tibio-femoral resections. All the resections were made with a cutting block. The leg's position was digitalized in flexion and extension. Using this information, the navigation system was able to automatically calculate size and position of the implant. Prior to fixation of the tibio-femoral cutting block under navigation the pre-operative mechanical data regarding axis and slope had to be reconsidered. In the frontal plane, the line of resection of the medial tibial plateau is not always perpendicular to the mechanical axis (line A) [5, 13, 14, 18] (◘ Fig. 38.4).

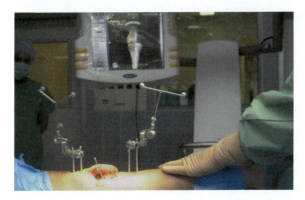

Fig. 38.1. The Vector Vision Uni-Knee System by BrainLab with the attached reference arrays. The skin incision was made and the joint had been balanced with the joint balancing shim.

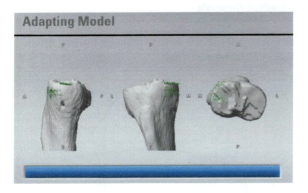

Fig. 38.2. Adapting registration 3D model (tibia). The position of the implant will be based on the acquired points and not on the model.

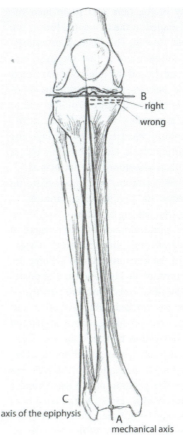

Fig. 38.4. The correct line of resection of the medial plateau. **A** Mechanical axis. **B** Joint line. **C** Epiphyseal axis

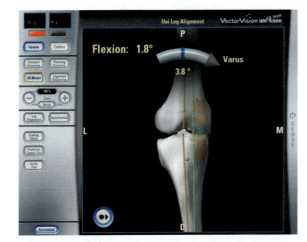

Fig. 38.3. Leg-alignment screen

The angle depends on the degree of varus-deformity of the tibial head. The tibial implant has to be concordant with the line of the lateral tibial plateau (line B). In presence of a tibia vara or degenerative varus deformity of the medial tibial plateau, the tibial osteotomy is not to be performed perpendicular to the tibial plateau, but right-angled to the axis of the epiphysis (line C). According to Cartier, the angles were measured with the patient standing. Deviations of the line of resection from the perpendicular line of the mechanical tibial axis should not be greater than 4°.

A = Mechanical axis of the tibia (centre of tibial plateau – centre of ankle joint)

B = Line parallel to lateral tibial plateau

C = Perpendicular line to line B (plane of resection)

The sagittal osteotomy of the tibia was performed diagonally and not right-angled to the tangential line at the dorsal aspect of the tibial plateau. The diagonal osteotomy had to be performed in such a way that impingement between the femoral condyle and the intercondylar notch was avoided. Trying to perverse the insertion point of the ACL, the beginning of the sagittal osteotomy was to be located as centrally as possible. In 110° of flexion the posterior femoral osteotomy was performed through the superior slot or the cutting block. Using the same block, the lower and sagittal tibial osteotomy was performed.

The slope of the tibial osteotomy had to be according to the anatomical situation and preoperative planning.

After the planning, the cutting block was positioned and fixed on the bone with guidance by the navigation system (Fig. 38.5). Performing the next step, navigation was used to flex in the knee in order to achieve the planned posterior cut position at 110 degrees. The posterior femoral cut and the tibial resection were performed (Fig. 38.6). The tibia was verified with navigation and after femoral reaming, trial prostheses were implanted under control of the navigation to check the leg alignment. By using the navigation system, position, function and stability of the implants in relation to the axis was monitored for any possible position of the leg. The size of the implant was chosen with respect to the tension of the ligaments. At flexion of 15–20° the medial joint-space should open under stress by 1–2 mm. With correctly position trial implants the femoral drill was reattached and wholes for the spikes of the femoral implant were drilled. To achieved rotational stability a cut is made through the femoral component. If an al-poly-onlay tibial component was used, further preparation of bone was not performed. When using metal backed tibial implants, a slot is made between the open space at the base of the tibial trial implant and the vertical osteotomy.

All implant were cemented. The cementing technique for anchoring the components of prothesis is particulary important because of the small weight-bearing surface area for the implant. In case the bone is sclerotic either on the tibial or the femoral side a number of 3.2 mm whole are drilled down to the subchondral bone-layers in order to achieve better anchoring of the cement. The bone has to be dry and free of tissue and blood (jet lavage) before implantation.

Statistical Analysis

The Kolmogrof test was used. Criteria for t testing with a p value of 0.05 were also met.

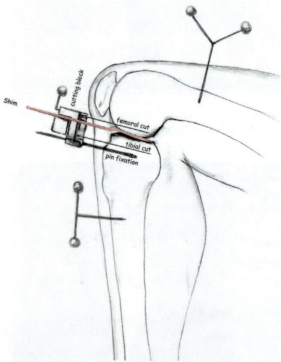

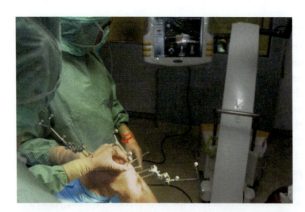

Fig. 38.5. The femoral and tibial cutting block adapter is used to navigate the tibio-femoral cutting block to the planned resection plane (*arrow*)

Fig. 38.6. The tibio-femoral cutting block is pushed over the shim. Before making the femoral and tibial saw cuts a slope adapter and the femoral and tibial cutting block adapter is placed on the cutting block

38

Results

Mechanical Leg Axis

In both groups the mechanical axis of the leg had improved significantly after operation. The improvement in the group having the standard procedure varied from 5.23°–0.77° with a mean value of 4.46° and a standard deviation of 1.62°.

In the computer-assisted group these value were 4.18°–0.54°, 3.64° and 2.03°, respectively.

No statistical difference could be shown between the two groups.

Frontal Plane Alignment

In group 1 the pre-operative angle of the implant in relation to the longitudinal axis of the tibia was 88.84° on average (SD: 2.81°, variation 85°–99°). Post-operatively it was 86.91° (SA = 2.52° Range 82.0–92°).

In group 2 the average pre-operative angle was 87.13° with an SD of 1.82° and a variation of 83.0–89.0°). Post-operatively this angle measured 87.13° on average (SA 1.82 Range 83.0–89.0°)

Sagittal Plane Alignment (Slope)

In group 1 the average slope was measured as 6.17° (SD: 1.97°, variation 2°–10°) pre-operatively and 5.09° (SD: 3.25°, variation 0°–12°) post-operatively. In group 2 the pre-operative angle was 6.90° on average (SD: 3.09°, variation 1.0°–12.9°) and the post-operative one was 6.38° (SD: 2.63, variation 1–10.9°).

Discussion

In the meantime, results from various studies on minimally invasive implantation of unicompartmental knee replacements have been published [7, 16, 20, 22, 23, 25].

Repicci followed up 136 cases with minimally invasive implanted unicompartmental knee replacements for 8 years. 7% of those had to be revised and in 3 of the revised cases revision was necessary due to technical error.

Price and al. prospectively compared the minimally invasive operation technique (short medial skin incision without dislocation of the patella) for unicompartmental knee replacement with the standard procedure (»long« access, standard arthrotomy with dislocation of the patella) used in unicompartmental knee replacements and total knee replacements [15]. Rehabilitation in respect to walking stairs, straight-leg elevation and achieving 70% of knee flexion took half the time in the »minimally invasive operated and unicompartmental group« in »comparison to the standard procedure and unicompartmental group« and on third in the »minimally invasive operated and unicompartmental group« in »comparison to the standard procedure and total knee replacement group«. Post-operative x-rays did not show any difference between the two groups regarding the correct implant position.

Müller et al. post-operatively compared 35 patients who had minimally invasive surgery with 38 patients who had received an Oxford-knee replacement in standard technique [12]. Each group had surgery in a different hospital. Functional outcome in the »minimally invasive group« was better. Patients of this group had a post-operative HSS score of 92 on average. The average score for those who had the standard procedure done was 78 points. Knee flexion was almost equal in both groups: post-operatively 113° in the minimally invasive operated group and 107° in the group with the standard technique.

In our population of 26 patients who had 28 Accuris unicompartmental knee replacement implanted, the HSS score was 87.4 and flexion was 123° on average. On follow-up appointments, 78.8% of patients rated the outcome as being excellent and 22.2% as good [3].

The implant position and the achieved axis are the main parameters responsible for long-term results. An extensive tissue release must not be performed, since this can result in overcorrection. After correction of pre-operative deformities they still should be slightly recognizable on post-operative radiological assessment. It should be aimed at an undercorrection of 1°–2° depending on ligamental tension. Mahlfeld, Thermann and Wirtz recommend moderate to physiological correction of the axis depending on the anatomical and pathological situation [12]. Eventually, it is only possible to stress the medial ligamental structure as far as their original length allows. The original length of the medial collateral ligament can be assessed after resection of exophytes situated at the tibial and femoral margin of the joint. Additionally, lateral ligamental laxity has to be considered when bringing the trail plateaus. Differentiation between medial ligamental laxity due to ipsilateral gonarthrosis and due to increased contralateral ligamental tension is difficult. Stress X-rays are a good option to assess and interpret ligamental structures.

Extensive overcorrection with valgus deformity can lead to subluxation of the tibio-femoral compartment, to intense tension of the ligamental structures, medial instability and increased lateral pressure followed by potentially early secondary degeneration of the lateral compartment. False implantation led to early failure. The external calibration systems of many unicompartmental knee-replacements systems do not always offer the chance of exact positioning. Rates of incorrect implantation of more than 30% are reported for conventional surgical techniques. Minimally invasive implantation includes the risk of false implantation due to limited visibility resulting in possibly false calibration of the axis. Fischer et al. compared unicompartmental knee replacement implanted with the minimally invasive technique and under standard procedure [8]. They found a great variation of the position of the axis for minimally invasive operated cases and also a significant number of mal-positions of the tibial and femoral implant. On the other hand, Price and Müller could not show any significant difference in technical outcome when comparing the two techniques. Müller describes identical quality of implantation for both groups, but also mentions that in both groups he found a great number of implants positioned outside the ideal range [16]. Jenny et al. report significantly higher number of correctly implanted prostheses in all planes when using the Orthopilot systems [10]. In 60% of the replacements implanted with computer-assisted navigation, the position of the axis was sufficient and only in 20% of the case implanted conventionally this was the case. Regarding the femuro-tibial angle Jenny reports a range of 5° varus to 4° valgus when using computer-assisted navigation and 10° varus to 10° valgus for the conventional technique.

Perlick et al. found a varus axis of 2° in 95% in patients operated on with minimally invasive technique and varus axes of 0°–4° in 70% for »conventional« cases [19].

Comparison of Pre-operative and Post-operative Results

The leg axis improved significantly in both groups. On average the leg axis was improved by 5.23°–0.77° = 4.46° in group 1 and 4.18°–0.54° = 3.64° in group 2. The difference between the two groups is non-significant.

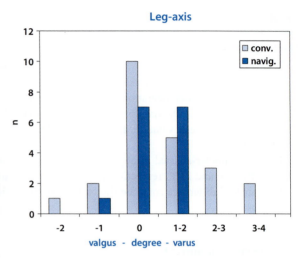

■ Fig. 38.7. Distribution of achieved leg axes between the two groups

To sum up it may be said, that computer-assisted navigation provides a better chance to reach position »0« (range of deviation -1.0° to +1.9°) compared to the conventional technique (range of deviation –2.0° to +4.0°) (**■** Fig. 38.7).

According to our findings and to studies by Jenny as well as Perlick, the use of computer-assisted navigation and minimally invasive techniques for implantation of unicompartmental knee replacements allows more precise positioning and axis calibration [10, 19]. We found that there is no statistical difference to conventionally implanted replacements. The computer-assisted navigation offers better visualization when calibrating the axis. It can help to avoid overcorrection especially. Therefore, the navigation system seems to be an additional feature to help to improve implantation techniques and long-term results.

References

1. Berger RA et al. (1999) Unicompartmental knee arthroplasty. Clin Orthop 367: 50–60
2. Buckup K (2005) Langzeitergebnisse lateraler Schlittenprothesen. In: Buckup K (Hrsg) Die unikondyläre Schlittenprothese Pro & Contra. Steinkopff, Darmstadt
3. Buckup K (2006) Die minimalinvasive Implantation eines unikondylären Kniesystems. Minimally Invasive Implantation of a Unicondylar Knee System. Operat Orthop Traumatolog 2: 135–152
4. Cartier P et al. (1996) Unicompartmental knee arthroplasty surgery, 10-year minimum follow-up period. J Arthroplasty 11: 782–788

5. Chao EYS et al. (1994) Biomechanics of malalignment. Orthop Clin North Am 25: 379–393

6. Cooke, TDV et al. (1987) The use of standardized radiographs to identity the deformities associated with osteoarthritis. In: Noble J, Galasko CSB (eds) Recent developments in orthopedic Surgery. Manchester University Press, Manchester

7. Endres S et al. (2005) Minimalinvasiv implantierte unikondyläre Knieendoprothese Typ Stryker-Osteonics mit metal-backed Tibia-komponente. Ein 5-Jahres-Follow-up. Z Orthop 143: 573–580

8. Fisher DA et al. (2003) Implant position in knee surgery: a comparison of minimally invasive, open unicompartmental, and total knee arthroplasty. J Arthroplasty 18: 2–8

9. Jenny JY et al. (2003) Accuracy of implantation of a unicompartmental total knee arthroplasty with 2 different Instrumentations: a case-controlled comparative study. J Arthroplasty 17: 1016–1020

10. Jenny JY et al. (2003) Unicompartmental knee prosthesis implantation with a non-image-based navigation system: rationale, technique, case-control comparative study with a conventional instrumented implantation. Knee Surg Sports Traumatol Arthrose 11: 40–45

11. Kißlinger E et al. (1998) Infektionsraten bei Knie-Endoprothesen unterschiedlicher Größe – Vorteile der unicompartment-Schlittenprothese (1977–1996). In: Rabenseifer L (Hrsg) Knieendoprothetik. Steinkopff, Darmstadt

12. Mahlfeld K, Thermann H, Wirtz DC (2005) Statements. In: Buckup K (Hrsg) Die unicondyläre Schlittenprothese Pro & Contra. Steinkopff, Darmstadt

13. McLeod WD et al. (1977) Tibial plateau topography. Am J Sports Med 5: 13–18

14. Mikulicz J (1878) Ueber individuelle Formdifferenzen am Femur und an der Tibia des Menschen. Archiv f A u Ph, Anat Abteilg 1: 351–404

15. Mielke RK et al. (2001) Navigation in knee endoprosthesis implantation-preliminary experiences and prospective comparative study with conventional implantation technique. Z Orthop Ihre Grenzgeb 139: 109–116

16. Müller PE et al. (2004) Influence of minimally invasive surgery on Implant Positioning and the functional outcome for medial unicompartmental knee arthroplasty. J Arthroplasty 2004; 19: 296–301

17. Murray DW et al. (1998) The Oxford medial unicompartmental arthroplasty, a ten year survival study. J Bone Joint Surg Br 1998; 80: 983–989

18. Paley D et al. (1994) Deformity planning for frontal and sagittal plane corrective osteotomies. Orthop Clin North Am 25: 425–465

19. Perlick L et al. (2004) Minimally invasive unicompartmental knee replacement with a nonimage-based navigation system. Intern. Orthopaedics 28; 4: 193–197

20. Price AJ et al. (2001) Rapid recovery after Oxford unicompartmental arthroplasty through a short incision. J Arthroplasty 16: 970–976

21. Sparmann M et al. (2003) Positioning of total knee arthroplasty with and without navigation support. A prospective randomised study. J Bone Joint Surg Br 85: 830–835

22. Repicci JA et al. (1999) Minimally invasive surgical technique for unicondylar knee arthroplasty. J South Orthop Assoc 8: 20–27

23. Repicci JA et al. (2004) Minimally invasive unicondylar knee arthroplasty for the treatment of unicompartmental osteoarthritis: an outpatient arthritic bypass procedure. Orthop Clin N Am 35:201–216

24. Robertson O et al. (1999) Use of unicompartmental instead of tricompartmental prostheses for unicompartmental arthrosis in the knee is a cost-effective alternativ. Orthop Scand 70: 170–175

25. Romanowski MR et al. (2002) Minimally invasive unicondylar arthroplasty. Eight year follow-up. J Knee Surg; 15: 17–22

26. Rosenberg TD et al. (1988) The forty-five-degree posterior-anterior flexion weight-bearing radiograph of the knee. J Bone Joint Surg Am 1988; 70: 1479–1483

27. Windhagen H (2005) Das Navigationskonzept. Prozessoptimierung in der navigierten Knieendoprothetik. Orthopäde 35: 1125–1130

Part III   Anterior-Cruciate Ligament Reconstruction

Image-Free Navigation in ACL Replacement with the OrthoPilot System

H.-J. Eichhorn

Introduction

In many areas of surgery, ever smaller approaches are being sought to reduce soft tissue traumatisation in minimally invasive operating techniques. This is associated with the danger that the surgeon will lose an overview of the topography of the structures as a whole. Computer-assisted navigation promises to remedy this. Computer-assisted surgery began in the 1990s with intracranial neurosurgical operations and the implantation of pedicle screws in spinal surgery, using CT and MRI imaging. Today however, there are other solutions which do not require pre- and intra-operative X-rays. One of these solutions is offered by the OrthoPilot navigation system (◘ Fig. 39.1). One problem in cruciate ligament surgery has arisen because, whilst it is certainly true that the number of cruciate ligament operations has substantially increased, there has at the same time been an over proportional rise in the number of surgeons performing these operations. In fact, approximately 85% of cruciate ligament operations are conducted by surgeons or orthopaedic surgeons who perform fewer than 10 cases a year, and who can thus gather relatively little experience. Responsible government departments and insurance companies are therefore now thinking out loud about establishing process and quality controls similar to those which exist for osteosynthesis. According to such a scheme, the operation may only be performed if the site of the tunnels, and therefore the site of the ACL replacement, is documented. Monitoring the tunnel site with an image converter is now being recommended at the various cruciate ligament congresses. However, there are problems associated with image converter monitoring: the patients are exposed to a not inconsiderable dose of radiation, and the position of the image converter must be altered several times in order to obtain an image in two planes.

The main problem in cruciate ligament surgery is correct tunnel placement. Computer-assisted navigation can represent a solution to this problem, as it can determine and document the tunnel site without CT scans or intra-operative X-rays. For this reason, software was developed for OrthoPilot to allow the optimum tunnel sites to be defined by navigation.

Methods

The objectives for the OrthoPilot system are as follows:
- the additional operation time caused by navigation should be reduced to a minimum (max. 10–15 min);
- intra-operative X-raying of the patient should be avoided;
- the extremely time-consuming, CT- or MRI-based pre-operative planning required by other navigation systems should not be necessary;
- fixation of sensors (rigid bodies) to record the anatomical landmarks in the knee and the knee kinematics should only be associated with minimal traumatisation for the patient;
- the entire system should be so user friendly that it can be operated by surgeons and theatre nurses without any problems.

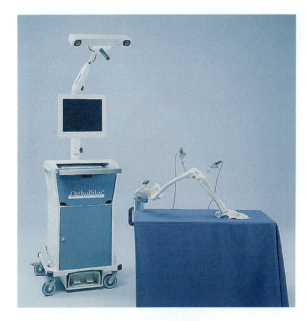

◻ **Fig. 39.1.** Setting- up the OrthoPilot system

Criteria for Tunnel Placement

The ACL navigation software contains the experiences and opinions of experts drawn from a great many publications in anatomical and surgical orthopaedics.

Criteria for anatomical placement of the tibial tunnel: The tibial exit point on the tibial plateau should satisfy the following criteria:

- 7 mm distance from the anterior margin of the posterior cruciate ligament with the knee joint in approx. 80° flexion,
- center between the anterior horn of the lateral meniscus and the spine of the medial tibial tubercle,
- 44% of the coronary width of the tibial plateau beginning from the most medial position.

If the navigation is being used for a double tunnel technique, only the antero-medial bundle is navigated. In this case the distance from the posterior cruciate ligament changes to 9 mm.

For tibial tunnel placement it is also important to project the silhouette of the femoral intercondylar fossa in extension onto the tibial surface, in order to show any possible impingement situation here.

If the intercondylar fossa overlaps the navigated, anatomically optimum target circle partially or completely, the surgeon has the alternative of either moving the tibial tunnel site in a dorsal direction or of performing a suitable notch plasty to avoid impingement.

Criteria for anatomical placement of the femoral tunnel: The femoral entry point in the notch should satisfy the following criteria:

- 3–5 mm distance from the posterior margin of the fossa,
- Placement of tunnel in
  - left knee: 12.30–01.30 o'clock position,
  - right knee: 10.30–11.30 o'clock position.

The main mistakes in planning the femoral tunnel occur through a placement which is too high (towards a 12 o'clock position) and/or too ventral. OrthoPilot shows a section between 10.30–11.30 o'clock for the right knee and 12.30–01.30 o'clock for the left knee during navigation. This is particularly important, since even slight distortion of the camera horizon can lead to a false interpretation of the fossa topography.

As the posterior margin of the fossa is palpated and recorded in the computer, OrthoPilot permanently displays the relation between the tip of the femoral pointer and the posterior outlet of the fossa. From this the surgeon can determine the distance according to the operating technique used.

Since OrthoPilot also records the kinematic data of the knee joint, the isometric relation between both selected target points (tibial exit point/femoral entry point) is given as useful additional information. Furthermore, an impingement check is conducted and recorded depending on the thickness of the graft across the entire flexion range of the knee up to extension.

Performing the Computer-Assisted, Image-Free Cruciate Ligament Operation

Preparing the Navigation

Firstly, the OrthoPilot is positioned next to the arthroscopy tower on the opposite side from the surgeon. Care must be taken to ensure that neither the arthroscopy tower nor any other instrumentation or people are standing in the camera's observation field. The ideal distance of the camera from the knee is 2 m ± 20 cm. The leg should be placed in a leg support.

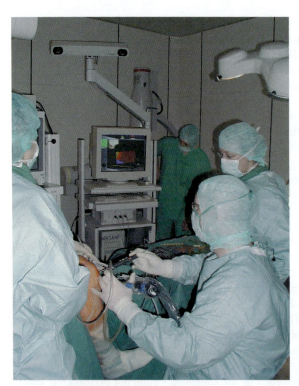

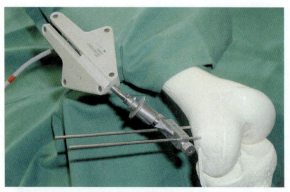

Fig. 39.3. Femoral rigid body fixation

Fig. 39.2. Position of OrthoPilot during a cruciate ligament reconstruction

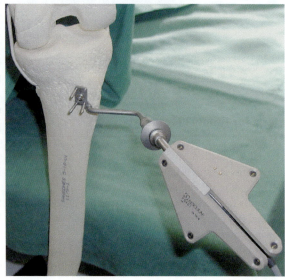

After the leg has been washed and draped in a leg holder and the arthroscopy equipment has been made ready, arthroscopic joint revision is first performed. It is important to rectify any additional damage to the cartilage surfaces and the menisci before the rigid bodies are attached. If an obviously very narrow notch is found to exist before a secondary stabilization procedure, a notch plasty should already be performed at this point. The rigid bodies should only be fixed into position when these operation steps have been completed (**Fig. 39.2**).

Fig. 39.4. Tibial rigid body fixation

Fixing the Rigid Bodies in Position

The peak of the medial epicondyle is palpated and a 2.5 mm Kirschner wire is inserted approx. 2 cm into the condyle. This site has been chosen because no nerves, vessels or sensitive capsule structures are injured with the knees in flexion. After the fixation has been put into

place a second Kirschner wire is set somewhat proximally through the fixation.

Screwing the fixation tight just above the skin gives the Kirschner wires an overhang, which guarantees that the femoral rigid bodies are firmly fixed into position (**Fig. 39.3**).

The fixation on the tibia close to the tuberosity or as an alternative approx. 10 cm distal from the tendon har-

39

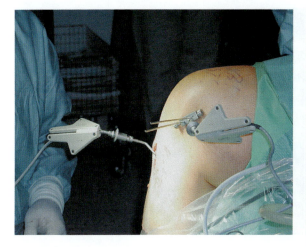

■ **Fig. 39.5.** Position of rigid bodies

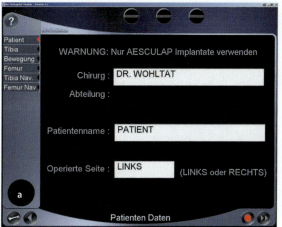

vest site, follows the procedure of femoral fixation, with 2 Kirschner wires in the area of the ventral margin of the tibia (■ Figs. 39.4 and 39.5).

Entering Patient Data

The following data are subsequently input into the system: patient's name, the side of the operated knee joint, surgeon's name, graft type and the graft thickness (■ Fig. 39.6).

Acquisition of Extraarticular Landmarks

The extraarticular reference points, tuberosity, ventral tibial margin, medial and lateral side of the tibial plateau are acquired using a navigated pointer (■ Figs. 39.7 and 39.8).

Acquiring the Knee Kinematics

After the leg position has been established in 90° flexion and maximum extension, the kinematic data of the knee joint are recorded in the computer by letting the leg sink from the extension position to 90° flexion (■ Fig. 39.9).

Acquisition of Intraarticular Landmarks

After the extraarticular landmarks have been acquired, the arthroscope is inserted into the knee joint and the

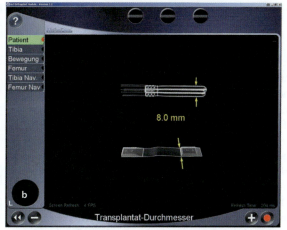

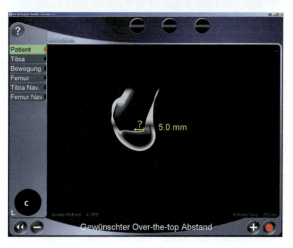

■ **Fig. 39.6a–c.** Data input, such as patient's name, graft type and thickness

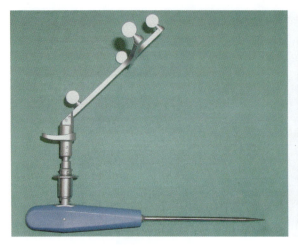

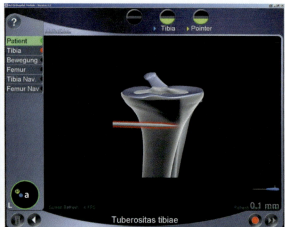

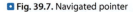
Fig. 39.7. Navigated pointer

intraarticular reference points are recorded. To do this, the anterior margin of the posterior cruciate ligament, the anterior horn of the lateral meniscus and the medial spine of the intercondylar tubercle are first recorded.

Acquisition of the notch data begins with palpation of the medial notch wall at 9 o'clock (left knee) or 3 o'clock (right knee), respectively. Following this, the contour of the ventral margin of the fossa is recorded with at least 10 points. This should be done starting from a medial position and moving to a lateral position. After the lateral notch wall has been acquired at 9 o'clock (left knee) or 3 o'clock (right knee), the wall is extensively palpated, also with at least 5 points (■ Fig. 39.10).

The posterior margin of the fossa is then palpated. This is one of the most important and sensitive steps of the acquisition. The posterior margin must be fully freed from soft tissue using the shaver and the curved raspatory if necessary, and well exposed to view.

The navigated hooked pointer must be carefully inserted, making sure that it sinks completely behind the fossa (■ Fig. 39.11). Now it is pulled very slowly in a ventral direction until the margin is palpated with the palpation hook. First of all the extreme cranial point (12 o'clock »over the top« position) is palpated and recorded.

Subsequently the extreme lateral point (1.30 o'clock for the left knee and 10.30 o'clock for the right knee) is established in the same way.

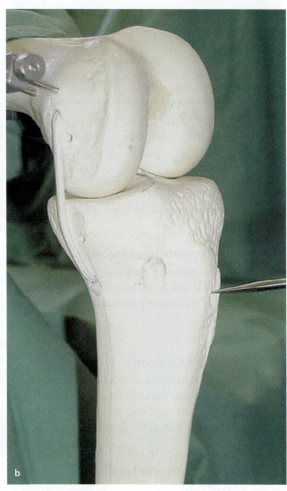

Fig. 39.8a,b. Palpation of extra-articular landmarks

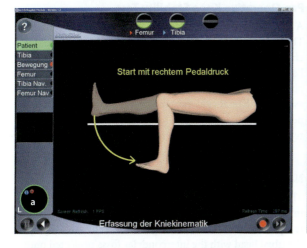
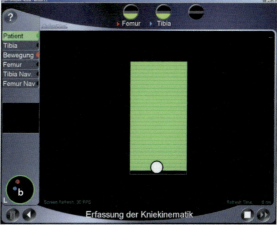

Fig. 39.9a,b. Recording the kinematics of the leg

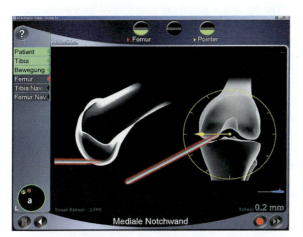
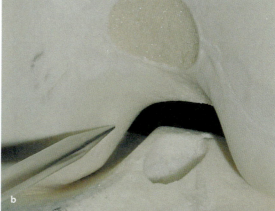
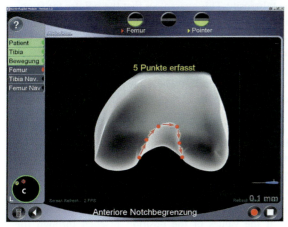
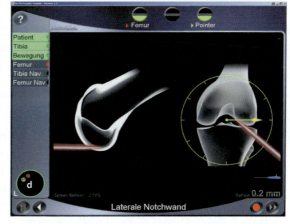

Fig. 39.10a–d. Acquisition of notch topography

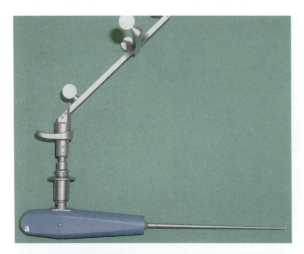

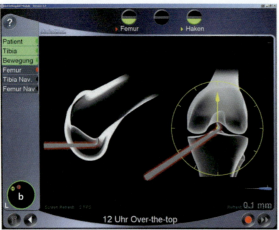

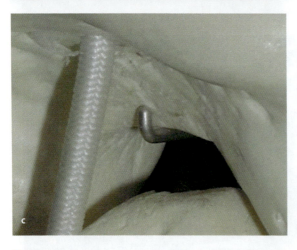

Fig. 39.11a–c. Navigated hooked pointer, 12 o'clock over the top position

Pre-Operative Knee Stability Test

A pre-operative knee stability test can be performed. The investigation under anesthetic is performed pre-operatively with the navigation equipment. This allows the Lachman test (corresponding to the KT 1000 test), the pivot shift phenomenon, and medial and postero-medial as well as lateral and postero-lateral instability components to be documented. The same investigation is then repeated after the operation is completed.

Navigation of the Tibia

The tibial pointer fitted with the mobile rigid body is introduced through the medial port lying close alongside the patellar tendon. The navigation screen now displays the tibial head with the intercondylar fossa projected onto it in full knee extension.

The tip of the pointer is now moved backwards and forwards on the tibial plateau until the blue circle, whose center represents the target point of the pointer, converges with the green circle (on the navigation screen; Fig. 39.12) and the color changes to green. Now the distance from the posterior cruciate ligament and the coronal width distance (medial/lateral) is checked – here expressed in percentages. Thus OrthoPilot completes the missing dimension of the image and the incomplete overview of the entire topography which is a result of the tunnel vision of arthroscopy.

After the intraarticular target point has been fixed on the tibial plateau with the tip of the tibial pointer, it must be ensured that the extra-articular attachment on the medial top view of the tibial plateau is far enough away from the tuberosity. This guarantees that the pointer for femoral navigation can also reach the desired target points. Consequently an angle of between 25 and 30 degrees in the frontal plane should be chosen.

Once the target wire has been set, OrthoPilot records the data of this position. The guide wire is now overdrilled according to the size of the graft.

Navigation of the Femur

The navigated femoral punch is introduced transtibially. The insertion area registered previously is approached at approximately 90° flexion. During this procedure the navigation screen informs the surgeon permanently about the values of the position reached through the »clock position«, and about the distance from the poste-

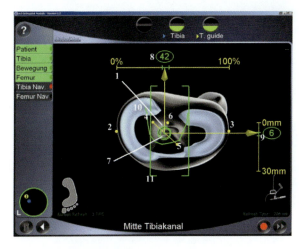

Fig. 39.12. Tibia navigation screen

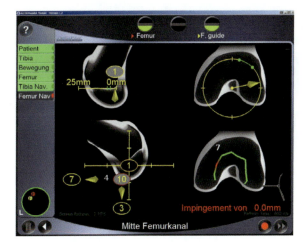

Fig. 39.13. Femur navigation screen

also registered in the navigation system and thereby documented.

The drilling wires can be subsequently overdrilled according to the operating procedure selected. The tibial and femoral rigid body fixations are removed. After the tunnels have been set the operation is continued in the usual manner (◘ Fig. 39.13).

Post-Operative Knee Stability Test

This test shows the improvement in stability achieved during the operation in relation to the preoperative test results. These values are documented and can thus prove the quality of the operation performed. Checks can also be made as to whether for instance a postero-lateral additional instability component could be adequately reduced through the central stabilization, or whether an additional extra-capsular operation is necessary.

Summary

As a precondition for the safe use of ACL navigation it is necessary to master precise diagnostic arthroscopy and the precise use of the hooked pointer, since the result of the navigation depends crucially on the quality of the acquisition of anatomical landmarks.

During development the navigated points were checked with the Fluoroscope (C-Arm) and mechanical isometric measuring equipment (Isotac). A high level of accuracy and reproducibility of the navigation results was documented.

The experience gained has shown that the use of the computer assisted navigation system permits highly accurate placement of tunnels for cruciate ligament reconstruction and avoids tunnel placement errors, regarded as the main cause of graft failure.

Future Prospects

Now that image-free navigation has proved its worth in anterior cruciate ligament surgery, we are working on further indications for which this technology can be used.

Work is actually being done on surface mapping (anatomic fitting) of cartilage surfaces, which allows the surfaces to be treated by osteochrondal transplantation to be precisely defined, or the areas for autologous chon-

rior margin of the fossa. Isometric data and any threatening impingement situations are also given as additional information for every point palpated with the tip of the femoral pointer.

After the target point has been optimized, the pointed tip of the pointer is fixed into the bone with light hammer blows and the drilling wire is set. This position is

drocyte transplantation to be calculated. In future there will also be navigated surgical instruments; it will be possible for example to avoid divergent tunnel screw sites by using navigated screwdrivers. Retrograde drilling of an osteochondrosis dissecans in the condyle and talus will also be possible; these areas are often difficult to depict by image converter.

Expanding the indications will mean that computer-assisted navigation in arthroscopic surgery will increasingly gain in significance.

PRAXIM ACL Navigation System using Bone Morphing

S. Plaweski, A. Pearle, C. Granchi, R. Julliard

Introduction

Primary Anterior Cruciate Ligament (ACL) reconstruction is the sixth-most common procedure in orthopedic surgery with nearly 75,000–125,000 procedures performed per year. While the procedure remains highly successful, there remains a 10–15% failure rate in most series. The etiology of ACL failure can be classified as failures due to a) surgical technique b) graft incorporation and c) trauma [5].

Background

Among failures due to surgical techniques, the most common technical error is poor tunnel placement [6, 13]. Anisometric graft positioning can cause graft stretch and poor control of knee rotational or translational stability. For example, anterior femoral tunnel placement produces strain in flexion and laxity in extension while posterior femoral tunnel placement produces strain in extension and laxity in flexion and risks back wall »blow out«. Anterior tibial tunnel placement results in strain in flexion and possible impingement in extension. Posterior tibial tunnel placement places strain on the graft in extension and possible PCL impingement. Medial or lateral tibial tunnel positioning can cause impingement conflicts with the PCL and femoral condyles.

Current surgical techniques rely on anatomic criteria, intra-operative fluoroscopy, and alignment jigs to create an isometric, non-impinging, and appropriately positioned graft. However, arthroscopic landmarks may be variable and inaccurate, fluoroscopic monitoring is cumbersome, and conventional transtibial approaches jigs such as the over-the-top guide can affect the femoral and tibial positioning (femoral tunnel tends to be anterior and vertical and tibial tunnel tends to be posterior) [5].

Surgical navigation offers an additional means of supervising tunnel positioning. In addition to anatomic criteria, quantitative isometric and impingement criteria can be used to plan tunnel positioning. This provides the surgeon with increased control in choosing tunnel position to optimize graft placement for the individual knee anatomy.

This chapter represents a summary of some recent research and clinical experience carried out at our institutes with the PRAXIM ACL navigation system. Below, a brief history and detailed description of the system is provided. Three recent studies related to the technical and clinical evaluation of the system, as well as to its use in revision procedures, are then presented, followed by a brief discussion.

History of the Praxim ACL Navigation System

ACL reconstruction surgery aims to restore normal knee stability and function, for a patient population that is typically young and active. Since our early studies performed in 1992, the development of our computer assisted ACL system focused on:

1. Improving joint function with precise measurement of knee kinematics,

2. Implementing an accurate registration procedure without exposing the patient to pre- or per-operative radiation,
3. Providing an effective and convenient procedure for use in clinical routine.

The resulting system does not require the use of any pre- or intra-operative imaging modalities such as CT, C-Arm fluoroscopy, radiography, or MRI, and it can be used without changing the surgical approach or the instrumentation. This unique technique of CT-less navigation for orthopedics was developed, patented and published for the first time in 1993 [8]. In 1994, Dr R. Julliard performed the first computer-assisted ACL surgery. This technique was first reported by Dessenne et al. in 1995 [3].

This early experience revealed that three major criteria had to be considered to correctly place the graft:
1. the joint anatomy,
2. the ligament isometry, and
3. impingement in the notch.

The results of this work were commercialized in an efficient Computer-Assisted Surgical Protocol on the Praxim platform. The system included tunnel-placement navigation based on the above criteria, and immediately appeared to be a significant help for the surgeon. More recent improvements to the system included accurate knee stability evaluation, a bendable 3D ligament model to simulate realistic graft behavior, and refinement of the protocol for increased safety, convenience and flexibility [1]. The system is now recognized as a comprehensive, accurate and proven solution for ACL reconstruction surgery [10, 11].

Methods

System Description

The Praxim surgical system is an image-free system that integrates *Bone Morphing*® technology to reconstruct the anatomy of the patient under arthroscopy. The ACL navigation system includes: a station, a small set of instruments and image-free per-operative software.

Station and Instruments

The Praxim *Surgetics*® station, an open platform system independent of implant companies, is a proven standard which has supported more than 10,000 surgeries. For added convenience, the ACL application is also supported by the portable Praxim NANO station, and the integrated digital operating room platform, which allows side-by-side placement and picture-in-picture integration of the arthroscopic video display and the navigation screen directly in front of the surgeon for optimal ergonomics.

The system is based on an accurate infrared optical tracking system. There is no keyboard or mouse; the main interaction is performed by the surgeon, pressing a blue foot pedal to go forward and a yellow foot pedal to go backward in a linear protocol. A tactile screen is used to enter patient demographics and to select options at the beginning of the procedure, such as particular stability tests to be performed. Patient information can be recorded and stored in the post-operative report on the individual patient's CD-ROM.

The set of instruments include 6 rigid bodies (or reference markers), 2 universal fixations for the instruments and 2 bone fixation devices. Wireless passive reference markers are constructed in shapes that are easily differentiable (□ Fig. 40.1), and are tracked by the optical localization system.

The system has been designed for easy integration into the classical clinic and normally does not require any significant changes in the routine procedure or in the instrumentation. To ensure the accuracy of the system, the instruments and the pointer are calibrated at the beginning of the protocol using a calibrator reference marker.

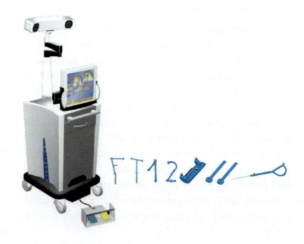

□ **Fig. 40.1.** Surgetics station and instruments set. F and T reference markers respectively fixed on the femur and on the tibia, 1 and 2 rigidly attached to the classical drill guides

Image-Free Per-Operative Software

In ACL reconstruction, a universally optimal position for the femoral tunnel has not yet been determined. More often than not, it is placed deep and high in the notch, far from the center of the anatomical attachment site. There is general agreement that the aim of ACL reconstructive surgery is to stabilize the knee by obtaining correct isometry and absence of impingement.

- Anisometry is defined as the maximal variation of distance between the tibial and femoral attachment sites during flexion of the knee. The anisometry profile is the curve of this distance with respect to the flexion angle, from extension to flexion. Therefore, a decreasing profile will result in a tight knee in extension and a lax knee in flexion.
- Impingement is defined as contact between the graft and the notch in extension. A virtual graft is drawn between the insertion sites. If there is impingement, the distance of penetration of this cylinder into the notch defines the impingement values.

The image-free software uses bone-morphing® technology to reconstruct the exact anatomy of the patient in 3D. The resulting models are used to (1) display in real-time a bendable graft model, (2) evaluate the impingement, and (3) construct the ligament anisometry profile for a planned set of tunnel placements.

Surgical Protocol

The following surgical protocol for ACL reconstruction surgery has been designed based on surgeon practice and experience. This system is designed to be integrated and adapted to most of the classical approaches and instrumentation, including most innovative procedures.

Installation

The navigation system does not require any specific arrangement in the operating room. The Praxim station is installed next to the arthroscopic tower so that the surgeon can see both screens at the same time, and the optical cameras can have an unobstructed view of the reference markers.

Once the patient's leg is washed and draped, the surgeon installs the reference markers on the tibia and on the femur. Fixation requires the use of either a one or a two pin external fixation device. The one pin fixation is a triangular shaped pin which has been specifically designed for this surgery by one of the authors. The pin can be preset and installed quickly and percutaneously for minimum invasiveness. The preparation of the graft and the arthroscopic examination of the notch are then performed.

Data Acquisition

Anatomical Points

The acquisition sequence is performed arthroscopically and on the patient skin (depending on the landmark) using the specially designed pointer (reference marker P). On the tibia:

- the center of the ankle is determined by computing a point between the skin over the lateral and medial malleoli,
- the medial and lateral tibial spines are acquired to constitute an anatomical reference,
- the middle of the medial and lateral tibial plateaus are digitized in order to quantify the translational laxity in each compartment,
- the middle of the anterior inter-meniscus ligament is used as a reference for the pivot shift test measurements

Kinematic Acquisition

The reference markers F and T on the femur and tibia are used to acquire the specific kinematics of the patient.

- A passive flexion-extension motion is performed by the surgeon. This dynamic acquisition is aimed at calculating the anisometry values and profiles of the graft.
- If requested by the surgeon, it is possible to acquire the centre of the femoral head by performing a conic movement in order to calculate a true hip-knee-ankle angle in the sagittal plane [12]. This option is useful in cases of knee flexion contracture.

3D Anatomy Reconstruction

Bone morphing consists in computing the accurate morphology of the patient's knee from a deformable statistical model, without use of CT, radiography or fluoroscopy. Several hundred scattered points are acquired quickly by the surgeon, by »painting« the cartilage and bone surface with the probe. These points are matched with the statistical model using a 3D/3D registration algorithm [4]. The

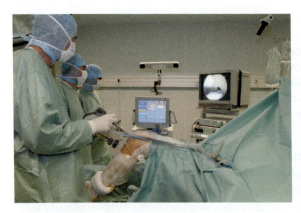

Fig. 40.2. Clinical set-up of the system. Surgeon acquiring the femoral bone morphing area. Visualization of the arthroscopic view and the Surgetics at the same time

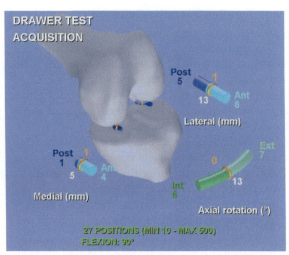

Fig. 40.3. Display of the medial and lateral translation laxity and rotation during a drawer test. The stability for each compartment can be assessed in real-time

bone model displayed on the screen is formed in real-time, to adapt to the knee of the patient.

Through this procedure the femoral notch and the tibial inter-spinal areas are reconstructed. The intra-operative 3D anatomy allows real customization of the procedure to each patient as shown on ◘ Fig. 40.2.

Pre- and Post-Operative Stability Evaluation

Although various clinical tests exist for assessing the integrity and function of the ligaments in the knee, objectively incorporating clinical test results into the surgical plan can be illusive. We have therefore been working to effectively integrate knee instability measurements into the protocol for guiding both intra-articular and extra-articular ligament reconstructions. The quantitative laxity measurements can be performed at various stages in the procedure, for pre- as well as post-reconstruction evaluation. Upon review of the various clinical tests for assessing knee injuries and instabilities, we selected four protocols for intra-operative evaluation:

- Drawer test,
- Varus-Valgus stability test,
- Lachman test,
- Pivot shift test.

For each test, the landmarks previously acquired are used to determine the rotation and translation of the medial and lateral compartment individually. ◘ Figure 40.3 shows the screen during the acquisition.

The system guides the surgeon in performing each test by displaying the 3D anatomical models in real-time, along with the flexion angle, the landmark point trajectories and their maximum displacements in the relevant planes/directions.

At the end of the stability exam, the summary screen gives a global appreciation of the knee stability in three dimensions at 0, 30 and 90 degrees of flexion. With this unique tool the instability of the knee can be objectively characterized and interpreted, and the knee properly reconstructed [2].

Interactive Planning and Navigation
Anatomical References

The radiological features of the tunnels are well known by the surgeon, and their positions are defined in relations with different landmarks such as the Blumensaat's line, the over the top limit and the tibial spines. The projection of the femoral notch on the tibia in the direction of the Blumensaat's line helps the surgeon to position the tibial tunnel as anterior as possible while avoiding notch impingement whereas the tibial spines displayed on the tibia gives a conventional arthroscopic reference.

The over the top limit display allows the surgeon to make the compromise between anatomical and isometric placement of the femoral tunnel.

40

Graft Simulation and Notch Impingement

In order to correctly guide graft placement, an advanced graft-simulation algorithm has been integrated into the system. A bendable ligament model is calculated and displayed in real-time as a function of the position and shape of the femoral notch and the planned fixation points. The simulation is based on a non-linear energy criterion that monitors collisions with the 3D bone surface during the kinematics measurements. The renderings aid visualization of the ligament trajectory, by depicting how the virtual ligament glides overtop of the 3D bone surface models as the knee is flexed and extended.

Using this graft simulation, any notch impingement can be identified and its intensity evaluated dynamically. A red zone appearing on the femoral surface reveals the presence of potential impingement between the virtual graft and the notch. The displayed distance represents the maximum penetration distance of the virtual ligament inside the notch for the entire range of flexion measured (■ Fig. 40.4).

Graft Anisometry Profile Description

The anisometry is globally defined as the maximal variation of the graft fiber length during flexion-extension. A single value of anisometry displayed on the screen for a single graft fiber would make the tunnel placement process long and non intuitive. The system therefore computes for a given tibial point an anisometry color map painted directly on the external femoral notch surface. The locations corresponding to minimum anisometry are displayed in green and the maximum value is represented in red. The resulting map is superimposed in the femoral bone model as presented in ■ Fig. 40.4. While moving the pointer on the bone, the potential graft insertion point is displayed as a circle and the surgeon can check at the same time the anisometry of the anterior, central and posterior fibers.

For any given pair of Femoral and Tibial insertion sites (F and T) selected by the surgeon, an anisometry curve is represented and defines the graft profile. A favorable profile characterizes a fiber that loses tension during flexion, whereas a non-favorable profile characterizes a fiber that stretches in flexion.

Optimization Strategy

A possible strategy for the planning consists in
1. First choosing a point on the tibia with respect to the anatomical references given by the system;

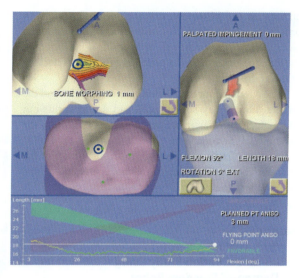

■ **Fig. 40.4.** Interactive planning on tibia and femur. The blue circles correspond to the insertion points of the tunnels – the red area on the right image of the femur shows the potential impingement area between the graft and the notch for the selected centre of the tunnels. The anisometry map on the femur is color-coded: green indicates an anisometry value less than 2 mm; yellow, 2–4 mm; orange, 4–6 mm; and red more than 6 mm. Blumensaat's line is represented by a dotted line. The over-the-top limit is represented by a pink line on the femur. The anisometry curve is illustrated in green; it is computed in real time as the surgeon selects new insertion sites

2. The system displays the anisometry map for the given tibial point on the femur. The anisometry curve is represented in real-time as the pointer is moved on the potential femoral insertion point. If it can't be ideal, the anisometry must be positive but not too high as that would leave a pathological laxity in flexion;
3. The surgeon adjusts the tibial point to prevent any conflict for the given femoral point, and checks the corresponding anisometry profile.

Navigation of Tunnels

Currently different surgical approaches on placement of the tunnel as well as fixation of the graft exist. As such a tool should respond to most of these techniques, the system has been designed to be very flexible, interactive but also intuitive for the surgeon. Using any standard instrumentation for drilling the tunnels, one reference marker is fixed on the conventional tibial guide and one on the femoral guide, and the guides are calibrated. The navigation of the tibial tunnel consists in placing the guide on the tibia and follows the virtual guide on the screen in order to reach the target previously recorded. During this part of the navigation the axis of the guide is projected on the femur in order to have a preview of the final trajectory of the graft.

The operation for the femoral tunnel is similar and the femoral tunnel may be navigated and drilled inside-out (through the medial arthroscopic portal or through the tibial tunnel) or outside-in.

After the fixation of the graft, individual fibers of the graft are checked in order to validate the isometry and impingement.

Results

Technical Validation Study Using a 6 Degree-of-Freedom Robot

One of the exciting aspects of the Surgetics navigation system is the ability to quantify multiplanar knee translations and rotations (coupled motions) during knee stability examination. Traditionally, clinical examination, the cornerstone of clinical decision making in knee instability, remains empirical and may be confusing in the setting of multiplanar knee instability. We have assessed the accuracy of a navigated knee stability examination in cadaveric knees subjected to varus loading with and without external rotation loading in intact and posterolateral corner deficient knees. In this injury pattern, there is multiplanar instability with an increase in both varus and external rotation.

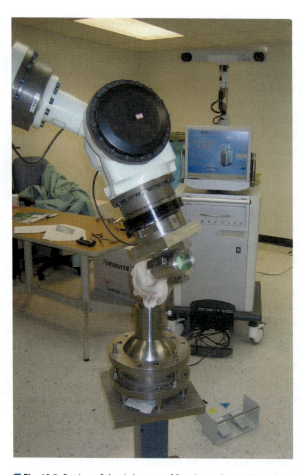

Fig. 40.5. Setting of the 6 degrees of freedom robot with the knee mounted and the Surgetics system on the side

Methods. Six cadaveric knees were mounted on a 6 Degree-of-Freedom (DOF) robotic manipulator/positional sensor (Kawasaki ZX 165U, Kawasaki Heavy Industries, Japan). The knees were taken through a full range of motion and then subjected to 9 Nm of varus stress at 0°, 30° and 60°. The procedure was then repeated with the 9 Nm varus stress and 4 Nm external rotation force at the same flexion angles. This protocol was used in both intact knees and the same knees after sectioning of the postero-lateral corner.

The testing system, composed of a 6-DOF robotic manipulator and a 6-DOF universal force-moment sensor (ATI DAQ F/T Multi-Axis Force-Torque Sensor System, ATI Apex, North Carolina), allowed for quantification of unidirectional knee translations and rotations. This surgical navigation system was used to quantify coupled knee motion and characterize translation and rotation in both the medial and lateral compartments of the knee (Fig. 40.5).

Accuracy of the surgical navigation system compared to the robot was assessed using the intraclass correlation coefficient. Wilcoxon Rank Sum Test (paired nonparametric test) was used to determine differences in knee rotations.

Results. Intraclass Correlation Coefficients (ICCs) between the robotic sensor and the navigation system for varus and external rotation at 0, 30, and 60 degrees were all statistically significant at <0.01. The overall ICC for all tests was 0.99 (p<0.0001).

40

This study demonstrated Praxim ACL navigation system is a highly accurate means of dynamically quantifying knee stability examination and may help identify pathologic multiplanar or coupled knee motions, particularly in the setting of complex instability patterns [11].

Clinical experience

Comparative Study on 96 Patients

In 2000, Menetrey et al. [9] proposed an innovative method for comparing the positioning of the tibial and femoral tunnel using computer assisted ACL surgery as a gold standard. The study compared the accuracy and reproducibility of 5 different conventional guides on 5 cadaveric knees looking at the positioning with respect to the anatomical original position, the notch impingement, and the elongation of the graft. The »Aimer« and transtibial guides appeared the more reproducible and reliable positioning.

Today about 300 ACL reconstructions were performed using this system in our center. Based on this study and our previous experience [10], we compared in-vivo in a group of 96 patients the placement using manual instrumentation with the result given by the system.

Methods. All patients received a ligament reconstructive surgery using the same technique: semi-tendinosus tendon using BioRCI tibial screw fixation (Smith and Nephew, Andover, MA USA) and femoral endo-button. The manual guides used: Acufex PCL related (Smith and Nephew, Andover, MA USA) for the tibia and In/Out femoral guides.

The positioning given by the ancillary was first blindly chosen by the operator and recorded using the navigation system. The reconstruction objectives were to get a tibial tunnel as anterior as possible avoiding notch impingement, and which minimize the anisometry with a favorable curve.

Results. The operating time was increased by 17 min (10–30); no per or post operative complications were noticed. On the tibia, the tunnel selected using the manual instrumentation appears too posterior in all cases. The navigation tool changed the positioning of the tibial tunnel giving a more anterior and medial. These modifications were possible and secured in all case by the visualization of the projection of the notch on the tibia

and the real-time display of the conflict. On the femur the manual instrumentation proposed a good position with respect to the anisometry in 60% of the cases, a favorable anisometry curve in 15% of the case, and a non-favorable position for the other cases. The operator changed the original position proposed by the manual guides in 40% of the case avoiding 15% of femoral tunnel misplacement.

This system allowed to safety place the tibial tunnel more anterior increasing the anterior stability of the knee. The navigation tool was also useful in 40% of the case helping the positioning of the femoral tunnel.

Clinical Study of 30 ACL Revision Reconstructions

The clinical utility of the navigation system has also been evaluated for ACL revision procedures.

Methods. The study included 30 patients with previous history of ACL repairs (2 synthetical grafts, 17 semi-tendinosus grafts and 11 patella tendons). The repairs consisted in 13 quadrupled semi-tendinosus grafts and 17 patella tendon reconstructions.

The failed center position of the tibial and the femoral tunnel were analyzed and recorded using the system: the anisometry curve of the initial plasty were computed. The operator reconstructed the ACL following standard navigation (◻ Fig. 40.6).

Results. In 20 knees, the authors reported an initial malpositioning of the tunnels (66% of the cases). 8 tibial tunnels were positioned too anterior leading to anterior conflict with the femoral notch, 10 tibial tunnels were too posterior with an anisometry superior to 8 mm and only 12 tunnels was reported correctly placed. In 60% of the cases (18 knees), the defavorable anisometry curve were due to the mal-positioning of the femoral tunnel.

Discussion. The main difficulty appeared to us in the analysis of the failure and the realization of new tunnels. The system allowed us to understand the reason of the first failure and to avoid reproducing any mal-positioning of the new tunnels. The use of the Praxim ACL navigation system appeared to be a valuable tool but also essential as medicolegal justification. The multiple ACL reconstruction methods and the choice of the fixation system associated with the use of the navigation greatly simplified the ACL revision surgery in our practice.

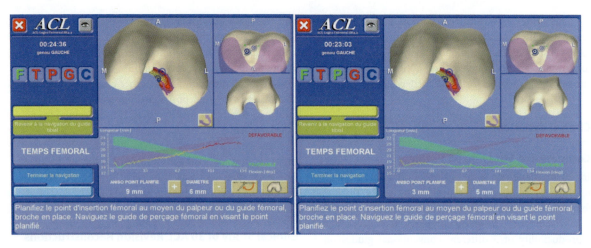

■ **Fig. 40.6.** Example of ACL revision. *Left image*, the first stage: The femoral tunnel is located in non-favorable anisometry area and the tibial tunnel is positioned too anterior: The anisometry is 9 mm with a non-favorable curve profile. *Right image*, the second stage: The chosen femoral point is in a favorable area with an anisometry of 3 mm. The tibial tunnel center point is more anterior without notch conflict. The anisometry curve is horizontal

Discussion

Anterior Cruciate Ligament (ACL) reconstruction is the treatment of choice for young, active individuals with an ACL deficient knee and symptoms of instability. While this procedure is widely performed, estimated rates of revision surgery are as high as 10–20%, which has prompted a search for modified techniques such as the double bundle ACL reconstruction. While failure to recreate knee stability may result in early failures, ACL reconstruction is also associated with a late risk of the development of osteoarthritis. Both modes of failure may be associated with the surgeon's inability to properly recreate the normal knee kinematics. Surgical navigation offers the potential to not only navigate the position of the graft by supervising the placement of graft tunnels, but also the opportunity to interrogate the multiplanar kinematics of the knee before, during, and after ACL reconstruction.

While we have demonstrated that navigated knee examination is accurate and provides real-time multiplanar visualization and kinematic data, inter and intra-observer variation in the application of clinical tests remains problematic. In addition, standard pitfalls of surgical navigation systems, such as landmark and mechanical errors, increased surgical time, and line-of-site issues, must be recognized when applying this technology clinically [7].

Surgical navigation offers the opportunity to monitor multiple aspects of knee ligament reconstructions dynamically. An inherent difficulty in ACL reconstruction is choosing the correct position for the placement of the graft so as to create an isometric graft that best reproduces the knee's normal kinematics. Navigated knee stability examination may help surgeons tailor the knee reconstruction to the patient's particular pattern of knee instability. In addition, the ability to integrate isometry and impingement criteria with arthroscopic landmark criteria allows the surgeon to refine the planning and execution of tunnel placement in accordance with the individual pattern of knee instability.

Acknowledgements. The authors wish to thank Dr Allard, Dr Warren, Dr Kirchmeier, Stephane Lavallée PhD, and Lionel Carrat for their contributions to the work presented in this paper.

References

1. Colombet P, Allard M (2004) Computer-assisted surgery of the anterior cruciate ligament. Rev Chir Orthop Reparatrice Appar Mot 90: 3S21-28
2. Colombet P, Allard M, Granchi C, Plaskos C, Lavallée S (2005) Anterior Cruciate Ligament Reconstruction using knee joint laxity measurements and a bendable ligament model. In CAOS Annual Meeting Helsinki Finland

3. Dessenne V, Lavallée S, Julliard R, Orti R, Martelli S Cinquin P (1995) Computer-assisted knee anterior cruciate ligament reconstruction: first clinical tests. J Image Guid Surg 1: 59–64

4. Fleute M (2001) Shape reconstruction for computer-assisted surgery based on non-rigid registration of statistical models with intraoperative point data and X-ray images. TIMC IMAG Laboratory

5. Harner CD (2005) Controversies in ACL Surgery. AOSSM 2005 Annual Meeting, Keystone, CO

6. Harner CD, Giffin JR, Dunteman RC, Annunziata CC, Friedman MJ (2001) Evaluation and treatment of recurrent instability after anterior cruciate ligament reconstruction. Instr Course Lect 50 : 463–474

7. Langlotz F (2004) Potential pitfalls of computer aided orthopedic surgery. Injury 35 (Suppl 1): S-A17–23

8. Lavallée S, Julliard R, Orti R, Cinquin P, Capentier E (1993) Anterior Cruciate Ligament reconstruction: computer assisted determination of the most isometric femoral attachment point. Orthop Traumatol 3: 87–92

9. Menetrey J, Suva D, Genoud P, Sati M Fritschy D, Hoffmeyer P (2000) Validation de differents guide de visee utilises dans la reconstruction du LCA par le systeme CAOS. Communication. Congres de la Societe Francaise d'arthroscopie, Annecy

10. Plaweski S, Cazal J, Rosell P, Merloz P (2006) Anterior cruciate ligament reconstruction using navigation: a comparative study on 60 patients. Am J Sports Med 34(4):542–552

11. Solomon D, Pearle A, Lenhoff M, Granchi C, Wickiewicz T, Warren R (2006) Evaluation of coupled knee motions and force on the ACL with varus loading in posterolateral corner deficient knees. ORS 52nd Annual Meeting, Chicago

12. Stindel E, Gil D, Briard JL, Merloz P, Dubrana F, Lefevre C (2006) Detection of the center of the hip joint in computer-assisted surgery: an evaluation study of the Surgetics algorithm. Comput Aided Surg 10(3): 133–139

13. Wirth CJ, Kohn D (1996) Revision anterior cruciate ligament surgery: experience from Germany. Clin Orthop Relat Res 325: 110-115

14. Julliard R., Cinquin Ph., Lavallee S., La surgétique du ligament croise antérieur. La navigation sans imagerie. Revue Chirurgie Orthopédique, 2002, 88, pp 1S88–1S90

15. Fleute M, Lavallee S, Julliard R. Incorporating a statistically based shape model into a system for computer-assisted anterior cruciate ligament surgery. med Image Anal. 1999 Sep;3(3):209–22

16. R. julliard, S. Lavallee, and V. Dessenne. Computer Assisted Anterior Cruciate Ligament Reconstruction. Clinical Orthopaedics and Related Research, (354):57–64, September 1998

17. V. Dessenne, S. Lavallee, R. orti, R. Julliard, S. martelli, and P. Cinquin. Computer assisted knee anterior cruciate ligament reconstruction: first clinical tests. J. of Image Guided Surgery, 1(1):59–64, 1995.

18. R. Julliard, S. Plaweski, S. Lavallee. ACL Surgetics: an effecient Computer-assisted technique for ACL reconstruction. In Navigation and robotics in total joint and spine surgery. Springer edit 2003. Chapitre 57. P 405–411

Fluoroscopic-based ACL Navigation

S. Shafizadeh, Th. Paffrath, S. Grote, J. Hoeher, Th. Tiling, B. Bouillon

Introduction

With the increasing importance of sport activities and with better diagnostics, the recognized incidence of anterior cruciate ligament (ACL) ruptures has risen in the past years Increasing numbers of ACL reconstructions have been registered in Europe and the USA [1]. ACL reconstruction has become a popular surgical technique to restore knee stability, allowing the patient to resume participation in sports.

The goal of ACL reconstruction is to restore physiological joint biomechanics in order to prevent secondary cartilage and meniscal lesions.

Despite greater knowledge of the knee anatomy, biomechanics and improved reconstruction techniques, increasing numbers of patients with failed ACL reconstructions have been observed. With a rather positive publication bias, success rates following ACL reconstruction are reported to be between 75–92% [2–4]. In addition to factors such as patient selection, surgeon experience, graft choice, graft fixation or rehabilitation, there is general agreement that correct anatomical tunnel positioning is fundamental to successful ACL reconstruction and long term stability [5].

According to publications, the rate of revision surgery following failed ACL reconstruction is reported to be as high as 10–20%. Radiological studies indicate that approximately 10–40% of drill holes in primary ACL reconstructions have been incorrectly placed [6–10]. An error analysis study of failed ACL reconstructions showed that incorrectly-placed tunnel positions caused graft failure in 73.5% [11].

Increasing rates of ACL revision surgery demonstrate that there remains considerable room for improvement [12, 13].

Anatomical and Biomechanical Aspects of the ACL

Anatomical understanding of the ACL is crucial in order to understand its stabilizing function and is the key to improve techniques for reconstruction. The complex anatomy of the ACL is characterized by fan shaped insertion areas on the tibia and femur with the ligament fibers running an oblique torn course through the interconylar fossa. The tibial insertion is described as an oval or triangular area between the medial interconylar eminence and the anterior horns of the menisci covering a mean area of 136 ± 33 mm^2. The femoral insertion area has been described as an ovoid, semicircular or circular area complementing the dorsal curvature of the condyles. It covers an area of 113 ± 27 mm^2 on the inner wall of the lateral condyle. Relative to the insertion areas on tibia and femur, the midsubstance area is found to be 3.5 times smaller.

Based on the insertion site and tensioning patterns during flexion and extension of the knee, the ACL can be divided into at least two anatomically distinct bundles, with the antero-medial (AM) bundle being more taut in flexion and the postero-lateral (PL) bundle being more taut in extension [14–16]. This principle of flexion-depending fiber recruiting allows the complex interplay between stability and motion. In addition, it is essential for the primary function of the ACL; to prevent anterior tibial translation and to be a passive restraint for internal rotation.

Significance of Tunnel Positioning in ACL Reconstruction

Looking at the complex fiber architecture of the ACL, which allows a complex interplay between stability and motion, it is obvious that current reconstruction techniques using autografts can only achieve these capabilities to a certain degree.

As studies show, tunnel positions have important influence on results following ACL reconstruction. Abnormal tunnel positioning is related to functional limitations. At the tibia anterior tunnel, positioning is associated with loss of extension and impingement at the femoral notch, which leads to chronic graft damages and subsequently to graft failure [17–21]. Posterior tibial tunnel positions may cause an impingement with the posterior cruciate ligament (PCL) and limitations in the flexion of the knee [22, 23]. Femoral tunnel positions that are too anterior result in a graft that is tight in flexion and lax in extension with a loss of stability control [24, 25].

The ACL is the most frequently studied ligament of the musculoskeletal system and many researchers have described tunnel positions in ACL reconstruction. There is common sense that anatomical tunnel positioning is fundamental to long term stability following ACL reconstruction. But how to achieve these tunnel positions has been widely debated and remains difficult due to several reasons:

- A variety of recommendations on tunnel positions exist [26, 27].
- Intra-operative arthroscopic identification of the correct insertions is difficult, because there are no landmarks, which allow reproducible identification of the footprints.
- The application of the theoretical anatomical knowledge to the actual surgical procedure remains difficult.
- The anatomy of the ACL itself makes tunnel positioning difficult, since the insertion areas at tibia and femur allow many different anatomical tunnel positions.

- Restricted local arthroscopic view with 30° endoscopes, lens distortions and the 2-dimensional view make orientation of the intercondylar anatomy challenging.

To achieve best tunnel positions, offset guides, aiming devices and fluoroscopically assisted techniques [28] are recommended by many experts [29, 30] to increase accuracy. However, even for advanced arthroscopic surgeons correct tunnel positioning can be a problem as Kohn et al. showed in a cadaver study [31]. In an own cadaver study, we analyzed inter- and intra-observer variability of tunnel positions in order to evaluate accuracy and consistency. Thirteen orthopaedic surgeons with different levels of experience (6 experts and 7 beginners) were asked to define the tunnel positions on the femur and tibia with a navigated hook in a test-retest scenario. Screenshots of the tunnel positions were analyzed to compare the tunnel positions. Independent of the surgeon's experience there was a high intra-and intra-observer variability of 6 mm (Range 4–8 mm) for the femoral and tibial tunnel positions. This amount of inaccuracy indicates the significant clinical implication between tunnel positions and clinical results in ACL reconstruction.

How Can Navigation Systems Enable Improvements in ACL Reconstruction?

Although several studies and recommendations on tunnel positioning in ACL reconstruction exist, the optimal tunnel positions will remain controversial as long as there are no reliable methods to compare and analyze the long term clinical outcome of tunnel positions.

Currently there are no methods available that allow reproducible tunnel positioning and documentation to evaluate the long term influence of tunnel positions on anterior-posterior (AP) and rotational stability.

Recently, navigation systems have been introduced to enable improvements in ACL reconstruction by providing substantial anatomical information to surgeons. Computer aided navigation systems use infrared camera systems and minimally invasive markers that display the position of surgical instruments relative to the knee with a precision of <1 mm and <1°.

The fluoroscopy-based ACL navigation technique described in this paper is a hybrid technology that combines

41

image-guided surgery based on fluoroscopic images with intra-operative acquisition of surface landmarks.

The system allows reproducible planning of tunnel positions based on reliable radiological planning methods, precise k-wire drilling for tunnel positioning and AP and rotational stability analysis before and after graft implantation. The following sections describe the principles of this technology and its implementation in the operating theatre.

Basic Principle of Fluoroscopic Navigation

The system is based on a commercial wireless navigation system (Vectorvision®, Brainlab, Heimstetten, Germany). Unlike other navigation systems, this system does not require cables, batteries, or foot switches. Instead, the system uses two infrared Polaris® cameras which emit infrared flashes which are reflected by passive marker spheres that are attached to the patient's distal femur and proximal tibia and to the navigation instruments. For image acquisition, a registration kit containing reflective marker discs is attached to the c-arm of the fluoroscope (◘ Fig. 41.1a). The cameras digitize the infrared reflection image which is created by reflecting the infrared flashes from the cameras. Image acquisition with the registered c-arm position data allows the software to calculate the three-dimensional position of the fluoroscopic image. Tracked by the infrared camera, the position of the surgical instruments can now be accurately determined and is displayed real-time on the fluoroscopic images (◘ Fig. 41.1b). According to radiographic measurement methods, tunnel positions can be reproducibly planned (◘ Fig. 41.1c) and precise navigation-controlled tunnel drilling can be performed (◘ Fig. 41.1d).

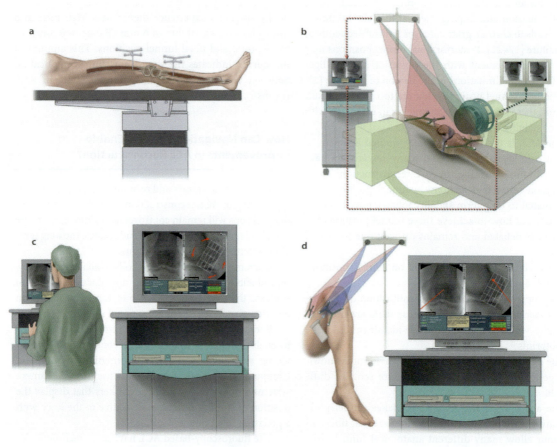

◘ **Fig. 41.1.** Principle of fluoroscopic navigation

Setup

The technical equipment needed for fluoroscopic-based ACL reconstruction requires a careful setup. The patient, the navigation system with the camera and the c-arm must be positioned in such a way that the cameras have an unobstructed view on the marker spheres at all times during the surgical procedure. We prefer to position the navigation system contralateral to the knee to be operated on with the camera positioned above the patient's head. The c-arm of the fluoroscope and the arthroscopic tower are positioned on the ispsilateral side (■ Fig. 41.2).

Before image acquisition and patient registration can be performed, the registration kit must be attached to the c-arm of the fluoroscope, and reference arrays must be attached to the patient's distal femur and proximal tibia using small incisions with two K-wires or with one Schanz screw (■ Fig. 41.3). The femoral reference array (Y geometry) is attached to the anterolateral aspect of the femur, approximately 15 cm above the joint line and the tibial reference array (T geometry) is attached to the antero-medial aspect of the tibia, approximately 20 cm below the joint line of the knee. For all further steps, it is important that the femoral and tibial reference arrays are detected by the infrared camera in full extension, and in 30°, 90° and 120° flexion. Tracked positioning data are transferred to the navigation system and displayed on the touchscreen.

Fluoroscopic Acquisition

Once the reference arrays are attached, the user can proceed with the acquisition of the fluoroscopic images (■ Fig. 41.4). For reproducible evaluation of the AP tunnel positions, a standardized AP notch view projection of the knee with the free projection of the tibial plateaus is needed. Next, lateral X-rays of the femur and the tibia must be acquired.

For reproducible planning and evaluation, it is essential that all acquired images are of good quality and that they are acquired in the correct projection.

Bone Morphing

Using navigation pointers, the insertion areas of the ACL on the femoral and tibial side are roughly digitized under arthroscopical control. Soft tissue can result in unprecise surface morphs. Therefore, soft tissue from the inner surface of the lateral condyle must be removed with a shaver. Since removing soft tissue does not make sense on the tibia, we cut the soft tissue with a scalpel in order to allow bony contact during the bone morphing process on the tibia.

The morphed bone surface is projected on the registered fluoroscopic image and provides detailed information on the planned tunnel positions (■ Fig. 41.5).

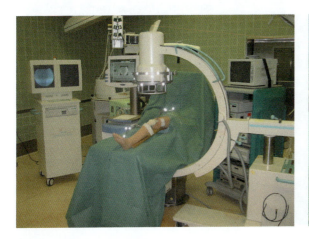

■ **Fig. 41.2.** Setup

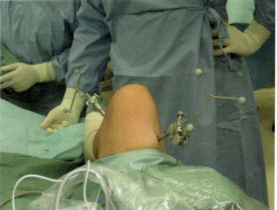

■ **Fig. 41.3.** Fixation of the reference arrays

41

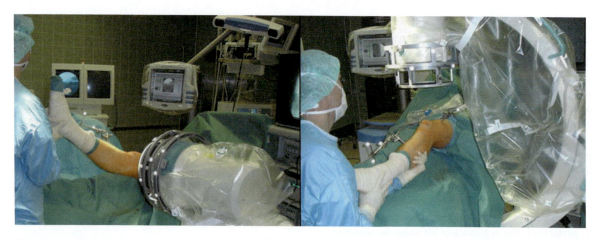

■ **Fig. 41.4.** Image Acquisition

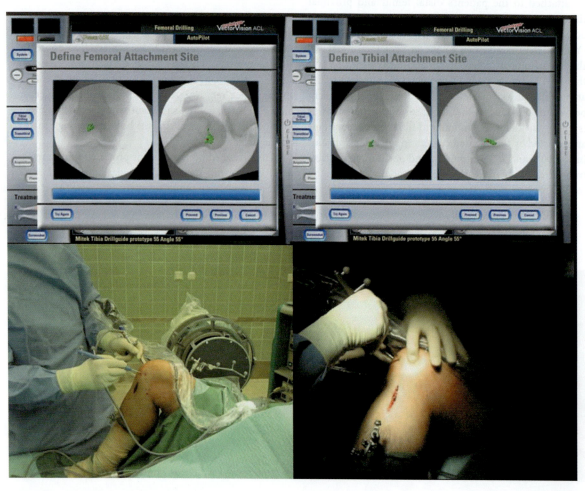

■ **Fig. 41.5.** Bone morphing

Planning of the Tunnel Positions

Once the images are acquired and the bone surface has been morphed, the surgeon can plan the femoral and tibial center of the tunnel positions on the touchscreen of the navigation system according to the »Quadrant method« for the femur [32] and Stäublis method for the tibia [33]. Both methods are considered to be reliable for planning and evaluation of tunnel positions (◘ Fig. 41.6).

Virtual Impingement Control and Stability Analysis

Once the tunnel positions have been planned, virtual impingement control can be performed previous to drilling. The surgeon must enter the graft diameter on the touchscreen, the graft is then virtually displayed on the images. Notch impingement can then be identified by bringing the lower leg into extension. In the Lachman position,

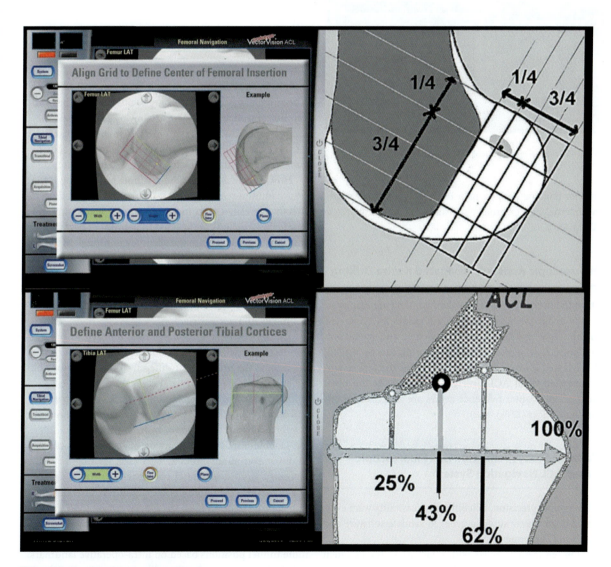

◘ **Fig. 41.6.** Planning of the tunnel positions

41

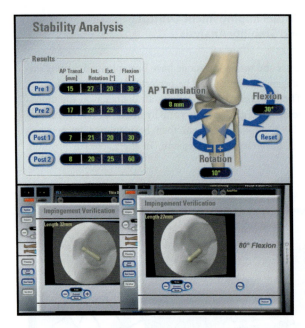

Fig. 41.7. Virtual Impingement control and stability analysis

anterior tibia translation can be tested and flexion, depending internal and external tibial rotation, can be analyzed (● Fig. 41.7).

Arthroscopic Assisted, Navigated K-wire Drilling

Once the tunnel positions are defined, they are displayed on the images as target points. Drill guides are navigated to the target points. Under arthroscopic and navigation guidance, K-wires for tunnel positioning can be drilled. A navigated 2.4 mm drill tube is used for the femur, and a navigated tibial ACL drill guide is used for the tibia. Instrument adapter reference arrays are attached to both aiming devices (● Fig. 41.8).

Cadaver Study: Validation of a Fluoroscopic-based ACL Navigation System

The system's precision, reliability and feasibility were evaluated in a cadaver study in order to validate software and hardware components.

On ten fresh cadavers with intact ACL's the ligament was arthroscopically removed. In line with the steps de-

scribed above, tunnels were planned and their placement navigated. Once the K-wires had been successfully navigated, their position at the femoral and tibial osteochondral surface was compared with the planned drill hole centre. In all 20 cases (10 femoral, 10 tibial) the tip of the K-wire was exactly in the centre of the planned drill hole. The radiological planning methods allowed reproducible tunnel positioning. The average time required for navigated tunnel positioning was approximately 20 min. The system thus enabled both simple and efficient ACL reconstruction. No software or hardware faults were observed.

Discussion

Although reconstruction techniques in ACL surgery have improved considerably, graft failure rates are still reported to be as high as 8–25%. According to publications the most common reason for graft failure following ACL reconstruction is wrong positioning of tunnels. Also increasing numbers of revision surgery indicate that there remains considerable room for improvements in ACL reconstruction.

How can we do better? Since tunnel positioning is the most common reason for graft failure and graft failure is directly correlated with incorrect tunnel positioning, reproducible methods are needed to determine best tunnel positions and to increase the accuracy of tunnel positioning in order to restore the normal ACL anatomy as closely as possible.

Recently navigation systems have been proposed to provide precise and reproducible results for tunnel positioning in ACL reconstruction.

Unlike other navigation systems, the hybrid navigation technology, described in this paper, enables surgeons to evaluate the influence of different tunnel positions on AP and rotational stability and clinical results.

In context with double-bundle ACL reconstruction and other approaches to restore the anatomy of the ACL as closely as possible, navigation systems are of special interest. Double-bundle reconstruction makes ideal tunnel positioning even more difficult, since even for single bundle reconstruction ideal tunnel positions are neither defined nor evaluated. Therefore double-bundle ACL reconstruction appears to be an ideal use for navigation [34].

In contrast to fluoroscopic-based ACL navigation systems, image free ACL navigation systems [35–37] determine tunnel positions based on intra-operative landmark acquisition. Those systems are like conventional methods

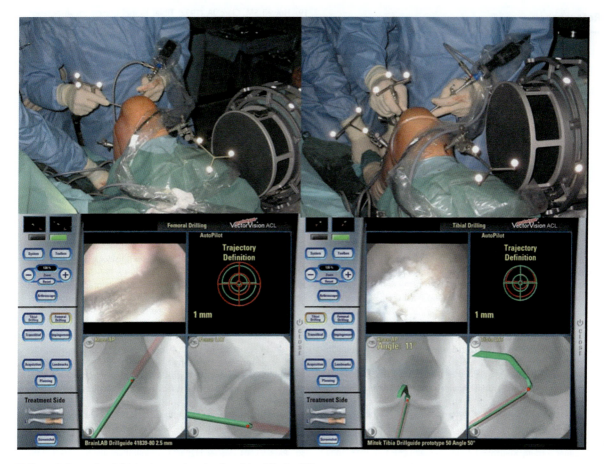

□ Fig. 41.8. Femoral and tibial arthroscopic assisted, navigated K-wire drilling

restricted to arthroscopic problems and result therefore in a considerable inter-observer and intra-observer variation since they do not allow reproducible and precise identification of landmarks. With a variability of 6 mm, arthroscopic identification of landmarks, as a basis for tunnel position calculation, does not seem to be reliable. Also image free ACL navigation systems do not allow describing the individual tunnel positions, since there is no reliable way to document and compare tunnel positions.

At the time of this writing, a first clinical feasibility study using the fluoroscopic-based ACL navigation system was finished. 25 patients were included. The system was found to be feasible in the OR with an additional time of 14 min (9–45 min) and an X-ray time of 72 s (12–145 s). The system allowed reproducible planning and comparison of tunnel positions. The technical equip-

ment needed in the OR has to be critically discussed, since it is essential for the intra-operative workflow. All patients showed 6 months postoperatively a free range of motion with stable knees in arthrometer analysis.

As far as results are analyzed at this point of time, the results are encouraging to initiate further comparative clinical studies to evaluate the benefit of this method.

Conclusion

Fluoroscopic-based ACL navigation allows reproducible planning and precise anatomical positioning of tunnels in ACL reconstruction. It is a reliable method to compare tunnel positions in ACL reconstruction and to evaluate the influence of tunnel positions on AP and rotational stability.

References

1. Paessler HH, Hoeher J (2004) Intraoperative quality control of the placement of bone tunnes for reconstruction of the anterior cruciate ligament. Unfallchirurg 107: 263–272

2. Holmes JG, James SL, Larson RL et al. (1991) Retrospective direct comparison of three intraarticular anterior cruciate ligament reconstructions. Am J Sports Med. 19: 596–600

3. Howe JG, Johnson RJ, Kaplan MJ et al. (1991) Anterior cruciate ligament reconstruction using quadriceps patellar tendon graft, part I: long term follow up. Am J Sports Med 19: 447–457

4. Panni AS, Milano G, Tartarone M et al. (2001) Clinical and radiographic results of ACL reconstruction: a 5-7-year follow-up study of outside-in versus inside-out reconstruction techniques. Knee Surg Sports Traumatol Arthrosc. 2: 77–85

5. Khalfayan EE, Sharkey SF, Alexander HA et al. (1996) The relationship between tunnel placement and clinical results after anterior cruciate ligament reconstruction. Am J Sports Med 24/3: 335–341

6. Sati M, Bourquin Y, Stäubli H, Nolte LP (2000) Considering anatomic and functional factors in ACL reconstruction: New technology. Presented at the 4th CAOS Meeting, Pittsburgh, PA, June 2000: 121–123

7. Shelbourne KD et al. (1995) Ligament stability two to six years after anterior cruciate ligament reconstruction with autogenous patellar tendon graft and participation on accelerated rehabilitation program. Am J Sports Med. 23: 575–579

8. Hefzy et al. (1986) Sensitivity of insertion locations on length pattern of anterior cruciate ligament fibers. J Biomed Engl 108: 74–82

9. Jaureguito J, Paulos L (1996) Why grafts fail. Clin Orthop Relat Res 325: 25–41

10. Oettl GM, Imhoff AB (1998) Revisionschirurgie bei fehlgeschlagener vorderer Kreuzbandplastik. Zentralbl Chir 123: 1033–1039

11. Paessler H.: Revisionseingriffe nach vorderer Kreuzbandoperation und neuerlicher Instabilität: Ursachenanalyse und taktische Vorgehen. Hefte zu »Der Unfallchirurg« 268: 447–450

12. Fu FH (2005) Editorial. Anatomical anterior ligament reconstruction: The next evolution. Operat Techn Orthop 15: 1

13. Eriksson E (2005) Preface. Do we need to perform double bundle anterior cruciate ligament reconstructions? Operative Techniques in Orthopaedics 15: 4

14. Girgis FG, Marshall JL, Monajem A (1975) The anterior cruciate ligaments of the knee joint. Anatomical, functional and experimental analysis. Clin Orthop 106: 216–231

15. Gabriel MT, Wong EK, Woo SL, Yagi M, Debski RE (2004) Distribution of in situ forces in the anterior cruciate ligament an its bundles in response to rotatory loads. J Orthop Res 22: 85–89

16. Sakane M, Fox RJ, Woo SL, Livesay GA, Li G, Fu FH (1997) In situ forces in the anterior cruciate ligament and ist bundles in response to anterior tibial loads. J Orthop Res 15: 285–293

17. Yaru NC, Daniel DM, Penner D (1997) The effect of tibial attachment site on graft impingement in anterior cruciate ligament reconstruction. Am J Sports Med. 20: 217–220

18. Romano VM, Graf BK, Keene JS, Lange RH (1993) Anterior cruciate ligament reconstruction. The effect of tibial tunnel placement on range of motion. Am J Sports Med 21: 415–418

19. Howell SM, Clarc JA (1992) Tibial tunnel placement in anterior cruciate ligament reconstruction and graft impingement. Clin Orthop 283: 187–195

20. Howell SM, Taylor MA (1993) Failure of reconstruction of the anterior cruciate ligament due to impingement by the intercondylar roof. J Bone Joint Surg Am 75:1044–1055

21. Howell SM, Clark JA, Farley TE (1992) Serial magnetic resonance study assessing the effects of impingement on the MR image of the patellar tendon graft. Arthroscopy. 8: 350–358

22. Allen CA, Giffin JR, Harner CD (2003) Revision anterior cruciate ligament reconstruction. Orthop Clin North Am 34: 79–98

23. Howell SM, Wallace MP, Hull ML, Deutsch ML (1999) Evaluation of single-incision arthroscopic technique for anterior cruciate ligament replacement. A study of tibial tunnel placement, intraoperative graft tension and stability . Am J Sports Med 27: 284–293

24. Allen CA, Giffin JR, Harner CD (2003) Revision anterior cruciate ligament reconstruction. Orthop Clin North Am 34: 79–98

25. Lo JC, Fukuda Y, Tsuda E, Steadman RJ, Fu FH, Woo SL (2003) Knee stability and graft function following anterior cruciate ligament reconstruction. Comparison between 11o'clock and 10 o'clock femoral tunnel placement. Arthroscopy 19: 297–304

26. Lintner DM, Dewitt SE, Moseley BJ (1996) Radiographic Evaluation of native anterior cruciate ligament attachments and graft placement for reconstruction. Am J Sports Med 24/1: 72–78

27. Musahl V, Burkart A, Debski RE, Scyoc A, Fu FH, Woo SL (2003) Anterior cruciate ligament tunnel placement: comparison of insertion site anatomy with the guidelines of a computer-assisted surgical system. Arthroscopy 19/2: 154–160

28. Goble EM, Downey DJ, Wilcox TR (1995) Positioning of the tibial tunnel for anterior ligament reconstruction. Arthroscopy 11: 688–695

29. Lobenhoffer P, Bernard M, Agneskircher J (2003) Quality assurance in cruciate ligament surgery. Means of assessing the drill holes in anterior cruciate ligament repair. Arthroskopie 16: 202–208

30. Paessler HH, Hoeher J (2004) Intraoperative quality control of the placement of bone tunnes for reconstruction of the anterior cruciate ligament. Unfallchirurg 107: 263–272

31. Kohn D, Beusche T, Caris J (1998) Drill hole position in endoscopic anterior cruciate ligament reconstruction. Results on an advanced arthroscopy course. Knee Surg Sports Traumatol Arthrosc 6/1: 13–15

32. Bernard M, Hertel P (1996) Intraoperative and postoperative insertion control of anterior cruciate ligament-plasty. A radiologic measuring method (quadrant method). Unfallchirurg 99: 332–340

33. Staeubli HU, Rauschnig W (1994) Tibial attachment area of the anterior cruciate ligament in the extended knee position. Knee Surg Sports Traumatol Arhtrosc 2: 138–146

34. Amis AA, Bull AMJ, Lie DTT (2005) Biomechanics of rotational instability and anatomic anterior cruciate ligament reconstruction. Operat Techn Orthop 15/1: 29–35

35. Muller-Alsbach UW, Staubli AE (2004) Computer aided ACL reconstruction. Injury 35/1: S65–67

36. Degenhart M (2004) Computer-navigated ACL reconstruction with the OrthoPilot. Surg Technol Int 12: 245–251

37. Sati M, Staubli H, Bourquin Y, Kunz M et al. (2002) Real-time computerized in situ guidance system for ACL graft placement. Comput Aided Surg 7/1: 25–40

Part IV **Total Hip Arthroplasty**

Part IV A **Navigation: Total Hip Arthroplasty**

Validation of Imageless Total Hip Navigation

J.B. Stiehl, D.A. Heck

Introduction

Optimal acetabular component orientation in total hip arthroplasty is a complex three dimensional problem with failure leading to increased wear and instability [1–6]. Although the exact frequency of acetabular component mal-position and the quantitative linkage to hip re-operation is uncertain, it is clear that at least some re-operations could be avoided through more reliable acetabular component positioning at the time of surgery. Extremes of component mal-position are associated with an increased risk of dislocation and loosening. In Lewinnek's investigation, the acetabular cup »safe zone« was radiographically identified as 15 degrees of anteversion and 40 degrees of opening angle in the performance of routine hip arthroplasty. The risk of dislocation increased from 1.5% to 6.1% if the cup was placed outside of the two degree of freedom, described »safe zone« [7]. The tolerance associated with optimal cup positioning was thought to be similar for both anteversion and opening angle at +/– 10 degrees. Computed tomography studies of post-operative cup insertions have shown that a large percentage of cases have an unacceptable positioning when depending on free-hand or conventional mechanical instrumentation [8, 9]. According to a recent European investigation of total hip arthroplasty cups positioned using manual instrumentation and evaluated using CT, it was found that only 27/105 (26%) fell within Lewinnek's safe zone [10].

Computer-assisted orthopaedic surgery has been recently defined as the ability to utilize sophisticated computer algorithms to allow the surgeon to determine three dimensional placement of total hip acetabular implants in situ. Computer-assisted navigation for acetabular cup placement requires a registration that defines the anterior pelvic plane. McKibbin et al. first defined the anterior pelvic plane as a plane connecting the ventral surfaces of the anterior superior iliac spines and the pubic tubercles of the pubic rami [11]. Basically, a cadaver pelvis was placed »table down« with these points contacting the table. Inclination and anteversion of the acetabulum were then measured in relation to this plane.

From the beginning, computed tomography was the most accurate and reliable imaging modality to define these three dimensional relationships and has a proven precision of about one millimeter or one degree [12–15]. Other methods have been sought due to the amount of resources and time required to utilize computed tomography for navigation. One promising alternative is imageless registration where simple anatomical referencing can be done at the time of the operation [16–21]. However, the laboratory validation of this clinical application is lacking. This study compared the precision, repeatability and reproducibility of these methods against known metrological and computed tomography standards.

Methods

Eight surgeons were asked to clinically evaluate the position of acetabular components after having been inserted using an anterolateral, minimally invasive surgical technique. Each surgeon was asked to clinically estimate the cup position in relationship to the anterior pelvic plane (APP). For purposes of this investigation, the APP was defined as the plane defined by the most anteriorly prominent aspect of the two anterior superior iliac spines and the most prominent, anterior portion of the symphysis pubis. The origin of the APP was defined as the midpoint of the line defined by the two ASISs. A right hand coordinate system with positive X directed toward the right acetabulum (resurfaced with prosthetic cup), positive Y directed anteriorly and positive Z directed superiorly was arbitrarily chosen (⬛ Figs. 42.1 to 42.3).

On a single reference cadaver eight surgeons then used the Medtronic Treon Plus[1] system and a custom software package to measure the component position. For the assessment of repeatability and reproducibility, each surgeon was randomly asked to re-reference the APP and to determine the position of the acetabular cup with eight independent repetitions. The cadaver was then assessed clinically using computed tomography (CT). Each cadaver was repositioned prior to each scan. CT scanning was performed using a Phillips' Brilliance 16 series computerized tomographic machine. One millimeter thick slices were obtained at 0.5 mm. increments. The machine was set at 140 KVP and 450 MAS. 3D reconstruction was carried out using the image reconstruction filter B, prior to measurement. During measurement, the CT images

were positioned such that the two reference planes were perpendicular to the plane of the monitor. This isolated the measurement plane to that being viewed (⬛ Figs. 42.4, 42.5) The Phillips angle and ruler image tools were used

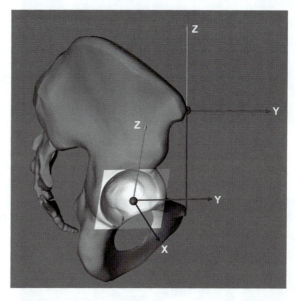

⬛ **Fig. 42.2.** Schematic pelvic diagram demonstrating calculation of anterior pelvic plane and the acetabular inclination and anteversion from lateral view

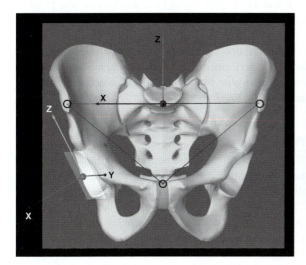

⬛ **Fig. 42.1.** Schematic pelvic diagram demonstrating calculation of anterior pelvic plane and the acetabular inclination and anteversion from anterior posterior view

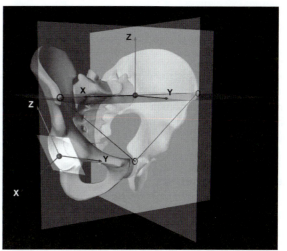

⬛ **Fig. 42.3.** Schematic pelvic diagram demonstrating calculation of anterior pelvic plane and the acetabular inclination and anteversion from oblique view

42

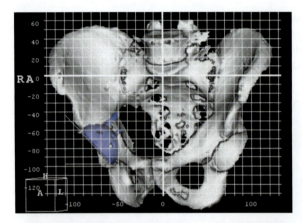

Fig. 42.4. Grid used for assessment of CT reconstruction for measuring acetabular inclination

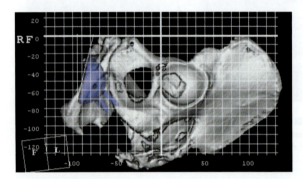

Fig. 42.5. Grid used for assessment of CT reconstruction for measuring acetabular anteversion

for measurement. This strategy allowed the direct measurement of independent DOFs without the need for projectional or magnification correction. A single trained, observer performed these multiple measurements in a masked fashion.

Surgeon Characteristics

The surgeons, who participated in the trial, ranged in age from 39 to 55 years of age. All surgeons were male. They averaged 19 (2–32) years from completion of their residency training. Four (44%) of the surgeons had previously used CAOS techniques previously. Seven of the eight American Board of Orthopaedic Surgery (ABOS)

eligible surgeons were certified by the American Board of Orthopaedic Surgery. One of the surgeons had completed Osteopathic training and was not ABOS certified. Seven of the eight respondents used minimally invasive surgical techniques in the performance of total hip arthroplasty. The surgeons stated that they had performed 84 (30–250) total hip arthroplasties and 123 (30–290) total knee arthroplasties in the past year.

Statistics

Descriptive statistics were calculated using Excel 2003 and Minitab version 14.2. A probability of less than 0.05 was selected for statistical significance. Process capability analysis was done with a threshold of Cp>1.3; Cpk>2.0. This method is described elsewhere.

Results

Absolute Assessment Measures and Variability

For eight surgeon, assessment of clinical cues from the conventional instruments yielded mean acetabular inclination of 44° (SD = 5.35°) and anteversion of 12.29 (SD = 1.06°). Using the imageless optical tracking referencing surgical navigation, mean acetabular inclination was 43.59° (SD = 3.56°) and anteversion was 17.03° (SD = 1.01°). For one observer with 3D computed tomography, acetabular inclination was 44.05° (SD = 1.07) with anteversion of 12,8° (SD = 0.087°). Based upon the modeling performed, the variations were most dependent upon the surgeon performing the assessment and ranged from 0.877 to 7.63.

Process Capability

Using the data from this experiment and clinical component specification limits associated with the avoidance of dislocation, C_p and C_{pk} were determined. (Table 42.1) The only process that consistently approaches very high quality manufacturing process capability is that using 3D CT for assessment of cup position. With 3D CT in the assessment of acetabular inclination the C_{pk} was 2.81. In the assessment of anteversion C_{pk} was 4.38. The optical tracking system (C_{pk} = 2.73) was six sigma process capable in the assessment of acetabular component anteversion.

▣ Table 42.1. Data from assessment of acetabular inclination and anteversion with process capability analysis. (Note: Upper and lower limits of +/– 10º; acceptable limits: Cp.1.3; Cpk>2.0) * Denotes below of process capability

Technique	Attitude	Standard Deviation	Mean	UCL	LCL	Cp	Cpk
Clinical	Inclination	5.35	40	50	30	0.62*	0.56*
	Anteversion	1.06	15	25	5	3.14	1.11*
Optical Tracking	Inclination	3.566	40	50	30	0.93*	0.88*
	Anteversion	1.01	15	25	5	3.30	2.73
3D CT	Inclination	1.065	40	50	30	3.13	2.81
	Anteversion	0.31	15	25	5	10.75	4.36

Surgeons, as a group, using visual cues alone, were unable to meet process specification associated with current definitions of high quality, rigorous manufacturing processes. The point picking surgical navigation technologies did not improve the surgeons' capabilities in the determination of acetabular inclination.

Discussion

Computed tomographic assessment of both acetabular inclination and anteversion was found to be process capable for the specification limits associated with dislocation avoidance based upon the measurements taken by one observer. The imageless referenced optical tracking surgical navigation system was process capable in the assessment only of acetabular anteversion. Unfortunately, when using clinical assessment alone, the participating surgeons' were not able to meet the rigorous process capabilities as used in other industries to address Lewinick's criteria for dislocation avoidance associated with cup mal-position. If more rigorous specification limits, such as those that have been proposed to avoid edge impingement, were set as boundary conditions, surgeons and imageless hip CAS applications are currently unable to achieve the desired level of accuracy or process capability.

It is possible that with improvements in the definition and determination of the pelvic plane, additional surgeon training and experience, that the effectiveness of these assessment systems may improve. It is also probable that with additional technical innovation, especially in approaches that will allow referencing improvement, that these systems may be able to have further improvement in their process capabilities. If the surgeon had a wider field of view, such as that associated with more extensile surgical approaches, it is possible that the ability to assess position might have been improved. However, based upon the single report of using conventional open surgical approaches in-vivo, it was found that the use of a CT based CAOS was required to improve both of the two degree of freedom accuracy and process capability in acetabular inclination and anteversion [22].

The findings of our current study are consistent with other recent work with imageless applications for the hip, and that is that point picking is problematic, especially for determining the transverse plane of the pelvis [16–19]. Anatomically, the anterior superior iliac spine is a relatively broad zone, and hitting a point that matches on both sides is difficult. Additionally, certain currently available systems have recommended that superficial skin surface point matching is suitable for referencing. We would disagree based on our current study. Recent studies have suggested that the error from these superficial methods approaches 0.5 degrees for one millimeter of discrepancy. For the pubic symphysis with a layer of fat that approximates 10 millimeters, this could for an error of at least 5°.

In conclusion, we believe that computer-assisted surgical applications will be needed to improve the overall precision of acetabular component positioning. From our analysis, computed tomography applications for CAS are currently process capable and this remains consistent with recent prior literature that confirms a precision of 1°/1 mm of reproducibility measures with these systems. We found determination of cup anteversion to be process capable for imageless hip applications but not for determining cup inclination. This most likely reflects the inability to accurately establish a transverse plane from point picking of the anterior superior iliac spines, at least done by current methodologies. In the future, it is possible that combinations of technologies will be needed to accurately reference the target anatomy.

References

1. Bader RJ, Steinhauser E, Willmann G, Gradinger R (2001) The effects of implant position, design, and wear on the range of motion after total hip arthroplasty. Hip International 11: 80–90
2. Giurea A, Zehetgruber H, Funovics P, Grampp S, Karamat L, Gott-sauner-Wolf F (2001) Riskfactors for Dislocation in cementless Hip arthroplasty- A statistical analysis: Z Orthop 139: 194–199
3. Jolles BM, Zangger P, Leyvraz PF (2002) Factors predisposing to dislocation after primary total hip arthroplasty. J Arthroplasty 17: 282–288
4. Kennedy JG, Rogers WB, Soffe KE, Sullivan RJ, Griffen DG, Sheehan LJ (1998) Effect of acetabular component orientation on recurrent dislocation, pelvic osteolysis, polyethylene wear and component migration. J Arthroplasty 13: 530–534
5. Kummer FJ, Shah S, Iyer S, DiCesare PE (1999) The effect of acetabular cup orientations on limiting hip rotation. J Arthroplasty 14: 509–513
6. Schmalzried TP, Guttmann D, Grecula M, Amstutz HC (1994) The relationship between the design, position and articular wear of acetabular components inserted without cement and the developement of pelvic osteolysis. J Bone Joint Surg 76A: 677–688
7. Lewinnek GE, Lewis JL, Tarr R, Compere CL, Zimmermann JR (1978) Dislocations after total hip replacement arthroplasties. J Bone Joint Surg Am 60: 217–221
8. Saxler G, Marx A, Vandevelde D et al. (2004) The accuracy of free-hand cup positioning: A CT based measurement of cup placement in 105 total hip arthroplasties. Int Orthop 28: 198–201
9. DiGioa AM, Jaramaz B, Plakseychuk AY, Moody JE, Nikou C, LaBarca RS, Levison TJ, Picard F (2002) Comparison of a mechanical acetabular alignment guide with computer placement of the socket. J Arthroplasty 17: 359–364
10. Seki M, Yuasa N, Ohkuni K (1998) Analysis of optimal range of socket orientations in total hip arthroplasty with use of computer-aided design simulation. J Orthop Res 16: 513–517
11. McKibbin B (1970) Anatomical factors in the stability of the hip joint in the newborn. J Bone Joint Surg 52B: 148–159
12. Leenders T, Vandervelde D, Nahiew G, Nuyts R (2002) Reduction in variability of acetabular cup abduction using computed assisted surgery: Prospective and randomized study. Comput Aided Surg 7: 99–106
13. Sugano N, Sasama T, Sato Y, Nakajima Y, Nishii T, Yonenobu K, Tamura S, Ochi T (2003) Accuracy evaluation of surface-based registration methods in a computer navigation system for hip surgery performed through a posterolateral approach. Comput Aided Surg 6: 195–203
14. Khadem R, Yeh C, Sadeghi-Tehrani JM (2000) Comparative tracking error analysis of five different optical tracking systems. Comput Aid Surg 5: 98
15. Widmer K-H, Zurfluh B (2004) Compliant positioning of total hip components for optimal range of motion. J Orthop Res 22: 815–821
16. Kalteis T, Handel M, Bäthis H, Perlick L, Tingart M, Grifka J (2006) Imageless navigation for insertion of the acetabular component in total hip arthroplasty: Is it as accurate as CT based navigation. J Bone Joint Surg 88B: 163–167
17. Kalteis T, Handel M, Herold T et al. (2005) Greater accuracy in positioning of the acetablular hip by using an image-free navigation system. Int Orthop 29: 272–276
18. Kalteis T, Beckmann J, Herold T, Zysk S, Bathis H, Perlick L, Grifka J (2004) Accuracy of an image-free cup navigation system. An anatomical study. Biomed Tech (Berlin) 49: 257–262
19. Nogler M, Kessler O, Prassl A, Donnelly B, Streicher R, Sledge JB, Krismer M (2004) Reduced variability of acetabular cup positioning with use of an imageless navigation system.Clin Orthop Relat Res 426:159–163
20. Grutzner PA, Zheng G, Langlotz U, von Recum J, Nolte LP, Wentzensen A, Widmer (2004) C-arm based navigation in total hip arthroplasty-background and clinical experience. Injury 35 (Suppl 1): S-A90–5
21. Zheng G, Marx A, Langlotz U, Widmer KH, Buttaro M, Nolte LP (2002) A hybrid CT-free navigation system for total hip arthroplasty. Comput Aided Surg 7(3): 129–145
22. Haaker R, Tiedjen K, Ottersbach A, Stiehl JB, Rubenthaler F, Shockheim M (2006) Comparison of freehand versus computer assisted acetabular cup Implantation. J Arthroplasty (accepted)

Cup and Stem Navigation with the Orthopilot System

H. Kiefer, A. Othman

Introduction

Navigation systems are designed to measure and display several parameters of implant position to support the surgeon during bone preparation and implant alignment. The introduction of navigation systems for hip arthroplasty started in the late 90-ties. Image based systems [1–5] and non-image-based systems [6–10] have shown that the basic principles of hip-implant alignment can be measured and monitored. Independent from navigation technology, the surgeon's individual experience has to be encountered, too [11].

The kinematic principles of the CT-free Orthopilot navigation system for hip arthroplasty were first presented in 2001 [6]. Since 2004 also the stem position can be navigated using additional femoral references [12, 13].

Methods

The Orthopilot navigation system references the instruments with a 3-dimensional infrared camera with passive tracking technology. Bone landmarks are acquired by pointer palpation, the hip center is acquired kinematically. ◻ Table 43.1 and ◻ Fig 43.1 summarize the Orthopilot THA navigation 2.0 workflow with referencing and surgery steps:

The acetabular bone sensor reference is fixed at the iliac crest. The femoral sensor is fixed with a special c-clamp to the proximal femur. The sensors are modular and can be removed for different surgical steps. Both sensors are necessary for initial hip joint alignment recording. The acetabular sensor is only needed for the workflow steps 2–9, the femoral sensor for the steps 10 to 12 (◻ Fig. 43.2 and 43.3).

Values for cup inclination and anteversion are referenced to the transcutaneous palpation of the anterior

◻ Table 43.1. OrthoPilot® THA navigation 2.0 workflow referencing and surgery steps

1. Initial hip joint alignment
2. Anterior acetabular plane registration
3. Medial wall registration
4. Hip joint center reference
5. Patella reference
6. Ankle reference
7. Navigated reaming of the acetabulum
8. Navigated cup implantation
9. Referencing of new acetabular center
10. Navigated femoral box osteotome positioning
11. Navigated femoral rasp positioning
12. Measurement femoral implant position

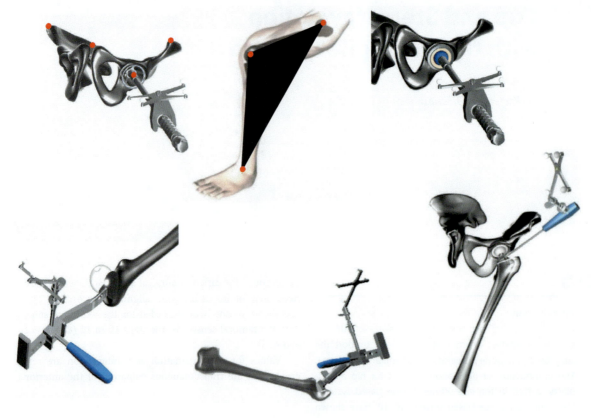

☐ **Fig 43.1.** OrthoPilot® THA navigation 2.0 referencing and basic surgery steps

pelvic plane. Antetorsion values of the femoral stem implant are computed by hip joint center reference, patella and ankle reference in flexed knee position. Changes of leg length and femoral offset are calculated from the difference to the initial hip-joint alignment. All changes of the functional hip center by acetabular reaming and cup implantation are displayed in 3 dimensions. The antetorsion position of the box osteotome, rasp and hip stem are displayed at any time of femoral preparation. Implant-related range-of-motion data is computed for the selected implant components.

Values of implant or instrument position are displayed as relative or absolute data in mm or degree. The accuracy is influenced by the palpation of bony references. Implant and instrument positions are chosen by the surgeon according to the pre-operative plan and the intra-operative situation.

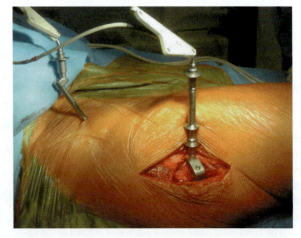

☐ **Fig 43.2.** Acetabular and femoral bone sensors (iliac screw and c-clamp)

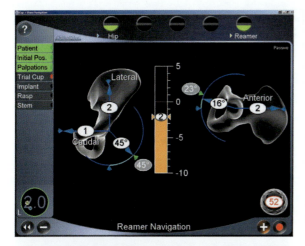

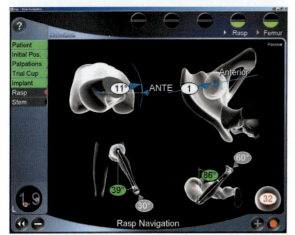

Fig 43.3. Examples of the OrthoPilot® THA 2.0 navigation sceens (Step 7 – navigated reaming of the acetabulum, Step 11 – navigated femoral rasp positioning)

Acetabular Cup Center

Relative three-dimensional data (mm) based on a trial cup registration of the unreamed acetabulum compared with the reamed situation.

Reamer and Cup Inclination and Anteversion

Absolute data (degree) based on the palpation of the anterior pelvic plane. The intra-operative decision for a

certain value of inclination and anteversion must include the consideration of the pelvic tilt position pre-operatively and post-operatively and the palpation accuracy at the symphysis.

Femoral Implant Position (Rotation)

Relative data (alignment) based on the acetabular center after cup implantation and the measurement of femoral rotation (i.e. torsion indicated as antetorsion or retrotorsion). Absolute data (degree) is displayed as the deviation from the sagittal femoral plane (defined by hip joint, patella and ankle joint)

Leg-length Differences Pre- and Intra-Operatively

Relative data (mm) of the pre- and intra-operative hip-joint situation. Pre-operative plan of necessary corrections of leg-length discrepancies are needed to choose the preferred implant position.

Femoral Offset Values Pre- and Intra-Operatively

Relative data (mm) of the pre- and intra-operative joint situation. Intra-operative data is referenced to the initial registration of hip joint alignment.

Range of Motion Values

Absolute data (degree) computed by the impingement free range of motion as a function of implant position and implant selection. Implant component data is available within the data file for the selected implant components.

Cup and stem positioning data of 80 consecutive total hip replacements with complete data and X-ray records were analyzed using the Orthopilot 2.0 THA application. The patients received navigated THA between 04/2005 and 12/2005. Patient position was supine, and cementless THA implant components were implanted with a standard transgluteal approach in all cases. A non-navigated control group was not defined during this series.

Cup position was analyzed on standard AP X-rays using the method of [14] for the cup anteversion value. The

43

axial hip stem position was analyzed by changes of leg length (X-ray examination). X-rays (supine patient position) were taken at time of hospital discharge and compared with the Orthopilot data records (cup inclination and anteversion, leg length and femoral offset difference pre-/post-operatively).

Results

80 navigated THA records were analyzed. The average patient age at time of THA was 69.4 years. Average time of THA surgery was 110 min and hospital discharge at 15.3 days. There was no early implant related post-operative complication as dislocation or implant instability at time of hospital discharge.

77 (96%) acetabular cups were positioned inside a target safe zone of 42.5±10 degrees radiological inclination and 12.5±10 degrees radiological anteversion (■ Fig 43.4). 2 cups were positioned with zero degree anteversion and one cup with 31 deg inclination. No cup was found in a retroverted position.

Data of femoral stem position was complete for 80 THA but 2 records were excluded because of non-consistent navigation values of changes for leg length and femoral offset. The remaining data records showed an average leg lengthening of 7.1 mm (min. −4.5 mm max. 22 mm). The maximum values of changes of femoral offset medialization or lateralization were 20 mm (■ Fig 43.5).

The comparison of intra-operative (Orthopilot data record) and post-operative data (X-ray measurements) was found to differ with different standard deviation for cup inclination (3.66 degrees), cup anteversion (6.86 degrees) and leg length (4.58 mm). The average data difference values for inclination (1.20 degrees) and stem length (0.22 mm) was smaller because of positive and negative data differences. The average data difference values for anteversion was mainly positive and the 6.86 degrees standard deviation higher compared to inclination (■ Table 43.2).

Discussion

The presented image-free navigation system is in routine use in our institution since 2001. The positioning of cup implants has shown reproducible results in terms of our safe-zone definitions of ±10 degrees, even if our

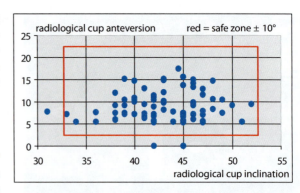

■ **Fig 43.4.** Acetabular cup inclination and anteversion values (X-ray measurements)

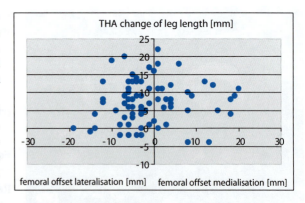

■ **Fig 43.5.** Intra-operative values for changes of leg length and femoral offset (OrthoPilot® data record)

investigation on routine standard X-rays contains certain inaccuracies.

Also existing inaccuracies of manual pelvic palpation do not lead to mal-positioning of cup components. These inaccuracies are ±3 degrees (±6 degrees) inclination for 10 mm (20 mm) palpation inaccuracy and +4 degrees to +12 degrees anteversion for 10 to 30 mm. The navigation inaccuracies for femoral stem position are mainly given by the stability of femoral bone reference fixation.

As we are aware of the excellent technological accuracy of the Orthopilot system, and we try to improve our manual skills of bone referencing, as well as the understanding of pathological and physiological changes of the pre- and post-operative pelvic tilt situation.

Our data for stem positioning shows the individual change of leg length which was achieved in the study

◻ Table 43.2. Data differences Orthopilot values minus X-ray measurement values

	Cup n=80	Cup n=80	THA n=78
	Inclination [degrees]	Anteversion [degrees]	Leg length [mm]
Average	1.20	7.00	0.22
Standard deviation	3.66	6.86	4.58

series. The comparison of X-ray and navigation data was within an acceptable accuracy. The values of femoral offset change represent realistic values for the straight stem implant which was used. However these values cannot be measured or validated on X-rays.

Conclusion

We are using the THA navigation technology as a routine procedure in our institution, and the confidence for acetabular cup position is well established during more than 1000 procedures. The navigation of the femoral stem component is at the beginning and the measured values are not all understood in order to optimize the placement of THA implant components. As the presented THA navigation system measures certain parameters the surgeon must be able to select the appropriate ones for the individual patient situation.

References

1. Bernsmann K, Langlotz U, Ansari B, Wiese M (2001) Computer-assisted navigated cup placement of different cup types in hip arthroplasty – a randomized controlled trial. Z Orthop 139(6): 512–517

2. Leenders T, Vandevelde D, Mahieu G, Nuyts R (2002) Reduction in variability of acetabular cup abduction using computer assisted surgery: a prospective and randomized study. Computer Aided Surg 7(2): 99–106

3. Hube R, Birke A, Hein W, Klima S (2003) CT-based and fluoroscopy-based navigation for cup implantation in total hip arthroplasty (THA). Surg Technol Int 11: 275–280

4. Gruetzner PA, Zheng G, Langlotz U, von Recum J, Nolte LP, Wentzensen A, Widmer KH, Wendl K (2004) C-arm based navigation in total hip arthroplasty-background and clinical experience. Injury 35 (Suppl 1): A90–95

5. Saxler G, Marx A, Vandevelde D et al. (2004) The accuracy of freehand cup positioning – a CT based measurement of cup placement in 105 total hip arthroplasties. Int Orthop 28(4): 198–201

6. Richolt JA, Mollard B, Leitner F, Reu G, Graichen H, Froehling M (2001) A simplified Navigation System for Hip Cup Implantation System Description and Report of first Cases. Poster presented at International CAOS Symposium, February 7–10, Davos, Switzerland

7. Kiefer H (2003) OrthoPilot cup navigation – how to optimize cup positioning? Int Orthop 27 (Suppl 1): 37–42

8. Stipcak V, Stoklas J, Hart R, Janecek M (2004) Implantation of a non-cemented acetabulum with the use of a navigation system – (Article in Czech). Acta Chir Orthop Traumatol Cech 71(5): 288–291

9. Nogler M, O Kessler, O Prassel, B Donnelly, RM Streicher, M Krismer (2004) Reduction variability of acetabular cup positioning using an imageless navigation system: a cadaver study. Clin Orthop 426: 159–163

10. Kalteis T, Handel M, Herold T, Perlick L, Baethis H, Grifka J (2005) Greater accuracy in positioning of the acetabular cup by using an image-free navigation system. Int Orthop 29(5): 272–276

11. Honl M, Dierk O, Gauck C, Carrero V, Lampe F, Dries S, Quante M, Schwieger K, Hille E, Morlock M (2003) Comparison of robotic-assisted and manual implantation of a primary total hip replacement. A prospective study. J Bone Joint Surg 85A(8): 1470–1478

12. Kiefer H, Othman A (2005) OrthoPilot total hip arthroplasty workflow and surgery. Orthopedics 28(10 Suppl): s1221–1226

13. Lazovic D, Kaib N (2005) Results with navigated Bicontact total hip arthroplasty. Orthopedics. 28(10 Suppl): s1227–1233

14. Pradhan R (1999) Planar anteversion of the acetabular cup as determined from plain anteroposterior radiographs. J Bone Joint Surg Br 81: 431–435

Imageless Cup and Stem Navigation in Dysplastic Hips with the Navitrack and Vector Vision Systems

J. Babisch, F. Layher, K. Sander

Introduction

Total hip arthroplasty performed for developmental dysplasia of the hip has a higher incidence of complications than total hip arthroplasty for primary degenerative arthritis [8]. The poorer results appear to correlate with the severity of the hip deformity and thus with the misalignment of the hip prosthesis. With an incidence of between 1% and 10% in primary and in revision total hip replacements, dislocations and fractures are second in frequency only to aseptic loosening as a cause for revision surgery [9, 16]. Contrary to knee replacements, where deformities of the joint axis of only 10° are clinically apparent, mal-positions of one or both components of a stable, non-dislocated hip are difficult to recognize. Nevertheless, they are important factors influencing the incidence of impingement, polyethylene wear and aseptic loosening of hip endoprostheses [5, 10, 15].

In the past 10 years, computer-assisted surgery has been introduced for hip replacement [4]. The aim is even more precise placement of the prosthesis. The necessity of pre-operative computed tomography (CT) scans in CT-based navigation has been a deterrent to practical application. For this reason, we have been involved in the development of the imageless navigation systems Navitrack (Orthosoft/Zimmer) and Vector Vision (Brainlab). These systems are intended to provide the surgeon with information not only about the anteversion and inclination of the cup, but also about the anteversion of the stem, changes in femoral offset and the resulting leg length.

Technique of Imageless Navigation

In the CT-free technique of optoelectronic navigation, the following basic principles must be observed:

1. Even with imageless navigation, the goal of surgery must be defined in the course of *pre-operative planning*. Particularly in hip dysplasias, joint geometry has to be designed a new with repositioning of the center of rotation and compensation of any difference in leg length. Despite the 3D navigation we still use X-ray images for conventional 2D planning by means of X-ray templates. Even more precise is computer-aided planning on X-ray images using the MediCAD system, which not only helps select the appropriate implant size but enables biomechanical evaluation of the chosen joint geometry by means of a 12-point score (biomechanics score, BLB score) [1].

2. In the next step, calibration of the special *surgical instruments* is required. For the stem navigation the tool set consisting of pointer, reamer and cup impactor is extended by a »femoral canal digitizer« (Navitrack) and a navigated broach handle. A reference star on these tools with three infrared light-reflecting spheres enables the 3D tracking of the instruments.

3. Using 5-mm Schanz screws or percutaneous threaded pins, the *dynamic reference base* (DRB) has to be securely fixed to the pelvis and, with a separate 5-mm skin incision, to the middle third of the femur.

4. Both image-based and image-free navigation systems use the anatomic anterior pelvic plane (PAP) as a uniform reference. The frontal plane is defined anatomi-

cally by the bilateral anterior superior iliac spines and the pubic tubercle. These points are digitized during the process of *pelvic registration* using a registration pointer. If there is a thick fat pad over the bone, this pointer should puncture the skin.

5. During *femur registration* the frontal plane of the femur is determined by taking points from the medial and lateral femoral condyle and additional points from the tip of trochanter major (Vector Vision and Navitrack) or from the malleoli of the ankle and from the femoral canal with a femoral canal digitizer (Navitrack). Additionally, we register three points in the plane of the operating table to obtain information about the tilt of the pelvic frontal plane in relation to the table (◻ Fig. 44.1 and 44.2).

6. The main difference of the CT-free technique from CT-based navigation is the registration and virtual representation of the anatomy of the hip joint. The surgeon requires a realistic *virtual illustration of the individual anatomical bone structures*, particularly in the presence of secondary deformities of the acetabulum and femur. The contours of the bone and the axis of the femur can be visualized by touching bone landmarks with a pointer. The 3D shapes of the acetabulum and femur are represented as a individual mosaic model (Navitrack) or as a virtual statistical bone model (Vector Vision) on the screen. The Navitrack-registration locates the old center of rotation (CR) with 16 points on the inner surface of the acetabulum. The Vector Vision system calculates the CR using a kinematic registration technique. Additional intra-operative fluoroscopy is not required.

7. We usually begin with the navigation of the cup. During reaming und impaction of the press-fit cup the navigation system shows not only inclination and anteversion but also mediolateral and craniocaudal displacement of the CR. During stem navigation, with each impacting of the rasp the position of the rasp itself, together with the varus or valgus position and anteversion of the stem, can be followed on the screen. As a result of the combined cup and stem navigation the leg length and femoral offset changes are monitored in real time while the femoral canal is prepared.

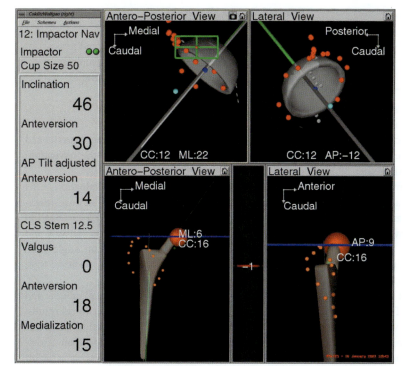

◻ **Fig. 44.1.** Cup and stem navigation (Navitrack)

44

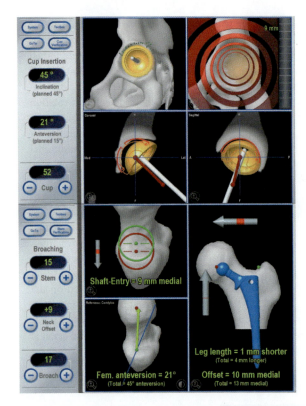

Fig. 44.2. Cup and stem navigation (Vector Vision)

Material and Methods

Clinical investigations with the imageless navigation began in February 2002 (Navitrack) and July 2004 (Vector Vision). Initially the development was characterized by upgrades of the software and stepwise improvements in the instruments to the actual level. Altogether 88 hip endoprostheses were implanted using combined stem and cup navigation. With experience of CT-based and CT-free navigation, and after overcoming the learning curve, we extended the indication for imageless navigation of THA to dysplastic hip arthritis.

With the hypothesis that computer-assisted planning and navigation of the THA would be more accurate and yield better clinical results we started a controlled prospective randomized study comparing CT-free navigation with the conventional surgical technique of THA. The examinations were accepted by the ethics commission responsible for our department. Informed consent was obtained from all patients. Patients with unilateral coxarthrosis secondary to congenital diseases such as dysplasia of the hip were enrolled into the study and randomly divided into two groups.

Navigation Group (Group 1)

Thirty-seven patients were randomly assigned to:
- computer-assisted planning and biomechanical analysis of the pre-operative hip geometry with determination of the optimal THA position using planning software MediCAD [1];
- imageless cup and stem navigation (10 THA with Duraloc press-fit cup and Vision 2000 stem implanted with Vector Vision navigation, 27 THA with Allofit press-fit cups and CSL stem with Navitrack navigation);
- supine position of the patient; lateral transgluteal approach.

All operations were performed by two experienced surgeons.

Control Group (Group 2)

Thirty-seven patients were randomly assigned to:
- conventional planning of THA using templates;
- conventional »free-hand« surgical technique;
- supine position of the patient;
- lateral transgluteal approach.

All operations were performed by three experienced surgeons using the same implants as in the navigation group.

At 6–8 months after surgery, detailed evaluation of the clinical results was performed. The data from post-operative CT scans of the pelvis were loaded into the navigation workstation. Using the CT-based navigation software and Murray's radiological definition of the cup angle [12], the cup position and pelvic tilt in supine position were measured.

The Harris hip score [7] and the Merle d'Aubigne and Postel score [11] were used to evaluate the clinical results. This outcome assessment was accompanied by measures of general health-related quality of life (36-Item Short-Form Health Survey, SF-36) and of disease-specific health

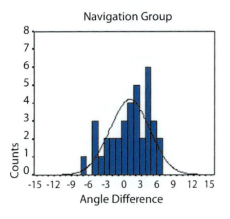

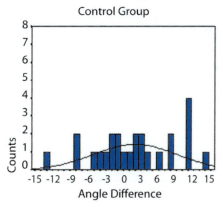

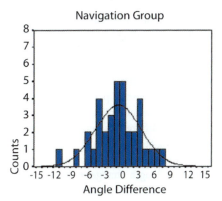

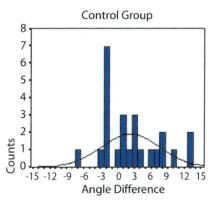

Fig. 44.3. Differences between the postoperative acetabular orientation as measured on CT scans and the optimal orientation

(Western Ontario and McMaster Universities Osteoarthritis Index, WOMAC score) [3,17].

Statistical analysis was performed with SPSS software using Student's *t*-test or the Mann–Whitney *U*-test after testing the distribution of the data by means of the Shapiro–Wilk test. Values of $p<0.05$ were regarded as significant.

Results

Experience with CT-based and also with imageless navigated total hip replacements (THR) in dysplastic hip arthritis has demonstrated high inter-subject variability and a trend towards anterior rotation of the iliac spines relative to the os pubis (pelvic flexion, anterior tilt of pelvic plane) with the patient standing and lying supine. In hip dysplasia we measured in this study a mean pelvic tilt angle of –13.8° (SD 6.1°, range –27° to –3°) Pelvic tilt variances should be taken into consideration in acetabular component positioning. The Lewinnek »safe zone« of cup alignment recommends 40° inclination and 15° anteversion in relation to the operating table in supine position [10]. If the surgeon aligns the cup with 15° anteversion relative to the anterior pelvic plane, even in cases with high anterior pelvic tilt (anterior flexion of the pelvis), the result is inaccurate cup alignment. The cup would show a low anteversion/retroversion with regard to the table plane, corresponding to a higher risk of hip dislocation [2]. Therefore we used tilt-adjusted cup anteversion

◻ Table 44.1. Results of post-operative CT analysis

	Navigation group (n=37) (Navitrack 27, Vector Vision 10) Post-operative CT (n=35) (Navitrack 26, Vector Vision 9)	Control group (n=37) Post-operative CT (n=25)
Inclination	Outliers in postoperative CT: Navitrack 0 Vector Vision 0	Outliers in postoperative CT: 6
Anteversion	Outliers in postoperative CT: Navitrack 0 VectorVision 1	Outliers in postoperative CT: 2
10° PE liner	1	6
Dislocations	0	1

Deviations of cup angle of more than 10° from the optimum are defined as outliers

and inclination with higher anteversion in cases of pelvic flexion. The Navitrack system calculates this adjusted inclination and anteversion after measuring the pelvic tilt angle. Using the Vector Vision system we developed a nomogram for calculation of tilt-adjusted cup angles. Deviation of the pelvic tilt of 1° of flexion/extension from the neutral 0° position leads to an increase/decrease in the optimal anteversion of about 0.75° and in the optimal inclination of about 0.3°.

◻ Table 44.1 shows the post-operative CT measurements.

The CT measurements of deviation from optimal cup position showed a wider distribution of cup angles in group 2 than in the navigated cups in group 1 (◻ Fig. 44.3).

Post-operative biomechanical analyses with the MediCAD planning system also demonstrated successful re-creation of biomechanically favorable joint geometry despite the pre-existing deformity. The difference in biomechanical score between the two groups is significant and seems to indicate superiority of the exact planning enabled by the MediCAD system and the successful realization of the planning by means of hip navigation (◻ Fig. 44.4).

The HHS and Merle d'Aubigne and Postel score also indicated a significantly better outcome of the patients after navigated THR; however, the SF-36 and the WOMAC score showed no statistically relevant differences between the two groups (◻ Fig. 44.5).

Only combined cup and stem navigation enables digital monitoring of changes in leg length. Differences in

leg length of over 3 cm are frequently found in unilateral grade 2 or 3 hip dysplasia according to Crowe classification. In such cases leg lengthening to compensate this difference in full would greatly increase the risk of nerve lesions. In this study, therefore, the safely attainable degree of leg lengthening was planned preoperatively and discussed with the patient. Lengthening of more than 3 cm was not planned. The differences between planned and achieved leg lengthening are shown in ◻ Fig. 44.6. The results are a testimony to the superiority of the precise real-time calculation of leg length change in the navigation system over the conventional manual technique in group 2.

Discussion and Conclusions

Mal-position of one or both components and soft tissue imbalance are important factors influencing the incidence of impingement, dislocations, polyethylene wear and aseptic loosening of hip endoprostheses [5, 10, 15]. To overcome the inaccuracy of conventional free-hand cup and stem implantation and to translate the pre-operative planning exactly into the surgery, hip navigation systems supporting not only the acetabular cup impaction but also the stem implantation were developed. Our study is not yet complete, but the results seem to confirm the hypothesis that the advantages of this computer-assisted technology outweigh the disadvantages for hip navigation. Our results and experiences can be summarized as follows:

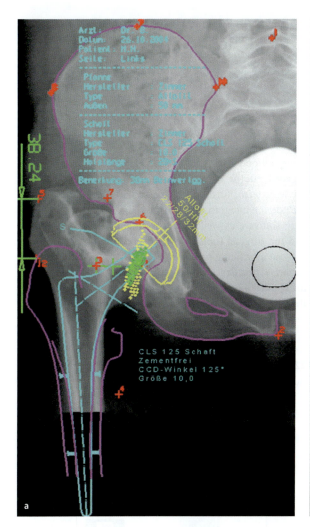

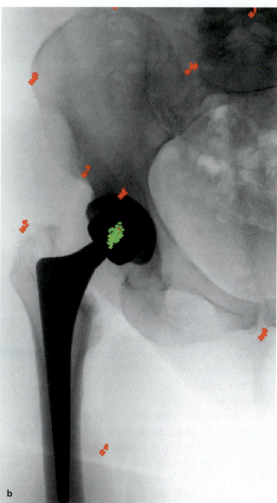

■ **Fig. 44.4a–c.** Biomechanical assessment in MediCAD. **a** Pre-operative joint geometry and planning, **b** post-operative joint geometry, **c** pre- and post-operative BLB-Scores

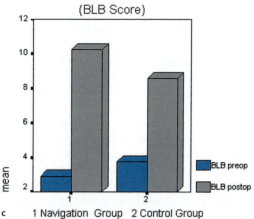

44

1. Imageless combined hip navigation requires precise determination of the pre-operative center of rotation. The CR serves as a reference point for calculation of changes of position of cup and stem. Notwithstanding the deformation of the acetabulum and femoral head in hip dysplasia, the CR could be ascertained with sufficient accuracy in all patients. The precondition for CR determination is the digitization of 16 points on the acetabulum, avoiding large bony defects (Navitrack), or a kinematic analysis (Vector Vision) before the resection of the stabilizing joint capsule.

2. All previous navigation systems used the anatomical anterior pelvic plane as reference for cup alignment, but this can lead to mal-positions in the case of a high pelvic tilt angle, particularly in hip dysplasia. The results of other studies on pelvic tilt must therefore be given greater consideration than has previously been the case [13]. The Navitrack system is the first to feature tilt-adjusted cup navigation. With the above-mentioned correction of the inclination and anteversion angles we attained acetabular stability in all patients in group 1. In this group there were no dislocations, in only one patient was an extended 10° PE liner used, and only 1 outlier were detected on postoperative CT.

3. The stem navigation requires absolutely stable fixation of the femur tracker distal to the stem components, so there is no danger of it hindering the subsequent preparation of the stem. The visualization of stem anteversion, resulting leg length and resulting femur medialization on the screen during the impaction of the femoral broach proved to be the greatest advantage of the stem navigation. In most cases a trial reduction is not necessary.

4. High anteversion of the proximal femur cannot be adequately corrected unless modular shafts are used. Especially in arthritis secondary to dysplasia, however, an additional reduction of the anteversion of the acetabular component can in some cases be advantageous. The navigation can provide the surgeon with the necessary information.

5. The potential of optoelectronic cup navigation with respect to reduced variability and greater precision of acetabular positioning have already been described [6, 14]. Our results also show for the first time the advantages of combined cup and stem navigation in accomplishing the planned biomechanical joint ge-

ometry. To this end, the hip navigation must register not only the implant angle, but also the 3D displacements of the cup, alterations in femoral offset and the cranio-caudal position of the stem.

6. The investigations described here were accompanied by analyses of gait before and 6 months after surgery by means of the Vicon system. However, evaluation of the data is not yet complete.

If the full potential of navigation is to be realized and the survival rate or comfort of the prosthesis improved in the long term, further refinements are necessary. These include the integration of biomechanically oriented planning software as well as improvements in the workflow and the surgical tools in order to reduce operating time without sacrificing precision. Similarly to CT-based navigation, a practical, simple technique must be developed for application of imageless hip navigation with the patient in the lateral position, which is required for the posterior surgical approach and the MIS approaches.

Acknowledgement. This study is part of project BA 2229/1–1 and 2229/1–2 supported by the Deutsche Forschungsgemeinschaft (DFG).

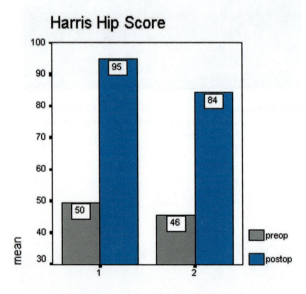

◘ Fig. 44.5. Differences in Harris hip score

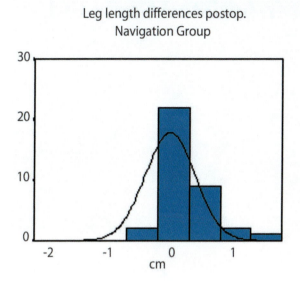

Fig. 44.6. Differences from the planned postoperative leg length

References

1. Babisch J, Layher F, Venbrocks RA, Rose I (2004) Biomechanisch fundierte Hüftoperationsplanung mit Hilfe des Softwaremoduls EndoMap (MediCAD). Electromedica, 70/1: 39–46
2. Babisch J, Layher F, Venbrocks RA (2004) Computer assisted planning and navigation using the Navitrack and MediCAD System. In: Stiehl JB, Konermann WH, Haaker RG (eds) Navigation and robotics in total joint and spine surgery. Springer, Berlin Heidelberg New York
3. Bellamy N, Buchanan W, Goldsmith CH, Campbell J, Stitt LW (1988) Validation study of WOMAC: A health status instrument for measuring clinically important patient relevant outcomes to antirheumatic drug therapy in patients with osteoarthritis of the hip and the knee. J Rheumatol 15: 1833–1840
4. DiGioia AM, Jaramaz B, Blackwell M, et al (1998) Image guided navigation system to measure intraoperatively acetabular implant alignment. Clin Orthop 355:8–22
5. Dorr LD, Wan Z (1998) Causes of and treatment protocol for Instability of total hip replacement. Clin Orthop 355: 144–151
6. Dorr LD, Hishiki Y, Wan Z, Newton D, Yun A (2005) Development of imageless computer navigation for acetabular component position in total hip replacement. Iowa Orthop J 25: 1–9
7. Harris WH (1969) Traumatic arthritis of the hip after dislocation in acetabular fractures: treatment by mold arthroplasty. J Bone Joint Surg Am 72: 737–735
8. Jasty M, Anderson MJ, Harris WH (1995) Total hip replacement for developmental dysplasia of the hip. Clin Orthop 311: 40–45
9. Lachiewicz PF, Soileau ES (2005) Changing indications for revision total hip arthroplasty. J Surg Orthop Adv 14(2): 82–84
10. Lewinnek GE, Lewis JL, Tarr R, Compere CL, Zimmermann JR (1978) Dislocations after total hip replacement arthroplasties. J Bone Joint Surg Am 60A: 217–220
11. Merle d'Aubigne R, Postel M (1954) Functional results of hip arthroplasty with acrylic prosthesis. J Bone Joint Surg Am 36: 451–457
12. Murray DW (1993) The definition and measurement of acetabular orientation. J Bone Joint Surg. Br 75: 228–232
13. Nishihara S, Sugano N, Nishii T, Ohozono K, Yoshikawa H (2003) Measurements of pelvic flexion angle using three-dimensional computed tomography. Clin Orthop 411: 140–151
14. Nogler M, Kessler O, Prassl A et al (2004) Reduced variability of acetabular cup positioning with use of imageless navigation systems. Clin Orthop 426: 159–163
15. Paterno SA, Lachiewicz PF, Kelley SS (1997)The influence of patient-related factors and the position of the acetabular component on the rate of dislocation after total hip replacement. J Bone Joint Surg Am 79: 1202–1210
16. Turner RS (1994) Postoperative total hip prosthetic femoral head dislocations. Incidence, etiologic factors and management. Clin Orthop 301: 196–204
17. Ware JE, Sherbourne CD (1992) The MOS 36-Item Short-Form Health Survey (SF-36). Med Care 30: 473–483

Navigation of Computer-Assisted Designed Hip Arthroplasty

J.-N. Argenson, S. Parratte, X. Flecher, J.-M. Aubaniac

Introduction

Acetabular and stem component mal-position during hip arthroplasty increase the risk of dislocation, reduce range of motion and may cause long-term wear. Computer assisted preoperative planning for total hip arthroplasty is used in our institution since 1990 on the basis of computer-assisted designed custom femoral stem [1]. Due to the recent developments in computer intra-operative assistance, the logical evolution was to obtain three dimensional data for intra-operative cup positioning during total hip arthroplasty (THA). After the initial work of DiGioia [2], numbers of computer-assisted orthopaedic systems have been described based on CT-based navigation or on imageless navigation. CT-based navigation need an intra-operative matching witch increases blood loss and time for surgery [3]. Among the imageless systems, one is based on Bone Morphing® technology initially described by Stindel [4] for computer assisted knee arthroplasty and adapted for THA. The principle is based on plastic intra-operative modeling of a statistical model. Thus anterior pelvic plane is registered intra-operatively by percutaneous palpation and cup impactor navigated in order to reach Lewinnek goals for cup abduction and anteversion angles. These types of imageless system do not require any extra radiation exposure for patients, or any loss of time for intra-operative matching with pre-operative planning. However, the benefits of an imageless system based on Bone Morphing® technology over freehand techniques for cup positioning should be proven.

The purpose of this study was to present the concept and evaluate the performance of dedicated software for cup positioning combined to the computer-assisted pre-operative planning routinely used in our institution for total hip arthroplasty in a prospective and randomized controlled study.

Methods

The Concept of Computer-Assisted Designed Hip Arthroplasty

The concept of individual computer-assisted design (CAD) has been the consequence of the natural evolution of the authors in the field of total hip arthroplasty (THA), facing the unacceptable failure rate of conventional cemented stems as reported in the literature for young and active patients [5]

Basic studies showed that successful cementless fixation include proximal adaptation and avoidance of micro-movements in order to obtain an optimal load transmission to the bone [6]. This adaptation to the proximal femur is only possible when the stem can match the patient femoral anatomy. Several anatomical studies have shown the wide range of proximal femoral anatomy [7, 8]. The logic answer for the necessary adaptation to the proximal intra-medullary femoral anatomy combined to the obligatory corrections in the prosthetic neck for solving extra-medullary deformities was CAD of individual stem geometry. The design of a three-dimensional custom neck allows corrections in length, lever arm and anteversion. The clinical consequence of such design is the restoration of length, abductor function and proper lower limb rotation [1]. The appropriate anteversion of the neck may also contribute to reduce dislocation rate [9]. The intra-medullary stem design is a combination of CT-based reconstruction of the proximal femur anatomy and priority areas of contact to obtain stability in rotation. The distal diameter of the stem is reduced to avoid any cortical impingement distally, possible source of thigh pain with maximal canal fillings stems. It is thus of high importance to preserve all the cancellous bone around the whole stem from proximal to distal by the use of a smooth compactor of identical shape than the final prosthesis (Fig. 45.1).

3-D Pre-Operative Planning

Preoperative Data

X- Ray Data

The radiographic analysis is based on several X-ray views. A full view of the two limbs using scannography is needed to assess the global pelvis and limb anatomical status, and to evaluate the extent of disturbance of the pelvic balance by assessing bilaterally the position of the hip rotation centers (in the vertical axis). A frontal pelvic view is used to determine the extent of lever arm between the rotation centers and the corresponding femoral axis. Pre-operative planning included pelvic version analysis on M-L standing X-ray of the pelvis. Angle between

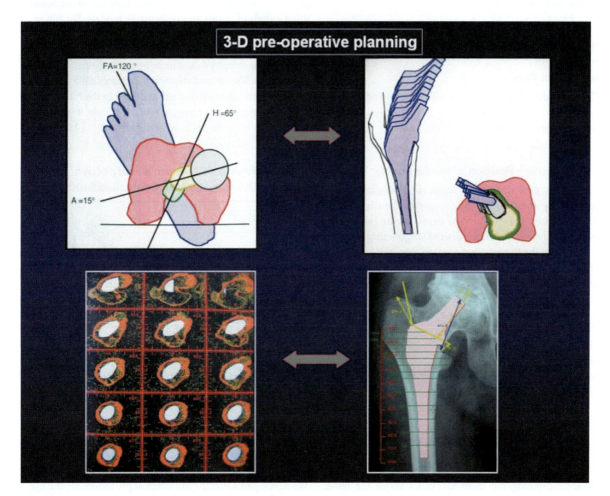

 Fig. 45.1. Computer-assisted pre-operative planning of computer-assisted designed hip arthroplasty

vertical plane and anterior pelvic plane was calculated pre-operatively for each patient.

CT Data

Data obtained from computerized tomography scanner are necessary both for the design of the intra-medullary femoral stem and for the planning of the extra-medullary part of the joint reconstruction. The intra-medullary femoral anatomy is assessed by CT-views taken every 5 mm from the top of the iliac crest down to the bottom of the lesser trochanter, then every 10 mm until the femoral isthmus. The extra-medullary planning requires CT views taken at the base of the femoral neck, at the knee level across the femoral condyles and at the foot level, by the second metatarsus axis.

Preoperative Planning

Acetabular Cup

The size is determined using the CT view passing through the center of the true acetabulum (witch allows furthermore assessment of bone stock).

Corresponding Position of the Femur

The future position of the femur (as determined for instance by the location of the greater trochanter) is determined on the frontal view based on the position of the acetabular socket, on the desired lengthening as determined from the scannogram, and on the neck lever arm. This position will determine the level of the femoral cut and assess the correct neck lever arm on the frontal view.

Neck Anteversion

The anteversion angle of the prosthesis neck must be set such as that normal gait anatomy can be restored. The normal gait anatomy requires three conditions:
1. foot axis showing 10°–20° of external rotation,
2. posterior bicondylar axis perpendicular to the gait direction,
3. anteversion of the femoral neck between 15° and 20° with respect to the bicondylar axis.

By superimposing the three CT views above the lesser trochanter and at the knee and foot levels, it is possible to calculate the correction angle to add (or substract) to the helitorsion angle such that a final prosthetic anteversion angle of 15°–20°, referencing the knee condylar axis, is achieved.

The Concept of Imageless Navigation Based on Bone Morphing for Total Hip Arthroplasty

We performed an adaptation of the Hiplogics Universal Protocol (PRAXIM Medivision™) for cup positioning control. This system is CT-free, based on Bone-Morphing Technology [4]. In an image-free-based concept, the goal is to obtain easily per-operatively a reliable 3D model. This 3D model is specific to each patient's anatomy. The 3D shapes of the bones are built from data collected with a 3D optical pointer in relative coordinate systems attached to the bones using clouds of points and deformable models. For hip arthroplasty, the first step was to obtain the patient pelvic 3D model by percutaneous palpation of anterior-superior iliac spines, pubic symphysis and intra-operative palpation of the acetabulum. The second step was to reference the acetabular reamer and the cup impaction device in the relative coordinate system. Then navigation of the acetabular reaming and the cup impaction will be performed (□ Fig. 45.2).

Cup Positioning Validation: a Prospective Comparative Randomized Controlled Study

Study Design

We performed a controlled, randomized matched prospective study including two groups of 30 patients with previous approval of French Ethic Committee. In the first group, cup positioning was assisted by computer-assisted orthopaedic system (CAOS group). Inclusion criteria were: age >20 years and <80 years, weight <100 kg, primary hip arthroplasty, antero-lateral approach, same surgeon (JNA), same cementless cup. Exclusion criteria were: trochanterotomy or revision. In the control group, a free-hand cup placement was performed by the same surgeon, using the same implant.

Surgical Procedure

We developed a specific hip surgical procedure for the use of an imageless cup positioning computer-based naviga-

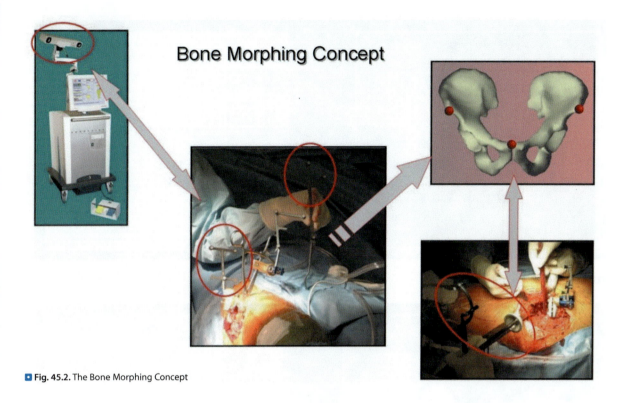

Bone Morphing Concept

◘ Fig. 45.2. The Bone Morphing Concept

tion system trough an antero-lateral approach, the patient in supine position. The acetabular component was a cementless socket and the femoral stem was a custom made prosthesis. All the patients have been operated through an antero-lateral approach by the same surgeon under general or rachi-anesthesia. Patient was draped in such a way that both anterior-superior iliac spines and pubic symphysis could be palpated. An iliac rigid-body was positioned in the acetabular roof trough the conventional exposure. Lewinnek plane [10] was obtained by percutaneous palpation of anterior-superior iliac spines and pubic symphysis with a special palpation device. Pre-operative pelvic version angle was registered on the computer. Then an acetabular bone morphing was realized. After this first step of spatial pelvic reconstruction, reamer navigation was performed (◘ Fig. 45.3). Finally, we performed cup impactor navigation in order to control per-operative cup anteversion and abduction angles (◘ Fig. 45.4). Angular goals were 40° of abduction and 15 ° of anteversion. The standard definitions of cup orientation (anteversion and abduction angles) in operative, radiographic and anatomic referentials of Murray [11] were used.

Post-Operative Evaluation

Cup positioning was evaluated post-operatively for each patient in the two groups by an independent observer on CT-scan with a special cup evaluator soft-ware (◘ Fig. 45.5). Full pelvic CT-scans were performed one month after surgery for all patients with the same protocol in the same center. We performed a 3-D reconstruction for each patient with the special post-operative evaluator software. Then Lewinnek plane [10] was registered on the 3-D model and pre-operative pelvic version integrated. Cup anteversion and abduction angles were measured in operative, radiographic and anatomic referential of Murray [11].

Results

There were 16 males and 14 females in each group, 14 right hips and 16 left. Mean age was 61 years (24–80) and mean Body Mass Index was 24 (17–37). The mean pelvic version angle measured pre-operatively on the standing M-L pelvic X-ray was –1.72° (–15°/14°). Mean acetabular

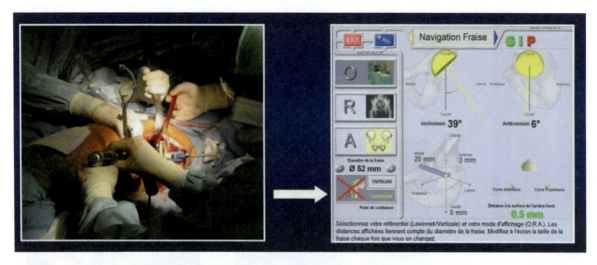

Fig. 45.3. Reamer Navigation

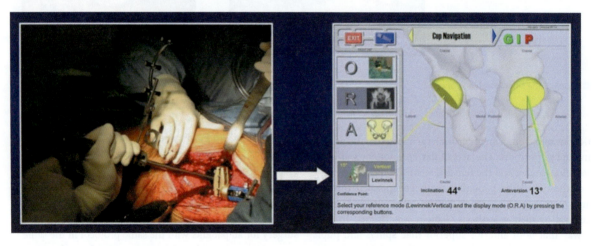

Fig. 45.4. Cup impaction navigation

cup diameter was 52 mm. We never needed additional skin incision. Mean additional time for the CAOS procedure was 12 min (8–20). Intra-operative subjective agreement by the surgeon with the computer guidance system demonstrated a high correlation in 23 cases, weak correlation in 6 cases and a poor correlation in 1 case.

The results of the post-operative angles in the two groups are detailed in Table 45.1. The differences between the intra-operative values and the post-operative values were in 95% of the cases less than 5° for the abduction angles and less than 10° for the anteversion angles. The differences were mainly found in obese patients.

Table 45.1. Results of the postoperative angles in the CAOS group and in the Control group

	Abduction (°) CAOS/Control	Anteversion (°) CAOS/Control
Operative mode	30 (25–46)/32 (21–48)	14 (0–25)/17 (0–37)
Radiologic mode	35 (25–47)/34 (23–50)	13 (0–26)/15 (0–35)
Anatomic mode	36 (27–47)/38 (22–55)	19 (0–27)/22 (0–39)

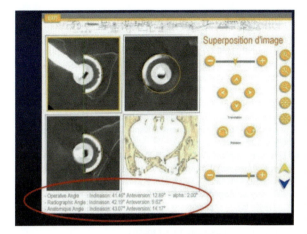

Fig. 45.5. 3D scannographic post-operative evaluation

There was no statistical difference between the CAOS group and the Control group for the abduction and inclination angles.

Discussion and Conclusion

Stem Positioning Validation

The next step of the protocol will be the validation of computer-assisted guidance of stem introduction by performing a prospective randomized controlled study. The computer-assisted measurement of intra-medullary stem placement according to the pre-operative planning should be evaluated as well as the extra-medullary parameters like neck anteversion, varus-valgus and neck lever arm. Navigation of the cup alone is not sufficient for optimizing hip range of motion after THA [12]. Thus computer-assisted per-operative control of both intra and extra-medullary stem parameters have to be achieved.

Limits of the System

Cutaneous Lewinnek Plane

During the procedure, a percutaneous bony landmark registration is performed. Considering that the anterior pelvic plane registration is modified by subcutaneous fat tissue, we call it the »Cutaneous Lewinnek plane«. Thus the poor correlation between intra-operative and post-operative measurements for obese patients observed in

our study was probably due to the limits of the percutaneous registration of the Lewinnek plane [10]. This point is probably one of the most obvious limitation of the imageless anatomical navigation system [13, 14] based on Bone Morphing® in THA.

Pre-operative Individual Pelvic Motion Analysis

Analysis of the pelvic version in our study has shown important inter-individual differences witch should be considered pre-operatively to provide the best anteversion angle intra-operatively. Furthermore, a few studies [15, 16] considering motion analysis of the pelvic tilt have shown important variations according to the patient's position or the patient's thoracic cage motion. Considering pelvic tilt in standard standing position as we have done in the current study seems to be not reliable enough. A kinematic analysis of the pelvic tilt could allow the surgeon to define preoperatively a functional anteversion angle goal to reach during intra-operative computer-assisted cup positioning.

Future of the System

Echo-Morphing™

Alternative solutions for percutaneous palpation could be realized by intra-operative echographic morphing of the anterior pelvic plane. Reproducibility and accuracy of the percutaneous registration of the Lewinnek plane and the echographic morphing have been studied during an anatomical study (Fig. 45.6). Echo-morphing™ could

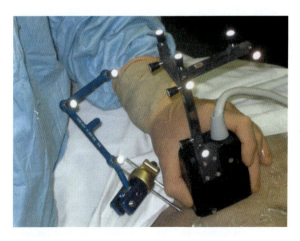

Fig. 45.6. Cadaveric study for echo-morphing evaluation

represent a good alternative to percutaneous palpation and should be tested in vivo.

Difficult Cases: Revision, Dysplastic Hip

Validation studies were necessary to confirm the usefulness of both computer-assisted designed and computer-assisted positioning in THA for conventional cases. Then we will be able to adapt the concept to revision or dysplasia. The system may be very helpful for reconstruction of the original patient anatomy in a reproducible way for theses difficult cases.

Conclusion

The results of this study are in accordance with the recent ones published on the same subject showing less variability for cup positioning when using a navigation system [17–20]. Whether the definition of correct acetabular orientation is still debated, the effects on hip stability and optimal range of motion are proven [9]. The next steps will be the potential for reducing error analysis by using echo-morphing instead of skin reference planes, and the validation of computer-assisted guidance of stem introduction either standard or custom.

The combination of an optimal cup positioning to a three-dimensional designed prosthetic neck may provide the best conditions for adequate range of motion after THA while reducing the risk of potential dislocation. Further research in the biomechanical field including the evaluation of the patient hip function before and after THA using gait analysis, stereoradiography, fluoroscopy, or accelerometry during everyday or sport activities will be also necessary in order to improve our knowledge in patient's quality of life and hip function after THA.

References

1. Argenson JN, Pizzeta M, Essinger JR, Aubaniac JM (1992) Symbios custom hip prosthesis: Concept, realization and early results. J Bone Joint Surg [Br] 74-B (Suppl 2): 167
2. DiGioia AM, Jaramaz B, Blackwell M et al. (1998) The Otto Aufranc Award. Image guided navigation system to measure intraoperatively acetabular implant alignment. Clin Orthop 355: 8–22
3. Widmer KH, Grutzner PA (2004) Joint replacement-total hip replacement with CT-based navigation. Injury 35–1S: 84–89
4. Stindel E, Sinquin P, Lavalée S (2002) Bone morphing: 3D morphological data for total knee arthroplasty. Comput Aided Surg 7–3: 156–168
5. Boeree NR, Baniister (1993) Cemented total hip arthroplasty in patients younger than 50 years of age. Clin Orthop 287: 153–159
6. Robertson DD, Walker PS, Hirano SK (1988) Improving the fit of pressgits stems. Clin Orthop 228: 134–140
7. Argenson JN, Ryembault E, Flecher X, Brassart N, Parratte S, Aubaniac JM (2005) Three-dimensional anatomy of the hip in osteoarthritis after developmental dysplasia. J Bone Joint Surg [Br] 87-B:1192–1196
8. Husmann D, Rubin PJ, Leyvraz PF, Deroguin B, Argenson JN (1997) Three-dimensional morphology of the proximal femur. J Arthroplasty 12: 444–450
9. Kennedy JG, Rogers WB, Soffe KE, Sullivan RJ, Griffen DG, Sheehan LJ (1998) Effect of acetabular component orientation on recurrent dislocation, pelvic osteolysis, polyethylene wear, and component migration. J Arthroplasty 13–5:530–534
10. Lewinnek GE, Lewis JL, Tarr R, Compere CL, Zimmerman JR (1978) Dislocation after total hip-replacement arthroplasties. J bone Joint Surg [Am] 60-A: 217–220.
11. Murray DW (1993) The definition and measurement of acetabular orientation. J Bone Joint Surg [Br] 75-B: 228–232
12. Gotze C, Vieth V, Meier N, Bottner F, Steinbeck J, Hackenberg S (2005) CT-based accuracy of implanting custom-made endoprostheses. Clin Biomech 20–8: 856–862
13. Tannast M, Langlotz U, Siebenrock KA, Wiese M, Bernsmann K, Langlotz F (2005) Anatomic Referencing of Cup Orientation in Total Hip Arthroplasty. Clin Orthop 436:144–150.
14. Wolf A, Digioia AM 3rd, Mor AB, Jaramaz B (2005) Cup alignment error model for total hip arthroplasty. Clin Orthop 437: 132–137
15. Harrison DE, Cailliet R, Harrison DD, Janik TJ (2002) How do anterior/posterior translations of the thoracic cage affect the sagittal lumbar spine, pelvic tilt, and thoracic kyphosis? Eur Spine J 11: 287–293
16. Lembeck B, Mueller O, Reize P, Wuelker N (2005) Pelvic tilt makes acetabular cup navigation inaccurate. Acta Orthop 76: 517–523
17. Dorr LD, Hishiki Y, Wan Z, Newton D, Yun A (2005) Development of imageless computer navigation for acetabular component position in total hip replacement. Iowa Orthop J 25: 1–9
18. Jolles BM, Genoud P, Hoffmeyer P (2004) Computer-assisted cup placement techniques in total hip arthroplasty improve accuracy of placement. Clin Orthop 426:174–179.
19. Leenders T, Vandevelde D, Mahieu G, Nuyts R (2002) Reduction in variability of acetabular cup abduction using computer assisted surgery: a prospective and randomized study. Comput Aided Surg 7: 99–106
20. Nogler M, Kessler O, Prassl A, Donnelly B, Streicher R, Sledge JB, Krismer M (2004) Reduced variability of acetabular cup positioning with use of an imageless navigation system. Clin Orthop 426: 159–163

Computer-assisted Hip Resurfacing

Comparison of Fluoroscopic and Landmark-Based Technique with the Vector-Vision System

H. Bäthis, L. Perlick, M. Tingart, T. Kalteis, J. Grifka

Introduction

In the 1970s the early results of surface arthroplasty of the hip with metal-on-polyethylene bearing surfaces showed high failure rates due to polyethylene wear between 5 to 10 year after implantation with the procedure being abandoned [10].With the introduction of metal on metal bearings in hip resurfacing arthroplasty, this procedure has gained new interest in the treatment of hip arthritis especially for younger patients [3, 16, 20]. Several advantages have been advocated in the use of surface replacement of the hip compared to traditional total hip replacement. This procedure has been reported with superior results in terms of conservation and restoration of the natural anatomy and biomechanical function of the hip [11].

On the other hand, hip resurfacing is a technical demanding procedure. The preparation of the acetabulum is performed with the femoral head and neck in place and there have been concerns about possible complications, in particular fracture of the neck of the femur following this procedure [21]. Moreover, follow-up data have shown an increased rate of revision surgery in a patient cohort, where the stem-shaft axis of the femoral implant showed a varus inclination [5].

At the time surface replacement was introduced at our department in early 2003, no navigation system, specialized for the use in a hip resurfacing procedure, was available. At this time, in our department, navigation techniques have been already used in various orthopaedic procedures like total knee replacement or spinal surgery regularly [4, 17].

So the idea came up to provide additional intra-operative information for the hip-resurfacing procedure and to improve the surgical accuracy by introducing navigation technique. The procedure is technically demanding and technical errors in the preparation of the femoral head like notching may lead to early femoral fracture. Looking for improvements in our technique, a usability of a standard fluoroscopic technique of computer-assisted surgery was developed and tested in a feasibility study which will be presented. We subsequently embarked on a development effort to assess a »fluoro-free« landmark based technology. In both presented techniques the Vector-Vision®-Navigation-System (Brainlab AG, Heimstetten, Germany) has been used. The navigation system has an optical tracking unit, which detects passive, reflecting marker spheres by an infrared camera. It is controlled by a touch-screen monitor. Both surgical navigation procedures are described and the results of the first experience are presented.

Fluoroscopic-assisted Navigated Surface Replacement of the Femoral Head (Vector-Vision Spine Module – Off-Label Use)

The available Spinal surgery application (Spine 5.0) of the Vector-Vision® Navigation System, which provides the ability of surgical navigation within different fluoroscopic images simultaneously, was tested for its capability in the hip-resurfacing procedure. Previously, good results were already gained with the use of the spine software package in femoral head screw fixation in children with slipped femoral capital epiphysis and in navigation based removal of pelvic screws [18, 19].

The usability of the system in a hip-resurfacing procedure was tested in several sawbone and cadaver sessions before. This surgical technique is comparable to the technique of biplanar fluoroscopy in the treatment of femoral neck fractures with internal fixation like dynamic-hip screws (DHS) or proximal femoral nails (PFN).

Surgical Technique

For femoral head resurfacing, the patient is positioned in a lateral position. The preparation of the hip joint is performed in the standard posterior approach, and the femoral head is dislocated. A standard reference array of the navigation system is attached to the femur in a position of good visibility to the camera in different rotation positions of the leg. Two fluoroscopic images of the femoral head and neck in an anterior-posterior and lateral view are acquired and processed to the navigation system (■ Fig. 46.1).

The accuracy of these fluoroscopic images can be verified using the navigation pointer on top of the surface of the bone.

After verification of the accuracy, the surgeon has the possibility of planning a drilling canal centrally within the femoral head and neck according to the pre-operative planning. Finally, the navigation is used for drilling the central K-wire in the femoral neck using a pre-calibrated navigation probe according to the planning proposal. This

is facilitated within the two different fluoroscopic images presented at the navigation screen simultaneously and the virtual rod displayed in both images according to the position of the navigation probe (■ Fig. 46.2).

In our series, in all patients the final position of the central K-wire was verified using standard fluoroscopy before preparation of the femoral head.

Feasibility Study Data

In 2003 and 2004, a series of 20 patients has been operated on in our department using this fluoroscopic based computer assisted technique.

The mean time for surgery was 85 min (range 70–110 min) including fluoroscopic verification. In 17 cases the primary navigation based position of the central K-wire was used for further preparation without any change of position.

In two cases, due to poor fluoro-image quality, the placement of the central K-wire was additionally guided by the conventional guiding system (BMI >38 m²/kg). In one case we observed a deviation in only one of the fluoro-images, which was found to be associated with a bending of the reference array during image acquisition. In all cases the final implant position was evaluated on post-operative radiographs with no signs of femoral notching.

Landmark-based Technique of Computer-assisted Hip Surface Replacement (Vector-Vision HipSR)

Based on our experience with the fluoroscopic assisted technique, we joined in a development cooperation to set up a specialized software application for the hip-resurfacing technique. One of the major aims was to develop a surgical tool, without the need of an additional intra-operative fluoroscopy. Comparable to the technique of the CT-free knee software, the intra-operative data acquisition is based on a surface matching technique with a navigation pointer. Further, in this software, positioning of the acetabular component can be performed computer assisted using the software module from the CT-free hip application.

Surgical Technique

The patient is placed in supine or lateral position, as convenient for the surgeon. After standard lateral or posterior

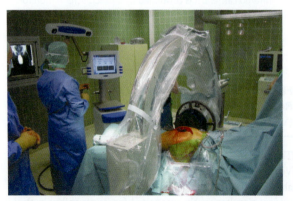

■ **Fig. 46.1.** Intra-operative setup of the fluoro-based technique. Acquiring of two fluoro-images of the proximal femur and automatic transfer to the navigation system

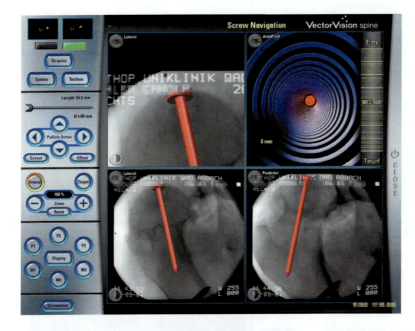

Fig. 46.2. Planning screen for screw-position centrally within the femoral neck

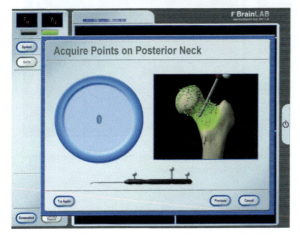

Fig. 46.3. Digitizing the bone surface of the femoral neck using a navigation pointer

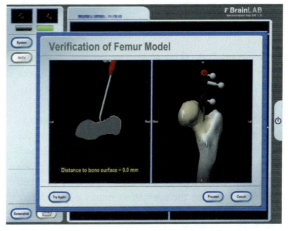

Fig. 46.4. Verification of the virtual bone model

approach and dislocation of the hip, a reference array is attached to the femur. Different landmarks as well as surface information of the femur have to be digitized using the navigation pointer. For the definition of the femoral anatomic axis and the anteversion of the femoral neck, the piriformis point and the midpoint between the distal femur epicondyles are used.

Bone-surface information of the femoral head and the superior, anterior posterior and inferior femoral neck sur-

face are digitized with the navigation pointer (Fig. 46.3). Even if the hip has to be moved in different positions for optimal access to the neck regions, this process is very comfortable for the surgeon and takes about 4–5 min at all.

Based on this data, the system calculates an adapted bone model and the specific axes of the femur (stem-shaft angle, femoral neck anteversion). The surgeon is able to verify the adapted bone model using the navigation pointer (Fig. 46.4). Placing the pointer on top of the

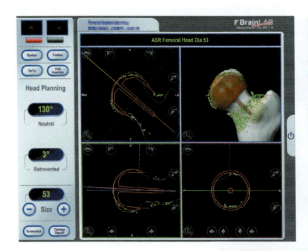

Fig. 46.5. Planning of the femoral implant size and position

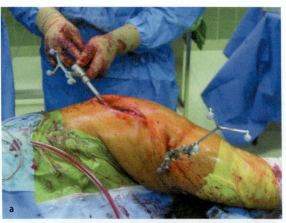

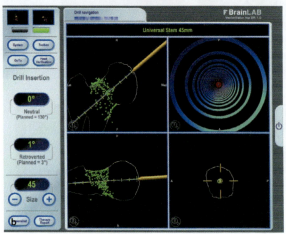

Fig. 46.6a,b. Navigation-based drilling of the K-wire. Intra-operative view with the navigation drill-probe

digitized neck region, the system displays the offset/distance between the pointer tip (= true bone surface) and the virtual bone model.

Within the bone-model, the system provides a planning proposal for the optimal position of the femoral resurfacing implant (Fig. 46.5). The surgeon is able to identify possible regions of notching the femoral neck during preparation and he can readjust the implant position in different views.

With the correct planning of the implant position, a k-wire is placed centrally within the femoral neck using the computer system. This is performed in the same method, as in the fluoroscopy based technique. A navigation probe is used as a drilling guide and the position of the drill guide is displayed on the navigation monitor in different perspectives (Fig. 46.6a,b).

In both computer-assisted techniques, the conventional instruments can be used to control the position of the central k-wire before final bone preparation.

Study Design and Patients

In a prospective study 30 hip-surface replacements were performed. 16 male and 14 female were included in the study. The mean age was 53 years (range: 37–66 yrs).

In all patients, the same implants (cemented femoral component and cementless porous coated acetabular component) and instrumentation were used (ASR®, DePuy Inc., Warsaw, USA). All operations were performed by one team (L.P. and H.B.) experienced in computer-assisted and conventional hip resurfacing.

Component alignment and the variation of the femoral offset were evaluated on standardized a.-p. and axial pre-operative and post-operative radiographs and compared to the pre-operative radiographic plan.

Results

Surgical procedure data: In 28 cases the computer-assisted procedure was used for the placement of the guide-wire centrally within the femoral neck. In two cases there was an insufficient femoral model due to a limited access to all necessary femoral neck areas and the surgery was completed with the conventional instrumentation guide. The mean time for surgery (skin to skin) was 78 min (SD 12 min) No complications (e.g. infections, fractures) occurred due to the fixation of the reference array attachment.

Frontal Plane Alignment. In the pre-operative X-rays a mean shaft-neck angle (CCD-angle) of 129 degrees was measured. In the pre-operative planning, the mean shaft-neck angle was set to a relative valgus-position of the implant with a range of 129 to 144 degree. The mean post-operative femoral implant to shaft angle was 137 degrees, ranging from 127 to 146 degrees. Compared to the pre-operative planning, the mean deviation in the frontal plane was 2.1 degrees (SD 1.9°). There was no notching of the cranial and the caudal aspect of the femoral neck.

Axial Plane Alignment. The mean deviation from the ideal placement in the axial plane was 2.9 degrees with a standard deviation of 1.8°. There was no notching of the anterior or posterior cortex.

Discussion

While hip resurfacing arthroplasty was used during the 1970s and early 1980s with discouraging results, there has been a resurgence of interest in the past years. The concept of surface arthroplasty for the treatment of advanced arthritis of the hip in young and active patients has many attractive features, because of its ability to preserve femoral bone [1].

Several authors reported reliable results with fewer complications when using an uncemented acetabular component and a cemented femoral component for resurfacing the hip [7, 14, 16]. Treacy et al. reported an overall cumulative survival at five years of 98% and an aseptic survival rate of 99% [23].

Certain technical considerations must be fulfilled when performing hip resurfacing. The amount of bone resected from the femoral head can be altered and this affects the offset and length of the femur. Varus alignment of the femoral component increases the femoral offset and the tension on the femoral neck increasing the risk of fracture [8]. The femoral component should therefore be placed in either neutral or valgus alignment while avoiding notching of the lateral cortex of the femoral neck [5, 15].

Fracture of the neck of the femur has long been recognized as a major complication [6, 16]. It has been assumed that the majority of fractures occur within the first six to eight weeks after implantation of the prosthesis [22]. Shimmin and Back reported an incidence of 1.46% with the Birmingham Hip Resurfacing System, while notching of the superior aspect of the neck of the femur was seen on the radiographs taken after operation in 46.6% of the patients who subsequently fractured. They found that none of the fractures occurred when the femoral component had been placed in valgus compared with the pre-operative neck-shaft angle [22].

Alignment guides of the conventional instrumentation sets of the various resurfacing implants are created in a comparable method. Particularly, in cases with a short femoral neck or reduced access to the femoral head and neck region non-optimal femoral implant positions may occur. Moreover, there is no intra-operative control of the shaft-neck axis. Therefore, the introduction of computer-assisted technique seems reasonable. Already for standard total hip replacement a significant improvement of component alignment and post-operative leg length has been reported when using a navigation system [12, 13]. There are only a few studies available reporting on the use of navigation in hip resurfacing. With our experience in using the fluoroscopic technique of the Vector-Vision Spine application, the feasibility of this technique within a standard intra-operative procedure for hip resurfacing is presented. Hess et al. have published a comparable computer-assisted hip-resurfacing technique using a different navigation system. They also reported a good feasibility of this comparable technique. Their analysis showed a high reproducibility between intra-operative data and post-operative X-ray measurements [9].

One of the major advantages of the presented landmarked-based technique compared with the fluoroscopic one is the improved intra-operative accuracy without the additional use of the fluoroscopy equipment. Our first experience has shown very promising data concerning the accuracy of the implantation.

The combination of large head sizes and the metal-on-metal bearing in surface arthroplasty of the hip makes wear and dislocation less of a concern than they are with conventional total hip replacement [2, 14]. Nevertheless, one should focus on the problems that might occur from the larger diameter of the residual neck compared to a femoral component of a standard total hip replacement. Due to this aspect, in cases of mal-positioning of the acetabular component, impingement and also dislocation even with large head components are possible. Therefore, the combined use of navigation on the acetabular side as well, as for the femoral head is recommended. The newly available software package is the first one offering this opportunity.

Conclusion

The computer-assisted technique in surface replacement of the hip improves the intra-operative information for the surgeon and enables a precise implantation technique. Possible reasons for complication like femoral notching and varus mal-positioning of the femoral component may be reduced.

References

1. Amstutz HC, Beaule PE, Dorey FJ, Le Duff MJ, Campbell PA, Gruen TA (2004) Metal-on-metal hybrid surface arthroplasty: two to six-year follow-up study. J Bone Joint Surg Am 86-A: 28–39
2. Amstutz HC, Grigoris P (1996) Metal on metal bearings in hip arthroplasty. Clin Orthop Relat Res 329: S11–S34
3. Amstutz HC, Su EP, Le Duff MJ (2005) Surface arthroplasty in young patients with hip arthritis secondary to childhood disorders. Orthop Clin North Am 36: 223–230
4. Bathis H, Perlick L, Tingart M, Luring C, Zurakowski D, Grifka J (2004) Alignment in total knee arthroplasty. A comparison of computer-assisted surgery with the conventional technique. J Bone Joint Surg Br 86: 682–687
5. Beaule PE, Lee JL, Le Duff MJ, Amstutz HC, Ebramzadeh E (2004) Orientation of the femoral component in surface arthroplasty of the hip. A biomechanical and clinical analysis. J Bone Joint Surg Am 86-A: 2015–2021
6. Bell RS, Schatzker J, Fornasier VL, Goodman SB (1985) A study of implant failure in the Wagner resurfacing arthroplasty. J Bone Joint Surg Am 67: 1165–1175
7. Daniel J, Pynsent PB, McMinn DJ (2004) Metal-on-metal resurfacing of the hip in patients under the age of 55 years with osteoarthritis. J Bone Joint Surg Br 86: 177–184
8. Freeman MA (1978) Some anatomical and mechanical considerations relevant to the surface replacement of the femoral head. Clin Orthop Relat Res137: 19–24
9. Hess T, Gampe T, Kottgen C, Szawlowski B (2004) Intraoperative navigation for hip resurfacing. Methods and first results. Orthopade 33: 1183–1193
10. Howie DW, Campbell D, McGee M, Cornish BL (1990) Wagner resurfacing hip arthroplasty. The results of one hundred consecutive arthroplasties after eight to ten years. J Bone Joint Surg Am 72: 708–714
11. Itayem R, Arndt A, Nistor L, McMinn D, Lundberg A (2005) Stability of the Birmingham hip resurfacing arthroplasty at two years. A radiostereophotogrammetric analysis study. J Bone Joint Surg Br 87: 158–162
12. Kalteis T, Beckmann J, Herold T, Zysk S, Bathis H, Perlick L, Grifka J (2004) Accuracy of an image-free cup navigation system--an anatomical study. Biomed Tech (Berl) 49: 257–262
13. Kiefer H (2003) OrthoPilot cup navigation--how to optimise cup positioning? Int Orthop 27 Suppl 1: S37–S42
14. Knecht A, Witzleb WC, Gunther KP (2005) Resurfacing arthroplasty of the hip. Orthopade 34: 79–89
15. Loughead JM, Chesney D, Holland JP, McCaskie AW (2005) Comparison of offset in Birmingham hip resurfacing and hybrid total hip arthroplasty. J Bone Joint Surg Br 87: 163–166
16. McMinn D, Treacy R, Lin K, Pynsent P (1996) Metal on metal surface replacement of the hip. Experience of the McMinn prothesis. Clin Orthop Relat Res 329 (Suppl): S89–S98
17. Perlick L, Bathis H, Perlick C, Luring C, Tingart M, Grifka J (2005) Revision total knee arthroplasty: a comparison of postoperative leg alignment after computer-assisted implantation versus the conventional technique. Knee Surg Sports Traumatol Arthrosc 13: 167–173
18. Perlick L, Tingart M, Lerch K, Bathis H (2004) Navigation-assisted, minimally invasive implant removal following a triple pelvic osteotomy. Arch Orthop Trauma Surg 124: 64–66
19. Perlick L, Tingart M, Wiech O, Beckmann J, Bathis H (2005) Computer-assisted cannulated screw fixation for slipped capital femoral epiphysis. J Pediatr Orthop 25: 167–170
20. Schmalzried TP, Fowble VA, Ure KJ, Amstutz HC (1996) Metal on metal surface replacement of the hip. Technique, fixation, and early results. Clin Orthop Relat Res 329 (Suppl): S106-S114
21. Shimmin AJ, Back D (2005) Femoral neck fractures following Birmingham hip resurfacing: a national review of 50 cases. J Bone Joint Surg Br 87: 463–464
22. Shimmin AJ, Bare J, Back DL (2005) Complications associated with hip resurfacing arthroplasty. Orthop Clin North Am 36: 187–193
23. Treacy RB, McBryde CW, Pynsent PB (2005) Birmingham hip resurfacing arthroplasty. A minimum follow-up of five years. J Bone Joint Surg Br 87: 167–170

Navigation for Hip Resurfacing

T. Hess

Introduction

Hip resurfacing is a special procedure different from THR in planning and surgery. In recent years, this method has experienced a revival of interest in Europe, Asia and Australia, due to the development of a new generation of implants. These systems differ from the previous generation in their use of advanced metal-on-metal bearings and an instrumentation allowing accurate positioning of the femoral component [1]. There are, however, special risks and complications reported for this procedure, such as femoral neck fracture for several reasons and ventral impingement due to improper positioning of the implants with respect to the unfavorable neck – head ratio of this system [2–4]. Moreover, most of the systems available for hip resurfacing demand a larger exposure compared to THR. Navigation in hip resurfacing is expected to simplify the positioning procedure, reduce the amount of the abovementioned specific complications and help introducing less invasive procedures.

Material and Methods

For preparation of the femoral side in hip resurfacing, a guide wire is inserted into the femoral head in the position and orientation of the later implant pin. This wire is then over-drilled and replaced by a pin, over which all other instruments for the preparation of the implant are placed. This pin is later replaced by the final implant pin.

With navigation, the first guide wire is inserted using the navigation system.

Pre-operative planning is done as usual using an antero-posterior X-ray of the hip in slight internal rotation. Templates are used to determine size and position of the femoral component. We always attempt to achieve a marked valgus position of the component. Also, the natural CCD angle (the femoral neck-shaft angle) and the angle between implant axis and femoral shaft (»Shaft – neck – angle«, SNA), which are used later during surgery, are measured and noted.

We use the Birmingham Hip Resurfacing system with a standard posterior approach as recommended by the system developer. Generally, a dissection of the gluteus maximus tendon is not performed. The navigated insertion of the guide is done after the dislocation of the joint and before the preparation of the acetabular cup. The reference frame for the navigation system is attached with a 6-mm Steinmann pin which is drilled monocortically into the lesser trochanter. Thus the drillhole can be used later for the suction cannula during the cementation of the femoral cap.

To perform an imageless navigation, a three-dimensional model of the femoral neck and head must be generated by the navigation system. This is done by so-called morphing, which is the adaptation of predefined bone models to the actual patient-specific bone anatomy by means of imageless navigation software. The data for the patient-specific model are registered by digitizing the bone surface with pointers (Fig. 47.1). Here, the model is built by digitizing 6 regions of the upper femur:

- the femoral head is digitized with 150 points,
- the anterior, posterior, superior and inferior outlines of the femoral neck are each digitized with 40 points,
- the so-called notching zone (the anterior – superior part of the femoral neck) is digitized with an additional 20 points.

The computer then collects these data and calculates a patient-specific model of the upper femur. The accuracy of this model can be verified by touching the bone with the pointers while the computer displays the calculated distance from the bone (where any value different from zero means inaccuracy).

The representation of the bone model appears as a three-dimensional animation (◘ Fig. 47.2). Three split images are displayed: one in the antero-posterior plane, a second one in the axial plane and a third sagittal split image analogous to a coronal CT-view. The level of the sagittal split image is indicated on the other two images by a red line and can be changed on the touchscreen. The navigation system then uses the outlines of the femoral head to position a correct sized implant in a neutral position, i.e. in the direction of the calculated neck axis. The surgeon can adjust the size and position of the implant in any direction. If, through mal-positioning or incorrect dimensioning, the planned position could lead to femoral notching, the system will give a warning and indicate the affected areas with red points.

When the surgeon is satisfied with the indicated implant size and position, he can continue to the next surgical step. From this point on, the screen will only display the planned implant axis in two planes, a cross hair and a canal to aid in targeting the guide wire. With the aid of a navigated drill guide, the surgeon now inserts the guide wire and checks its position based on the preplanned values. When the position of the guide wire is satisfactory, the navigation is ended and the rest of the operation can be performed in the usual manner.

For navigation of the socket, the procedure as well as the software module are identical to those of THR: a reference frame is mounted to the pelvis and the pelvis planes are recorded by taking landmarks from the anterior superior iliac spine and the pubic frame on both sides. This can be done with the patient already in a lateral position before mounting the fixation device, so the patient can be turned back slightly for referencing the contra-lateral iliac spine. Later, after exposition of the acetabulum, further points are recorded from the inner

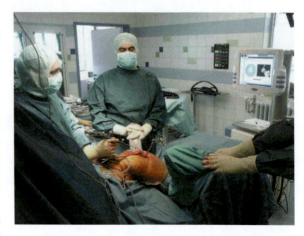

◘ **Fig. 47.1.** Intra-operative setup during registration of landmarks

contour of the acetabulum. The system then calculates a morphed image of the acetabulum. With a navigated impactor, positioning of the socket can be controlled during impaction both by figures indicating anteversion and inclination and by visualization of its position within the acetabulum (◘ Fig. 47.3).

The stability, functionality and accuracy of the Vector Vision navigation system were tested on bone models and cadavers in the laboratories of BrainLAB, the system manufacturer, before starting clinical trials on humans. The first clinical trials on humans were performed at the Orthopaedic Department of the Dreifaltigkeitshospital in Lippstadt, Germany. In the first 20 cases a navigated hip resurfacing procedure was performed by only two surgeons under the supervision of the Ethical Committee of the Kaiser-Wilhelm-Universität in Münster, Germany. Before the surgery, the patients were informed about the experimental character of the navigation system and its possible risks and they had given their consent to the use of such a procedure.

The implant planning and the insertion of the guide wire were performed as previously described. The criteria for an optimal implant positioning had been defined as follows:

1. The implant axis-femoral shaft angle is more valgus than the natural CCD angle.
2. There is no erosion of the femoral neck during reaming.
3. There is an adequate bone preparation all around the femoral head.

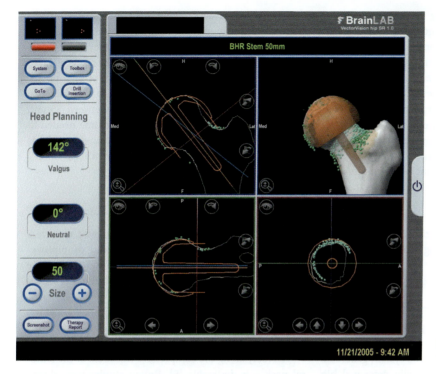

■ **Fig. 47.2.** Display for planning the femoral component.

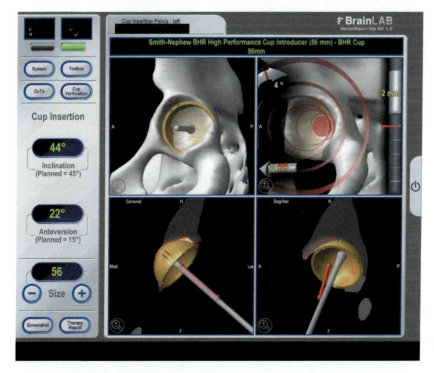

■ **Fig. 47.3.** Display for planning the acetabular component

These criteria were fulfilled by using the navigation system for the implant planning. Then, the guide wire was inserted and the validity of the above mentioned criteria was tested with the aid of conventional mechanical alignment guides.

The following points were evaluated:

1. The fulfillment of the abovementioned criteria.
2. The difference between the intra-operatively defined and the postoperatively measured shaft – neck angle (indicating the accuracy of intra-operative the SNA – values measured by the system).
3. The deviation of the axial implant axis from the axial femoral neck axis (indicating the accuracy in the axial plane).
4. The difference between the preoperatively measured CCD angle and the postoperatively measured shaft – neck -angle (the degree of valgization).

Results

The hip-resurfacing procedure was performed in 67 consecutive cases.

During the experimental phase, the system generated an unusable bone model in two heavily deformed hip cases. After changing the calculating algorithm, this error was no longer observed in the next 57 cases.

The three criteria were fulfilled in 64 of the 67 cases. In the three remaining cases only criteria 1 and 2 were fulfilled. The third criterion, the overall bone preparation of the femoral head, was missed in an antero-superior area of the head. In all three cases, this criterion was then fulfilled by slightly repositioning the implant axis-femoral shaft angle. Femoral notching was not observed in any of the navigated cases.

The accuracy of the model was checked by digitizing the femoral head and neck on four points each, which resulted in differences between 2.01 mm (upper femoral head) and 1.40 mm (upper femoral neck) in average. In 35 cases, the CCD angle that had been calculated by the system differed from the preoperatively defined value by more than 3%. In these cases, the CCD angle was adjusted to the predefined value. The shaft neck angle, which was calculated intra-operatively by the system, differed by 2.8 degrees from the value, which was measured post-operatively with an antero-posterior x-ray. This postoperative angle had a more valgus position of 7.0 degrees in average in comparison with the pre-operative measured CCD angle (◘ Fig. 47.4).

In none of the 67 cases were there complications directly or indirectly related to the navigation system. General complications appeared in two cases (reversible sciatic nerve palsy). No fracture of the femoral neck, erosion of the femoral neck, infection or dislocation of the implant occurred. The time needed from attaching the reference frames to inserting the guide pin took between 55 and 18 min. This must be compared with the time needed to perform all necessary steps in hip resurfacing procedures using conventional mechanical alignment guides.

Discussion

The new hip-resurfacing systems are believed to have a longer life span than former models because of improvements in design and implanting procedure. One of the latter is the possibility of an accurate positioning of the femoral component.

Already in 1994, Freeman reported that a neutral positioning of the femoral component in hip resurfacing is not sufficient, and that a significant valgus placement – preferably along the compressive trabecula of the femoral neck – is desireable [5]. Recent studies have shown that a varus positioning of the cap had a negative outcome on the life span of implants [3, 6]. These results confirm the speculation that a valgus placement of the femoral component reduces the risk of femoral neck fractures or implant loosening.

On the other hand however, the valgus placement of the femoral cap exposes the hip to the danger of femoral neck erosion during reaming. This complication, which is known as femoral notching, has been implicated as another main cause of postoperative femoral neck fractures in hip resurfacing [4, 7]. In a multicenter study in Australia, Shimmin reported 50 fractures in 3497 resurfacing hips. In 85% of the fractures either femoral notching, significant varus placement of the femoral cap or other intra-operative technical problems were present [3].

A valgus position for the femoral component by placing it more proximal, thus avoiding femoral notching, may lead to an insufficient bone stock, as the superior part of the femoral head will not be reamed sufficiently. This may lead to an inadequate fixation and subsidence of the implant.

The difficulty in achieving a good femoral component positioning thus lies in the contradiction of targeting a more valgus position, while at the same time avoiding

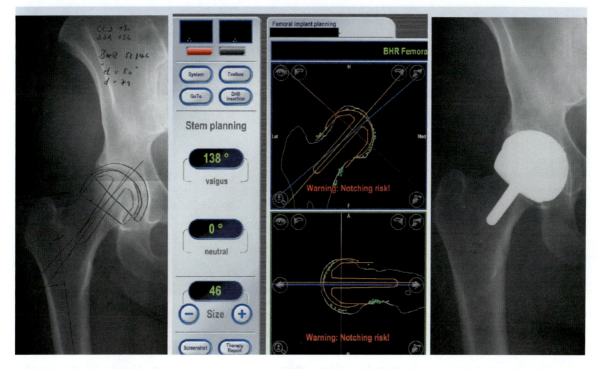

◻ Fig. 47.4. Planning, intra-operative display and result of an hip resurfacing, ap view: notice the marked valgus position of the femoral component

femoral notching and guaranteeing an adequate bone preparation all around the femoral head.

The implant positioning in the antero-posterior plane and the implant size, finally, also influences the mobility of the new hip. As a resurfaced hip generally shows a unfavorable head-neck ratio, a significant posterior position of the cap may lead to early impingement of the neck in internal rotation. A neutral or slight anterior position reduces this risk (◻ Fig. 47.5). Femoral impingement, together with the accompanying pains in flexion or internal rotation is a common problem in the otherwise successful hip resurfacing technique. Besides a correct implant positioning in the antero-posterior plane, the risk of femoral impingement could also be reduced by choosing a large diameter femoral component. However, this entails the need of a larger acetabular cup, which in its turn often leads to resection of excessive bone stock in the pelvic area. Therefore, a most accurate determination of the implant position and size is a highly important factor in hip resurfacing.

Until recently, surgeons only disposed of mechanical alignment guides and templates to address the above-mentioned problems of positioning and size determination. We often experienced difficulties in using these device. The introduction of highly accurate measuring systems such as navigation therefore seems very helpful for advanced hip resurfacing. Some of the benefits are the immediate, intra-operative visualization of the implant position and the possibility to simulate different implant positions and sizes.

We assessed the relation between the pre-operative planning data and the intra-operative position by comparing the femoral stem-shaft angle and the CCD angle. The difficulty in using these angles is that they are sensitive to rotation of the femur. In particular, small errors are inevitable, as the intra-operative computer representation on screen is always adjusted and presented without an anteversion projection error. We attempted to adjust this error on the pre-operative and post-operative X-rays through internal rotation of the femur. Still, the error

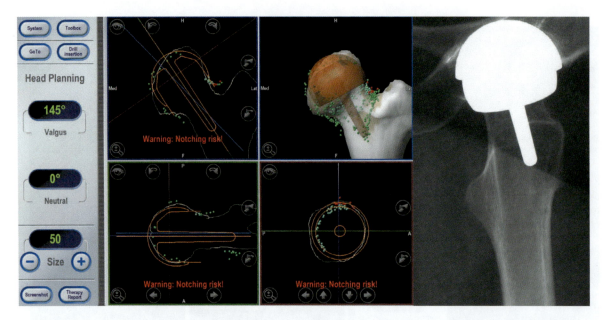

Fig. 47.5. Intra-operative display and result of a hip resurfacing, axial view: notice the marked anterior offset of the femoral component

could not be fully compensated, as the exact and individually different anteversion was not known and can only be established through additional X-rays or a CT-scan. But, as the pre-operative planning should serve as a reference value and the navigation system represents the exact, real intra-operative situation, we consider the projection error in the planning to be defensible. In the original procedure described by the implant designer, the relation between the preoperative planning data and the intra-operative position is assessed by transferring the distance from the tip of the trochanter to the exit point of the implant axis to a straight line. This procedure is sure to be free from rotation errors, however, sensitive to magnification errors. According to our own calculations, the inaccuracy resulting from such magnification errors can augment to a difference of up to 12 degrees in the femoral stem-shaft angle. This is a lot more than the presumed projection error of different rotations on the pre-operative X-ray.

A procedure to represent the entire upper femur had to be especially developed for the resurfacing navigation through modeling from the database and outline data. With 1.40 to 2.01 mm, the accuracy of the incurred models in our study was sufficient. However, in future, the error algorithm on the outlines of the femoral head and neck area should be aimed at less than 2 mm through fur-

ther improvement of the system. Already with the current models, the three criteria for a reliable use of the system were fulfilled in 64 out of 67 cases. In the other two cases, an insufficient reaming of the bone in the femoral head had occurred. This error was corrected by decreasing the femoral stem-shaft angle. In both cases, the navigation system indicated adequate femoral bone preparation, which in reality would not have taken place. The cause for this mis-interpretation lies in an insufficient accuracy of the model in the femoral head area. This error especially occurred, when there was a heavy deformity of the femoral head, particularly since the point density of 150 points for the entire femoral head is not very high. The most important area to avoid errors, however, remains the superior femoral neck. Because of the higher point density in this area, the accuracy of the model was at its highest there and no errors occurred here.

The representation of the model on screen is intuitive and self-explaining. The axial orientation in different, selectable planes is especially helpful to establish a correct implant positioning. This orientation offers valuable additional information, particularly in the notching zone. In this zone, the crucial bone side on the antero-superior surface of the femoral neck often does not provide a useful outline in the antero-posterior and axial plane, so that notching can not be detected by the representation of these two planes alone. As a result thereof, notching can not be avoided. Here, the imageless system seems to outperform the fluoroscopy-based navigation system, as the latter needs at least one additional oblique view to offer the same guarantee [8]. For the further navigation, however, a third additional oblique view is unfavorable, as this may complicate the surgeon's orientation.

The »fine adjustment« of the implant on the screen as a separate step in the procedure has proven to be useful in practice. Through such fine adjustment, factors such as angles, notching and adequate bone preparation needs no longer to be considered during the following drilling of the guide wire. This way, the surgeon can better focus on finding the correct insertion point and both alignment planes.

The accuracy of the intra-operatively assessed femoral stem-shaft angle was absolutely sufficient in comparison with the post-operatively established values, as only a slight measurement error due to femoral neck anteversion needed to be considered. In addition, the further conventional surgical steps (such as the over-drilling of the guide wire, the over-reaming of the guide pin etc.) still carry tolerances, which already needed to be considered during the navigation procedure.

Finally, a significant valgus placement of the femoral cap was achieved in all cases, thus avoiding femoral notching and achieving adequate femoral bone preparation. No femoral neck fracture occurred. In our opinion, the system herewith proves itself as reliable and useful. Of course, an increase in operation time could be observed. Yet, considering the benefits of the system, this additional time cost can easily be justified. It must be mentioned, however, that in the first cases, the increase in operation time was partly due to the surgeon's learning curve and the trialing of the system. The last 10 cases had an average navigation time of 22.5 min. This time includes the setting of the reference frames up to the insertion of the guide pin and must be compared with the corresponding surgical steps performed with a conventional system. In our experience, an additional time cost of about 15 min for navigation must be taken into account.

The navigation of the socket is identical to the procedure known from total hip replacement, using the same software already validated. After setting up the basic principles for this procedure (position of reference frame, design of impactor) we experienced no specific difficulties with this module and found the system to produce reliable information about implant positioning. This is especially true for an adequate anteversion, as this is important not only for proper implant positioning but also to avoid impingement of the femoral neck against a protruding anterior rim of the socket or irritation of the psoas tendon.

Summary

The imageless navigation in Birmingham Hip Resurfacing has proven to be a ready-for-use, reliable and user-friendly system for the positioning of the components. With this system, a reliable, significant valgus positioning of the femoral component was achieved without the risk of femoral notching. The possibility to simulate positions and sizes in real-time allows an optimal adaptation to patient-specific conditions. The socket can be placed reliably with correct inclination and anteversion. In our opinion, these benefits clearly weigh against the disadvantage of an additional time cost of about 15 min.

References

1. McMinn D (2003) Development of metal/metal hip resurfacing. Hip International 13: 43–51
2. De Smet KA (2005) Belgium experience with metal-on-metal surface arthroplasty. Orthop Clin North Am 36: 203–213
3. Shimmin AJ, Bare J, Back DL (2005) Complications associated with hip resurfacing arthroplasty. Orthop Clin North Am 36: 187–193
4. Treacy RB, McBryde CW, Pynsent PB (2005) Birmingham hip resurfacing arthroplasty. A minimum follow-up of five years. J Bone Joint Surg Br 87: 167–170
5. Freeman MA (1994) The complications of double-cup replacement of the hip. Churchill Livingstone, Philadelphia
6. Beaule PE, Lee JL, Le Duff MJ, Amstutz HC, Ebramzadeh E (2004) Orientation of the femoral component in surface arthroplasty of the hip. A Biomechanical and clinical analysis. J Bone Joint Surg Am 86: 2015–2021
7. Amstutz HC, Campbell PA, Duff MJL (2004) Fracture of the neck of the femur after surface arthroplasty of the hip. J Bone Joint Surg Am 86: 1874–1877
8. Hess T, Gampe T, Köttgen C, Szawlowski B (2004) Einsatz der Navigation beim Oberflächenersatz des Hüftgelenkes – Methodik und erste Ergebnisse. Orthopäde 33: 1183–1193

Cup and Stem Navigation with the OrthoPilot System

D. Lazovic

Introduction

The aim of navigation in THA is to achieve a higher accuracy in the placement of all components witch should result in a better clinical outcome. The outcome is judged for short term and long term results [1].

Short term clinical results are a good function and a low rate of complications. Both are not only depending on the correct placement of the THA but also of soft-tissue and peri-operative management. The placement related function can be measured by a natural range of motion of the hip, a good muscular function and an equal leg length. By restoring the primary geometry, i.e. the center of rotation, the offset and leg length, the restoration of the muscular function should be eased and the rate of mechanical complications as impingement or dislocation should be excluded.

Different authors have evaluated the importance of a correct positioning of THA. Lewinnek (1978) [2] was the first to calculate the »safe zone« of the cup position in a larger series and Katz (2001) could proof the decreased dislocation rate with correctly positioned cups. In the long run it could prevent increased wear [3] and a higher revision rate [4, 5]. But not only the cup, also the position of the stem influences the leg length and may cause impingement and dislocations [6, 7].

These problems of mal-positioning of THA might even occur more often with »minimally invasive« procedures, as the site of surgery offers a reduced overview of anatomical landmarks [8].

As navigation of the cup position has already proved to increase clinical results it seems consequent that navigation of the stem position should increase these results again.

The Oldenburg Experience

In November 2001, we started with navigation of THA. First systems allowed only the navigation of the cup. In December 2003, navigation of the stem was introduced. Up to now over one thousand THA were implanted with the help of navigation.

The Navigation System

The navigation system (OrthoPilot, BBraun/Aesculap) underwent several technical changes and software releases. Mainly it is an image-free system based on kinematical calculations without the need of pre-operative scanning. The infrared tracking system changed from cable depended active sensors to a passive system, which made handling much more comfortable.

Surgical Technique

Surgical Approach

Surgery was done in a standardized manner, using a cementless titanium spray coated spherical pressfit cup (Plasmacup, BBraun/Aesculap) and a cementless titanium non-anatomical straight stem (Bicontact, BBraun/Aesculap), brought in by the lateral transgluteal approach according to Hardinge [9] and Bauer et al. [10] in supine position. Intra-operatively a c-arm X-ray imaging was used routinely to verify the position of the implants.

Parallel to this standard prosthesis, we use a short stem (Metha, BBraun/Aesculap) for patients younger than 55 years since November 2004. It is applied by a modified mini incision Watson-Jones approach [11].

We always start with the incision and exposure of the hip joint including the opening of the capsule. Then the rigid bodies are applied to the pelvis and the femur. Since 2006 we changed the pelvic rigid body from a pin fixation which was brought in by the main incision to a screw fixation which is done by an additional incision on the iliac crest. This allows shorter incisions in MIS technique. The femoral rigid body is fixed by a clamp on the major trochanter. The navigation system is then calibrated by reference points on both anterior superior iliac spines, the pubic symphysis, the center of the patella and the midpoint of the ankle, which is done in a 90° flexed position of the knee.

The surgical procedure continues with the dislocation of the hip joint and the femoral neck resection.

Cup Navigation

With the acetabulum exposed, the depth is measured with a pointer and the hip center is registered. These data allow now the guided reaming in depth and in the anterior and the lateral plane to achieve the »ideal position« of 45° of inclination and 15° of anteversion according to Lewinnek (1978). The spherical cup is inserted cementless to a safe press fit in the chosen planes and depth and the new center of rotation is registered (■ Figs 48.1 and 48.2).

In a small group of patients we evaluated the position which experienced surgeons would have chosen to ream and to place the cup prior to displaying the navigation values. This allowed an analysis of »free hand« vs. navigated cup position.

Stem Navigation

No reliable data exist on the ideal stem position [12]. So the main aim in placing the stem is to control leg length and offset and to restore a joint geometry which allows a maximum of free range of motion within a safe zone to dislocations by an individual antetorsion, which is depending also on the cup position.

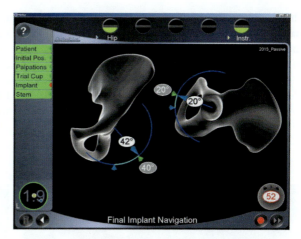

■ **Fig. 48.1.** Screen display of the angles of inclination and anteversion of the final cup implant

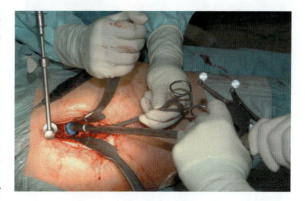

■ **Fig. 48.2.** Registration of the new center of rotation after implantation of the cup. The tracker is circled on a ball fitting the acetabular inlay

The stem preparation starts with a navigation guided box osteotome to open the femoral canal to the following raps. The screen displays real antetorsion of the osteotome and the differences to the former center of rotation of the hip joint.

A software release which also allowed the orientation to the axis of the femur was abandoned as the used straight Bicontact stem cannot be influenced in its position to the femoral axis.

With sequential insertion of the rasps to the final implant size, the screen displays essential predictive data. The expected safe-free range of motion is shown for external rotation with straight leg and for internal rotation in 90° flexion of the hip. The extent of the safe zone can be chosen and was determined to 60° external and 30° internal rotation. Achieving the safe zone can be influenced by modification of the stem antetorsion and by the diameter of the ball (■ Figs. 48.3 and 48.4).

The change of the leg length and the offset change are also displayed in dependence of the ball's neck length.

The short stem prosthesis has a modular cone with different options for ante- or retrotorsion, which allows for even more variations to influence the free range of motion (■ Figs. 48.5 and 48.6).

When the original stem implant is placed, the difference to the probe placement is measured with a pointer and can be taken into account. After the reduction of the hip joint finally the leg is placed in the neutral position in which the calibration of the system was done and the differences in leg length and offset are registered.

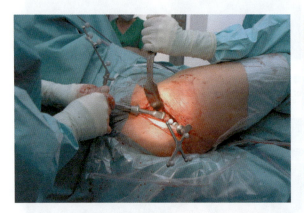

■ **Fig. 48.3.** After insertion of the stem (Short stem Metha) the implant position is registered to calculate the safe zone and the free range of motion

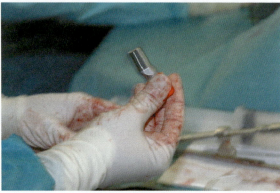

■ **Fig. 48.5.** The modular neck is chosen according to the given data of the navigation simulation

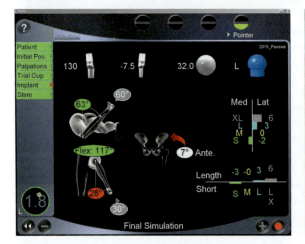

■ **Fig. 48.4.** Screen display after registration of the stem position. The simulation allows modification of antetorsion and CCD angle by choosing different modular necks and leg length and offset by the ball size and neck length

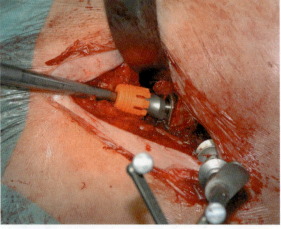

■ **Fig. 48.6.** The modular neck is inserted and connected to the stem prosthesis

Results

Since November 2001 to May 2006 we did 953 THA with cup navigation. THA with navigation of both cup and stem was done from December 2003 to December 2005 in 190 cases.

Additionally we did 17 cup navigation and 24 total THA navigation with the short stem system Metha since November 2004 (◘ Table 48.1).

The 190 cases with total THA navigation were evaluated in the same manner. For the acetabular cup the data of anteversion and inclination and the differences of the new compared to the anatomical center of rotation were registered. Additionally, the stem data for leg length and offset changes and the partially the antetorsion were documented.

Another point of interest was time consumption. We compared the overall time of THA surgery with and without navigation. In our first 110 navigated cups THA the mean time of surgery was 77 min which is 12 min more than without navigation. In the following series, with more routine, the overall time returned to 65 min.

Cup Results

We could already show a good precision of the cup placement by navigation [13] with only 3% of the cups out of a ±5° range to the ideal inclination and 7% out of a ±5° range to the ideal anteversion.

For inclination 100% of the cups were placed within a ±5° range and 85% within a ±2° range, for anteversion the ratio was 96% for the ±5° range and still 85% within the ±2° range (◘ Fig. 48.7 and 48.8).

The center of rotation showed a mean medialization of 2.1 mm and a cranialization of 1.7 mm.

Stem Results

The stem showed a mean leg lengthening of 5.2 mm which may be just the amount the center was cranialized

◘ **Table 48.1.** Numbers of navigated THA for the standard cementless »Bicontact« straight stem system and the cementless »Metha« short stem system, which was used for patients under 55 years since November 2004. Both THA were combined with the cementless »Plasmacup«

	Cup Navigation	Stem Navigation
»Bicontact« straight stem 11/2001–04/2006	953	190
»Metha« short stem 11/2004–04/2006	26	25

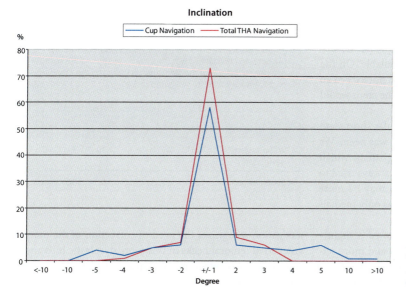

◘ **Fig. 48.7.** Mean deviation of cup inclination to the »ideal« inclination of 45° according to Lewinnek (1978), percentage of cups within the margins

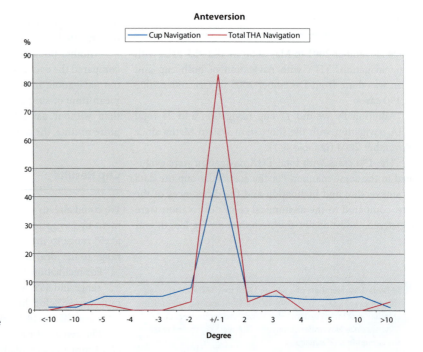

Anteversion

☐ **Fig. 48.8.** Mean deviation of cup ante-version to the »ideal« anteversion of 15° according to Lewinnek (1978), percentage of cups within the margins

by the arthritic wear. The maximum of 20.1 mm and the minimum of -19.4 mm were chosen voluntarily to compensate preexisting leg length discrepancies. A mean medialization of 8.1 mm could be observed. This is due to the geometry of the straight stem. Meanwhile a modified stem is offered, where a higher offset can be chosen to reduce the medialization.

The antetorsion had a mean value of 15°, but we stopped the evaluation, as we had to accept that no objective postoperative measurement was available. On the other hand changes of the antetorsion could not exceed an amount of near to 30° as the geometry of the stem would interfere with the femoral neck anatomy.

In the stem navigated group with modular short stem prostheses a mean elongation of 7.5 mm was seen. We think this due to the younger age of those patients which may have more dysplastic coxarthritis. We always tried to restore the ideal center of rotation, which may be more distal to the dysplastic center. The offset was only medialized to 3.4 mm mean value (☐ Table 48.2).

For the cone the navigated groups showed a slightly more varus CCD (132.5° vs. 135°, median) and more retroversion (−7.5° vs. 0°, median). This shows a tendency of more neutral estimation in free handed stems. The

☐ **Table 48.2**

	Lengthening	Medialization
Stem	10.8 mm	−4.9 mm
Femur	7.1 mm	4.0 mm

☐ **Table 48.3.** In the modular short stem prosthesis »Metha« the neck and ball choice was done by estimation in the series without navigation of the stem and according to the proposal of the simulation in the navigated series

	CCD	Antetorsion	Neck length		
			S	M	L
Without stem navigation	135°	0°	10	9	7
Stem navigation	130°	−7.5°	5	16	4

navigation recognizes the need of correction of the more anteverted femoral necks in this more dysplastic hips and can advise more retroversion within a calculated safe zone (☐ Table 48.3).

Clinical Evaluation

The common complications as thrombosis (0.7%) and 1 superficial infection without retrieval of the prosthesis were as low as in comparable groups.

The dislocation can commonly be seen as the major short term complication in THA. In the cup navigated group the we had 2 dislocations (0.3%) which is low compared to literature. Individual evaluation of those 2 dislocations documented a 20 mm stem subsidence in one case of a man with already the largest size of prosthesis available. In the other case of a woman no reason were found for the spontaneous dislocation. All measured parameters were in the desired range and no concomitant affections could be found. The reason for this dislocation remains unclear. Both dislocations could be treated successfully without further surgery.

In the group of total THA navigation no dislocation occurred, regardless of the stem design.

Conclusions

In our hands navigation of the cup in THA leads to good short term clinical results and to a more accurate implant placement which may lead to a better function and longevity of the prosthesis. With the use of total THA navigation the results even could be improved.

The handling got easier with newer software releases and the use of cable-free passive trackers. This leads to a straight workflow without measurable time delay.

The procedure is now done routinely by all orthopaedic surgeons in our hospital, including the residents. The navigation system forces them to be even more precise, as any deviation is displayed instantly.

Still, there remain some basic problems. First of all, we do not know which is the golden standard for cup inclination and anteversion. There seems to be a high variety in the natural position. We assume the safe zone of Lewinnek to be a good compromise until we get newer data for an individual cup position [14].

The second main problem is the accuracy of the landmark registration. If not done properly the data for the cup position will lack of precision, too [15].

The advantage of additional stem navigation in these cases is that the stem position is calculated in relation to the final cup position. Non-ideal cup positions lead to a modification of the stem position in antetorsion according to the needs of a still safe range of motion. Another advantage can be seen by the use of modular necks. The geometry can be restored to a good functional result without compromising the intra-medullar fixation of the stem. The stem can be placed ideally to the femur and the geometry is restored independently.

Total THA navigation is a useful tool in our hands. It reduces outliers in cup and stem position and leads to good clinical results which is promising a low dislocation and low revision rate and might lead to better long-term results by more accurate implant positioning.

References

1. Morrey BF (2000) Hip dislocation: it's later than you think. Orthopedics 23(9): 935–936
2. Lewinnek GE, Lewis JL, Tarr R, Compere CL, Zimmerman JR (1978) Dislocations after total hip-replacement arthroplasties. J Bone Joint Surg [Am] 60(2): 217–220
3. Del Schutte H Jr, Lipman AJ, Bannar SM, Livermore JT, Ilstrup D, Morrey BF (1998) Effects of acetabular abduction on cup wear rates in total hip arthroplasty. J Arthroplasty 13(6): 621–626
4. Malchau H, Herberts P, Ahnfelt L (1990) Prognosis of total hip replacement in Sweden. Follow-up of 92,675 operations performed 1978–1990. Acta Orthop Scand 64(5): 497–506
5. Malchau H, Herberts P, Eisler T, Garellick G, Sodermann P (2002) The Swedish Total Hip Replacement Register. J Bone Joint Surg [Am] 84A (Suppl 2): 2–20
6. DiGioa AM, Jaramaz B, Blackwell M et al. (1998) Image guided navigation system to measure intraoperatively acetabular implant alignment. Clin Ortho Relat Res 355: 8–22
7. Noble PC, Sugano N, Johnston JD, Thompson MT, Conditt MA, Engh CA Sr, Mathis KB (2003) Computer simulation: how can it help the surgeon optimize implant position? Clin Orthop Relat Res 417: 242–252
8. Woolson S.T. et al. (2004) Comparison of primary total hip replacements performed with a standard incision or a mini incision. J Bone Joint Surg 86-A: 1353–1358
9. Hardinge K (1982) The direct lateral approach to the hip. J Bone Joint Surg 64: 17–19
10. Bauer R, Kerschbauemer F, Poisel S, Oberthaler W (1979) The transgluteal approach to the hip joint. Arch Orthop Trauma Surg 85: 47–49
11. Watson-Jones R, Robinson WC (1956) Arthrodesis of the osteoarthritic hip joint. J Bone Joint Surg [Br] 38B: 353–377
12. Keppler P, Strecker W, Kinzl L (1998) Analysis of leg geometry – standard techniques and normal values. Chirurg 69(11): 1141–1152
13. Lazovic D, Kaib N (2005) Results with navigated Bicontact total hip arthroplasty. Orthopedics 28 s: 1227–1233
14. Kiefer H (2003) OrthoPilot cup navigation – how to optimize cup positioning? Int Orthop. 27 (Suppl 1): 37–42
15. Richolt JA, Rittmeister ME (2003) Is the palpation procedure in imagefree acetabular cup navigation truthful enough? A sonographic assessment. Presentation CAOS, Marbella

Cup and Stem Navigation with the VectorVision System

L. Perlick, T. Kalteis, M. Tingart, H. Bäthis, C. Lüring

Introduction

Over the last 40 years total hip arthroplasty has continued to evolve into a more predictable and refined procedure [20]. Nevertheless, it remains a technical demanding procedure. It is common view that mal-positioning of the acetabular cup in total hip arthroplasty (THA) might restrict the range of motion, that it is the most common cause of luxation and can lead to increased and premature wear and reduces patient's satisfaction [21]. Furthermore, leg-length inequality is still common after primary and revision THA which is also a primary cause for mal-practice liability lawsuits after THA in the United States and in Europe [2, 7, 23]. Therefore, assessing the correct 3-dimensional orientation of the acetabular cup for anteversion and inclination and the stem is the goal to achieve for long-term survivorship THA [13, 15, 16].

Even in experienced surgeons, cup positioning remains a problem when using the conventional operation technique. In a considerable degree the implanted cups exceed the »safe zone« (inclination 40°±10° and anteversion 15°±10°) defined by Lewinnek [3, 9, 11, 12]. The explanation proposed for this is the surgeon's lack of information about the actual and above all variable position of the patient's pelvis during the stages of the operation.

The inaccuracy might be enhanced by the growing interest among surgeons in minimally invasive surgery (MIS), which might provide an earlier recovery and a shorter hospital stay. However, MIS techniques for THR are difficult to perform, due to the limited visibility and therefore might result in a higher risk of implanting errors [23].

Computer-assisted technologies have the potential to solve some of the problems mentioned above. This chapter should present the different opportunities/modules of the Vector-Vision-System and their usage in the clinical routine.

Vector-Vision Workflow Principles

Since the launch of the first CT-based hip application for the Vector Vision in the year 2000, there has been a continuous development. At the current moment the Vector-Vision software 3.0 for total hip replacement consists of three applications. There are two image based modules, the CT-based und the fluoroscopic-based module and one image free module, which is based on intra-operative surface data acquisition only.

CT-Based Module

When using the CT-based module a pre-operative CT-scan of the acetabulum and parts of the femur has to be acquired following a special scan protocol. The data is transferred via CD-ROM to the planning station. After conversion of the data and adjustment of the gray scales several anatomic landmarks have to be defined. The frontal plane (Both spina iliaca anterior superior (ASIS) and most anterior pubic points) has to be fine tuned by the surgeon (Fig. 49.1).

After separation of the femur and the pelvis, which particularly needs some adjustment by the surgeon (Fig. 49.2), the system calculates the cup and stem posi-

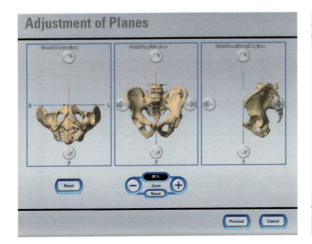

Fig. 49.1. Fine adjustment of the anterior pelvic plane

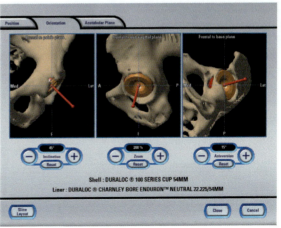

Fig. 49.3. 3D visualization of the planned cup while the surgeon can adjust inclination and anteversion

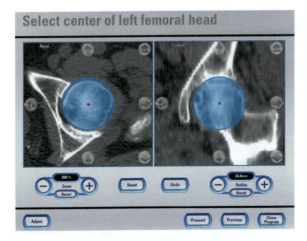

Fig. 49.2. The circumference of the femoral head is marked by the surgeon to ease separation of the bones

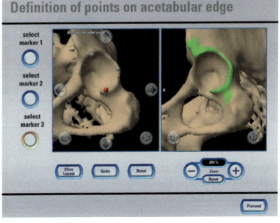

Fig. 49.4. Surface registration. The surgeon is asked to digitize points in the marked area

tion based on a 3-D reconstruction from the CT scan and offers the surgeon a first planning.

The implant position can be adjusted manually depending on the surgeon's preferences (■ Fig. 49.3). The planning can be transferred via network or ZIP-Disk to the Vector-Vision-Navigation system.

The registration process can be performed in two different ways. Paired-point matching takes prominent anatomical points that have been pre-determined and then intra-operatively uses a space digitiser (pointer probe), which identifies or 'matches' the same landmark. The computer algorithm then matches these points to a 'virtual' leg or pelvis built into the software system. Surface registration (■ Fig. 49.4) is a secondary referencing method where a small number of points may be digitized into the system to describe a surface contour such as the distal femoral condyle.

After successful registration the precision has to be verified by cross-referencing additional points on the real anatomy with the reconstructed 3D virtual object on the computer. From this information, the surgeon may judge the operational accuracy of the system.

49

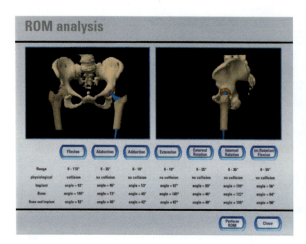

Fig. 49.5. ROM analysis. The system informs about pending collisions between components and bone

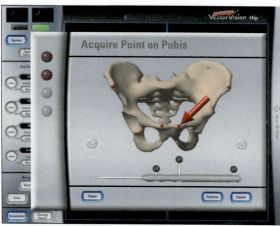

Fig. 49.6. Registration process of the imageless application. The surgeon is asked to digitize the landmarks for the anterior pelvic plane

This is followed by a virtual cinematic analysis of the planned components in which the system informs the surgeon about a possible impingent (▣ Fig. 49.5).

Image-Free Module

The imageless application has the advantage of instant use. It requires simply touch-pointing the anatomical landmarks, which are then registered from the computer. Firstly the anterior pelvic plane is defined by digitizing the ASIS points and two pubis points (▣ Fig. 49.6). Secondly the epicondylar axis and the highest point of the major trochanter are digitized, before the registration process is finished after collecting 30 points in the fossa acetabuli and a hundred points in the acetabulum (▣ Fig. 49.7). The precision of the artificial model can be controlled by placing he pointer on the bone and measurement of the deviation to the model.

Fluoroscopic-Based Module

Fluoroscopic applications suffer from the known problem that earth's magnetic forces might distort the image acquired. Therefore, this method requires a specific calibration to gain an adequate accuracy. The Vector-Vision System comes along with a calibrated grid with markers of known size and spatial relationship to create an accurate virtual portrayal on the computer. The necessary image

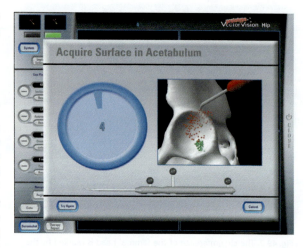

Fig. 49.7. Registration of the acetabulum. 30 points in the fossa (*green*) and a hundred points in the acetabulum have to be acquired

information for this application is acquired at the beginning of the operation.

A maximum of eight pictures is necessary, which includes two a.p. and one oblique view of the following regions: Pubis, spina iliaca on the treated side, femoral neck and femoral head. To generate the model fifteen points in the fossa acetabuli, 100 point in the acetabulum and the epicondylar axis have to be acquired by using the pointer. The femoral morphing, the femoral axis, caput-collum-diaphysis-angle (▣ Fig. 49.8) and the anterior pelvic plane

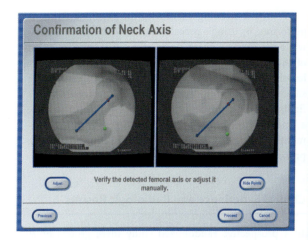

Fig. 49.8. The system automatically determines the CCD angle from the acquired image of the neck

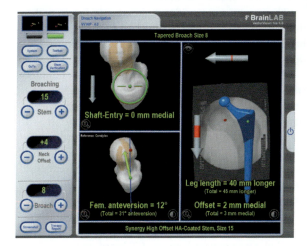

Fig. 49.9. Stem navigation using the fluoroscopic application. The surgeon gains additional information about the leg length, offset and varus/valgus alignment

are calculated automatically by the navigation system. Visualisation intra-operatively is done by an overlay of the acquired picture and the virtual objects (**Fig. 49.9**).

Surgical Procedure

In order to determine the exact spatial orientation of the patient and the surgical instruments, at least three non-collinear points on a fixed body (dynamic reference base

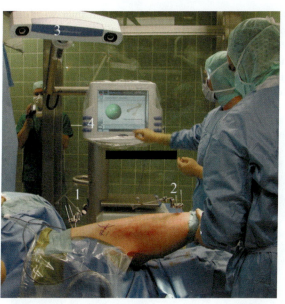

Fig. 49.10. Intra-operative setup for the posterior approach. Two DRBs are fixed by 3.0 mm k-wires (*1, 2*) to the femur and the tibia while the camera (*3*) and monitor (*4*) are positioned opposite to the surgeon

– DRB) must be recognized by a tracking system which then inputs data into the computer for »virtual« referencing. The camera systems of the Vector-Vision-System consist of two charged couple devices (CCDs) that pick up the light signal from the DRBs. The dedicated DRBs are equipped with passive reflector balls which reflect infrared light originating from the light source in the camera. By differentiating the sphere arrangements on the DRBs, the computer then detects the specific DRB on the distal femur or on the tibia.

The procedure can be performed either in a lateral or supine position. At the beginning of the procedure, the two DRBs must be rigidly attached to the pelvis and femur (**Fig. 49.10**). Care must be taken to place them within the camera's line of sight during all steps of the procedure.

The two reference stars and a pointer tool are used to reference the patients anatomy to the computer model or the reconstructed data set following the application specific workflow.

The skin incision is performed and data acquisition on the femur completed. The surgery continues with femoral head resection. Then the registration is completed by gathering the necessary points in the acetabulum. When a sufficient precision is achieved, the acetabulum is prepared by using a pre-callibrated reamer which is constantly guided in terms of inclination and anteversion according to the visualized angles and position on the monitor (■ Fig. 49.11). After the placement of the cup, the final achieved position can be verified, thus revealing how close this position matches the previous plan.

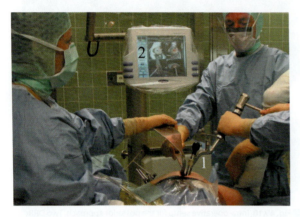

■ **Fig. 49.11.** Application of the acetabular component using a pre-calibrated inserter (*1*) while the system (*2*) is informing about inclination and anteversion

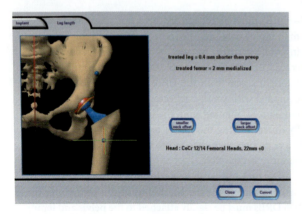

■ **Fig. 49.12.** Stem verification. The surgeon gains additional information about the variation of leg length and offset

Then the reaming process of the proximal femur is performed by using a precalibrated broach handle. Meanwhile the surgeon is informed about the actual position of the broach in the 3D-model, the offset and the leg length. When the desired position is achieved and a stable situation is gained the original stem is implanted and the final position is documented (■ Fig. 49.12). Furthermore a kinematic analysis is performed to exclude an impingement. Then the reference frames are removed and the procedure is finished.

Clinical Experience and Radiologic Results

In a prospective randomized study three groups of 30 patients each were compared to evaluate the precision of the imageless application versus the CT-based application and the conventional technique.

There were no significant differences between the three groups with regard to blood loss. During early rehabilitation there was only one complication as one hip dislocated in the conventional group.

The operation time was increased by 17 minutes when using CT-based navigation compared with the conventional technique and by eight minutes with imageless navigation.

Focussing on Lewinnek's save zone of 40° inclination (SD 10°) and 15° anteversion (SD 10°) 16 of the 30 components (53%) were outside when using the conventional technique, In the CT-based group, five of the 30 components (17%) were outside the safe zone, as were two of the 30 components (7%) using imageless navigation (■ Table 49.1). The smaller variation in the positioning of the acetabular component between CT-based and imageless navigation compared with conventional freehand surgery was indicated by the lower standard deviations in the computer assisted study groups, especially for anteversion.

In a further study using a minimal invasive posterior approach we focussed on the precision of leg length re-

■ **Table 49.1.** Deviations in the three groups

	Inclination	Anteversion
Conventional	43.7° (29° to 57°; SD 7.3°)	22.2° (1° to 53°; SD 14.2°)
CT-based	41.6° (34° to 53°; SD 4.0°)	10.7° (1° to 23°; SD 5.3°)
Imageless	43.2° (33° to 50°; SD 4.0°)	15.2° (5° to 25°; SD 5.5°)

construction using the imageless application versus the conventional technique. The mean variation of leg length was 2.6 mm (+/–3.4 mm) in the navigated and 4.2 mm (+/– 4.5 mm) in the conventional group. There were five outliers in the conventional group which exceeded a deviation of more than 10 mm and of these two had a lengthening of the treated leg of more than 2 cm.

Discussion

The purpose of total joint arthroplasty of the hip and knee is to safely and effectively relieve pain, restore motion, and improve function. As a result, total joint arthroplasty has become one of the most successful and widely acclaimed procedures of the modern operative procedures [17]. Nevertheless, some complications like post-operative dislocation after total hip replacement remained with an overall incidence of 2–3% [14].

The most common cause of failure, however, is an insufficient orientation of the acetabular component [1, 14].

Keeping in mind, that a hip that dislocates because of cup mal-positioning requires further open surgery in up to 71% [4] and this surgical correction is approximately successful in only 80% [14].

Surgical navigation systems have been developed for THA to allow a more precise component implantation compared to the traditional technique [6].

This thesis is supported by our data which showed that the use of the computer assisted technique [CT-based (p=0.003) and imageless navigation (p<0.001)] compared to the freehand procedure resulted in a significant reduction in component placements outside the safe zone, whereas no significant difference was seen between CT-based and imageless navigated acetabular component insertion (p=0.23).

Focussing on the different applications CT-based navigation enables a significant improvement in the accuracy of positioning of the acetabular component, but it was not established in clinical routine, due to the additional operative time, expense and exposure of the patient to radiation [3, 6, 11]. The advantage of this application is that it provides a highly accurate 3D data set for creating a patient specific virtual model in the computer. Therefore, the CT-based application is primarily used at our department for cases of congenital and post-traumatic deformities.

Hube and co-workers compared the precision of a CT-based system and a fluoroscopy-based system. Mean vari-

ation of the post-operative abduction angle to the pre-operative planning was 2.7 (0–8) after CT-based navigation and 3.9 (0–9) after fluoroscopy-based navigation. After the first 30 surgeries with each system, the operating time was extended by 9 min using the CT-based system and by 13 min with the fluoroscopy-based system compared to the traditional technique [5]. Tannast and co-workers analyzed the accuracy of fluoroscopy-guided acetabular cup placement. The variability of cup placement could be reduced for cup inclination but not substantially for cup anteversion. An error analysis of inaccurate landmark reconstruction revealed that the registration of the mid-pubic point with fluoroscopy was a potential source of error [19]. Again the additional OR-time will limit the usage of this application. It might be of use in cases with a minimal approach where it is particularly difficult to digitize the anatomic landmarks through the limited approach.

Imageless navigation may provide a viable alternative. In this procedure, alignment of the implant is based only on landmarks (ASIS, pubic tubercles) acquired intra-operatively by the surgeon using a reference pointer. Imageless navigation is a reliable technical tool, which significantly reduces the variation and inaccuracies of conventional freehand placement of the acetabular component in hip arthroplasty. Nogler and co-workers showed that computer-assisted cup positioning using a non-image-based hip navigation system allows a more consistent placement of the acetabular component in a cadaver study. Kalteis showed as mentioned above, that it is as accurate as the CT-based method, resulting only in a clinically tolerable deviation in cup anteversion and cup inclination [10].

Up to now, it has remained difficult for the imageless application to determine the valgus/varus alignment of the stem correctly. Digitizing the intra-medullary channel seems to be a step in the right direction. Furthermore, the orientation of anteversion is critical when it is only based on the short epicondylar axis [8]. This problem might be enhanced by the fact that the anteversion of the majority of stems follow the natural anatomy. Therefore, it is worthwhile to convert the surgical procedure into a femur first workflow, because the cup adjustment offers more variability for the surgeon.

There are potential pitfalls while using computer-assisted techniques. Problems may occur during different steps of the procedure such as imaging, planning, data collection, tracking, registration and surgical performance. For imageless navigation, surgeons need to be aware that the system cannot determine whether the collected data are correct or incorrect. The accuracy depends on the experience and performance of the surgeon while collecting the data. This scenario can be summarized as »rubbish -in – rubbish-out«. Other errors may occur during the tracking process when the fixation pins of the tracking targets loosen during the registration und tracking. The precision of the optical tracking process might be influenced by operating room lights. Richolt and co-workers focus on the bias of soft-tissue distribution affecting anteversion. Measuring the soft-tissue thickness in 72 patients by ultrasound, they were able to calculate the expected misinterpretation of the anteversion given by a navigation system. Their calculations suggest that a navigation system would have underestimated the anteversion on average by 2.8 degrees +/– 1.8 degrees [18].

Conclusion

The Vector Vision Hip software offers a package of applications which help the surgeon to deal with all kinds of hip from the instant use of the imageless software to the high sophisticated planning module of the CT-based application. Our results show that component alignment can significantly be improved compared to the conventional technique. Nevertheless, the higher precision is connected to extra costs for the hard- and software and a lengthening of the OR-time.

References

1. Biedermann, Tonin A, Krismer M, Rachbauer F, Stockl B, Eibl G (2005) Reducing the risk of dislocation after total hip arthroplasty: the effect of orientation of the acetabular component. J Bone Joint Surg Br 87: 762–769
2. Bose WJ (2000) Accurate limb-length equalization during total hip arthroplasty. Orthopedics 23: 433–436
3. DiGioia AM, Jaramaz B, Blackwell M et al. (1998) The Otto Aufranc Award. Image guided navigation system to measure intraoperatively acetabular implant alignment. Clin Orthop 355: 8–22
4. Dorr LD, Wan Z (1998) Causes of and treatment protocol for instability of total hip replacement. Clin Orthop Relat Res 355: 144–151
5. Hube R, Birke A, Hein W, Klima S (2003) CT-based and fluoroscopy-based navigation for cup implantation in total hip arthroplasty (THA). Surg Technol Int 11: 275–280
6. Jaramaz B, DiGioia AM, III, Blackwell M, Nikou C (1998) Computer assisted measurement of cup placement in total hip replacement. Clin Orthop 354: 70–81
7. Jasty M, Webster W, Harris W (1996) Management of limb length inequality during total hip replacement. Clin Orthop Relat Res 333: 165–171
8. Jerosch J, Peuker E, Philipps B, Filler T (2002) Interindividual reproducibility in perioperative rotational alignment of femoral components in knee prosthetic surgery using the transepicondylar axis. Knee Surg Sports Traumatol Arthrosc 10: 194–197
9. Jolles BM, Genoud P, Hoffmeyer P (2004) Computer-assisted cup placement techniques in total hip arthroplasty improve accuracy of placement. Clin Orthop Relat Res 426: 174–179
10. Kalteis T, Handel M, Herold T, Perlick L, Paetzel C, Grifka J (2005) Position of the acetabular cup-accuracy of radiographic calculation compared to CT-based measurement. Eur J Radiol 58: 294–3000
11. Leenders T, Vandevelde D, Mahieu G, Nuyts R (2002) Reduction in variability of acetabular cup abduction using computer assisted surgery: a prospective and randomized study. Comput Aided Surg 7: 99–106
12. Lewinnek GE, Lewis JL, Tarr R, Compere CL, Zimmerman JR (1978) Dislocations after total hip-replacement arthroplasties. J Bone Joint Surg Am 60: 217–220
13. McCollum DE, Gray WJ. Dislocation after total hip arthroplasty. Causes and prevention. Clin Orthop Relat Res 261: 159–170
14. Morrey BF (1997) Difficult complications after hip joint replacement. Dislocation. Clin Orthop Relat Res 344: 179–187
15. Paterno SA, Lachiewicz PF, Kelley SS (1997) The influence of patient-related factors and the position of the acetabular component on the rate of dislocation after total hip replacement. J Bone Joint Surg Am 79: 1202–1210
16. Pierchon F, Pasquier G, Cotten A, Fontaine C, Clarisse J, Duquennoy A (1994) Causes of dislocation of total hip arthroplasty. CT study of component alignment. J.Bone Joint Surg.Br. 76: 45–48
17. Ranawat CS, Ranawat AS (2003) Minimally invasive total joint arthroplasty: where are we going? J Bone Joint Surg Am 85-A: 2070–2071
18. Richolt JA, Effenberger H, Rittmeister ME (2005) How does soft tissue distribution affect anteversion accuracy of the palpation procedure in image-free acetabular cup navigation? An ultrasonographic assessment. Comput Aided Surg 10: 87–92
19. Tannast M, Langlotz U, Siebenrock KA, Wiese M, Bernsmann K, Langlotz F (2005) Anatomic referencing of cup orientation in total hip arthroplasty. Clin Orthop Relat Res 436: 144–150
20. Waldman BJ (2003) Advancements in minimally invasive total hip arthroplasty. Orthopedics 26: s833–s836
21. Widmer KH, Zurfluh B (2004) Compliant positioning of total hip components for optimal range of motion. J Orthop Res 22: 815–821
22. Woolson ST, Hartford JM, Sawyer A (1999) Results of a method of leg-length equalization for patients undergoing primary total hip replacement. J Arthroplasty 14: 159–164
23. Woolson ST, Mow CS, Syquia JF, Lannin JV, Schurman DJ (2004) Comparison of primary total hip replacements performed with a standard incision or a mini-incision. J Bone Joint Surg Am 86-A: 1353–1358

49

Part IV B Minimally Invasive Surgery: Total Hip Arthroplasty

Total Hip Arthroplasty with the Minimally-Invasive Two-Incisions Approach

R. Berger

Introduction

Minimally invasive surgery has the potential for minimizing surgical trauma, pain, and recovery time. These attributes are especially appealing in total hip replacement, which historically has had a protracted recovery. To achieve the rapid recovery that these minimally invasive techniques can afford, the entire peri-operative pathway needs to be revised. Combining a minimally invasive total hip arthroplasty, where no muscle or tendon is damaged as part of the surgery, with a new pathway, which expedites that entire recovery process, outpatient total hip replacement is possible. In fact, outpatient total hip replacement but is currently routinely performed at our institution daily.

These minimally invasive techniques in total hip replacement include single incision and two-incision techniques. Most of the single incision minimally invasive techniques for total hip replacement are modification of traditional total hip replacement techniques. However, a new minimally invasive technique for total hip replacement was developed that uses two-incision. This new minimally invasive technique avoids transecting muscle or tendon, thereby minimizing morbidity and recovery. This chapter describes this new minimally invasive hip replacement procedure performed with two-incisions; one incision is for acetabular preparation and placement; the other is for the femoral preparation and placement. Unique instruments have been developed to facilitate this technique. Since the patient is supine with this technique, fluoroscopy can be used to aid in many steps in this process to ensure the proper starting points for the incisions and accurate component position and alignment. Standard implants are used to maintain the present expectation for implant durability.

Indications and Contraindications

As in most surgical procedures, female patients who are thin and not muscular with a small bone structure and atrophic changes are the easiest to perform this procedure. These patients are best to begin your experience. As experience is gained, the surgeon can progress to more challenging patient type. The most difficult patients are males who are heavy and muscular with a large bone structure and hypertrophic changes. However, I have found that this two-incision approach is the easiest of the minimally invasive approaches to perform on the heavy, muscular male patients. Unlike all of the other minimally invasive THA approaches that require significant mobilization of the leg during the procedure, which is especially difficult in the heavy, muscular male patient, during this two-incision approach the leg remains in one of two anatomic positions during the entire case.

While this procedure was found to be safe and practical to most patients who are candidates for traditional THA, there are conditions that are not amenable to the minimally invasive two-incision procedure at this time. Cadaveric work has shown that this two-incision procedure is very challenging in morbidly obese patients. Additionally, patients with very marked abnormal hip joint anatomy, significant prior surgical scaring, or complete hip dislocation may be better candidates for an alternate total hip arthroplasty approaches. Today, with these exceptions, there is no significant difference in patients receiving a minimally invasive two-incision approach compared to a more standard approach in my practice.

Pre-Operative Planning

The importance of pre-operative planning and templating cannot be overemphasized. This is particularly true in the case of this minimally invasive total hip arthroplasty approach since visualization of extra-articular landmarks is limited. The objective of pre-operative planning is to enable you to gather anatomic parameters that will allow accurate intra-operative placement of the femoral and acetabular implants. Optimal femoral and acetabular component fit, the level of the femoral neck cut, the prosthetic neck length, and the femoral component offset can be evaluated through pre-operative radiographic analysis. Pre-operative planning also allows the surgeon to have the appropriate implants available at surgery.

Determining pre-operative leg length is essential for restoration of the appropriate leg length during THA. As in all total hip arthroplasties, pre-operative templating using an anterior/posterior (A/P) view of the pelvis is usually the most accurate method of determining proper leg length. Only in extremely unusual cases is a scanogram or CT evaluation of leg length helpful. From the clinical and radiographic information about leg lengths, determine the appropriate correction, if any, to be achieved during surgery.

Although rare, it may not be possible to restore offset in patients with an unusually large pre-operative offset or with a severe varus deformity. In such cases, lengthening the limb can increase the tension in the abductor muscles. This method is especially useful when the involved hip is shorter than the contra-lateral hip. However, in these cases there is usually no choice but to lengthen the hip and leg. With lengthening, patient dissatisfaction my result; however, in some uncommon cases where stability and leg length cannot be optimized, it is more important to achieve hip stability than leg-length equality.

The initial templating begins with the A/P radiograph. Superimpose the acetabular templates sequentially on the pelvic X-ray film with the acetabular component in approximately 45 degrees of abduction. Assess several sizes to estimate which acetabular component will provide the best fit for maximum coverage. Mark the acetabular

size and position, and the center of the head on the x-ray films. Note the superior coverage of the acetabular component in 45° of abduction, reproduce this during surgery to assure proper component abduct and avoid vertical positioning. Next, select the appropriate femoral template. To estimate the femoral implant size, assess both the distal stem size and the body size on the A/P radiograph, and then check the stem size on the lateral radiograph. The stem of the femoral component should fill, or nearly fill, the medullary canal in the isthmus area on the A/P X-ray film. Next, assess the fit of the stem body in the metaphyseal area. The medial portion of the body of the component should fill the proximal metaphysis as fully as possible.

After establishing the appropriate size of the femoral component, determine the height of its position in the proximal femur. If the leg length is to remain unchanged, the center of the head of the prosthesis should be at the same level as the center of the femoral head of the patient's hip. This should also correspond to the center of rotation of the acetabulum. To lengthen the limb, raise the template proximally. To shorten the limb, shift the template distally. Once the height has been determined, note the distance in millimeters from the collar or most proximal aspect of the porous surface to the top of the lesser trochanter.

Surgical Approach

The patient is placed in the supine position with a small bolster under the ischium on the effected side. This allows better visualization of the acetabulum as the femur falls posteriorly after the femoral head is resected. A radiolucent operating room table is used. The entire leg and hip are prepped and draped. The fluoroscope is used to define the femoral neck. A metallic instrument is used to mark the midline of the femoral neck from the junction of the head and neck distally to the inter-trochanteric line. In addition the interval between sartorius medially and tensor fascia lata laterally should be palpated. Most of the incision should be lateral to this interval, avoiding the lateral femoral cutaneous nerve. The anterior incision is made directly over the femoral neck from the base of the femoral head distally about 1.5 inches to the inter-trochanteric line. The fascia of sartorius is present in the proximal-medial incision whereas the tensor fascia lata lies at the distal-lateral portion of the incision. The sartorius muscle and tensor fascia lata can be seen beneath the fascia. Just medial to the edge of the tensor fascia lata, the fascia is incised longitudinally, parallel to the sartorius muscle and tensor fascia lata. This lateral fascial incision avoids the lateral femoral cutaneous nerve, which is located superficial to the sartorius muscle. Sartorius is retracted medially, and tensor fascia lata is retracted laterally; exposing the lateral border of rectus femoris. The medial retractor is repositioned to retract the rectus muscle medially (■ Fig. 50.1). This exposes the lateral circumflex vessels, which are coagulated with an electrocautery. The pericapsular fat then is retracted medially and laterally exposing the capsule over the femoral neck.

Two curved lit Hohmann retractors (part of the minimally-invasive two-incision instruments [Zimmer, Warsaw, IN]) are placed extra-capsularly around the femoral neck, illuminating the capsule. The capsule is incised in line with the femoral neck. This incision is made from the edge of the acetabulum distally to the inter-trochanteric line. The two curved lit Hohmann retractors are repositioned intra-capsularly exposing the femoral head and neck from the acetabulum to the inter-trochanteric line.

Since the muscles and tendons around the hip have not been disrupted, the hip cannot easily be dislocated. An in situ neck cut should be made. It is easier to remove the head in two pieces rather then one; therefore, two neck cuts are made. The initial neck osteotomy is made at the equator of the femoral head, as close to the acetabulum as possible, with an oscillating saw. A second cut is made 1 cm distal to this. The small 1 cm wafer of bone is removed using a threaded Steinmann pin. Next, a threaded Steinmann pin is placed into the femoral head and the head is removed. If the ligamentum teres is intact, a curved osteotome is used to transect the ligamentum teres. Then the final femoral neck osteotomy is made based upon pre-operative templating. Appropriate femoral neck resection is confirmed with fluoroscopy or by flexing and externally rotating the hip in a figure-of-four, which exposes the lesser trochanter.

Three curved lit Hohmann retractors are placed around the acetabulum, one anteriorly around acetabulum, a second posteriorly around the acetabulum, and the third directly superiorly over the brim of the acetabulum. This retracts the capsule and allows excellent visualization of the acetabulum (■ Fig. 50.2). The labrum is excised, exposing the entire peripheral bony rim of the acetabulum and the pulvinar.

The superior retractor is removed while the anterior and posterior retractors are left in place. Specially designed, low profile reamers (part of the minimally-invasive two-in-

cision instruments), which are cutout on the sides, are used to ream the acetabulum (■ Fig. 50.3). These reamers are aggressive with square cutting teeth; therefore, it is possible to start with a reamer that is close in size to the intended final reamer to avoid inserting and extracting many reamers. Furthermore, the open design of these reamers allows visualization of the acetabulum during reaming. With gentle traction on the leg, the reamer is inserted in line with the femoral neck, with the cutouts of the reamer aligned with the two retractors. The cut out reamer is seated to the floor

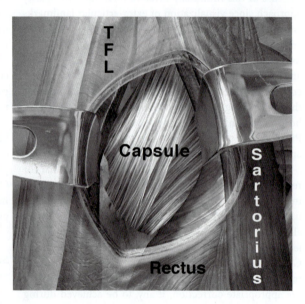

■ **Fig. 50.1.** Illustration shows the capsule exposed by retracting rectus femoris medially

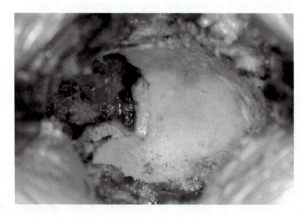

■ **Fig. 50.2.** Photograph shows lit Hohmann retractor placement and an excellent view of acetabulum

of the acetabulum. The acetabulum is reamed at 45° of abduction and 20° of anteversion. The fluoroscope can be used for visualization as the acetabulum is reamed. When the cut out reamers are rotating, they appear as solid reamers so that the fit and fill of the acetabulum can be assessed. The acetabulum is sequentially reamed until a healthy bleeding bed of cancellous bone is present throughout. The acetabulum component is selected that is 2 millimeters larger then the final reamer used.

A specialized dogleg acetabular inserter (part of the minimally-invasive two-incision instruments) with the supine positioner is used to place the chosen acetabulum shell. The anterior and posterior retractors are left in place, as gentle traction is placed on the leg. The bolster beneath the ischium is removed so that the patient's pelvis is parallel to the bed and floor. This can be confirmed with fluoroscopy. The acetabular component is inserted as the retractors keep the capsule from invaginating. The acetabulum is viewed with the fluoroscope as the cup is positioned in 45° of abduction and 20° of anteversion, following the native acetabulum. The cup is then impacted in place. The inserter is then removed and the final cup position is then confirmed. With the curved lit acetabular retractor in place around the acetabulum, the stability of the shell is assessed. If desired, supplemental screws are placed in the posterosuperior quadrant of the shell. Finally, a small curved osteotome is used to remove any osteophytes around the rim of the acetabulum and the polyethylene liner is impacted into the shell. All retractors are removed from the acetabulum and attention is turned to the femur.

The leg is adducted and placed in neutral rotation. A 1 to 1.5 inch incision is made in the posterior lateral buttocks, just posterior to a line colinear to the femoral canal. A Charnley awl is guided through the posterior incision, posterior to the gluteus medius and minimus and anterior to the piriformis fossa down the femoral canal. Fluoroscopy can aid this starting point and can be used to visualize the leg in a frog lateral position to confirm the entry point. Specially designed side-cutting reamers (part of the minimally-invasive two-incision instruments) are used to enlarge this starting hole and position the starting point laterally against the trochanteric bed so that the stem is in a neutral position. These side-cutting reamers are used sequentially through the posterior incision within the same track as the Charnley awl. If a distally coated stem is to be used, flexible reamers are used to ream the canal until cortical chatter is obtained. Subsequently, straight reamers with a tissue-protecting sleeve then are used to ream the

femoral diaphysis until good cortical chatter is obtained. If a proximally coated stem is to be used, proceed directly to broaching. (I recommend using a distally coated stem for this procedure.)

After reaming to the appropriate size, broaching is done. With visualization though the anterior wound, the rasp is rotationally aligned to the calcar. The rasp is fully seated. Rasps then are sequentially introduced and seated, finishing with appropriate size (◘ Fig. 50.4). When the final rasp is seated, care must be taken to visualize the

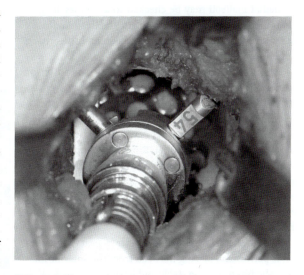

◘ **Fig. 50.3.** Photograph shows the acetabular reamer being placed into the anterior incision, between the two lit Hohmann retractors

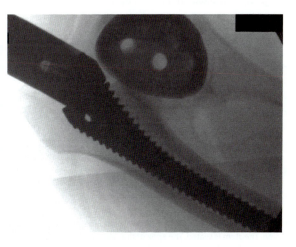

◘ **Fig. 50.4.** Fluoroscopic view shows the final femoral rasp seated

rotation of the rasp in the anterior wound to ensure alignment with the metaphysis.

A trial reduction may be performed. The trial neck and head are placed on the broach from the anterior wound. The hip is then put through a range of motion to assess stability. The hip should be stable in full extension with 90° of external rotation and 90° of flexion with 20° of adduction and at least 50° of internal rotation. The fluoroscope can be used to assess leg lengths by comparing the level of the lesser trochanters with the obturator foramen. In addition, with the patient in the supine position, the medial malleoli may be checked to assess leg length. When the trial reduction is complete, the head and neck are removed though the anterior incision and the broach are removed through the posterior incision.

Two Hohmann retractors are placed into the posterior wound, one anterior to the femoral neck, and one posterior to the femoral neck. These retract the soft tissue as the stem is placed into the femoral canal. The stem then is introduced into the femoral canal from the posterior incision. Once down the canal, the stem is impacted into place as the rotation is controlled. Visualization through the anterior incision ensures no soft tissue entrapment between the calcar and the collar and assures correct stem version (◘ Fig. 50.5). The final stem is seated and confirmed with fluoroscopy.

With the actual component in place, repeat trial reduction is performed, placing the head from the anterior incision. The hip should be stable and leg lengths equal. With the hip in external rotation and the bone hook around the neck, the actual metal head is then placed on the neck and gently impacted in place. The hip is located with

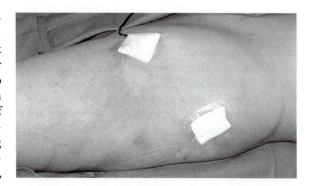

◘ **Fig. 50.6.** Photograph shows the final two 2 x 2 inch bandages cover the incisions on a patient who had a minimally invasive two-incision THA.

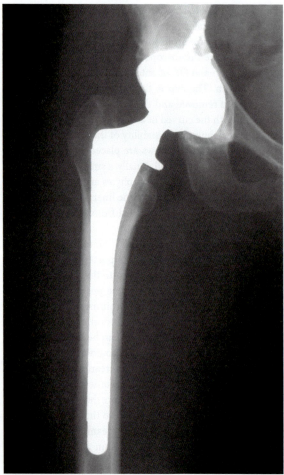

◘ **Fig. 50.7.** Post-operative radiographs show with the minimally invasive two-incision THA reconstruction

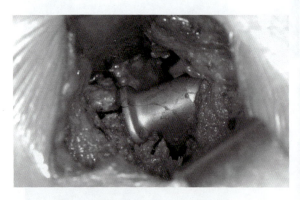

◘ **Fig. 50.5.** Photograph shows the femoral component in the anterior incision. The stem is seated. The apex of the calcar and the apex of the stem are marked, showing the stem in the correct version

gentle traction and internal rotation. The capsule is then closured. The fascia between the sartorius and the tensor fascia lata is closed, followed by closure of the anterior and posterior incisions. Two 2×2 inch bandages are used to cover the incisions (◘ Fig. 50.6). ◘ Figure 50.7 demonstrates the post-operative radiographs of this case example.

Avoiding Common Intra-Operative Error

Complications of the minimally invasive two incision total hip replacement are similar to traditional total hip replacement. The most common intra-operative complication is femoral fracture resulting from either varus alignment or excessive anteverting during femoral preparation or stem insertion. Outlined are commonly made mistakes and how to avoid them.

Anesthesia: Regional anesthesia will result in increased muscle tone compared to general anesthesia and will make every step of the procedure more difficult. It is preferable to start with general anesthesia, as this allows maximum muscle relaxation and facilitated the procedure, and then when more experience is gained, regional techniques may be used.

The anterior incision: A common mistake is to make the anterior incision too medial – especially on heavier patients. The incision should be centered over the TFL and extend just to the lateral boarder of sartorius. The interval between TFL and sartorius can usually be palpated prior to the incision. Alternately, the incision should be made lateral to a line that extends from the ASIS to the center of the knee. Medial placement of the incision will cause the lateral aspect of the incision to be over stretched and possible torn when preparing and placing the acetabulum. Furthermore, if the incision extends over the body of sartorius, the lateral cutaneous nerve my be encountered and injured.

The lateral femoral cutaneous nerve: It is not advisable to explore or dissect the lateral cutaneous nerve; this may result in scaring of the nerve with subsequent hypoesthesia of the thigh.

The femoral head resection: First, a common mistake is to have the side edge of the saw either cut into sartorius, TFL, or the skin. This is avoided by proper retractor placement. Second, there is a tendency to not see the acetabulum prior to cutting the head. This results in a neck cut that is too low, making it very difficult to remove the femoral head since the resection will not be intra-capsular. The femoral head should be exposed until edge of the acetabulum is seen. Once the acetabular is seen, the first neck cut is made as high on the head as possible, close to the edge of the acetabulum. Another common mistake is to not cleanly osteotomize the head so that irregular edges remain, subsequently making head removal more difficult. After making the proximal cut, the second resection cut is made 1 cm distal to the proximal cut. It is common to use the saw so that the anterior aspect of the intercalary thinner than the posterior aspect; this results in inability to remove the intercalary segment. The second femoral osteotomy must be made so that the anterior aspect of the intercalary piece is thicker than the posterior aspect; this allows the intercalary segment to be removed.

Acetabular reaming: As the acetabulum is reamed in the correct version, the reamer can be levered on the femur forcing the reamer anteriorly. This is especially true if the femoral neck osteotomy results in a long remaining neck. This tendency to ream anteriorly can be counteracted by posterior pressure on the reamer during reaming.

Acetabular positioning: It is common to overly anteverted the acetabular component. Make sure the acetabular component is anatomic with the native acetabulum.

The posterior incision: It is common to mark the posterior incision too anterior, colinear with the femoral canal. This will result in piercing and injuring the abductor. The posterior incision must be made posterior to a line colinear to the femoral canal. Then, the femoral awl is introduced posterior to the abductors.

Entering the femoral canal: Allowing the starting awl to enter the femoral canal too medial, into the cancellous bone of the osteotomy, is a common mistake. If this starting hole is placed medial, varus stem positioning or femoral fracture will likely result. This will be avoided if the femoral canal is initially entered at the most lateral aspect of the canal.

Broaching and stem placement: The broach and stem will initially seem retroverted when properly rotated. In other words, the common mistake is to overly anteverts the broach and stem; this can result in femoral fracture.

Stem insertion: In some cases, particularly with a larger stem or an extended offset stem, the femoral neck may get caught the lateral edge of the acetabulum during insertion. Less adduction of the leg can alleviate this impingement. Alternately, bringing the leg into a neutral position and applying traction will deliver the collar and neck trough the capsule. This maneuver is most effectively done when the stem is about 1 cm from fully seated.

Postoperative Management

During the procedure and post-operatively, the patient was keep well hydrated to prevent postoperative hypotension and nausea. The Foley catheter is discontinued in all patients 2 hours postoperatively. Twenty milligrams of OxyContin are given orally 2 hours post-operatively and the epidural is removed 4 hours post-operatively. The intravenous tubing is removed and the intravenous catheter was maintained with a heparin lock five hours post-operatively.

Occupational and physical therapy are initiated at 5 to six 6 post-operatively. Patients are weight bearing as tolerated on the surgically treated extremity. All patients are first taught bed and chair transfers. They receive teaching for ambulation; first with crutches, then with a cane, and finally without any assistive device the day of surgery. Lastly patients are taught chair ascent and descent; first with crutches and then without any assistive. Patients are discharged from the hospital once strict criteria were met including the ability to independently transfer out of and into bed from a standing position, rise to and from a chair to a standing position, ambulate 100 feet, and ascend and descend a full flight of stairs.

Upon discharge, patients continue taking Celebrex, 200 mg daily for at least 2 weeks, and gradually decreased their dose of OxyContin as needed; hydrocodone is taken as needed for breakthrough pain. Starting the evening of surgery, all patients receive aspirin for deep venous thrombosis prophylaxis for three weeks.

Patients are encouraged to start activities as soon tolerated. They are allowed to drive when off all narcotics. Home physical therapy is used until the patient could drive; then outpatient physical therapy is started. The patient and therapist are encouraged to advance as quickly as possible. No hip precautions are emphasized. Patients progressed to a cane as tolerated. They are encouraged to use a cane until they could ambulate without a limp, and then to discontinue the use of the cane. Patients also are encouraged to resume activities as tolerated. Patients who work are encouraged to return to work as soon as they feel comfortable.

Results

In a study 200 consecutive patients were carefully selected from 571 otherwise healthy patients undergoing primary total hip replacement. A comprehensive peri-operative management pathway was developed and implemented around preoperative teaching, regional anesthesia, and preemptive oral analgesia and antiemetic therapy. A rapid rehabilitation pathway with full weight bearing was implemented within few hours after surgery. If standard discharge criteria were met the day of surgery, the patient had the option of discharge to home the day of surgery.

One hundred ninety-two (96%) of the 200 patients were discharged to home the day of surgery. In the four patients that received general anesthesia instead of regional anesthesia, two developed post-operative orthostatic hypotension and consequently were unable to achieve the discharge criteria the day of surgery (p < 0.05). Post discharge, there were no readmissions for pain, nausea, or hypotension. There was one readmission 10 week for a traumatic peri-prosthetic fracture and one stress fracture at the end of the stem was treated conservatively.

These newer anesthetic and rehabilitation protocols allow outpatient total hip arthroplasty to be done in carefully selected, healthy patients. Of the 200 patients enrolled in this comprehensive outpatient protocol, 96% were discharged the day of surgery. The use of regional anesthesia was statistically related to patients being discharged the day of surgery. Furthermore, as the team became more responsive to early signs of nausea and hypotension, acting swiftly, a larger percentage of patients were discharged the day of surgery.

Conclusion

Minimally invasive surgery has the potential to minimize surgical trauma and pain while improving functional recovery in patients having total hip replacement. The minimally invasive two-incision total hip technique described here, where muscle and tendon trauma is minimized, shows substantial short-term pain and functional improvement over traditional hip replacement. While this minimally invasive two-incision technique shows great promise; this technique requires meticulous surgical technique, specialized instrumentation, and special instruction. Therefore, specialized training is strongly recommended for surgeons interested in this new technique to minimize complications and ensure success.

50

Direct Lateral Approach in Minimally Invasive Surgery Total Hip Arthroplasty

A.V. Lombardi Jr., K.R. Berend

Introduction

During the past several years there has been an increasing interest in reducing iatrogenic surgical trauma while performing arthroplasty via a minimization of the surgical dissection required to achieve a satisfactory total hip arthroplasty. Concomitant with less invasive surgical approaches has been the development of rapid recovery protocols, which facilitate an earlier return to activities of daily of living [1, 2]. Therefore, the ability to streamline postoperative recovery has been an effective marriage of minimally invasive surgery with detailed postoperative rehabilitation protocols. Rapid recovery protocols have been defined as multi-factorial. They involve the development of a culture of healing. At the onset there must be an alignment of expectations of the surgeon, the patient and the family. Preoperative education of patient and family combined with preoperative physiotherapy and rehabilitation serve to allay peri-operative stress and anxiety and facilitate a more rapid return to function. Optimization of the patient's preoperative medical status facilitates a smoother postoperative course which allows the patient to participate immediately in physiotherapy and rehabilitation. Effective multimodal pain management strategies have been shown to assist patients in earlier attainment of postoperative milestones [3, 4]. Critical pathways focused on early mobilization and discharge have also been shown to enhance outcomes. When rapid recovery outcomes are combined with minimization of surgical trauma via minimally invasive surgery, incremen-tal improvement in the early postoperative phase has been demonstrated.

The direct lateral or anterolateral abductor splitting approach has been a traditional workhorse in total hip arthroplasty [5–7]. As with many surgical techniques, numerous variations have been described. At the essence of all of these modifications is a partial release of the confluence of the vastus lateralis, and gluteus medius and minimus from the anterolateral attachment to the femur, which facilitates an anterolateral approach to the hip joint. The virtues of the direct lateral approach have been excellent visualization of the acetabulum and proximal femur for appropriate alignment and orientation of both the acetabular and femoral components. This approach has also been touted as a safer approach with respect to minimization of the incidence of dislocation. While this may represent its primary virtue, it comes at the expense of a slightly prolonged postoperative rehabilitation course to eliminate the initial limp. The author's experience with the anterolateral abductor splitting approach through a standard incision has been previously summarized [5,6]. The skin incision utilized was a straight laterally based incision, centered over the trochanter and lateral aspects of the femur commencing at the approximate level of the anterior superior iliac spine extending across the greater trochanter and distally for 10–15 centimeters. Overall length of the incision was not considered critical. The incision in the fascia of the gluteus maximus and the iliotibial band was made along the line of the incision. The deeper dissection commenced in the posterior vastus lateralis several centimeters distal to the vastus tubercle, extended proximally to the vastus tubercle and curved anteriorly along the anterolateral aspect of the femur to the anterolateral tip of the trochanter (■ Fig. 51.1). Dissection into the gluteus medius, minimus and capsule proceeded along the line of the femoral neck thereby detaching the anterior one-third of the gluteus medius, minimus complex and leaving the posterior two-thirds intact. Therefore, the most significant variation from the most popularized variation by Hardinge of the direct lateral approach involved minimization of the detachment of the gluteus medius and minimus [7]. We initially described the utility of this modification and demonstrated excellent recovery of the abductor function with gait lab analysis [5]. In a study of 1518 total hip arthroplasties in 1262 patients the authors reported the efficacy of this approach with respect to postoperative stability and minimal dislocation, reporting a dislocation rate of 0.25% in a subset of 1205 total hips in patients with a diagnosis of osteoarthritis [6]. Low dislocation rates were also reported in patients with high risk diagnoses for dislocation such as patients with developmental dysplasia of the hip or a preoperative diagnosis of subcapital hip fracture. More recently, we have studied our experience with this approach in revision total hip arthroplasty involving isolated liner exchange [8]. We noted a significant reduction in the incidence of dislocation when compared to other reports of the same procedure performed via posterior approach. Our findings have been confirmed by several other authors [9,10].

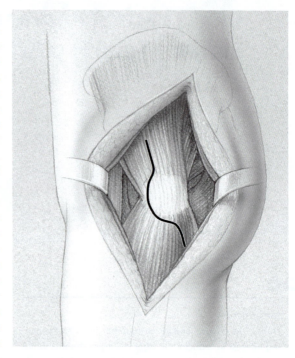

■ **Fig. 51.1.** Illustration shows the dissection into gluteus medius and minimus utilized with the traditional direct lateral approach. (Reproduced with permission of Joint Implant Surgeons, Inc. ©2006)

Surgical Technique

Based on our long-term excellent experience with the anterolateral abductor muscle-splitting approach and our commitment to rapid recovery, combined with a growing patient expectation for rapid return of function, we have adopted a modification to this approach which involves a minimization of surgical dissection (■ Fig. 51.2). The essentials of this modification are avoidance of dissection into the vastus lateralis insertion into the proximal femur, a limit in the proximal dissection of the gluteus medius to 1–2 cm, and an attempt to spare the majority of the gluteus minimus insertion. It is the authors' impression that concentration on these details constitutes the core meaning of minimally invasive surgery.

To facilitate exposure during minimally invasive surgery, manufacturers have assisted by developing a number of specialized instruments. In addition to a variety of retractors, curved reamers, curved acetabular and femoral inserters, and brooch handles have been designed. Visualization has also been enhanced by the use of light sources incorporated into the helmets of personal isolator suits and lighted retractors.

The actual surgical procedure commences with proper preoperative planning. An antero-posterior (AP) radiograph of the pelvis to include both hips is extremely useful to assist in determination of leg length discrepancy. An AP of the involved hip with appropriate magnification markers will assist in the correct placement of templates. Determination of the proper placement of the center of rotation and the resection level of the femur to restore the center of rotation are two critical aspects of pre-operative planning. It is important to determine the placement of the femoral component with respect to both the lesser trochanter and the tip of the greater trochanter.

The patient is positioned in the lateral decubitus position with the operative hip facing the operative field. It is imperative to palpate and determine bony landmarks, specifically the lateral aspect of the femur and the most

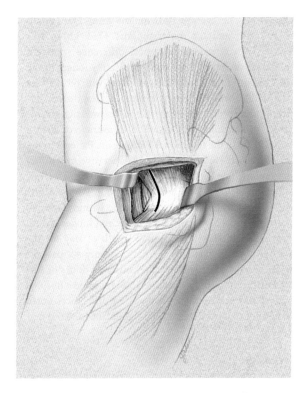

◘ **Fig. 51.2.** Illustration shows the muscle dissection used for the minimally invasive direct lateral approach. Note that the skin incision has evolved to a slightly more anterior to posterior direction compared with the more inferior to superior incision used in the traditional approach. (Reproduced with permission of Joint Implant Surgeons, Inc. ©2006)

superior aspect of the greater trochanter. A spinal needle is used to assist in localization of the tip of the greater trochanter. The incision is then outlined, which is two thirds proximal and one third to this point. This incision should be biased approximately 30 degrees posteriorly with the superior aspect being posterior to the greater trochanter and inferior aspect being slightly anterior to greater trochanter. In this fashion, the distal portion of the wound is used to ream and prepare the acetabulum, while the proximal portion of the wound is used to ream and prepare the femur.

The incision is carried down through the skin and subcutaneous tissue, which is released from the underlying fascia. The fascia is then incised along the line of the incision. This allows for exposure of the lateral aspect of the femur, and specifically the greater trochanter. Abduction and external rotation of the femur by the assistant

will facilitate exposure. Beginning at the vastus ridge distally, and moving proximally, the anterior attachment of the gluteus medius is released from the proximal femur. The authors prefer to utilize electrocautery, which allows hemostasis, while the entire sleeve of soft tissue is released from the anterior cortex of the femoral neck. As the dissection proceeds proximally, the assistant continues to externally rotate the extremity, allowing for further release from the anteromedial neck. The soft tissue sleeve includes the distal insertion of the gluteus medius and capsule, and release occurs from the proximal aspect of the lesser trochanter across the femoral neck and head. Proceeding from distal to proximal, release is carried out to the antero-superior aspect of the greater trochanter. The gluteus medius is bluntly separated from the gluteus minimus. A fatty tissue plane exists between the gluteus medius and minimus. A blunt retractor is placed superiorly, reflecting the gluteus medius off of the gluteus minimus. This allows for visualization of the femoral head and neck with the overlying capsule and gluteus minimus. The inferior-most aspect of the neck is also identified, and the gluteus minimus and capsule are split along the line of the femoral neck. The superior blunt retractor is now placed beneath the gluteus minimus and capsule and retracted postero-superiorly. A pointed Hohmann is then placed anteriorly and the remaining capsule and minimus are retracted anteriorly. The split in the minimus and capsule is carried proximally to the labrum. This allows for visualization of the femoral head and neck. The capsule can be partially released anteriorly and posteriorly from the labrum of acetabulum if required.

Dislocation is usually performed with a flexion, external rotation and adduction maneuver. In the case of difficulty dislocating the femoral head, the femoral head and neck can be resected *in situ*. The authors recommend the placement of special retractors around the femoral neck. A high subcapital resection followed by a second resection 5–8 mm distal to this proximal resection is performed. This produces a »napkin ring« of bone, which is removed to facilitate extraction of the femoral head from the acetabulum. The resection of the femoral neck is then modified according to preoperative templating using landmarks such as the tip of the greater trochanter and the lesser trochanter.

Attention is now focused on the acetabulum. The extremity is placed on the operating table in approximately 35 to 45 degrees of flexion and slight external rotation. A pointed 90-degree retractor is placed anteriorly. A posterior retractor is placed at the level of the ischium just posterior to the labrum, displacing the posterior capsule posteriorly. The labrum is excised and the condyloid notch is debrided. The acetabulum is reamed sequentially. The initial reamers are directed medially to the medial wall, and then the orientation of the reamers is changed to the anatomic position of abduction of approximately 45 degrees and anteversion of approximately 10 to 15 degrees. Reaming continues until a tight press fit is achieved. The definitive component is placed after a trial component is inserted to confirm appropriate size and orientation. The landmarks used for positioning of the acetabulum are the ilium, ischium and pubis.

Once the acetabular component is placed, attention is focused on the proximal femur. The hip is flexed to 45 to 70 degrees, maximally externally rotated, and adducted. A wide elevating retractor is placed under the greater trochanter in an effort to elevate the proximal femur out of the surgical wound. A pointed retractor is placed in the piriformis fossa, displacing the abductor postero-laterally. The femoral canal is now reamed and broached according to the specific technique for the individual implant being utilized. The skin is protected with appropriate wound protecting sleeves. After appropriate trial reduction to determine leg length equality and stability, the final implant is placed and the definitive head and neck unit.

The hip is reduced and attention is now focused to closure. Heavy, non-absorbable suture is used first to approximate the split in the gluteus minimus and capsule, then to repair the gluteus medius. This repair is over-sown with absorbable suture. Drill holes in the tip of the greater trochanter can facilitate this repair. The fascia is then repaired with an absorbable suture followed by the subcutaneous tissue and a running monofilament suture for the skin.

Safety and Efficacy of Minimally Invasive Anterolateral Approach

Between August 2003 and April 2004, 99 primary total hip arthroplasties were performed with the minimally invasive anterolateral abductor split approach (◘ Fig. 51.2). In this group of patients, the incisions were between 7.5 and 12 cm in length. These patients were compared to an age and gender matched series performed between January 2003 and July 2003 of 127 primary total hip arthroplasties via the traditional anterolateral abductor split approach

(◘ Fig. 51.1). The average BMI for the mini-THA group was 29 kg/m^2 and for the traditional THA group was 30 kg/m^2. There was no statistical difference (p>0.05). The average operating time was significantly longer in the mini-THA group at 80 minutes compared with 68 minutes in the traditional THA group (p<0.001). Despite this significantly longer operative time, blood loss was significantly lower in the mini-THA group at an average of 204 ml versus 251 ml in the traditional THA group. Patients in the mini group achieved immediate postoperative milestones more rapidly than those in the traditional group. The hospital length of stay for the traditional group averaged 2.65 days. One patient was discharged home within 24 hours of surgery and 13 patients (10%) required longer than a 3-day length of stay. The hospital length of stay for the mini-THA group averaged 2.1 days. Twenty-six patients (26.2%) were discharged to home within 24 hours of surgery. Furthermore, only 5 patients (5%) required a hospital length of stay greater than 3 days. These differences noted in length of stay were statistically significant (p<0.001).

Discussion

The efficacy of the direct lateral approach in total hip arthroplasty has been well documented. Masonis and Bourne performed an extensive literature review [11]. They identified 260 clinical studies between 1970 and 2001. Fourteen studies involving 13,203 primary total hip arthroplasties met their inclusion criteria. The combined dislocation rate for these studies was 1.27% for the trans-trochanteric approach, 3.23% for the posterior approach, 2.18% for the anterolateral approach (the interval between the gluteus medius and rectus femoris), and 0.5% for the direct lateral approach. These authors also identified 8 studies involving 2455 primary total hip arthroplasties, which evaluated postoperative limp. The incidence of postoperative limp for the lateral approach was 4% to 20% of patients, while the posterior approach had a reported incidence of limp of 0 to 16%. The authors concluded that larger prospective studies were required to investigate the potential benefits of the posterior approach, especially in lieu of the 6 times greater dislocation rate than with the direct lateral approach.

Our own personal experience with the direct lateral approach has also shown minimal postoperative limp with satisfactory return of abductor function, and a dislocation rate of less than one percent in 1,518 total hip arthroplasties [6]. Similarly, in a study 1,515 total hip arthroplasties performed via the direct lateral approach, Demos et al noted an 11.6% incidence of moderate to severe limp, 2.5% heterotopic ossification, and a 0.4% dislocation rate [12]. Clearly the literature documents the efficacy of the direct lateral approach in primary total hip arthroplasty.

The current question is whether all the benefits of the traditional direct lateral approach will be transferred to a minimally invasive direct lateral approach. To date we have found no reason to believe that these inherent benefits will not apply to the minimally invasive approach. Our patients have obtained a more rapid return of function and have had no adverse effects. Demonstrating that these results are not related to the length of the skin incision, de Beer et al noted that the same direct lateral approach performed through either a 10 cm length incision or a standard length incision resulted in no significant differences, and therefore restricting the length of the skin incision did not afford any clinical advantages to the patient [13]. However, Howell et al demonstrated that total hip arthroplasty can be performed safely through a minimal incision anterolateral approach [14 l]. The major benefit of this approach was a reduction in hospital length of stay. Berger suggested that surgeons should gradually diminish the length of the skin incision and the deep surgical dissection [15]. He advised that specialized instruments and retractors were required to effectively perform mini-incision surgery. The benefits of the less invasive approach were shorter length of stay, reduction in pain, rapid recovery and improved cosmesis. Therefore, it may concluded that the minimally invasive direct lateral approach will improve the immediate peri-operative period for patients undergoing total hip arthroplasty, and hence improve patient satisfaction.

References

1. Lombardi AV Jr; Berend KR, Mallory TH (2005) Perioperative management – Rapid recovery protocol. In: Breusch SJ, Malchau H (eds) The well cemented total hip arthroplasty – theory and practice, Springer, Heidelberg, pp 307–312
2. Berend KR, Lombardi AV Jr, Mallory TH (2004) Rapid recovery protocol for peri-operative care of total hip and total knee arthroplasty patients. Surg Tech Int 13: 239–247
3. Mallory TH, Lombardi AV Jr, Fada RA, Dodds KL, Adams JB (2002) Pain management for joint arthroplasty: preemptive analgesia. J Arthroplasty 17(Suppl 1): 129–133
4. Mallory TH, Lombardi AV Jr, Fada RA, Dodds KL (2000) Anesthesia options: Choices and caveats. Orthopedics 23(9): 919–920
5. Frndak PA, Mallory TH, Lombardi AV Jr (1993) Translateral surgical approach to the hip: The abductor muscle »split«. Clin Orthop Relat Res 295:135–141
6. Mallory TH, Lombardi AV Jr, Fada RA, Herrington SM, Eberle RW (1999) Dislocation after total hip arthroplasty using the anterolateral abductor split approach. Clin Orthop Relat Res 358: 166–172
7. Hardinge K (1982) The direct lateral approach to the hip. J Bone Joint Surg Br 64-B(1):17–19
8. Smith TM, Berend KR, Lombardi AV Jr, Mallory TH, Russell JH (2005) Isolated liner exchange using the anterolateral approach is associated with a low risk of dislocation. Clin Orthop Relat Res 441: 221–226
9. O'Brien JJ, Burnett RS, McCalden RW, MacDonald SJ, Bourne RB, Rorabeck CH (2004) Isolated liner exchange in revision total hip arthroplasty: clinical results using the direct lateral surgical approach. J Arthroplasty 19(4): 414–23
10. Wade FA, Rapuri VR, Parvizi J, Hozack WJ (2004) Isolated acetabular polyethylene exchange through the anterolateral approach. J Arthroplasty 19(4): 498–500
11. Masonis JL, Bourne RB (2002) Surgical approach, abductor function, and total hip arthroplasty dislocation. Clin Orthop Relat Res 405: 46–53
12. Demos HA, Rorabeck CH, Bourne RB, MacDonald SJ, McCalden RW (2001) Instability in primary total hip arthroplasty with the direct lateral approach. Clin Orthop Relat Res 393: 168–180
13. de Beer J, Petruccelli D, Zalzal P, Winemaker MJ (2004) Single-incision, minimally invasive total hip arthroplasty: length doesn't matter. J Arthroplasty 19(8): 945–950
14. Howell JR, Masri BA, Duncan CP (2004) Minimally invasive versus standard incision anterolateral hip replacement: a comparative study. Orthop Clin North Am 35(2):153–162
15. Berger RA (2004) Mini-incision total hip replacement using an anterolateral approach: technique and results. Orthop Clin North Am 35(2):143–151

Minimally Invasive Surgery Anterolateral Approach in Total Hip Arthroplasty

D.S. Garbuz, C.P. Duncan

Introduction

In recent years there has been increasing interest in the concept of limited incision or minimally invasive hip replacement. The proposed advantages include reduced blood loss, shortened operative time, decreased pain, reduced morbidity, shortened hospital stay and accelerated recovery. While there has been a lag in the collection of scientific evidence in support of these proposals, the concept has been enthusiastically received by patients and hip joint replacement through limited incisions is now widely practiced in North America.

A variety of classification systems have been proposed (eponymous, approach to the hip, number of incisions etc.) to describe a variety of surgical techniques. One that has attracted attention, because of its potential influence on morbidity and speed of recovery, is the classification of approaches into: a. intermuscular; and b. transmuscular or transtendinous [1]. Examples of the transmuscular or transtendinous approach, in which muscles are detached for exposure and reattached during closure, include the limited incision direct lateral [2] and the limited incision or mini postero-lateraL as popularized by Dorr and by Sculco [4,5]. Examples of the intermuscular approach include the two-incision technique popularized by Mears and Berger [6] although recent cadaveric studies have revealed substantial damage to the muscles and tendons underlying the posterior incision of this surgical technique [7] A more recent proposal has been the adaptation of a limited incision through the natural interval between the posterior border of the tensor fascia lata and anterior border of glu-

teus medius. This anatomic approach, first described by Sayer in 1876, was popularized by Watson-Jones in 1936 for the management of fractures of the proximal femur, and modified by Roettinger in 2000 for its use in total hip replacement [8].

This truly intermuscular approach has a number of advantages, with particular reference to the two-incision approach developed by Mears and Berger:

- Patient positioned lateral, not supine.
- Single incision, not two.
- Muscle dissection not blind.
- Lateral cutaneous nerve not injured.
- Lateral femoral circumflex vessels not in field.
- Femoral preparation under direct vision
- Trial reduction with broach in place.
- Fluoroscopy not required.
- Incision easily extended if needed.

Indications

This is a suitable surgical approach for hemiarthroplasty following subcapital fracture or total hip replacement. It is recommended that, while developing experience with the approach, the surgeon choose straightforward cases such as idiopathic osteoarthritis or avascular necrosis in patients of standard or slight build. With increasing experience, the indications can be extended to include protusio acetabuli and more stiff cases such as post traumatic degeneration and ankylosing spondylitis. Caution should be exercised in the use of this approach in patients who are morbidly obese (unless the obesity does not extend below the inguinal ligament – a common clinical occurrence) and in heavily muscled patients, until the surgical team is fully familiar with the nuances of the technique. It should not be used as the approach of choice in the presence of anterior soft tissue scarring (after burns, or a previous Smith-Peterson approach with heterotopic bone formation), in the presence of significant deformity (such as dysplasia requiring acetabular segmental bone augmentation or osteotomy of the femur), when dealing with significant deformity of the proximal femur after injury or osteotomy, or if fixation hardware needs to be removed. The nature of the soft tissue dissection is such that the construct is very stable after reduction of the hip and it is therefore unwise to choose this approach if the surgeon wishes to lengthen the limb more than 15–20 m0 mm. The circumferential tension of the soft tissues, which are not released during the procedure, may render the construct irreducible, or reducible but not dislocatable after trial reduction.

Surgical Technique

A number of distinct steps need to be given attention in preparation for and during the procedure:

- Modified table
- Patient positioning
- Draping
- Team positioning
- Abduction stand
- Landmarks
- Incision
- Deep dissection
- Bone referencing
- Neck division
- Cup preparation
- Femoral preparation
- Trial reduction
- Closure

The lower end of the surgical table needs to be split longitudinally and the posterior support removed (■ Fig. 52.1). This will create a posterior well into which the operative limb will be positioned during preparation of the femoral canal. This can be accomplished with a Maquet or Jupiter table, or standard table with custom modification.

The patient is positioned laterally, affected side up, with the pelvis and underlying trochanter just above the split of the table, positioned anteriorly so that the limbs

are supported on the anterior portion of the split lower table which was not removed (■ Fig. 52.2). It is critical that the pelvis be rigidly supported so as to avoid a change in position during preparation of the femur.

Draping is standard, taking care to ensure that the anterior superior iliac spine remains visible or easily palpable, as well as the greater trochanter. These are the

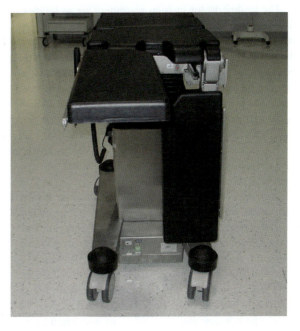

■ **Fig. 52.1.** Demonstrates split table needed to perform femoral preparation

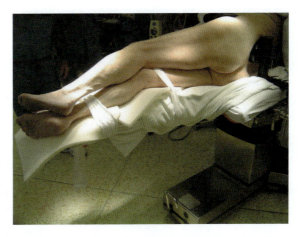

■ **Fig. 52.2.** Patient positioned to side of table. The surgeon will is anterior and assistant(s) are posterior

landmarks required for correct incision placement. A posterior sterile bag, incorporated in the drape, or added to it, is required to contain the leg while preparing the femur.

In contrast to other conventional surgical approaches, the surgeon is positioned anterior to the patient and the one or two assistants posterior. It is wise to prepare a sterile stand to help pull the limb in 20° abduction, again positioned posteriorly.

The landmarks for incision placement are as follows. First the anterior superior iliac spine and prominent lower end of the anterior edge of the greater trochanter are identified. A line between these marks outlines the anterior edge of gluteus medius. In most cases this anterior edge can be palpated. One fingerbreadth behind that line, starting at or just below the anterior edge of the greater trochanter, and extending for 3 inches proximally, is the ideal location of the surgical incision (◘ Fig. 52.3).

A 3-inch incision is made to the deep fascia, longer during the surgeon's initial cases or if the patient is above average in stature or size.

Deep dissection will begin with an incision of the deep fascia parallel with the skin incision, but extended for one or two cm above and below the superior and inferior edges of the skin incision. This facilitates deeper dissection and placement of instruments. The muscle protruding through the deep fascia is the gluteus medius if the incision was truly made behind the anterior edge of that muscle, as outlined on the skin markings.

The limb is now placed in 20° or 30° abduction (supported by the abduction stand) to relax the glutei and

single finger dissection is used to elevate the gluteus medius from the undersurface of the anterior edge of the deep fascia, then changing direction so that the tip of the dissecting index finger identifies the capsule of the hip. Modified Hohman retractors are placed around the superior and inferior surface of the capsule and gently separated. The limb is maintained in abduction (to avoid damage to the glutei). The capsule now comes into view. Two landmarks are useful at this point to confirm location. The medial surface of the greater trochanter can be palpated and seen at the lateral extent of the capsular attachment. The oblique head of rectus femoris can be found at the medial extent of the capsule; clearly indicating the edge of the acetabulum.

A longitudinal capsulotomy is next made from the lip of the acetabulum to the medial face of the greater trochanter, along the anterior surface of the femoral neck. The inferior retractor is placed inside the capsule around the inferior surface of the femoral neck and used to place the inferior capsule under tension. This will facilitate the important step of releasing the inferior capsule from the intertrochanteric line down as far as, or close to, the lesser trochanter. The lateral attachment of the superior capsule is also released from the greater trochanter back to the piriformis fossa. The superior retractor is now placed inside the capsule around the superior surface of femoral neck.

In this manner, an inverted T-shaped capsulotomy is completed, bringing the femoral head, neck and medial face of the greater trochanter into view.

In some cases of substantial dysplasia, it is possible to dislocate the hip anteriorly, but this is uncommon. Instead, the femoral neck needs to be divided into two locations, as follows:

First, the limb is placed in slight abduction, extension and maximum external rotation (placing the foot within the posterior sterile bag with the knee in 90 degrees flexion). This will sublux the femoral head and bring the head-neck junction and equator of the femoral head easily into view. Minor adjustment of the modified Hohman retractors may be necessary. The neck or equator of the head is divided at this point, being careful to make this osteotomy oblique so that it does not enter the acetabulum, posterior column or ischium. A broad osteotome is placed in this osteotomy and with the combined effort of traction and external rotation on the limb, along with leverage of the osteotome, the femoral neck will separate from the head and rise to a superficial position in the wound.

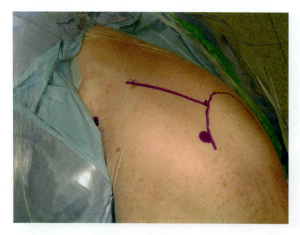

◘ **Fig. 52.3.** Skin incision using greater trochanter and anterior superior iliac spine as landmarks

52

The limb is again placed, as before, in slight abduction, extension and 90 degrees external rotation (now possible because the head and neck are disassociated), with the knee in 90 degrees flexion and the foot in the posterior sterile bag. This brings the femoral neck into a superficial location parallel with the ground.

Referencing for the precise distal femoral neck division is now possible.

The lowest point of the superior surface of the femoral neck, medial to the medial face of the greater trochanter, is now easily palpated and seen. We have coined the term »saddle« of the neck to describe this important reference point. On the preoperative templating, the distance below this saddle should have been measured, indicating the line of the definitive femoral neck osteotomy. This marks the line of the vertical osteotomy from the saddle to the anticipated level of the oblique definitive osteotomy and is made with a reciprocating saw. The final oblique osteotomy is made with an oscillating saw (Fig. 52.4).

The femoral neck is removed as a single piece. The limb brought out of the bag to lie on the underlying leg, the femoral head exposed by replacement of the retractors, and removed. We find it a useful maneuver to skewer the femoral head with a threaded Steinman pin placed through the sclerotic subchondral surface first. If the ligamentum teres is still intact (as is common in subcapital fractures, and in osteonecrosis), then a curved scissors or teres cutter may need to be employed to release the head.

The acetabulum is now ready for preparation.

The limb is allowed to lie on the underlying limb in a relaxed position and slight external rotation. Modified Hohman retractors are placed at the 4 o'clock and 8 o'clock positions on the clock face of the acetabulum and, in heavyset patients, a narrow retractor or smooth Steinman pin is placed through the outer table of the pelvis above the acetabulum to gently retract the anterior edge of gluteus medius in a postero-superior direction. This is retained for acetabular preparation alone and promptly removed after insertion of the socket.

The labrum is removed and it is commonly necessary to release (by incision or excision) a tight band of inferior capsule just lateral to the transverse acetabular ligament. This will allow the retractors to spread further apart, facilitating exposure.

It is wise to consider using a curved or offset acetabular reamer arm so as to avoid being forced into a position of excessive lateral opening or anterior opening by the femur and adjacent soft tissues. The floor of the acetabulum is identified by medial reaming, to the lateral cortex of the acetabular teardrop. The acetabulum is then sequentially reamed until the appropriate size is chosen. Under reaming of 1–2 millimeters is at the discretion of the surgeon, based on previous experience, quality of bone, and implant

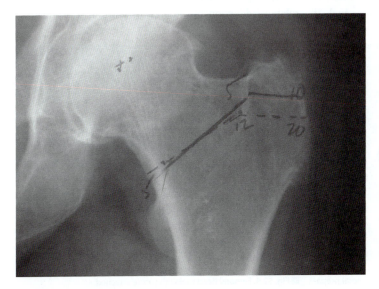
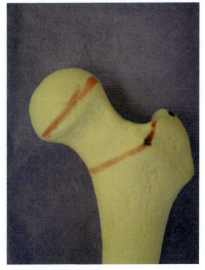

 Fig. 52.4. Outlines femoral head/neck cuts. The saddle is used for accurate neck cutting

to be used. The acetabular shell is introduced at this point, being careful to avoid excessive anteversion. Full seating and adequate fixation are confirmed. Screw fixation is added if required. The acetabular insert is placed at this point, unless potential instability is anticipated later in the case, in which circumstance a trial liner is inserted.

The acetabular retractors and the Steinman pin are removed, the limb now placed in flexion combined with external rotation and the lesser trochanter palpated or visualized. The distance above the lesser trochanter is now estimated and referenced to the preoperative templating so as to confirm the level of the femoral neck division.

Now comes the most challenging portion of the procedure; precise positioning of the limb and exposure of the femur for medullary canal preparation.

First, a specifically designed gluteal retractor is inserted. The tip of this retractor is over the tip of the greater trochanter while the cavity, at an angle of 40 degrees from the tip, is designed to remain parallel to the anterior edge of gluteus medius. The use of a standard or slightly modified Hohman retractor during this step will damage the anterior edge of gluteus medius (◘ Fig. 52.5).

Next the foot is placed in the posterior sterile bag and the limb placed in the combined position of 20 degrees extension, 90 degrees external rotation and 40 degrees adduction. It is held securely in this position by the assistant.

Finally, a pronged retractor, placed under the proximal posteromedial cortex of the femur (straddling the lesser trochanter) is used to elevate the femur into the wound and give clear access to its medullary canal. If

difficulty is encountered, retractor placement should be reviewed and a release of the capsule on the medial face of the posterior half of the greater trochanter released. Rarely will it be necessary to release the piriformis tendon insertion as well.

Next a series of four instruments are used to prepare the canal; modified box osteotome, modified awl, modified conical reamer, and sequential broaches on modified broach handles. The important role of the modified conical reamer, designed to place a trough in the medial face of the greater trochanter (to avoid varus stem placement) should not be overlooked. This is singularly important when dealing with large femurs and/or coxa vara.

The tip of the greater trochanter is now easily seen and used as a reference point for advancement of the broaches. After the broach of suitable size is inserted (judged by level of advancement and resistance to torque), the trial neck is attached and head, the leg taken out of the sterile bag, the joint reduced and its stability evaluated.

Because of the relative anterior placement of this incision and the deep dissection, it is easy for the trial femoral head to separate from the neck and become displaced under the ileopsoas; even into the iliac fossa. A worthwhile precaution is to add a retrieval suture to the trial femoral heads, which have been specially prepared for that function (◘ Fig. 52.6).

After confirmation of joint stability, leg length and horizontal offset in the standard fashion, the joint is dislocated, the limb replaced in the extension/external rotation/adduction position (with the foot in the bag),

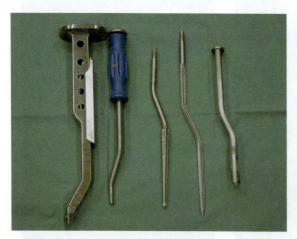

◘ **Fig. 52.5.** Modified instruments which facilitate safe femoral preparation

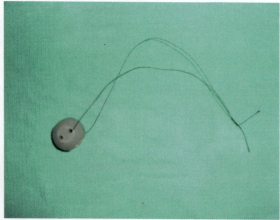

◘ **Fig. 52.6.** Femoral head trial with suture attached

the trial femoral components removed and the final stem inserted. The head is attached, with or without a further trial reduction, and the joint reduced.

The limb is next placed in abduction (on the abduction stand), the soft tissue is retracted to expose the capsule, the joint irrigated and the capsule closed with a single figure of eight absorbable suture. The muscles will now appose across their natural interval (tensor and glutei), and the wound may be closed in standard fashion in layers. The soft tissues may be infiltrated with local anesthetic at this time to facilitate postoperative pain control.

Post-Operative Management

If the contemporary multimodal method of managing pain, nausea and blood loss has been used, including preemptive intervention, then postoperative mobilization should be rapid and uneventful. The patient can be mobilized on the day of operation with an anticipated length of stay of one to two days. This will depend on preoperative education, body habitus, age and comorbidities. Many of the traditional postoperative restrictions can be relaxed, because no muscles or tendons were divided, and because the dissection and reconstruction are so stable. Weight bearing as tolerated can be permitted unless there is a concern regarding implant stability or a proximal fracture initiation not fixed with cerclage wire. It is common for these patients to progress rapidly from crutches to a single cane.

Discussion

This chapter describes the recent modification and application of a limited incision intermuscular approach to partial and complete replacement of the hip using the antero-lateral interval between tensor fascia lata and gluteus medius. The opportunity to use this approach to the hip was first described by Sayer over 100 years ago and was popularized by Watson-Jones 70 years ago. Its potential advantages, with particular reference to the two-incision approach, have been outlined already. It is expected that preservation of the posterior soft tissues should result in a lower risk of posterior dislocation when compared with the traditional or limited postero-lateral approach and that the avoidance of gluteal tendon separation from the greater trochanter will also avoid some of the drawbacks associated with a limited incision direct lateral approach.

While similar advantages, using the two incision approach, have been claimed by the proponents of that approach [6], substantial damage to the soft tissues underlying the posterior second incision has been recently documented in an independent study [7].

Similar principles associated with intermuscular exposure of the hip have been advanced by Keggi [9] and by Matta [10], but the former is difficult to complete in the absence of curved broaches and femoral stems, without making a separate transgluteal incision. And the approach proposed by Matta requires the use of an expensive traction table and potential complications associated with that approach.

This is not to suggest that the intermuscular single incision anterolateral approach outlined in this chapter is without difficulty or risk of complication. Positioning of the patient must be accurate and secure. Placement of the incision should be precise so that acetabular and femoral preparations are facilitated. Clear exposure of the acetabulum is a must to facilitate precise placement and orientation of the socket and the tendency to place the cup in excessive anteversion should be recognized and avoided. Preparation of the medullary canal should not commence until the proximal femur is completely visualized and the canal easily accessed. Else the risk of stem misplacement or fracture of the femur will rise steeply. The use of instruments that have been designed for this approach is strongly recommended so as to facilitate femoral preparation.

The learning curve to become familiar with this approach is steep but short. In our experience it is about 10 cases, for which reason we advise that patients of suitable anatomy and appropriate pathology be chosen during this learning curve. With time and experience the indications can be expanded with safety.

A final point relates to the critical role of limb positioning during each stage of this procedure. The assistant must be familiar and practiced in these positions if the case is to go smoothly. In closing, we will summarize those limb positions again:

- Limb lying on the underlying limb – while making skin markings s and as well as skin and deep fascial incisions.
- Limb in 20–30 degrees abduction and neutral rotation – during blunt dissection and exposure of the capsule
- Limb maintained in abduction and neutral rotation – while opening the capsule and placing retractors deep to capsule.

- Foot in posterior sterile bag and limb in slight abduction, extension, maximum external rotation – to visualize the head-neck junction and divide it at that point.
- Limb in slight flexion, external rotation and under traction – to separate the neck from the head using an osteotome as a lever.
- Foot back in the bag, with limb in slight abduction, extension and 90 degrees external rotation – to deliver the femoral neck superficially into the wound and orient it parallel to the floor. The distal precise neck cut is made at this point. The femoral neck is removed.
- Limb lying in a relaxed fashion on the underlying leg in slight external rotation – to expose and remove the femoral head and gain wide exposure of the acetabulum.
- Limb lying in same position – during preparation of acetabulum and placement of socket.
- Foot in bag, limb in 20 degrees extension, 90 degrees external rotation and 40 degrees adduction – to expose the femur, prepare the canal, place the broach, neck and trial head.
- Limb out of the bag – for trial reduction.
- Limb back in bag in same position – for removal of broach and placement of final component.
- Limb out of bag – final reduction.
- Limb back in abduction – for capsule and wound closure.

References

1. Duncan CP, Toms A, Masri BA (2006) Limited incision or minimally invasive hip replacement: classification and clarification. Instructional Course Lectures. American Academy of Orthopaedic Surgeons (editor Light T) Volume 55 (in press)
2. Hardinge K (1982) The direct lateral approach to the hip. J Bone Joint Surg Br 64(1): 17–19
3. Dall D (1986) Exposure of the hip by anterior osteotomy of the greater trochanter. A modified anterolateral approach. J Bone Joint Surg Br 68(3): 382–386
4. Inaba Y, Dorr LD, Wan Z, Sirianni L, Boutary M (2005) Operative and patient care techniques for posterior mini-incision total hip arthroplasty. Clin Orthop Relat Res 441: 104–114
5. Sculco TP, Jordan LC (2004) The mini-incision approach to total hip arthroplasty. Instr Course Lect 53: 141–147
6. Berry DJ, Berger RA, Callaghan JJ, Dorr LD, Duwelius PJ, Hartzband MA, Mears DC (2003) ally invasive total hip arthroplasty. Development, early results, and a critical analysis. Presented at the Annual Meeting of the American Orthopaedic Association, Charleston, South Carolina, USA, June 14, 2003. J Bone Joint Surg Am 85-A(11): 2235–2246
7. Mardones R, Pagnano MW, Nemanich JP, Trousdale RT (2005) The Frank Stinchfield Award: muscle damage after total hip arthroplasty done with the two-incision and mini-posterior techniques. Clin Orthop Relat Res 441: 63–67
8. Bertin KC, Rottinger H (2004) Anterolateral mini-incision hip replacement surgery: a modified Watson-Jones approach. Clin Orthop Relat Res 429:248–255
9. Kennon RE, Keggi JM, Wetmore RS, Zatorski LE, Huo MH. Keggi KJ (2003) Total hip arthroplasty through a minimally invasive anterior surgical approach. J Bone Joint Surg Am 85-A Suppl 4:39–48
10. Matta JM, Shahrdar C, Ferguson T (2005) Single-incision anterior approach for total hip arthroplasty on an orthopaedic table. Clin Orthop Relat Res 441:115–124

52

Posterior Minimally Invasive Surgery Approach for Total Hip Arthroplasty

T.P. Vail

Introduction

The popularity of the minimal incision posterior approach among many arthroplasty surgeons reflects the desire for an increasingly more tissue-preserving, rapid, and highly functional recovery after total hip replacement. Many surgeons have settled on the posterior approach after experience with other approaches. The surgical exposures for hip arthroplasty used over the years have included the direct lateral, the anterior, the antero-lateral with modifications, and the posterior approach. Each approach provided optimal access to the hip joint with the available instrumentation and implants of the time. The enduring feature of the posterior approach has been the easy access to the joint and a low incidence of limp due to the sparing of the abductor attachments [1]. The lateral Charnley approach facilitated the Charnley surgical technique, but was associated with occasional trochanteric non-union, dislocation, and a programmed slow recovery [2]. The anterior approach provided excellent acetabular exposure, but a more complicated access to the femoral shaft, particularly with the early straight-stemmed implants [3, 4]. The direct lateral and modified lateral approaches have been associated with an incidence of limp or abductor lurch and a slower recovery due to the need to protect the abductor mechanism [5]. The downside of the posterior approach historically has been a higher rate of dislocation [6, 7], especially when using a smaller prosthetic femoral head size. However, improvements in bearing function and refinement in surgical technique have brought the return of larger diameter articulations and recognition of the importance of capsular repair, allowing the posterior approach to evolve into a highly functional and highly stable approach for total hip arthroplasty [8].

The posterior approach to the hip was originally described as a technique for inserting a proximal femoral hemi-arthroplasty [9]. However, variations of the technique have also been useful for access to the sciatic nerve, the posterior column, the piriformis tendon, the lateral rim of the acetabulum, as well as the hip joint itself. Variously termed the posterior, Southern, dorsal, and posterolateral approach, related to nuances in the deeper dissection, the descriptions by all the names share the same pathway through the gluteus maximus muscle and behind the gluteus medius muscle in order to gain entry into the hip joint.

More recent evolution of the posterior approach centers on the development of smaller incisions, minimally invasive techniques, and rapid recovery [10–12]. The term »evolution« best describes the present status of the minimal incision posterior approach which has been adapted from the standard posterior exposure. The muscular and nervous interval is the same as the classic descriptions, with the exception of some subtle variation which will be described in this chapter. The size of the incision and the intentional preservation of soft tissue structures distinguish the minimally invasive posterior approach from a standard approach. The minimal incision approach eliminates all parts of the standard approach that are not necessary to perform a total hip arthroplasty with the use of lower profile instruments and modern total hip implants.

Methods

Positioning and Planning the Skin Incision

The surgical technique is performed with the patient in the lateral decubitus position. All downside pressure points are padded, and an axillary roll is placed under the thorax for additional protection of the shoulder and brachial plexus. Some type of pelvic positioning device is generally used to stabilize the pelvis which tends to shift when the patient is moved from a supine to a lateral position [13]. Once the patient is properly positioned on the operating table, the operative extremity is prepped and draped in the usual sterile fashion, preferably with an adhesive, bacterostatic covering over the operative site (◘ Fig. 53.1).

Placement of the skin incision is based upon palpation of the greater trochanter. The hip is flexed 45 degrees, and adducted 10 degrees during the planning of the skin incision. The incision is placed one-third below the tip of the trochanter, and two-thirds above the tip of the trochanter. The length of the incision will be dependant upon the depth of the subcutaneous fat, with a deeper fat layer requiring a longer incision in order to access both the acetabulum and the femoral shaft. The incision may start out short, and can be lengthened during the operation as needed in order to avoid tension on the skin edges during the preparation of the bone and introduction of the implants. The surgeon may choose to bring the incision across the trochanter toward the anterior edge of the vastus lateralis ridge at the base of the greater trochanter, or stay behind the trochanter parallel to the posterior border of the femur depending upon the position of the leg on the operating table. When the hip is more flexed, the skin incision will appear more posterior. With the hip in a more neutral position, the incision will cross the trochanter. In either case, the important consideration is to place the incision over the acetabulum, with the trochanter serving as a superficial landmark that one can palpate in order to orient and locate the incision properly. The direction of the skin incision is oblique, running perpendicular to the face of the acetabulum and thereby in line with the handle of the reamer that will be used to prepare the acetabulum at a later stage of the operation.

Skin and subcutaneous tissue are sharply divided down to the fascia overlying the gluteus maximus muscle. Avoid finger dissection and unnecessary trauma to the fat layer, as the fat can be easily devascularized with blunt

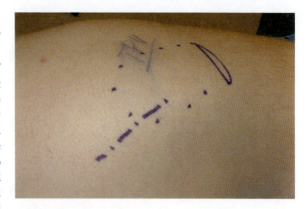

◘ **Fig. 53.1.** Skin incision

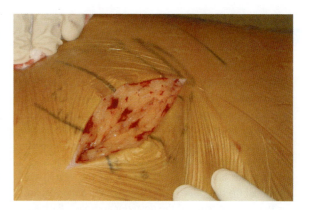

◘ **Fig. 53.2.** Muscle-tendon junction of the gluteus maximus

trauma. The investing fascia of the gluteus maximus is divided longitudinally in line with the direction of the fascial fibers and consequently, in line with the underlying gluteus maximus muscle fibers below the fascia. The fascial incision proceeds from the level of the sciatic notch proximally to the intersection of the tensor fascia distally. The sciatic notch can be palpated through the skin as a soft spot above the ischial tuberosity. The beginning of the tensor fascia corresponds with the muscle-tendon junction of the gluteus maximus muscle below the greater trochanteric ridge. There is no reason to extend the incision distally into the tensor fascia during the initial approach, as it has the potential to add to the morbidity of the recovery and may not be necessary for adequate exposure of the hip (◘ Fig. 53.2).

53

The Deeper Approach and Capsular Incision

The initial part of the deeper approach is really *trans-muscular* through the gluteus maximus muscle. The gluteus maximus muscle is divided bluntly in line with its fibers. It may be necessary to cut the investing fascia below the muscle with a scissors. Carefully control bleeding points within the muscle using electrocautery during the approach, but avoid cutting muscle fibers with electrocautery. Deeper exposure is achieved by placing a Charnley retractor carefully beneath the gluteus maximus muscle, applying the minimum tension required to provide visualization. In a small patient, a Charnley retractor may provide excessive soft-tissue pressure, especially with a particularly small incision. In such cases, it is wise to choose a smaller self-retaining device that applies less tension, or avoid a self-retaining retractor all together. Take care not to damage the gluteus medius muscle which lies below the gluteus maximus when placing a retractor into the incision.

The deeper dissection begins with reflection of the trochanteric bursa. The bursa is incised sharply along the posterior edge of the gluteus medius muscle from a point just above the trochanteric insertion of the medius tendon proximally to the top of the quadratus femoris muscle distally. The bursa is well vascularized, and will require coagulation of bleeding points as it is mobilized. Once incised, the bursa can be pushed posteriorly with a sponge, thereby exposing the short external rotators of the hip. Overlying the short external rotators and the hip capsule is often located a plexus of veins that will also require coagulation in order to minimize bleeding later during the capsular incision. The sciatic nerve can be palpated at this point in the operation, lying below the piriformis (with some variation in approximately 10% of cases) [14] and on top of the short external rotators and ischial tuberosity in most cases. The sciatic nerve is protected throughout the duration of the procedure. The piriformis, conjoint tendon (obturator internus, externus, and gemelli muscles), and the posterior hip capsule are tagged with a suture to facilitate exposure and later repair during closure.

Once the posterior capsule and external rotators are exposed, the next step in the exposure is the capsular incision (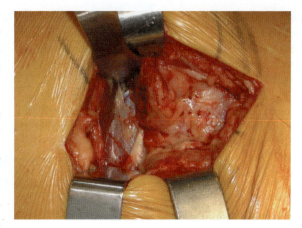 Fig. 53.3). The capsular incision is a watershed point in the operation that distinguishes the more commonly described posterior approach from a dorsal approach []15. Exposure is facilitated by placing a blunt Homan retractor beneath the gluteus medius muscle and on

⬛ Fig. 53.3. Capsular incision

top of the gluteus minimus muscle around the front of the femoral neck. The posterior border of the gluteus medius muscle is gently elevated, avoiding tension on the superior gluteal neuro-vascular pedicle emerging from the greater sciatic notch, thereby exposing the interval between the superior edge of the piriformis and the inferior edge of the gluteus minimus muscle. The dorsal approach uses this interval to access the femoral canal with the femoral head in situ. To continue the posterior approach, the capsule is incised along the top of the piriformis tendon proceeding from the acetabular rim down to the piriformis fossa, and then distally along the intertrochanteric line to the top of the quadratus femoris muscle. If possible, the dissection stops above the top of the quadratus femoris, which contains branches of the medial femoral circumflex artery. Coagulate bleeding points within the hip capsule during exposure. A capsulo-tendinous flap consisting of the posterior hip capsule and the short external rotators is then reflected posteriorly with the use of the previously placed suture, thereby protecting the sciatic nerve and exposing the hip joint. The author's preference is to tag the capsule and external rotators as a single layer, but a separation of these structures is also quite acceptable. The L-shaped capsulotomy as described here maintains the integrity of the ischio-femoral ligament, providing the strength of the posterior hip capsule and the resistance to dislocation when repaired [16].

With the capsule incised, the femoral head is dislocated by flexion and internal rotation of the joint. Tension on the sciatic nerve during hip dislocation is avoided by keeping the knee flexed at all times. The femoral neck is exposed by placing a slender retractor below the femoral neck to protect the posterior soft tissues. The neck of the femur is then osteotomized with an oscillating saw at a level determined by templating or navigation. The tip of the greater trochanter, the lesser trochanter, and the femoral neck are all clearly visible for registration within the surgical wound when computer navigation is utilized in conjunction with the mini-posterior approach. Once the femoral head is removed, the exposure of the acetabulum begins.

Acetabular Preparation and Exposure

The minimal incision posterior approach allows a complete view of the entire circumference of the acetabulum. The acetabular exposure is created by translating the femur forward through a combination of leg positioning and capsular elevation. Optimal leg positioning for acetabular exposure is achieve by placing the hip in a position of 45 degrees of flexion and 10 degrees of adduction, thereby relaxing the anterior hip capsule. A retractor is then placed under the femoral neck and over the anterior lip of the acetabulum. The anterior acetabular retractor and the proximal femoral elevator are the key instruments used during the mini-posterior approach (▣ Fig. 53.4). Translation of the femur is further facilitated by elevating the anterior hip capsule fibers off of the anterior rim of the acetabulum with the anterior retractor providing some degree of tension on the capsular fibers. This capsular elevation can be accomplished with the use of electocautery, or sharply with a knife. Additionally, a radial cut in the inferior capsule will provide further relaxation of the soft tissues required to translate the femur anterior to the acetabulum during more difficult exposures wherein capsular elevation alone is not satisfactory to mobilize the femur. The transverse acetabular ligament may be left intact when the inferior capsule is divided. Branches of the obturator artery travel from within the pelvis into the fovea of the hip over the inferior edge of the acetabulum, and may require coagulation during exposure or later during reaming.

With the anterior acetabular retractor in place, and traction on the posterior hip capsule, the entire acetabulum is in view. At this point the labrum is excised, the bony rim of the acetabulum is exposed, and osteophytes around the rim of the acetabulum can be removed. Li-

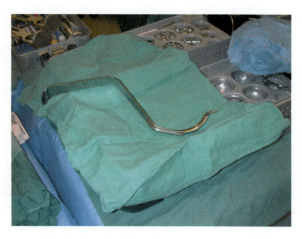

▣ **Fig. 53.4.** Anterior acetabular retractor

kewise, the medial osteophyte commonly covering the fovea in osteoarthritic cases can be removed prior to further preparation of the acetabulum. The acetabulum is prepared for the implant by sequentially reaming with spherical reamers. A modified curved, or S-shaped acetabular reamer allows reaming without tension on the skin and soft tissues. Likewise, a modified cup inserter allow impaction of the acetabular component with a minimum of soft tissue tension.

Femoral Preparation

The proximal femur is exposed by placing a narrow retractor beneath the femoral neck to elevate the proximal femur and protect the posterior soft tissues. Placement of a sponge between the retractor and the skin edge distributes the pressure of the retractor over a larger surface area and helps to protect the skin edge. Femoral preparation can then proceed with confidence as the surgeon is able to see the proximal femur in its entirety. With satisfactory visualization, the femoral broaches and reaming devices can be properly lateralized and anteverted to create a stable prosthetic articulation with the acetabular component. A cemented or cementless implant can be inserted using any combination of reaming and broaching. Careful movement of the proximal femoral elevator and the leg will allow better visualization of the piriformis fossa or calcar femorale, depending upon the wishes of the surgeon and the stage of the operation, thereby assuring appropriate fit

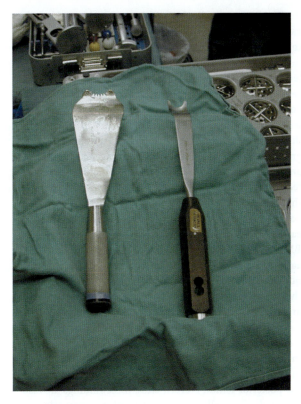

◘ **Fig. 53.5.** Proximal femoral elevator

and position of the implant while minimizing the risk of a calcar split or femur fracture (◘ Fig. 53.5).

Implant Insertion

It has been the habit of the author to obtain an intra-operative radiograph with the trial components in place prior to inserting the final components. The intra-operative radiograph can be used to determine that the implants chosen are appropriately sized, positioned, and matched to the desired amount of length, offset, and soft tissue tension. Additionally, the stability of the hip can be tested by removing all retractors with the trials in place, and checking the range of motion of the hip joint. If this assessment is performed during the operation, adjustments can be made prior to making the final choice of implants, thereby minimizing device wastage.

When inserting the implants it is critically important to keep them from touching the edges of the wound and

the skin. The skin, even when prepped, is a potential source of prosthetic bacterial contamination. Thus, it is worthwhile to make an effort to adjust retractors and move the leg in order to allow placement of the components within the operative site without running them across the skin edge in the process. The skin incision must be large enough to accommodate this process. Insertion of the femoral component may require flexion of the hip to place the component within the femoral canal initially, then once the trunion of the implant is within the wound, the implant is turned into the appropriate amount of anteversion to match the desired position of the component and the bone preparation. When using a particularly small incision, the neck of the prosthesis and the trunion may extend over the skin edge unless the implant is introduced into the wound in retroversion and then rotated to the appropriate position prior to the implant engaging the endosteum of the femur as it is pushed into the femoral canal.

Mechanical lavage of the wound using a water pick type device with antibiotic irrigation is performed liberally during the procedure, particularly after the use of broaches, reamers, and other processed or autoclaved instruments. Irrigation of soft tissues is done cautiously to avoid the possibility of injection injury from overly aggressive mechanical lavage. Additionally, irrigation of the bone bed prior to implant insertion will help to ensure that no component is placed into an inadvertently contaminated wound.

Closure

Wound closure is performed in an anatomic fashion by restoring the normal tissue relationships. Debridement of any devitalized tissue within the wound or along the edges of the skin helps to ensure timely healing, a better cosmetic result, and lower risk of infection. Closure starts with repair of the posterior hip capsule and short external rotators. The capsule-tendinous flap can be re-attached through drill holes in the trochanter, or by pulling the flap up underneath the posterior border of the gluteus medius muscle toward the piriformis fossa, pulling the sutures through the gluteus medius tendon, and then tying them over the top of the tendon. The remaining closure is performed in layers that include the fascia overlying the gluteus maximus and tensor fascia, the subcutaneous layer, and the skin. Skin closure can be done with a running subcuticular closure, interrupted suture, or staples. The author prefers interrupted suture due to the strength of the interrupted technique, and the more cosmetic appearance of the scar when a modified horizontal mattress suture is used, keeping the side opposite the knot beneath the skin in the subcuticular layer.

Important Tips

The following tips are of key importance to successfully accomplish total hip arthroplasty through a mini-posterior approach:

1. make the incision long enough to access both the femur and the acetabulum without undue tension on the skin,
2. do not hesitate to lengthen the skin incision during the procedure,
3. protect the soft tissues by moving the extremity and the incision to accommodate the field of view,
4. avoid the prolonged use of tensioned self-retaining retractors,
5. elevate the anterior hip capsule to mobilize the femur and expose the acetabulum,
6. do not let poor mobilization of the femur allow misdirection of the acetabular reamer or acetabular component,
7. do not let poor visualization of the proximal femur result in varus position or undersizing of the femoral component,
8. keep the implants away from the skin edge during insertion.

Results

While the literature on the results of all minimally invasive approaches remains quite limited, the available reports on the mini-posterior approach for total hip arthroplasty are the most numerous. The literature consists of a number of single surgeon case series, a few comparative studies, and fewer prospective evaluations. Most evaluations are short term, therefore not addressing the impact of the less invasive approach on the long term performance of the total hip procedure. The case series available in the literature serve to demonstrate that a total hip can be done safely through a minimal posterior hip incision in the hands of an experienced surgeon [17, 18].

The literature falls short of demonstrating a clear advantage of the minimal posterior hip incision compared to a standard posterior approach or any other minimal incision approach, beyond the cosmetic appeal of a smaller incision. The most comprehensive prospective, and randomized evaluation of the minimal posterior approach compares over 200 hips performed with either an incision less than 10 cm or an incision of 16 cm [19]. The deep dissection performed in the study was the same in both groups. Despite matching patients for age, co-morbidity, and body mass index (BMI), no differences were reported in the rate of transfusion, the assessment of pain, or the use of analgesic medication after surgery. Only the patient's age and preoperative hematocrit correlated with earlier discharge. The length of operation correlated with BMI, independent of the length of the incision. Likewise, early ambulation and optimal component position was not impacted by the length of the skin incision. While this study was very well designed and executed, one could argue that the 16 cm incision may not be representative of a standard incision or a more classical posterior approach which often utilized a much longer incision, sometimes including a more extensive and distal deep dissection that might take down the insertion of the gluteus maximus on the posterior femur. Nevertheless, these findings are also reflected in a smaller report of 60 patients comparing an 8 cm incision to a 15 cm incision [20]. While the minimal incision group had less intra-operative blood loss, total blood loss, and fewer limped at 6 weeks, there was no difference in operative time, transfusion rates, narcotic usage, length of stay, rehab milestones, cane usage, or rates of complications out to 2 years post-operatively.

Complications

Particularly important is the consideration of potential complications or unique hazards that might be introduced by the minimal incision approach. Several case reports have outlined the potential for improper reaming of the acetabulum, vertical cup placement, intra-operative fractures, and prolonged operative time, citing surgeon inexperience as a possible cause [21]. While those complications are not unique to the minimal incision approach, at least one study has suggested that the minimal posterior incision might be associated with a higher rate of complications than a standard approach [22]. In a comparison of a group of patients with a standard posterior approach

53

to a group with a minimal incision posterior approach, the minimal incision group had a higher incidence of wound complications and component mal-position. This finding was remarkable in light of the fact that the minimal incision group had a lower mean BMI. Finally, recent evidence has pointed to the fact that all minimal incision approaches for THA cause some damage to muscle. A dissection of 20 cadaver hip replacement procedures, divided between 10 mini-posterior approaches and 10 2-incision approaches revealed more damage to the gluteus medius and minimus muscle after the 2-incision technique, but no difference in damage to the gluteus tendon between the two groups [23].

Discussion and Conclusions

The minimal incision posterior approach for total hip arthroplasty represents an evolution of the standard posterior incision, focusing the exposure only on the pertinent anatomy required to perform a total hip replacement successfully. The minimal posterior approach can result in a highly functional early recovery and a cosmetic result, but it also has the potential to add complexity to the total hip replacement procedure. Success is linked to experience and meticulous soft-tissue management.

References

1. Roberts JM, Fu FH, McCain EF, Ferguson AB (1984) A comparison of posterolateral and anterolateral approaches to total hip arthroplasty. Clin Orthop 187: 205
2. Joshi A, Lee CM, Markovic L, Vlatis G, Murphy JCM (1998) Prognosis of dislocation after total hip arthroplasty. J Arthroplasty 13: 17–21
3. Kennon R, Keggi J, Zatorski L, Keggi K (2004) Anterior approach for total hip arthroplasty – beyond the minimally invasive technique. J Bone Joint Surg 86A (Suppl 2): 91–97
4. Light T, Keggi K (1980) Anterior approach to hip arthroplasty. Clin Orthop 152: 255–260
5. Hardinge K (1982) The direct lateral approach to the hip. J Bone Joint Surg 64B: 17–24
6. Lu-Yao GL, Keller RB, Littenberg B, Wennberg JE (1994) Outcomes after displaced fractures of the femoral neck: A meta-analysis of one hundred and six published reports. J Bone Joint Surg 76A: 15
7. Woolson ST, Rahimtoola ZO (1999) Risk factors for dislocation during the first 3 months after primary total hip replacement. J Arthroplasty 14: 662–668
8. Pellicci PM, Bostrom M, Poss R (1998) Posterior approach to total hip replacement using enhanced posterior soft tissue repair. Clin Orthop 355: 224–228
9. Moore AT (1957) The self locking metal hip prosthesis. J Bone Joint Surg 39A: 811–821
10. Vail TP (2004) Minimal Incision hip arthroplasty – the posterior mini-incision. Semin Arthroplasty 15(2): 83–86
11. Sculco T (2003) Is smaller necessarily better? Am J Orthopedics 32: 169
12. Berry D, Berger R, Callaghan J et al. (2003) Minimally invasive total hip arthroplasty – development, early results and a critical analysis. J Bone Joint Surg 85A(11): 2235–2246
13. McCollum DE, Gray WJ (1990) Dislocation after total hip arthroplasty. Causes and prevention. Clin Orthop 261: 159–170
14. Johanson NA, Pellicci PM, Tsairis P, Salvati EA (1983) Nerve injury in total hip arthroplasty. Clin Orthop 179: 214–222
15. Murphy SB (2004) Technique of tissue-preserving minimally-invasive total hip arthroplasty using a superior capsulotomy. Oper Tech Orthop 12: 94
16. Hewitt JD, Glisson RR, Guilak F, Vail TP (2002) The mechanical properties of the human hip capsule ligaments. J Arthroplasty 17(1): 82–89
17. Goldstein W, Branson J, Berland K, Gordon A (2003) Minimal-incision total hip arthroplasty. J Bone Joint Surg 85A: 33–38
18. Swanson T (2005) Early results of 1000 consecutive, posterior, single-incision minimally invasive surgery total hip arthroplasties. J Arthroplasty 20 (Suppl): 26–32
19. Ogonda L, Wilson R, Archbold P et al. (2005) A minimal-incision technique in total hip arthroplasty does not improve early postoperative outcomes – a prospective, randomized, controlled trial. J Bone Joint Surg 87A(4): 701–710
20. Chimento G, Pavone V, Sharrock N et al. (2005) Minimally invasive total hip arthroplasty – a prospective randomized study. J Arthroplasty 20: 139–144
21. Fehring T, Mason J (2005) Catastrophic complications of minimally invasive hip surgery. J Bone Joint Surg 87A: 711–714
22. Woolson ST, Mow C, Syquia J et al. (2004) Comparison of primary total hip replacements performed with standard incision or a mini-incision. J Bone Joint Surg 86A(7): 1353–1358
23. Mardones R, Pagnano M, Nemanich J, Trousdale R (2005) Muscle damage after total hip arthroplasty done with the two-incision and mini-posterior techniques. Clin Orthop 441: 63–67

The Medial Approach to the Hip Joint for Implantation of Prostheses

W. Thomas, L. Lucente, P. Benecke, C.L. Busch, H. Grundei

Introduction

The surgical approach to the hip joint for implantation of prostheses should be as direct as possible and yield a good overview of the operation site, so that the component parts of the implant can be placed in position safely and accurately. Blood loss should be kept to a minimum, and functionally important structures such as vessels, nerves and muscles should not be endangered. Moreover, the surgical incision should be small and should allow the patient to lie comfortably with minimal pain in the post-operative period. The most commonly used standard approaches (antero-lateral, lateral, posterior) are reported to be accompanied by typical complications in a significant proportion of patients: dislocation in up to 9.5% of cases, blood loss necessitating transfusion in up to 75%, and nerve damage, often permanent, in up to 75% [2, 3, 7–9, 11–13].

For these reasons we performed an anatomical study in which an alternative, median approach was tested and developed for clinical application.

Anatomical Study

After preliminary theoretical studies, in October 2001 we experimented on non-formalinized cadavers to establish a medial approach to the hip joint that would be suitable for clinical application. The work took place at the Anatomical Institute of the University of Lübeck, Germany.

With the cadaver's leg abducted and hip joint flexed (see »Operation Technique«), a transverse incision is made in the groin and the adductor longus muscle is dis-

sected or divided from its proximal insertion. This gives direct access to the hip joint.

The study revealed the following findings:

1. After division of the adductor longus muscle one regularly encounters the large deep ramus of the medial femoral circumflex artery, which stretches over the neck of the femur and has to be divided to assure a satisfactory overview.
2. The view of the hip joint is unusually good (❑ Fig. 54.1).
3. Any type of prosthesis can be implanted via this route.
4. No special instruments are necessary.
5. Revisions can be carried out. In one cadaver we had no difficulty in removing one prosthesis and inserting another.

Since January 2002 we have been using our medial route for implantation of hip prostheses in an increasing proportion of our patients [10].

Advantages

- Direct access to the hip joint.
- Good overview of the operation site.
- No special instruments necessary.
- Low blood loss.
- No damage to the lateral abductor apparatus (gluteal muscles, fascia lata) or the superior gluteal nerve.
- Enables lateral positioning of the patient immediately after operation.
- Inconspicuous scar.

Disadvantages

- Possible hematomas of groin and/or thigh.
- Potential transitory weakness of the adductor muscles.
- Learning curve because of unfamiliar approach.
- Unsuitable for patients with ankylosis of the hip.
- Any existing inguinal cutaneous infections have to be dealt with first.
- Additional reconstruction of the roof of the acetabulum in the case of severe dysplasia or dislocation is very difficult and is better achieved via the standard approaches.

Operation Technique

Under intubation or lumbar anesthesia, the patient is placed supine on an operating table that features abductable leg rests. The affected leg is sterilized, draped and placed in the greatest possible abduction and flexion. The operator stands between the patient's legs, while the principal assistant positions himself lateral to the leg to be operated on. He holds the leg in abduction and flexion throughout the operation and performs the later maneuvers. The second assistant stands at the other side of the table, next to the unaffected leg. The image intensifier is positioned lateral to the affected leg in case X-ray controls are necessary (Fig. 54.2).

With the leg abducted about 50° and the hip and knee joints flexed about 90°, the adductor longus muscle is visible and palpable in the groin (Fig. 54.3).

The cutaneous incision is made about 5 cm distal (lateral) to the inguinal fold. It is ca. 8–10 cm long and curves slightly laterally. The tendon of the adductor longus muscle lies in the middle of the incision. The leg is held in flexion and abduction throughout the operation. The lips of the wound are held apart with blunt hooks. The adductor longus muscle is dissected free, and its proximal tendinous insertion is provided with a holding suture and divided in »Z« fashion. The muscle is then held to the side. The pectineal muscle lies proximal to the route of access, the gracilis muscle and the short and great adductor muscles distal to it. If these muscles are particularly well developed, they are notched with the electric knife. The joint capsule is now visible and palpable with the femoral head and neck

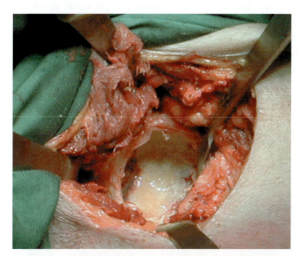
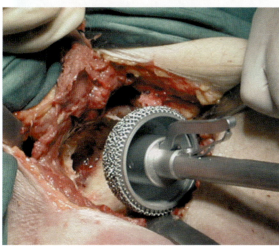

Fig. 54.1. Anatomical sketch of the medial approach

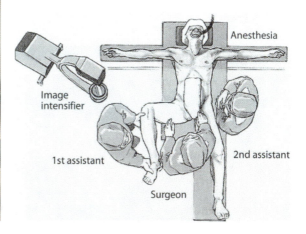

Fig. 54.2. Position of the patient and of the surgical team (from [10])

underneath it. The palpating finger ascertains the position of the femoral head, assisted by movement of the leg. The neck of the femur is worked around with Hohmann levers. The deep ramus of the medial femoral circumflex artery can now be discerned over the femoral neck. The artery is dissected free, two ligatures are applied, and the artery is divided. Both segments of the divided vessel are dissected away from the surrounding tissues. The joint capsule is opened by means of a double T-shaped incision and partially excised (■ Fig. 54.4).

The femoral head can now be dislocated antero-inferiorly by external rotation and abduction of the leg.

The femoral head is treated according to the type of prosthesis to be implanted:
1. For an epiphyseally fixed cap prosthesis, the head is prepared but not resected.
2. For a metaphyseally anchored femoral neck prosthesis, subcapital resection is performed.
3. For a diaphyseally fixed stem prosthesis, the head is resected near its base at the femoral neck.

First the acetabulum is worked around with three Hohmann levers. The inferior lever holds the proximal part of the femur away, yielding an excellent view of the acetabulum. The acetabulum is prepared with the appropriate burs, and the insertion instrument is used to fix the acetabular implant firmly in place. We favor the »Kapuziner« press-fit cup with cancellous–metal surface (Eska Implants, Lübeck) for cementless fixation (■ Fig. 54.5).

Next the femoral component of the prosthesis is implanted, using the appropriate instruments depending on prosthesis type. No special instruments are needed for this approach. When using the femoral neck prosthesis with cancellous–metal surface presented here (CUT 2000; Eska Implants) for cementless fixation in the metaphyseal segment of the femur, the proximal portion of the femur is prepared with the appropriate shaped rasps. The implant is then driven firmly into place and the modular femoral neck adapter and the prosthetic head are implanted (■ Fig. 54.6). The adapter can be set at various angles.

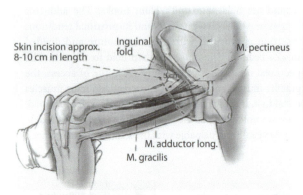

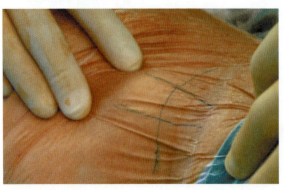

■ Fig. 54.3. The anatomical structures (adductor relief)

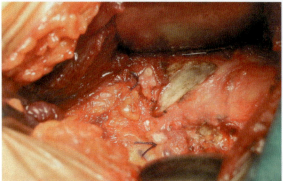

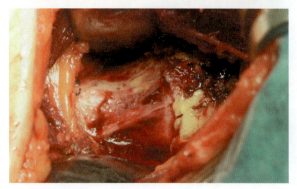

■ Fig. 54.4. Joint after vessel preparation and opening of the capsule

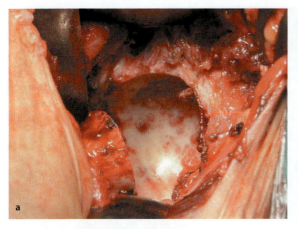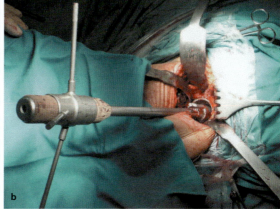

Fig. 54.5. a Overview of the acetabulum; **b** insertion of the prosthetic cup

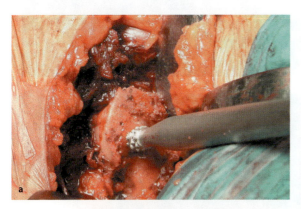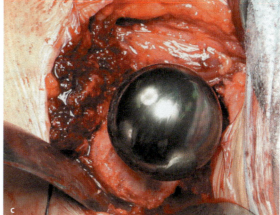

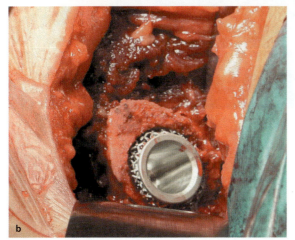

Fig. 54.6. a Preparation of the femoral shaft; **b** after implantation of the femoral component; **c** prosthetic femoral head in position (metal); **d** after repositioning (metal–metal coupling)

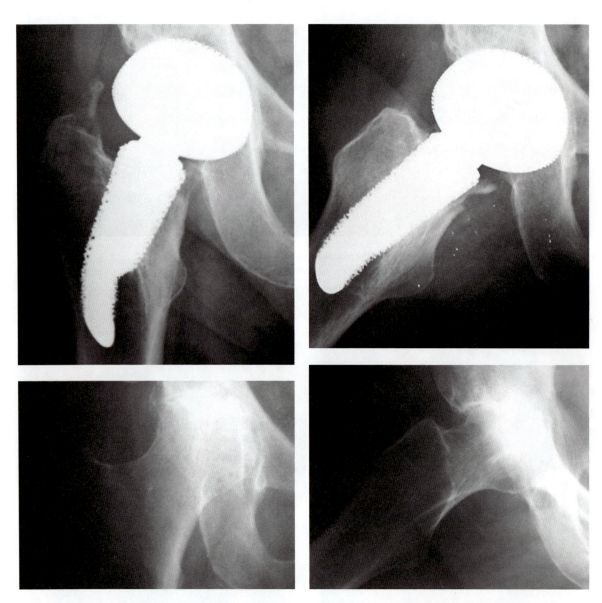

◘ **Fig. 54.7.** X-ray control at two levels

54

The size and exact positioning of the implants are determined during the preoperative planning.

After repositioning of the head of the prosthesis in the acetabulum, the operation site is rinsed with physiological saline solution, a Redon drain is placed, and the tendon of the adductor longus muscle is reattached with a suture. The final steps of the operation are closure of the wound layer by layer with single button vertical mattress sutures, application of a sterile wound dressing, neutral positioning of the leg, and control X-rays (◘ Fig. 54.7).

Post-Operative Care

The operated leg is placed in neutral position. A foam splint is not absolutely necessary. One dose of cephalosporin is given as prophylaxis against infection. The Redon drain is removed after 2 days.

A regimen of low-molecular-weight heparin, support stockings and foot exercises is used for 3 weeks to prevent thrombosis.

Mobilization begins on the day after operation. Partial weight-bearing (10 kg) is performed for 10 days. On the 10th day the cutaneous stitches are removed and loading is increased in increments of 10 kg every 2 days until full weight-bearing is achieved.

Clinical and X-ray follow-up is conducted at 6 weeks after surgery, after 3, 6, and 12 months, and annually thereafter.

Results

We began to implant prostheses via our new medial approach in January 2002. Here we report on 60 patients (62 hips) who were followed up for at least 18 months (range 18–42 months, mean 24 months).

Thirty-four left hips and 24 right hips were operated upon; two further patients underwent surgery on both hip joints in separate interventions. Thirty-five of the 60 patients were female, 25 male. Their age at the time of operation ranged from 27 to 74 years (mean 51 years).

The reasons for implantation were primary arthrosis (n=48), dysplastic arthrosis (n=6), rheumatoid arthritis (n=6), and femoral head necrosis (n=2) (▪ Table 54.1).

Various prostheses were used: CUT 2000 femoral neck prosthesis (n=34), cap prosthesis (n=12), diaphyseal stem prosthesis (n=16). All featured a cancellous–metal surface (Eska Implants) for cementless fixation.

The mean operating time was 70 min (range 45–130 min).

We used the cell saver in all cases for intra-operative recovery of blood, and transfusions were never necessary. The mean blood loss was 240 ml (range 120–430 ml).

Postoperative rehabilitation was uncomplicated in all cases, with no instances of infection, dislocation, or implant failure. As early as 3 months the patients reached their highest Harris score (mean 92 points). All patients displayed a hip-stable gait (Trendelenburg and Duchenne signs negative and adductor muscle strength normal) (▪ Table 54.2).

▪ **Table 54.1.** Epidemiology

Operations (n=62)	
Left	34
Right	24
Bilateral	2
Diagnosis (n=62)	
Arthrosis	48
Dysplasia	6
Arthritis	6
Femoralheadnecrosis	2
Gender (n=60)	
Female	35
Male	25
Follow-up	
No. of patients	58 (97%)
Mean duration, months	24 (range 18–42)

▪ **Table 54.2.** Results

Prostheses	
»CUT 2000« femoral neck prosthesis	34
»Penguin« stem prosthesis	16
Cap prosthesis	12
Operation time (min)	
Mean	70
Range	45–130
Blood loss [ml]	
Mean	240
Range	120–430
Harris hip score (mean)	
Pre-operative	48
Post-operative	
Three months	92
Six months	91
Twelve months	93
Last follow-up	92

In one case we observed impairment of the sensory conduction of the obturator nerve, but the deficit resolved spontaneously after 4 months.

All implants demonstrated radiologically correct and unchanged position and stability at all time points.

The patients appreciated the fact that they could lie on whichever side they chose directly after the operation, as well as the inconspicuous nature of the scar, which was practically invisible.

Discussion

Around 100 years ago Ludloff developed a medial approach to the hip joint for surgical treatment of congenital dislocation of the hip in infants [4–6]. This method quickly became widespread, but disappeared from the surgical repertoire with the advent of diagnostic ultrasound in pregnancy and the associated almost complete elimination of actual dislocations. On the basis of our own earlier good experience with this medial approach in infants, we initially decided to conduct an experimental anatomical study to test its applicability in adults. This investigation showed that the medial approach yields an excellent overview of the hip joint and endangers no important anatomical structures. We thus began to use this approach for implantation of prostheses in an increasing proportion of our patients. The results confirmed our positive impression from the anatomical study. This medial approach is not feasible in ankylotic hip joints because the affected leg cannot be placed in the required position.

Significant reconstruction of the lateral acetabular roof via this route is associated with severe difficulties. Surgery on particularly muscular patients may also require technically difficult and lengthy preparation. All patients operated on via this approach were pleased to be able to lie in almost any position they wanted with practically no pain, in contrast to patients operated on via other approaches. They could lie on the affected side with no danger of dislocation.

The fact that the scar was practically invisible (◘ Fig. 54.8) was particularly appreciated by the female patients.

Another significant advantage of our medial approach over the conventional standard routes is that the abduction apparatus (gluteal muscles and fascia lata) remains unaffected, giving high protection against dislocation and allowing immediate mobilization.

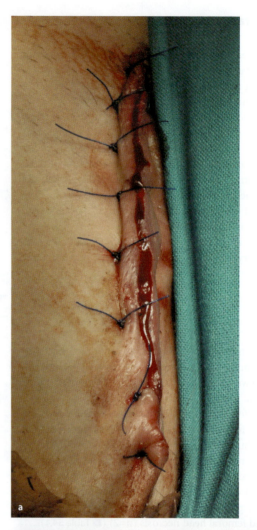

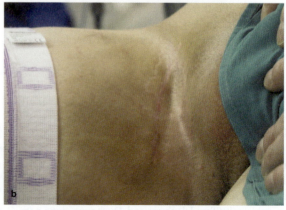

◘ **Fig. 54.8. a** Cutaneous suture; **b** scar 3 months after operation

Summary

Having first tested the clinical applicability of a medial approach to the hip joint in an anatomical study on fresh, non-formalinized cadavers, since 2002 we have been using this route in an ever-increasing proportion of our patients. After temporary division of the tendon of the adductor longus muscle, the medial approach affords direct access to the joint and yields an excellent overview of the acetabular and femoral parts of the implantation site without endangering any important anatomical structures. The operation can be performed using standard instruments. The operating time is no longer than with the conventional methods, and blood loss is low. The abductor apparatus (gluteal muscles and fascia lata) remains intact, enabling rapid rehabilitation with stable gait and no risk of dislocation. The patient can lie on the affected side. The inconspicuous nature of the scar is greatly appreciated.

References

1. Crowe JF, Mani VJ, Ranawat CS (1979) Total hip replacement in congenital dislocation and dysplasia of the hip. J Bone Joint Surg Am 61: 15–23
2. Grossman P, Braun M, Becker W (1994) Luxationen nach Hüft-TEP-Implantationen. Abhängigkeit vom operativen Zugang und anderen Faktoren. Z Orthop 132: 521–526
3. Kohn D, Rühman O, Wirt CJ (1997) Die Verrenkung der Hüfttotalendoprothese unter besonderer Beachtung verschiedener Zugangswege. Z Orthop 135: 40–44
4. Ludloff K (1908) Zur blutigen Einrenkung der angeborenen Hüftluxation. Z Orthop Chir 22: 272
5. Ludloff K (1913) The open reduction of the congenital hip dislocation by an anterior incision. Am J Orthop Surg 10: 438
6. Ludloff K (1914) Die Erfahrungen bei der blutigen Reposition der angeborenen Hüftluxation mit einem vorderen Schnitt. Zentralbl Chir 41: 156
7. Mulliken BD, Rorabeck CH et al. (1998) A modified direct lateral approach in total hip arhroplasty: a comprehensive review. J Arthroplasty 13: 737–747
8. Otto S, Gabel M, Trost E et al. (2000) Wird die Häufigkeit von Nervenläsionen nach totalendoprothetischem Hüftgelenkersatz unterschätzt? Orthop Prax 36: 696–699
9. Roberts JM, Fu FH, McClain EJ et al. (1984) A comparison of the posterolateral and anterolateral approaches to total hip arthroplasty. Clin Orthop 187: 205–210
10. Thomas W, Benecke P (2004) Der mediale Zugang zum Hüftgelenk zur Implantation von Endoprothesen. Operat Orthop Traumatol 16: 288–299
11. Vicar AJ, Coleman CR (1984) A comparison of the anterolateral, transtrochanteric, and posterior surgical approaches in primary total hip arthroplasty. Clin Orthop 188: 151–159
12. White RE Jr, Forness TJ, Allman JK et al. (2001) Effect of posterior capsular repair on early dislocation in primary total hip replacement. Clin Orthop 393: 163–167
13. Woolson ST, Rahimtoola ZO (1999) Risk factors for dislocation during the first 3 months after primary total hip replacement. J Arthroplasty 14: 662–668

Part IV C   Navigation and Minimally Invasive Surgery: Total Hip Arthroplasty

Cup and Offset Navigation with OrthoPilot System

R.G. Haaker, G. Trottenberg, A. Gleichmann

Introduction

Optimal acetabular component orientation in total hip arthroplasty is a complex three dimensional problem with failure leading to increased wear and instability. Recent publications have demonstrated a connection between the positioning of the prosthesis and the frequency of dislocation [1–7]. Lewinnek et al. noted an increase of the hip dislocation rate from 1.5% to 6.1% if a safe range of 15° +/–10° radiographic anteversion or 40° +/–10° acetabular abduction were exceeded [8]. Recent computer simulations have studied range of motion and concluded that the greatest range of motion was noted with acetabular anteversion of 20 to 25°, acetabular abduction of 45°, and femoral stem anteversion of 15° [1, 9, 10].

The positioning of the acetabular component during surgery is dependent on the orientation of the bony acetabulum and position of the patient's pelvis on the operating table. McCollum et al. have stated that patient positioning is not always reproducible in the lateral decubitus position and often leads pelvic mal-alignment with resultant improper cup alignment. Pelvic flexion and adduction are virtually unavoidable in this position placing greater demands on the surgical technique for satisfactory outcome [11, 12]. Therefore, improvement in cup implantation will occur if either the pelvis position can be standardized or a method of correctly localizing the anatomical orientation of the acetabulum can be created.

Computer-assisted orthpaedic surgery has been recently defined as the ability to utilize sophisticated computer algorithms to allow the surgeon to determine three di-mensional placement of total hip implants in situ [13, 17]. A rapid ongoing evolution of technical advances have allowed the ability to move from cumbersome systems requiring a pre-operative computed tomography of the patient's hip joint to more elegant systems that utilize image-free registration or the simple use of fluoroscopy at the time of surgery [18–20]. In total hip replacement, several reports have cited the accuracy with which implants can be placed using computer-aided robotic devices or surgical navigation [16, 17, 21, 22].

The OrthoPilot-system has been found to be reliable, and the accuracy of cup placement has been proven by several authors (Kiefer 2002; Ottersbach 2005). Since 2005 there is the opportunity to control stem position as well. In this special chapter the procedure of cup computer controlled placement combined with a movement mapping of a mayo-like neck prosthesis called Metha-stem is described.

Methods

The method of cinematic based computer controlled cup insertion is using the OrthoPilot system is described very well in the chapter 43 by *Kiefer*. The method of stem navigation using the same system is described by *Lazovic* in chapter 48. The introduction of spheric cups using a ventral minimally invasive approach needs a special angulated reamer. The acquisition of the preoperative rotational center is done first (◘ Fig. 55.1).

To insert a neck prosthesis type Mayo-stem is a so-phisticated procedure, because the femoral neck has to

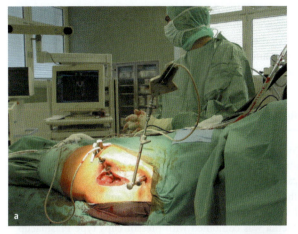

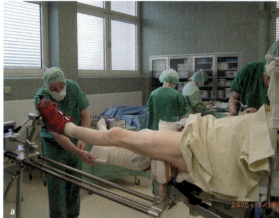

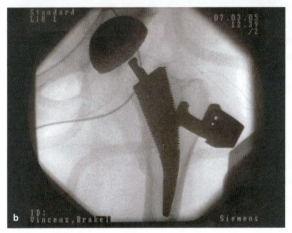

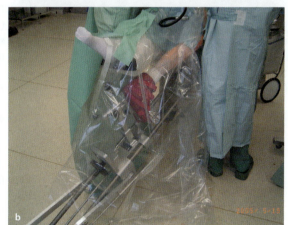

Fig. 55.1. a Acquisition of the in situ situation at the beginning of the procedure with rigid body fixed to the pelvic bone and to the greater trochanter with a special clamb. **b** Fluoroscopy intra-operativly with a reamer of the Metha stem in position and the clamp positioned at the greater trochanter

be conserved performing a cut of the femoral head right beneath the border of the head.

This results in narrow space for reaming the acetabulum. So a special extension frame for the minimally invasive ventral approach is useful (■ Fig. 55.2). During the reaming of the acetabulum the hip is in a neutral position and 3–5 cm extension is performed after high head resection. To insert the stem, the hip is turned in 90° external rotation, adduction and hyperextension so that the neck entrance comes up and the stem insertion can be made very easily.

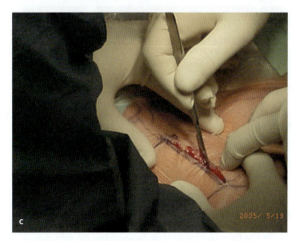

Fig. 55.2. a Extension frame for the cup placement using a ventral Judet-approach. **b** Leg position in external rotation and adduction for the stem placement in the frame. **c.** 7 cm ventral incision

Using a lateral minimally invasive approach the cup insertion can be done in a normal way using a straight reamer. The stem insertion is done by external rotation of the hip.

Using the computer navigation the neutral position of the leg is taken by the pointer tip on the patella and a rigid body fixed to the major trochanter by a clamp. After insertion of the stem the stem position is collected with the pointer on the base of the neck prosthesis type Metha. This compared to the saved data of the neutral position of the hip. Afterwards a special rigid body is introduced in the conus-hole of the modular stem (◘ Fig. 55.3). A move-

ment mapping then can be carried out on the computer screen with helps us to decide which anteversion or retroversion of the modular conus is the best according to the offset and the ROM of the hip in relation to the saved cup position (◘ Fig. 55.4).

Results

We performed the prosthesis in 20 cases and 19 patients since 01.01.2005 by now using the lateral approach in 11 cases and the ventral approach in 9 cases by the help of the extension frame. The 6 female and 13 male patients had an average age of 51.5 years. The neck prosthesis Metha was combined with pressfit cups type Plasmacup (Aesculap) in 15 cases and with pressfit cups type Versafit (Medacta) in 5 cases. The Metha stem was used 7 times in size 4, 4 times each in size 3 and 5, 3 times in size 2 and 2 times in size 1. Size 6 was never used.

The combined conus was in 6 times 7.5° anteversion and in 10 times 7.5° retroversion.

A neutral conus with 0° and 135° CCD-angle was used 4 times.

All the stems were implanted very well in the neck of the femur with contact of the distal tip of the stem to the lateral cortical bone right under the major trochanter (◘ Fig. 55.5). In one case we have seen a migration of the stem towards a lower position within 6 month (11 mm) but with very well bony integration in the deeper position and without clinical problems. The navigation was successful in all the 11 cases using the lateral approach. The ventral approach needs more adaptation of the navigation tools for the movement mapping of the stem. But the navigation of the cup was possible with a curved drill even in that cases.

Discussion

Acetabular component placement in total hip arthroplasty can be difficult with optimal placement required to prevent chronic instability, exaggerated wear, and implant migration [1–5, 7, 23, 24]. Recent investigators have sought to define the radiographic analysis of cup position in the clinical setting, prosthetic issues such as range of motion and component impingement, and technical issues at the time of surgery such as body position and how to place the prosthesis in the desired location [1, 6,

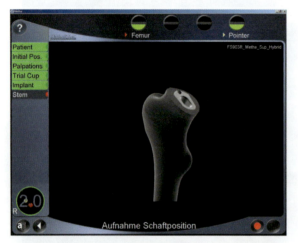

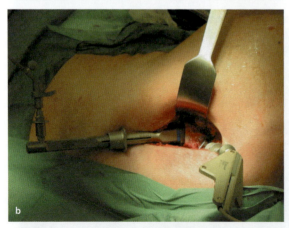

◘ **Fig. 55.3. a** Computer screen view demonstrates the collection of the stem position with the pointer. **b** Real collection of the stem position in the approach with a pointer armed with passive markers on a rigid body

9, 10, 25–30]. Computer-assisted navigation represents a new technology that can be used to deal with all of these problems [13, 14, 22, 31].

The spatial orientation of the natural acetabulum and prosthetic components placed at surgery is a complex three dimensional problem and most authors have attempted to describe a two dimensional radiographic answer [32–35]. Murray has provided the most complete insight into this problem by defining geometrically

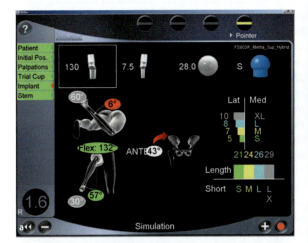

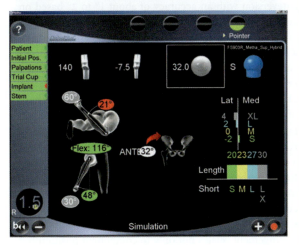

■ **Fig. 55.4. a** Computer screen »analysis« image after acquisition of the stem position like a movement mapping with the virtual use of 7.5° anteversion conus, a 28 mm head as well as 130° CCD-angle and the resulting ROM and alteration of the rotational center. **b** Computer screen with the alternative in the same case with 7.5° retroversion and a 32 mm head as well as 140° CCD-angle and the resulting ROM and alteration of the rotational center

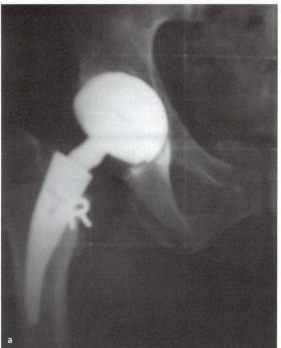

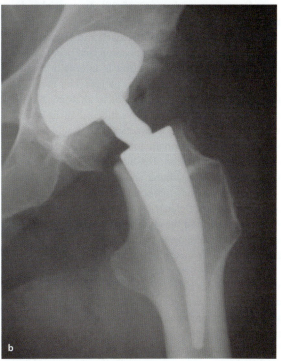

■ **Fig. 55.5a,b.** Post-operative X-rays in two planes of a Plasmacup and a Metha stem (**a** ap view, **b** Lauenstein view)

exactly what these solutions represent [36]. For simple comparison, the acetabular abduction is defined as the angle formed to the tranverse plane of the patient when the superior cup is tilted toward the longitudinal axis of the patient, or in the anatomical specimen a line drawn from the superior lip down to the inferior cotyloid notch on the anterior posterior radiograph. The more complex issue is how to determine the acetabular anteversion or flexion and three possibilities are possible based on how the cup is measured [17]. Operative anteversion occurs when the acetabular component is flexed in the coronal plane of the patient, essentially rotating about a line through the acetabulum which is perpendicular to the longitudinal axis of the patient. This is the maneuver accomplished by most freehand surgical guides and is the planar measurement made by determining the angulation of the cup in the frontal plane compared to the sagittal plane by looking at the coronal section CT scan [16, 17, 28]. Radiographic anteversion occurs when the anterior cup lip is rotated superiorly around the oblique transverse axis of the acetabulum which lies in the coronal plane of the patient. This measurement was typically used on cemented cups of known dimension that had wire radio-opaque markers [32, 35, 37]. A new trial to define the anatomical cup position in fluoroscopy postoperative controls is made by Ottersbach and Haaker [38]. Anatomical anteversion is the position that occurs when the abducted acetabulum position is internally rotated around the longitudinal axis of the patient. This measurement has been used to assess acetabular anatomical position in dysplasia. Murray has concluded that the operative anteversion is the most practical and should be used to describe cup position in total hip arthroplasty. For the computer application, DiGoia et al. have concluded that the operative acetabular abduction and anteversion measurements are the most straightforward reducing the conclusions to strict planar two dimensional terms [16]. We used this method for our abduction and anteversion measurements and have found no other variations in recent publications concerning computer navigation.

Lewinnek et al. were first to describe the concept of the anterior pelvic plane which is defined as a coronal slice passing through bilateral anterior superior iliac spines and the bilateral anterior pubic tubercles. In the normal standing position, this plane is usually parallel to the longitudinal axis of the patient [8]. McCollum et al. have shown that this plane may altered, especially if patients are placed in the lateral decubitus position, or there is hip flexion reducing the normal lumbar lordosis [12]. Lewinnek et al. employed a crude device with three legs and a bubble level applied to the pelvic crests and pubis to make certain that the pelvic plane was parallel to the plane of the table prior to taking their anterior posterior radiographs of the pelvis for anteversion measurement [8]. An important step in the registration procedure for computer assisted navigation is to define the anterior pelvic plane using the same references generating a standardized pelvic position [16, 17].

Numerous investigators have questioned the accuracy of standard radiographic methods for measuring cup position. For radiographic views, the X-ray beam must be carefully directed in a standardized fashion centered over the pelvis and the pelvis must be level with the beam perpendicular to the pelvic frontal plane in each case [8, 22, 35]. However, Ackland et al. stated that an error of as much as 5° could be introduced if the X-ray was centered over the symphysis pubis and not the hip joint itself [37]. Pelvic rotation certainly is an important consideration, and Thorén et al. demonstrated a 2.5° alteration of cup anteversion for 5° of pelvic rotation [34]. Herrlin et al. found that 5° of pelvic flexion or extension could introduce a maximum error of 8° in acetabular anteversion. Computed tomography assessments done with computer navigation on the other hand have been described as the »gold standard« for measuring cup abduction and anteversion with an accuracy of about 1° to 2° based on current methodologies [20, 22].

Optimum acetabular component orientation has been a subject of much debate, but most recent investigations conclude that the approximate position of 45° abduction or inclination and 20° radiographic anteversion is the ideal target. Obviously, retrospective studies such as those of Lewinnek et al. and Fontes et al. define a »safe« envelope or range about which hip stability after arthroplasty is much greater [8]. However, Barrack et al. have utilized a complex three-dimensional computer analysis to define the optimization to the above parameters and have shown that certain positions such as cup abduction below 25° or cup anteversion below 0° are clearly unsatisfactory for positions such as sitting or stooping. Acetabular stability and impingement relates not only to component position but also to prosthetic design dimensions and related femoral stem positioning [9, 25]. The average cup position after navigation in our study was acetabular inclination of 43° and cup anteversion of 22°, closely approximating the best position in the majority of cases (measured using the method of Ottersbach et al.).

DiGioia et al. used a computer-assisted navigation system similar to the method we used to study the problems of mechanical alignment in the conventional operative setting with the lateral decubitus position and with the use of typical freehand alignment guides. They found that the mean pelvic position was close to the desired anterior pelvic plane prior to dislocation, but after dislocation the pelvis tilted anteriorly causing a shift of the mean anteversion of the pelvis to 18°. Of 74 cups, 58 were placed outside the desired anteversion of 20° +/− 10° while only one cup was outside of the desired abduction of 45° +/− 10° [38]. In another study, they were able to determine that post-operative radiographs produced variable and inaccurate results compared to their precise intra-operative computer-generated measurements [17].

Concerning stem navigation, there exists only few experience and the most recent publication is made by Jerosch et al. [40] dealing with a kind of movement mapping to define the ROM after THR. Bader et al. [1, 25] could show that there is a problem of early impingement of the cone of the stem if the right anteversion and abduction of the cup is not achieved. Our first experience with the stem navigation of the Metha prosthesis shows sufficient results according leg length and range of motion as well as lateralization and offset. The anteversion of this special kind of neck prosthesis is oriented at the anatomical anteversion and does not need any navigation help. The Goal to use it together with a minimal invasive ventral approach is an important factor to introduce this method into modern hip surgery. Further investigations are necessary to determine the usefulness of the system.

References

1. Bader RJ, Steinhauser E, Willmann G, Gradinger R (2001) The effects of implant position, design, and wear on the range of motion after total hip arthroplasty. Hip International 11: 80
2. Fontes D, Benoit J, Lortat-Jacob A, Didry R (1991) Luxation of total hip endoprothesis. Statistical validation of a modelization of 52 cases. Rev Chir Orthop 77: 163
3. Giurea A, Zehetgruber H, Funovics P, Grampp S, Karamat L, Gottsauner-Wolf F (2001) Risk factors for Dislocation in cementless Hip arthroplasty- A statistical analysis: Z Orthop 139: 194
4. Jolles BM, Zangger P, Leyvraz PF (2002) Factors predisposing to dislocation after primary total hip arthroplasty. J Arthroplasty 17: 282
5. Kennedy JG, Rogers WB, Soffe KE, Sullivan RJ, Griffen DG, Sheehan LJ (1998) Effect of acetabular component orientation on recurrent dislocation, pelvic osteolysis, polyethylene wear and component migration. J Arthroplasty 13: 530
6. Kummer FJ, Shah S, Iyer S, DiCesare PE (1999) The effect of acetabular cup orientations on limiting hip rotation. J Arthroplasty 14: 509
7. Schmalzried TP, Guttmann D, Grecula M, Amstutz HC (1994) The relationship between the design, position and articular wear of acetabular components inserted without cement and the developement of pelvic osteolysis. J Bone and Joint Surg 76A: 677
8. Lewinnek GE, Lewis JL, Tarr R, Compere CL, Zimmermann JR (1978) Dislocations after total hip replacement arthroplasties. J Bone Joint Surg [Am] 60: 217
9. Barrack RL, Lavernia C, Ries M, Thornberry R, Tozakoglou E (2001) Virtual reality computer animation of the effect of component position and design on stability after total hip arthroplasty. Orthopaedic Clinics NA 32: 569
10. Seki M, Yuasa N, Ohkuni K (1998) Analysis of optimal range of socket orientations in total hip arthroplasty with use of computer-aided design simulation. J Orthop. Res. 16: 513
11. Hassan DM, Johnston GHF, Dust WNC, Watson G, Dolovich AT (1998) Accuracy of intraoperative assessment of acetabular prosthesis placement. J Arthroplasty 13: 80
12. McCollum DE, Gray WJ. Dislocation after total hip replacement. Clin Orthop: 159
13. Bernsmann K, Langlotz U, Ansari B, Wiese M (2000) Computerassistierte navigierte Pfannenplatzierung in der Hüftendoprothetik – Anwenderstudie im klinischen Routinealltag. Z Orthop 138: 515
14. Bernsmann K, Langlotz U, Ansari B, Wiese M (2001) Computerassistierte navigierte Platzierung von verschiedenen Pfannentypen in der Hüftendoprothetik – eine randomisierte kontrollierte Studie. Z Orthop 139: 512
15. DiGioia AM, Jamaraz B, Blackwell M et al. (1998) Image guided navigation system to measure intraoperatively acetabular implant alignment. Clin Orthop 354: 8
16. Di Gioia AM, Jamaraz B, Nikou C, LaBarca RS, Moody JE, Colgan S (2000) Surgical Navigation for total hip replacement with the use of HipNav. Operative Techniques in Orthopaedics 10: 3
17. Jarmaz B, DiGioa AM, Blackwell M, Nikou C (1998) Computer assisted measurement of cup placement in total hip replacement. Clin. Orthop 354: 70
18. Hofstetter R, Slomczykowski M, Bourquin Y, Nolte LP (1997) Fluoroscopy based surgical navigation. In HU Lemke, MW Vannier, K Inamura (eds.): Computer Assisted Radiology and Surgery. Elsevier Science B.V., Amsterdam, pp 956
19. Hofstetter R, Slomczykowski M, Sati M, Nolte LP (1999) Fluoroscopy as an imaging means for computer-assisted surgical navigation. Comput Aided Surg 4: 65
20. Zheng G, Marx A, Langlotz U, Widmer KH, Buttaro M, Nolte LP (2002) A hybrid CT-Free navigation system for total hip arthroplasty. Computed Aided Surgery 7: 129
21. Jolles BM, Genoud P (2001) Accuracy of computer-assisted placement in total hip arthroplasty. International Congress Series 1230: 314
22. Leenders T, Vandervelde D, Nahiew G, Nuyts R (2002) Reduction in variability of acetabular cup abduction using computed assisted surgery: Prospective and randomized study. Computer Aided Surgery 7: 99
23. Berry DJ (2001) Unstable total hip arthroplasty: Detailed overview. AAOS Instructional Course Lecture 50: 265

24. Del Schutte H, Lipman AJ, Bannar SM, Livermore JT, Ilstrup D, Morrey BF (1998) Effects of acetabular abduction on cup wear rates in total hip arthroplasty. J Arthroplasty 13: 621

25. Bader R, Willmann G (1999) Ceramic acetabular cups for hip endoprothesis: How do the position of the center of rotation and CCD-angle of the shaft modify range of motion and impingement? Biomed Tech (Berl) 44: 345–351

26. Demos HA, Rorabeck CH, Bourne RB, MacDonald SJ, McCalden RW (2001) Instability in primary total hip arthroplasty with the direct lateral approach. Clin Orthop 393: 168

27. Hirakawa K, Mitsugi N, Koshino T, Saito T, Hirasawa Y, Kubo T (2001) Effect of acetabular cup position and orientation in cemented total hip arthroplasty. Clin Orthop 388: 135

28. Mian SW, Truchly G, Pflum FA (1992) Computed tomography measurement of acetabular cup anteversion and retroversion in total hip arthroplasty. Clin Orthop 276: 206

29. Scifert CF, Noble PC, Brown TD, Bartz RL, Kadakia N, Sugano N, Johnston RC, Pedersen DR, Callaghan JJ (2001) Experimental and computaational simulation of total hip arthroplasty dislocation. Orthop Clin 32: 553

30. Scifert CF, Brown TD, Pedersen DR, Callaghan JJ (1998) A finite element analysis of factors influencing total hip dislocation. Clin Orthop 355: 152

31. Hu Q, Langlotz U, Lawrence J, Langlotz F, Nolte LP (2001) A fast impingement detection algorithm of computer-aided orthopaedic surgery. Computed Aided Surgery 6: 104

32. Herrlin K, Pettersson H, Selvik G (1988) Comparison of two- and three-dimensional methods for assessment of orienbtation of the total hip prosthesis. Acta Radiol 29: 357

33. Hoikka V, Hlikoski M, Eskola A, Santavirta S (1993) Inclination of the acetabular cup in erect posture radiographs. Orthopaedics 16: 1321

34. Thoren B, Sahlstedt (1990) Influence of pelvic position on radiographic mesurements of the prosthetic acetabular component. Acta Radiol 31: 133

35. Visser JD, Konings JG (1981) A new method for measuring angles after total hip arthroplasty. J Bone and Joint Surg 63B: 556

36. Murray DW (1993) The definition and measurement of acetabular orientation. J Bone and Joint Surg. J Bone and Joint Surg 75B: 228

37. Ackland MK, Bourne WB, Uhthoff HK (1986) Anteversion of the acetabular cup. J Bone Joint Surg 68B: 409

38. Ottersbach A, Haaker R (2005) Optimization of cup positioning in THA – Comparison between conventional mechanical instrumentation and copmuter-assisted implanted cups by using the OrthoPilot navigation system. Z Orthop 143: 611–615

39. DiGioa AM, Jaramaz B, Plakseychuk AY, Moody JE, Nikou C, LaBarca RS, Levison TJ, Picard F (2002) Comparison of a mechanical acetabular alignment guide with computer placement of the socket. J Arthroplasty 17: 359

40. Jerosch J, Steinbeck J, Stechmann J, Güth V (1997) Influence of a high hip center on abductor muscle function. Arch Orthop Trauma Surg 116: 385–389

55

Minimally Invasive Navigation-Guided Total Hip Arthroplasty in Practice

J.E. Brandenberg, C. De Simoni

Introduction

Since the publication by Di Gioia et al. 1998 [1], navigation-guided hip surgery has been on the increase. While in the early stages, CT of hips and pelvis was required, presently CT-free navigation systems [2, 3] are the preferred approach. Various studies demonstrate that navigation-guided implantation of the acetabulum is more precise than a free hand implantation [4–6]. The almost contemporaneous development of minimally invasive operation techniques puts further weight on the importance of navigation [7].

In 2003, Berger published the first 100 MIS cases [8]. A complication rate of 1% and significantly shorter hospitalization sojourns received much attention. Since then, reports about various MIS techniques have been positive as well as critical.

In Europe, the OCM access technique developed by Bertin and Roettinger [9] is widely used, its disadvantage is the lateral position of the patient on the operating table. Other techniques, such as Berger's two-incision technique, have the disadvantage of having to use fluoroscopic image monitoring during the operation.

Our SAL-technique allows for surgery in supine position without the requirement for fluoroscopic image monitoring and is suitable for navigation purposes.

Methods

Between February 2004 and December 2005, a total of 103 patients received 104 navigation-guided THA at our clinic.

The patients were aged between 43 and 85 years, the average age being 65.4 years. We had 52 female and 51 male patients. One male patient received THA on both sides.

Diagnoses:
- Osteoarthritis: 98
- Rheumatoid arthritis: 2
- Femur head necrosis: 4

In 64 cases we applied the SAL procedure (St. Anna Lucerne-Procedure) and navigation-guided surgery, 29 cases were carried out in the mini-transgluteal manner and in 11 cases we used the conventional approach.

Operation Technique

CT-free navigation system Galileo (Plus Orthopedic AG, Switzerland). In supine position, the navigation locators are fixed with two pins each bicortically at the iliac crest (■ Fig. 56.1) and monocortically at the distal femur at 45° to the frontal plane. They are fixed by way of minimally invasive incisions. The mobile locator (■ Fig. 56.2) explores the anterior pelvic plane (APP). The femoral head's centre of rotation is registered. Following the removal of the femoral head, the depth of the acetabulum, its inclination

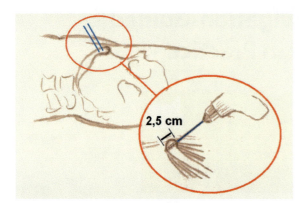

Fig. 56.1. Pin fixation on the pelvis crest

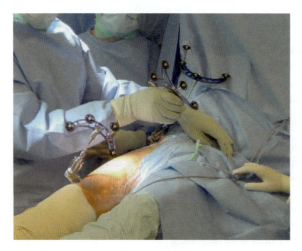

Fig. 56.2. Measurement of the APP (anterior pelvis plane)

and anteversion is registered on the navigation computer. The fraising of the acetabulum and the implantation of the press-fit cup are navigation-guided and carried out with bent instruments (Fig. 56.3). Following registration of femur antetorsion and stem direction, the femur medullary space is fraised open under navigation-guidance. ROM and stability is tested with test implants. Leg length is then examined under navigation-guidance. The supine position also permits a conventional clinical check of the leg lengths.

In the cases of SAL procedure (St. Anna Lucerne procedure) and mini-transgluteal access, a straight incision of 8–10 cm is made above the greater trochanter. We have abandoned the oblique incision between spina anterior superior and trochanter. Lancing of the tractus iliotibialis in longitudinal direction. In case of the SAL procedure, we use access according to a modified Watson-Jones approach in the interval between M. gluteus medius and M. tensor fasciae latae without resection of tendons. In the case of mini-transgluteal access, the tendon-periost layer is detached ventrally of the trochanter with the help of a scalpel. Both legs are individually rested on a newly developed operating table, so that the leg can be crossed over or underneath the non-operative leg (Fig. 56.4). A new dilating elevator with rounded edges was developed for safe protection of the anterior rim of the M. gluteus medius (Fig. 56.5).

After definitive implantation (EP-Fit cup, SL stem, Plus Orthopedics AG, Switzerland), follows closure of the Tractus ilio-tibialis. Drainage with cell saver intra-articularly and subcutaneously. Intra-cutaneous sewing with absorbable suture material.

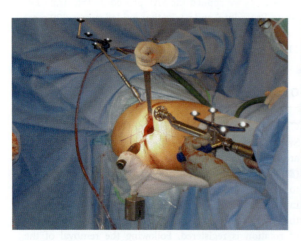

Fig. 56.3. Acetabulum fraising with navigated and angled reamer

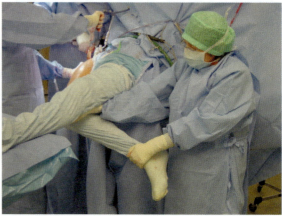

Fig. 56.4. Leg position crossed underneath the non-operative leg

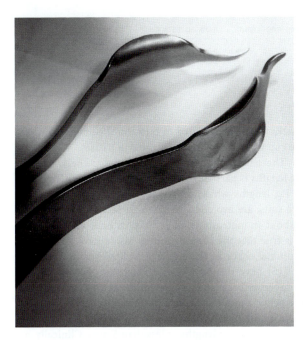

◻ Fig. 56.5. Elevator with rounded edges to protect the gluteus medius muscle

Post-operative Treatment

Mobilization from day one at full weight bearing up to threshold of pain. Walking training and instruction for safe day-to-day behavior. Discharge from hospital depending on individual subjective condition after 3 to 10 days following the operation. No physiotherapy required after discharge.

Results

92 patients who underwent 93 navigation-guided minimally invasive operations (SAL and mini-transgluteal) were involved in this study. A follow-up check was possible in 78 cases 3 months after surgery.

Duration of Surgery

Between 48–89 min, average of 63 min. Additional time required for navigation: an average of 10 min.

Hospitalization Period

Comparable group of patients: 2002–2003 undergoing conventional surgery. n=124. 67 female, 57 male patients, aged between 43 and 88 years, average age 67 years

MIS and Navigation N 78	total	5–13 d	Ø 9.6 d
	M < 65 y	5–10 d	Ø 7.9 d
Comparable group undergoing conventional surgery 2002–2003 N 124	total	9–15 d	Ø 12.2 d
	M < 65 y	7–12 d	Ø 10.3 d

Complications

Complication	n	Revision surgery
Prosthetic dislocation	2	1 cup replacement
Ectopic osteosis I	1	
Fractured trochanter	3	
Intra-operative stem perforation	1	
Intra-operative fracture of the femur	2	
Early infection	1	1 x irrigation, prosthesis was maintained
Total	10	2

Early-stage Clinical Results

Clinical check-up after 6 weeks by physiotherapist. Check-up by surgeon after 12 weeks and 6 months.

78 patients, 42 female, 36 male were evaluated after a period of at least 3 months after undergoing surgery.

All patients are extremely satisfied with the cosmetic results. The straight incision of 8–10 cm length above the trochanter shows more pleasant results than the oblique incision between spina anterior superior and trochanter. The incisions at the iliac crest and the distal femur are hardly recognizable after 12 weeks.

Pain			Limping		Trendelenburg+	Leg length [mm]			Walking distance		Walking aid		
none	slight	severe	start	permanent		0	+5	−5	>1 h	<1 h	0	1	2
63	12	3	12	3	5	73	2	3	70	8	73	3	2

Early-stage X-ray Results

12 weeks after surgery, an ap X-ray was taken of the pelvis with the patient standing in upright position. 78 X-rays were evaluated and being compared to the pictures taken prior to surgery as well as to the navigation records.

Leg Lengths

	<−10 mm	<−5 mm	−5 to +5	> +5	> +10 mm
Postop.	0	5	65	8	0

Acetabulum Inclination and Anteversion

<40°	40°–50°	50°–55°	>55°
1	61	11	5

A standard X-ray does not provide for a secure statement on the anteversion angle.

Stem

Correct	Varus	Too small
68	4	6

Discussion

Navigation guidance compensates for the inferior overall view provided by minimally invasive surgery. Navigation guidance optimizes the implantation of the acetabulum and avoids incorrect placement [4–6, 10]. In our study, too, 95% of the cup's inclination angles are situated in the target area of 45°. The advantage of a better guidance during implantation is particularly apparent when using a press-fit cup [11]. Standard X-rays do not provide for statements about the anteversion of the cup [12]. CT checks would be required to measure the anteversion of the cup which seems to be enlarged in 8 cases.

The navigation-guided intra-operative check of the leg lengths is particularly beneficial [13, 14]. Differences in leg lengths which can frequently result in malpractice suits, are avoided in a safe and secure manner and without an increasing number of prosthetic dislocations. It is true that the supine position also allows for a conventional check of the leg lengths, however, as Sarin et al. [15] have demonstrated, a navigation-guided check is superior because it is not influenced by changes of the pelvic and femoral position. A radiographic analysis three months following surgery in 95% of the cases shows differences in leg lengths of less than 5 mm. Clinically, a difference in leg lengths of +/−5 mm was identified in only 5 cases. There are no differences in leg lengths of 10 mm or more. An offset increase (lit) in 50% of cases required an offset-stem.

Fixing the locators by way of minimally invasive incisions outside the operating area, results in an excellent cosmetic outcome. Complications were not encountered, neither at the iliac crest nor at the distal femur. The duration of the operation is only slightly longer and is congruent with what is stated in other references [16].

The MIS technique has advantages as a number of authors have already stated. This is confirmed by our results. The faster rehabilitation after surgery reduces the hospitalization period [8, 17]. With regards to the latter, there is no difference in the procedures we used, i.e. the modified Watson-Jones access and the mini-transgluteal access.

Similar to the study involving 121 cases presented in 2004 (lecture at the annual Meeting of the Swiss Orthopedic Society September 24th 2004 in Montreux), there were no complications using the mini-transgluteal access. In particular, no symptoms were found to indicate abductor insufficiency.

The SAL procedure allows for the implantation of a total hip arthroplasty without detaching the tendons of M. gluteus medius and minimus. However, this technique is more demanding. Similar to other authors [18, 19] our learning curve with regard to operation technique and

56

patient selection resulted in a higher number of complications. We now know that muscular patients – mostly men – should not undergo surgery using the SAL procedure. The mini-transgluteal access should be used instead. Obesity with a BMI of more than 28 as well as previous surgery are generally regarded as disqualifying criteria for MIS, whereas the application of navigation guidance is particularly helpful in these cases.

The analyses of X-rays taken 12 weeks after surgery, in 18 cases show an osteotomy of the collum femoris that is too proximal (🔲 Fig. 56.6). This phenomenon exclusively appeared when the SAL procedure was applied. In the case of strong male bone this can lead to a premature stop to the rasping process which in 4 cases resulted in a varus position. In 6 cases it resulted into the fact that too small a stem was implanted. In one case, the patient suffered from pain during rotational movement 6 months after surgery, however, axial movement is not affected. Further observation will reveal whether stem loosening will appear. All the other cases are without symptoms. In the case of weaker female bones, too long a neck of the femur stem can result in intra-operative femoral fractures as has happened to two patients. In one case, access was extended with the help of cerclages, in the other case, a LISS plate with cerclages was used for osteosynthetic treatment. In view of the poor overall view provided by minimally invasive surgery access, particular attention must be placed on the resection of the collum femoris so that a post-resection of the calcar can be done in time.

Perforations of the dorso-lateral femur metaphysis with rasps as well as trochanter fractures are a result of insufficient relaxation of strong muscles. This hampers a sufficient extension and adduction of the femur and, as a consequence, a correct insertion of the rasps. An optimal muscle relaxation with the help of anesthetics is a mandatory precondition for MIS. If this fails, access must be extended by partially detaching the tendons at the point of attachment at the trochanter. In our case, this solved the problem of perforation intra-operatively. The healing process was not affected. The trochanter fractures were only diagnosed during the radiographic check. Only in one case, radiography showed a slight dislocation towards proximal and resulted in the clinical symptoms of positive Trendelenburg's sign as well as limping while the patient was free from pain. The other cases are without symptoms and show no dislocation on the X-rays, which is probably due to the intact insertion of the gluteal tendons at the trochanter.

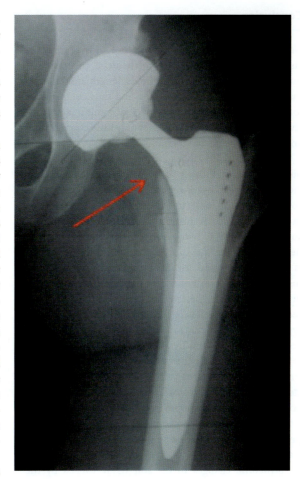

🔲 **Fig. 56.6.** The femur osteotomy too proximal

The MIS technique causes less postoperative pain which tempts particularly older patients to move beyond the ROM of the prosthesis. As in our case, this caused the dislocation of the prosthesis while the placement of the implant was correct. The patients must repeatedly be made aware of this danger.

The advantages of the MIS procedures become predominantly apparent during the early postoperative stage. However, Ogonda et al. [20] even queried these advantages. Our survey revealed that our patients did not place the main emphasis on hospitalization duration which could be due to the Swiss insurance system. To the patients it was rather important that the operation left only a small scar.

Conclusion

Navigation guidance is an excellent tool for the more precise implantation of hip endoprostheses. It ensures good intra-operative monitoring of the leg length and an optimal positioning of the acetabulum and thus compensates for the limited overall view provided by minimally invasive surgery. The technique causes only little complication and slightly extends the operation duration.

A minimally invasive access results in a faster rehabilitation and reduces hospitalization periods. In our view, the mini-transgluteal access also causes only little complications. In our study, we did not encounter the problem of adductor insufficiency. The modified Watson-Jones access is being carried out without tendon detachment when the special positioning of the patient is applied (We used the SAL method). An adductor insufficiency is thus not to be expected. However, this procedure has a higher rate of complications and thus requires a strict patient selection and the avoidance of typical pitfalls. Particular attention must be placed on the resection of the collum femoris, since an osteotomy that is too proximal can be the cause of intra-operative femur fractures, defective varus positions or the implantation of stem sizes that are too small. An insufficient muscle relaxation can foil the optimal external rotation and extension of the femur which can result in dorso-lateral stem perforations during the rasping process or in trochanter fractures respectively.

Structural changes to the soft tissue caused by the various access methods will be subject to further studies. Long-term results will reveal the effect of MIS and navigation-guided techniques on the survival rate of implants.

References

1. DiGioia AM, Jaramaz B, Blackwell M et al. (1998) The Otto Aufranc Award. Image guided navigation system to measure intraoperatively acetabular implant alignment. Clin Orthop Relat Res 355: 8–22
2. Wentzensen A, Zheng G, Vock B, Langlotz U, Korber J, Nolte LP, Grutzner PA (2003) Image-based hip navigation. Int Orthop 27 Suppl 1: S43–46
3. Dorr LD, Hishiki Y, Wan Z, Newton D, Yun A (2005) Development of imageless computer navigation for acetabular component position in total hip replacement. Iowa Orthop J 25: 1–9
4. DiGioia AM 3rd, Jaramaz B, Plakseychuk AY, Moody JE Jr, Nikou C, Labarca RS, Levison TJ, Picard F (2002) Comparison of a mechanical acetabular alignment guide with computer placement of the socket. J Arthroplasty 17: 359–364
5. Leenders T, Vandevelde D, Mahieu G, Nuyts R (2002) Reduction in variability of acetabular cup abduction using computer assisted surgery: a prospective an randomized study. Comput Aided Surg 7(2): 99–106
6. Nogler M, Kessler O, Prassl A, Donnelly B, Streicher R, Sledge JB, Krismer M (2004) Reduced variability of acetabluar cup positioning with use of an imageless navigation system. Clin Orthop Relat Res 426: 159–163
7. Stulberg SD (2004) The rationale for using computer navigation with minimally invasive THA. Orthopedics 27(9): 943–944
8. Berger RA (2003) Total hip arthroplasty using the minimally invasive two-incision approach. Clin Orthop Relat Res 417: 232–241
9. Bertin KC, Roettinger H (2004) Anterolateral mini-incision hip replacement surgery: a modified Watson Jones approach. Clin Orthop Relat Res 429: 248–255
10. Wixson RL, MacDonald MA (2005) Total hip arthroplasty through a minimal posterior approach using imageless computer-assisted hip navigation. J Arthroplasty 20(Suppl 3): 51–56
11. Bernsmann K, Langlotz U, Ansari B, Wiese M (2001) Computer-assisted navigated cup placement of different cup types in hip arthroplasty – a randomised controlled trial. Z Orthop Ihre Grenzgeb 139: 512–517
12. Kalteis T, Handel M, Herold T, Perlick L, Paetzel C, Grifka J (2005) Position of the acetabular cup-accuracy of radiographic calculation compared to CT-based measurement. Eur J Radiol 10
13. Kiefer H, Othman A (2005) OrthoPilot total hip arthroplasty workflow and surgery. Orthopedics 28(Suppl): 1221–1226
14. Lazovic D, Kaib N (2005) Results with navigated bicontact hip arthroplasty. Orthopedics 28 (Suppl): 1227–1233
15. Sarin VK, Pratt WR, Bradley GW (2005) Accurate femur repositioning is critical during intraoperative total hip arthroplasty length and offset assessment. J Arthroplasty 20(7): 887–891
16. Hube R, Birke A, Hein W, Klima S (2003) CT-based and fluoroscopy-based navigation for cup implantation in total hip arthroplasty (THA). Surg Technol Int 11: 275–280
17. Chung WK, Liu D, Foo LS (2004) Mini-incision total hip replacement- surgical technique and early results. J Orthopaedic Surg 12(1): 19–24
18. Archibeck MJ, White RE Jr (2004) Learning curve for the two-incision total hip replacement. Clin Orthop Relat Res 429: 232–238
19. Wohlrab D, Hagel A, Hein W (2004) Advantages of minimal invasive total hip replacement in the early phase of rehabilitation. Z Orthop Ihre Grenzgeb 142(6): 685–690
20. Ogonda L, Wilson R, Archbold P, Lawlor M, Humphreys P, O'Brien S, Beverland D (2005) A minimal-incision technique in total hip arthroplasty does not improve early postoperative outcomes. A prospective, randomized, controlled trial. J Bone Joint Surg Am 87: 701–710

Optimization of Cup Positioning in Total Hip Arthroplasty

Comparison Between Conventional Mechanical Instrumentation and Computer-assisted Implanted Cups by Using the Orthopilot Navigation System

A. Ottersbach, R.G. Haaker

Introduction

More than 150,000 total hip endoprostheses are implanted in Germany every year. Apart from tribological factors and the choice of the correct type of prosthesis with reference to the biological age of the patients, crucial elements for the functions of the artificial joint are exact positioning of the acetabular cup and the hip stem to reconstruct the rotation centre with optimum load transfer onto the pelvis, as well as restoration of the proper soft-tissue tension.

Incorrect positioning of one or both components increases the danger of early luxation. The frequency of luxation also depends on the surgical approach, the age of the patient and the offset of the prosthesis stem, or the resulting soft tissue tension. It is undisputed that a cup position that is too steep results in increased wear of the polyethylene inlay. The foreign bodies thus released can lead to local osteolysis with aseptic loosening of the entire implant [1–3, 6]. One of the essential preconditions for exact positioning of the cup is to establish the position of the pelvis on the operating table. Positioning aids used to date, such as the positioning aid according to Mittelmeier, have the disadvantage that the actual position of the pelvis on the operating table, in particular the pelvic tilt in the sagittal plane, is only approximately evaluated [23]. Since five years many computer systems are available in the German-speaking area for navigating the acetabular cup. Common to all these systems is the establishment of the so-called pelvic entry plane, which is defined by the two anterior iliac spines and the pubic tubercle. The significance of this anterior pelvic plane, as it is called, was already recognized by Cunningham in 1922 [4]. Inclination and anteversion are determined by the computer-assisted navigation systems in relation to this so-called reference plane. Since the lamina interna is also registered with the aid of a pointer, it is additionally possible to check the distance between the reamer and the acetabular floor.

Post-operative analysis of the cup position is difficult, since increased tilting in the view of the pelvis with the patient standing or lying causes substantial variations in the definition of the anteversion and inclination angle. According to the statistics gathered by the German Federal Office for Quality Assurance they vary between 1% and 10%.

Materials and Methods

First of all, our working group tried to find the simplest possible approach to taking standardized X-rays. This was implemented via a device constructed by the author containing two spirit levels at right angles and three adjustable legs that are placed or pressed onto the patient's symphysis and both anterior iliac spines directly after the operation. With the help of these spirit levels, the angle of the operating table is adjusted after surgery to horizontalize the anterior pelvic plane. Then it is possible to produce a standardized X-ray of the implanted hip joint.

The pelvis is horizontalized by adjusting the operating table, which can be tilted along the horizontal and vertical axis (☐ Fig. 57.1).

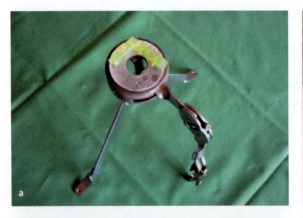

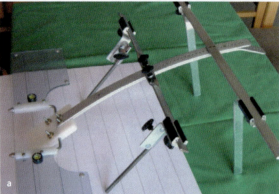

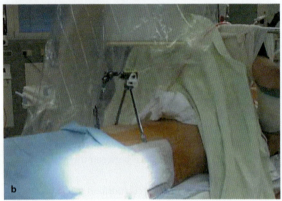

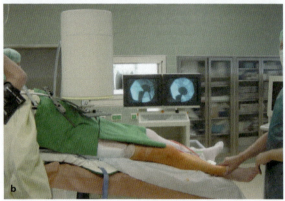

◘ **Fig. 57.1a, b.** Pelvis spirit level according to Ottersbach

◘ **Fig. 57.2a,b.** X-ray in neutralized pelvis position with »transverse referencing template« in place, the central radiation beam is directed at the midpoint of the hip joint

A template aligned parallel to the anterior iliac spines and equipped with an X-ray contrast stripe is brought into the radiation beam in order to determine the inclination angle exactly. The X-ray source and detector are setup in vertical alignment to the anterior pelvic plane, with the X-ray image intensifier positioned close up to the patient. The central radiation beam is directed at the midpoint of the hip joint (◘ Fig. 57.2).

Anteversion can be calculated using a sine function, as demonstrated by Pradhan in 1999 in J Bone Joint Surgery [22]. The data were established after the relevant measuring points were drawn directly onto the image intensifier printout by one and the same assessor (◘ Fig. 57.3).

Between October 2002 and November 2004, 100 patients were recorded prospectively for our study and treated with a hip endoprosthesis randomly with or without the help of a navigation system. The computer navigation system used, Orthopilot (Aesculap), is based on kinematic data and data obtained through surface registration. The average age of the patients at the time of implantation was 60.3 years (between 39 and 88 years) for the conventionally implanted group. The right side was treated 21 times and the left side 29 times in 28 female and 22 male patients. 45 non-cemented Plasmacup acetabular cups and 5 cemented PE cups were implanted. In the computer-navigated cases, the average age of the patients at the time of implantation was 59.2 years (between 27 and 80 years). The right side was treated 24 times and the left side 26 times in 33 female and 27 male patients. In this group 46 non-cemented Plasmacup acetabular cups and 4 polyethylene cups were implanted with the help of navigation.

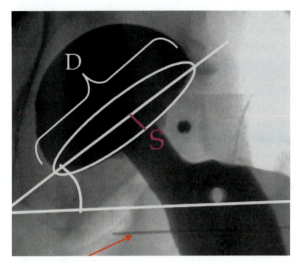

Horizontal reference line provided by x-ray contrast stripe to establish the inclination angle (a)

■ **Fig. 57.3.** Standardized post-operative X-ray. Determining the longitudinal and transverse diameter of the cup in order to establish antetorsion, according to Pradhan [22]: antetorsion = arc sin S/(D/2)

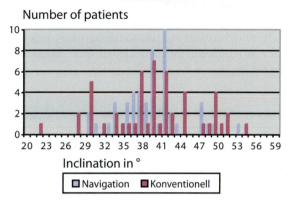

■ **Fig. 57.4.** Diagram: inclination

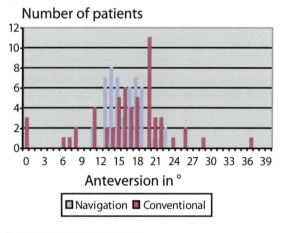

■ **Fig. 57.5.** Diagram: anteversion

Results

Inclination

The mean value of the conventionally implanted cups with regard to inclination was 40.3°, with a standard deviation of 7.4°. In comparison, the mean inclination of the cups implanted with computer assistance was 40.1° with a standard deviation of 5.0°. As expected, the confidence intervals were also narrower. 2 to 1.3 at a 95% confidence interval. 8 cases using the conventional operating techniques showed an inclination angle of 50° or over, compared to only 2 cups measured at more than 50° inclination in the control group of patients with computer-assisted implantations. An inclination of 30° or less was encountered only twice in the navigated group and 8 times in the freehand implantation group (■ Fig. 57.4).

Anteversion

The mean value of the conventionally implanted cups with regard to anteversion was 16° with a standard deviation of 6.9°. In comparison, the mean anteversion of the cups implanted with computer assistance was 16.3° with a standard deviation of only 2.8°. As expected, the confidence intervals here were even narrower than with the inclination angles. 0.7 to 1.9 at a 95% confidence interval. 4 cases treated with the conventional operating technique showed an anteversion angle of 25° or over, compared to the control group of patients with computer assisted implantations, where no anteversion values over 23° were measured. An anteversion of 10° or less was not encountered at all in the navigation group, but was found 7 times in the freehand implantation group (■ Fig. 57.5).

Early Luxation and Perforation of the Acetabular Floor

Whereas two luxations and two acetabular floor perforations were recorded in the control group, these complications did not arise in the navigation group.

Accuracy of the Orthopilot System

Following standardized application of the measuring procedure developed by Ottersbach, on a radiological basis, the deviation of the inclination values shown by Orthopilot from those of the X-ray control lies in 95% of the cases between -0.832° and 1.381°, with a mean deviation of 0.275°. The accuracy can be placed with 95% probability within a range of 2.213°. The mean deviation for anteversion is 2.373°. In 95% of cases the deviation lies between 1.567° and 3.178°. The accuracy can be placed with 95% probability within a range of 1.611°.

Discussion

The quality of the outcome after total hip arthroplasty treatment depends on various factors. The age of the patient at the time of implantation, the choice of implant, patient activity in dealing with the artificial joint, the tribological quality of the gliding pair and the offset geometry all have an essential influence on the survival time of the implant.

Giurea was able to show that the position of the cup is also an important factor [8]. The computer-navigation systems that have been in general use for some years must still provide evidence of adequate positioning accuracy in everyday use. Tanast et al. were able to show that the frontal plane of the pelvis when lying down does not run parallel to the frontal plane of the body [9]. This means that all external aids to positioning the acetabular cup can have only limited application.

CT-based navigation systems certainly allow the determination of the anterior pelvic plane, but are too much effort for standard use, and the radiation burden is also too high for the standard case. Whilst many publications exist on CT based navigation systems, publications on the kinematically based systems are rather sparse. One reason for this is to be found in the fact that post-operative determination of the implant position with the help of a CT

and the simultaneous use of special software requires a relatively high degree of effort. Moreover, a conventional post-operative CT scan merely to determine the position of the acetabular cup is not justifiable on radiation protection grounds. Because of these facts, the attempt was made to determine the cup position using a standardized post-operative X-ray, and the results were compared with the intra-operative information provided by the Orthopilot kinematic navigation system. It was possible to demonstrate an adequate level of accuracy. Using CT based navigation systems, the inclination and anteversion values in post-operative 3D CTs of the pelvis are very exact (standard deviation 0.99%), but this has not yet been proven for kinematically based navigation systems. As yet, there is no agreement on the optimum positioning of the acetabular cup. Regarded as reference points in the literature are the so-called »safe zone« recommended by Levineck et al. (inclination 40° plus or minus 10°, anteversion 15° plus or minus 10°) for minimizing the luxation tendency [13]. Thomas et al. drew attention to the increase in attritional force and surface strain on the components that results when the cup is incorrectly positioned in the sense of an excessively steep implantation [15]. The increased wear of the cup polyethylene that arises from this has been confirmed by several authors [1].

Hierakawa et al. were also able to show better long term results for cup inclination angles under 40° than for inclination angles above 45°. They found 90% mechanical failure rates after an implantation time of 15 years for a cup inclination angle of more than 45° [16].

Whilst the benefit of CT-based navigation systems could be demonstrated by Haaker et al. for hip dysplasia cases because of the possibilities for pre-operative position planning, as the results shown here reveal, the kinematically based system is obviously completely sufficient for the normal everyday acetabular cup implantation [11]. This is demonstrated by the very small standard deviations between intra-operatively established inclination and anteversion values and the postoperative values determined through standardized X-ray control, as well as by the narrow 95% confidence intervals.

Other systems, such as the cup positioning aid according to Mittelmeier [23], have not yet gained acceptance in everyday use [10,15]. The antetorsion check is not adequately registered, owing to the individual influence of the pelvic tilt. The method according to Graf [17] could possibly be regarded as a variation here. Whilst Bernsmann and Haaker found significant cup positioning differences in multicenter studies between conventional and computer-assisted cup implantations using CT based systems, it has been possible here for the first time to provide evidence that this significant difference also applies for kinematically based systems. Proof of reproducibility when using a kinematic navigation system of the same type has already been provided by Kiefer [21].

The decisive effect, in particular with regard to improving anteclination through navigation, could be proved for the first time in this study. During the practical application of the »pelvis spirit level«, involving adjusting the angle of the operating table, it became impressively clear how large the variation in individual pelvic tilts was. Precisely these individual pelvis positions make exact anteversion control difficult for the surgeon without navigation aids, as could be statistically demonstrated. But more consistent cup positions using navigation could also be achieved with regard to inclination.

Whereas in the control group two luxations and two acetabular floor perforations were recorded, these complications did not arise in the navigation group. Since the surgeon initially also registers the lamina interna with a pointer, the distance from the reamer to the acetabular floor can be checked during reaming, providing greater protection against acetabular floor perforations. To sum up, the improved accuracy in cup positioning when using computer assisted navigation systems must be accepted for both CT based and kinematic navigation systems. Whether the advantage of better cup positioning also influences the longevity of the implant must be established in clinical long term studies.

References

1. Bernsmann K, Langlotz U, Ansari B, Wiese M (2000) Computer Assisted Navigated Cup Placement in Hip Arthroplasty – Application Study in Clinical Routine. Z Orthop 138: 515–521
2. Amstutz HC, Campbell P, Kossovsky N, Clarke IC (1992) Mechanism and clinical significance of wear debris-induced osteolysis. Clin Orthop 276: 7–18
3. Mirra JM, Amstutz HC, Matos M, Gold R (1976) The pathology of the joint tissues and its clinical relevance in prothesis failure. Clin Orthop 117: 221–240
4. Willert HG (1977) Reactions of the articular capsule to wear products of artificial joint prostheses. J Biomed Mater Res 39: 222–226
5. Mittelmeier H, Mittelmeier W (2002) Die geschichtliche Entwicklung der Hüftendoprothetik. In: Konermann W, Haaker R (eds) Navigation und Robotik in Endoprothetik und Wirbelsäulenchirurgie, Springer, Berlin Heidelberg New York Tokio
6. Cunningham DJ (1922) Pelvis. In: Cunningham DJ (ed) Cunningham's textbook of anatomy, Hodder & Stoughton, London, pp 255–260
7. Pradhan R (1999) Planar anteversion of the acetabular cup as determined from plain anterio- posterior radiographs. J Bone Joint Surg [Br] 81:431–435
8. Giurea A, Zehetgruber H, Funovics P et al. (2001) Risk factors for Dislocation in cementless hip arthroplasty – A statistical analysis: Z Orthop 139: 194–199
9. Tannast M (2000) Die Berechnung von Anteversion und Inklination bezüglich der Beckenfrontalebene. Dissertation, Universität Bern
10. Bernsmann K, Langlotz U, Ansari B, Wiese M (2001) Computer assisted navigated cup placement of different cup types in hip arthroplasty – a randomised controlled Study. Z Orthop 139: 515–521
11. Haaker R, Tiedjen K, Rubenthaler F, Stockheim M (2003) Computer assisted navigated cup placement in primary and secondary dysplastic hips. Z Orthop 141:105–111
12. DiGioia AM, Jamaraz B, Blackwell M et al. (1998) Image guided navigation system to measure intraoperatively acetabular implant alignment. Clin Orthop 355: 8–22
13. Lewinnek GE, Lewis JL, Tarr T et al. (1978) Dislocations after total hip replacement arthroplasties. J Bone Joint Surg [Am] 60: 217–221
14. Fontes D, Benoit J, Lortat-Jacob A et al. (1991) Luxation of total hip endoprothesis. Statistical validation of a modelization of 52 cases. Rev Chir Orthop 77: 163–170
15. Thomas W, Schug M (1994) Über die Bedeutung der Position der Endoprothesenpfanne aus biomechanischer und klinischer Sicht – Vorschlag einer Klassifizierung. Biomed Tech 39: 222–226
16. Hirakawa K, Mitsugi N, Koshino T, Saito T, Hirasawa Y, Kubo T (2001) Effect of acetabular cup position and orientation in cemented total hip arthroplasty. Clin Orthop 388: 135–142
17. Graf R (2004) Der Pfannennavigator. In: Effenberger, Zichner, Richolt (Hrsg) Pressfitpfannen. Medical Corporate University, pp 93–97
18. Saxler G, Marx A, Vandervelde D et al. (2004) A comparison of freehand and computer assisted cup placement in total hip arthroplasty. A multi-center study. Z Orthop 142: 286–291
19. Saxler G, Marx A, Vabndervelde D et al. (2004) The accuracy of freehand cup positioning – a CT based measurement of cup placement in 105 total hip arthroplasties. Int Orthopaedics 28: 198–201
20. Haaker R, Tiedjen K, Ottersbach A, Rubenthaler F, Stockheim M, Stiehl JB (2005) Comparison of conventional versus computer assisted acetabular component insertion. J Arthroplasty (in print)
21. Kiefer H (2003) OrthoPilot cup navigation – how to optimize cup positioning? Int Orthopaedics 27 (Suppl 1): S37–S42
22. Pradhan R (1999) Planar anteversion of the acetabular cup as determined from plain anteroposterior radiographs. J Bone Joint Surg 81 B: 431–453
23. Mittelmeier H (2003) Herkömmliche Chirurgische Navigation und Bearbeitung des Prothesenlagers. In: Navigation und Robotic in der Gelenk- und Wirbelsäulenchirurgie. Springer, Berlin Heidelberg New York Tokio, pp 69–71

Computer-assisted Simulation of Femoro-acetabular Impingement Surgery

Concept and Preliminary Clinical Results

M. Tannast, M. Kubiak-Langer, S.B. Murphy, T.M. Ecker, M. Puls, F. Langlotz, K.A. Siebenrock

Introduction

In the past decade, sophisticated computer-assisted methods and simulations have been successfully introduced for various applications and questions in orthopaedic surgery [1]. Computerized imaging and visualization tools guarantee more accurate measurements which lead to more profound knowledge and to a better understanding of orthopaedic pathologies. They allow more accurately performed surgical interventions and differentiated, standardized evaluation of postoperative surgical outcome [2]. Moreover, virtual preoperative simulations were proven to simplify surgical planning procedures of orthopaedic operations.

Within the same time frame, femoro-acetabular impingement (FAI) has been detected as a novel major precursor of idiopathic 'primary' osteoarthritis in hip joints affecting predominantly young and active adults [3, 4]. Due to the simple mechanical collision concept of rigid bodies and newly posed questions for this new pathological entity and its treatment, FAI offers an ideal platform for application of computer-assisted methods. We describe a possible application of computer aided simulation for different unsolved clinically relevant questions in assessment and surgical treatment of this new entity.

Femoroacetabular Impingement (FAI)

Pathomechanical Concept

Hip pain in young patients has been associated with abnormal hip morphologies for decades. As an example,

hip dysplasia is well known as an underlying factor which leads (if untreated) to end stage osteoarthritis [5]. Recently, FAI was described as novel, purely mechanically based concept where subtle osseous prominences of the acetabulum and/or the femur can be another possible cause (◙ Fig. 58.1). The main concept describes an early pathological contact of bony prominences of the acetabulum and/or the femur during activities of daily living. Two types are distinguished: the *Pincer* and the *Cam* type. *Pincer* impingement represents the acetabular cause where a partial or general overcoverage leads to a linear abutment of the femoral head-neck junction with the excessive acetabular rim. *Cam* impingement as the femoral cause is due to an increase of the femoral head radius mismatching with the radius of the acetabulum. In this case, the head is jammed into the acetabulum. As a result of FAI, labral tears occur and early chondral signs of osteoarthritis could be found [4]. The proposed treatment of FAI consists of surgical removal of the osseous prominences [6] through a surgical hip dislocation [7] or a reorientation of the acetabulum with a peri-acetabular osteotomy [8].

Surgical Challenges in Operative Treatment of FAI

The overall aim of surgical interventions in impinging hips is the improvement of the clearance for hip motion and the alleviation of femoral abutment against the acetabular rim. For the acetabular side, a resection arthroplasty of the excessive part of the acetabular rim is performed. For the femoral side, the aspherical portion of the head-neck junction is excised using an osteotome. Although the basic principles of surgical remodeling of hips with FAI have been well described, an accurate method for anatomically based assessment of the severity of impingement with a quantitative definition of the femoro-acetabular range of motion (ROM) as well as quantified planning of the amount of required corrective surgery is absent. To the authors'

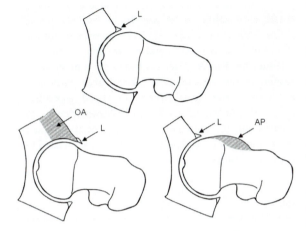

Fig. 58.1. *Top:* Normal hip with sufficient clearance for range of motion. *Bottom left: Pincer* impingement: The overcovering area of the acetabular rim (OA) leads to an early contact of the femoral head with the acetabulum. *Bottom right: Cam* impingement: The aspherical part (AP) of the femoral head is jammed into the acetabulum resulting in tears of the labrum (L) and considerable pre-arthrotic damage of the femoral and the acetabular cartilage. (Illustrations modified according to Lavigne et al. [6])

knowledge, there is no interactive visualization tool for non-invasive preoperative assessment of hips with FAI.

In this report, we describe our early experiences with a specifically developed software for femoro-acetabular impingement simulation including validation and the first clinical applications. Different aspects were addressed in detail including 1) the accuracy, reproducibility and reliability of the software; 2) the ROM pattern of hips with FAI in comparison to normal hips; 3) the specific impingement zones in hips with anterior FAI in comparison to previously reported intra-operative distribution of labral tears and chondral defects; 4) the effect of quantified surgical treatment for FAI on the resulting ROM.

System Description »HipMotion«

Software »HipMotion« was developed that is able to perform a computed-tomography (CT)-based three-dimensional (3D) kinematical analysis of any individual hip joint [9]. Computer hardware utilized was a SunBlade 100 workstation (Sun Microsystems, Volketswil, Switzerland). The CT scan of the patient's pelvis has to include approximately 10-cm of the proximal part of the femur and 4-cm of the distal femur covering both femoral epicondyles (□ Fig. 58.2). A slice thickness of 2 mm could be found to represent an acceptable compromise between data size and software accuracy. On the basis of the CT

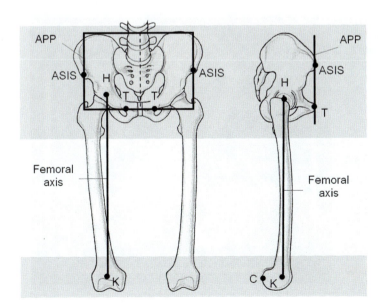

Fig. 58.2. Definition of the anatomical coordinate systems. The anterior pelvic plane (APP) as the pelvic reference is defined by both pubic tubercles (T) and the anterior superior iliac spines (ASIS). The femoral axis is constructed by the hip (H) and the knee (K) centers. A neutral femoral rotation is defined with the intercondylar axis (C) being parallel to the APP. The hatched area represents the regions to be covered by computed tomography

data a virtual 3D model of the patient's hip joint is created semi-automatically. A pelvic reference coordinate system based on the previously described anterior pelvic plane concept [2, 10] is established using both anterior superior iliac spines and the two pubic tubercles (◘ Fig. 58.2). On the femoral side, in order to calculate the anatomic coordinate system the strict geometrical definition presented by Murphy et al. [11] is applied, for which the posterior aspects of the two femoral condyles, the femoral head and the knee center are digitized within the CT data.

The acetabular contour is marked manually on the 3D model and is used to calculate the ROM within the individual virtual hip joint with a previously developed collision detection algorithm [12]. It enables fast and accurate calculation based on volumetric 3D models and can theoretically be used in any medical application to detect impingement between any anatomical structures and/or implant models. As a result, the individual ROM in terms of flexion/extension, abduction/adduction, internal/external rotation, and internal/external rotation in 90 degrees of flexion are displayed in a text field with the according normal mean values for comparison (◘ Fig. 58.3). The latter have been determined from the control group described later. Upon user request, any desired motion pattern can be displayed with visualization of the corresponding impingement point. The software also calcu-

lates and displays the location of all possible combinations of impingement points for a pre-defined range of motion, e.g. anterior or posterior FAI (◘ Fig. 58.4).

Quantified surgical maneuvers as trimming of the head/neck junction or the acetabular rim can be performed with HipMotion according to the current standards of treatment for FAI [6]. For the acetabulum, accurate localization of the segment to be trimmed is achieved with a superimposed clockwise system and the width of the resected rim in millimeter (◘ Fig. 58.5a). For the femur, head-neck offset is created by mm-stepwise removing of the non-spherical femoral neck portion in the antero-superior aspect of the femoral head-neck offset (◘ Fig. 58.5b). At last, taking the new volumetric data into consideration, the automatic simulation of the revised ROM of the hip joint is repeated and results are related to preoperative values.

Results

System Validation

System validation was performed with both the help of sawbones and in a cadaver setup [13]. The actual ROM determined with a commercially available navi-

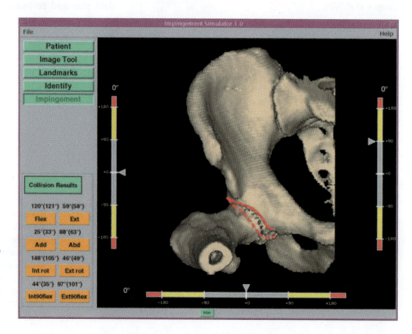

◘ **Fig. 58.3.** Interface of HipMotion. The actual range of motion of the individual hip joint is calculated and related to the mean values of normal hips (*brackets*). Upon user request, the hip can be rotated stepwise in any orientation with display of a possible femoro-acetabular impingement

58

gation system (Image-free hip version 1.0, BrainLAB, Heimstetten, Germany) was compared to the predicted ROM with HipMotion (◘ Fig. 58.6). A detailed study description and results were reported previously. Briefly, the same anatomical reference landmarks as determined on the virtual model were either digitized with a tracked pointer (all landmarks but hip joint center) or calculated kinematically (hip joint center). In summary, validation of the software with the sawbones revealed accuracy for the developed software of $-0.7° \pm 3.1°$ (range, $-9°$–$6°$) for all the 78 measured angles. Validation of the software with the cadaver hips revealed an accuracy of $-5.0° \pm 5.6°$ (range, $-19°$–$7°$). The accuracy of angle detection did not differ among the different motions neither for plastic bones (p=0.10) nor for cadaveric hips (p=0.28). The reproducibility and reliability were almost perfect for all motions except external rotation where only a moderate agreement could be found [14].

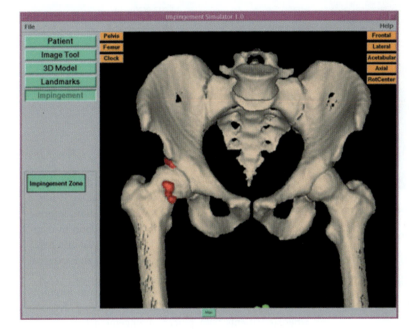

◘ **Fig. 58.4.** Dependent on the individual anatomy, the impingement zones are detected both for the femur and the acetabulum with localization on the virtual three-dimensional model

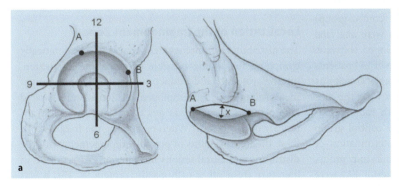
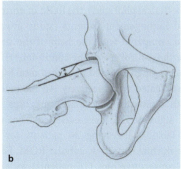

◘ **Fig. 58.5. a** Quantification of the acetabular segment to be trimmed is achieved with a superimposed clockwise system and the width of the resected rim in mm (x). **b** For the femur, head-neck offset is created by mm-stepwise removing of the non-spherical femoral neck portion (y) in the antero-superior aspect of the femoral head-neck offset

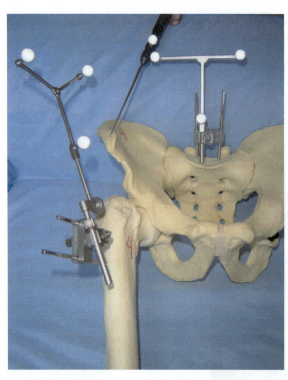

◘ Fig. 58.6. Validation setup with the help of a navigation system. The anatomical references are digitized with a pointer. The resulting, effective ROM determined with a navigation system was compared to the values predicted with the software

◘ Table 58.1. Exclusion criteria for the control group

Category	Specific criteria
Medical history	Total hip replacement
	Pain
	Previous hip surgery
Conventional radiographical criteria	Osteoarthritis grade > 0
	LCE < 25°
	Pistolgrip deformity
	Coxa profunda
	120° < neck shaft angle < 140°
	Acetabular retroversion
	Protrusio acetabuli
CT measurements	Alpha angle > 50°
	Femoral retrotorsion

Preliminary Clinical Results

Range of Motion of Normal and Impinging Hips

In a clinical pilot study, the ROM of normal (control group) and impingement patients (study group) were analyzed and compared with the help of the developed software. For the control group, the contra-lateral hip of 144 patients undergoing CT-based navigated total hip replacement was investigated retrospectively. All the painful hips, the hips with osteoarthritic changes and hips with radiographical signs of FAI were excluded from the control group (◘ Table 58.1), leaving 36 patients for determination of the normal femoro-acetabular ROM. For the study group, 24 consecutive hips (16 patients) with anterior FAI were recruited prospectively from the outpatient clinic of one of the authors (SBM). The impingement group consisted of 11 cam, 6 pincer and 7 combined pathologies.

It could be shown that there was no difference of ROM for any motion between men and women. Patients with FAI had a limited flexion, internal rotation, internal rotation in 90 degrees of flexion and abduction in comparison to the control group (p<0.001). No difference could be found for extension, adduction and external rotation in 90 degrees of flexion (◘ Fig. 58.7).

Among the study group, patients with cam impingement had a significantly increased internal rotation whereas patients with pincer impingement typically revealed a limited flexion.

Localization of the Impingement Zones

The distribution if impingement zones were automatically computed for all the possible combinations of flexion, internal rotation and adduction for the three impingement subgroups. The impingement zones were located antero-superiorly with various degrees of extension anteriorly or posteriorly. When comparing the frequency of these theoretical points of possible impingement with the distribution of labral lesions for anterior FAI reported in literature from other orthopaedic centers [8, 15], it was interesting to see that the theoretical impingement localization matches perfectly the location of intra-operatively observed labral and chondral lesions (◘ Fig. 58.8).

58

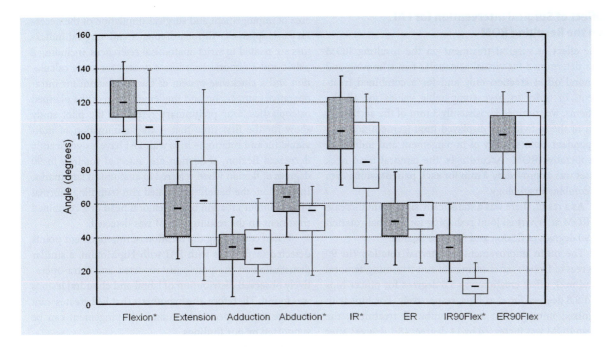

■ **Fig. 58.7.** Differences in range of motion for the control (*grey*) and the impingement (*white*) group. A statistically significant difference (*) was found for flexion, abduction, internal rotation (IR) and internal rotation in 90 degrees of flexion (IR90Flex). *ER* external rotation, *ER90Flex* external rotation in 90 degrees of flexion

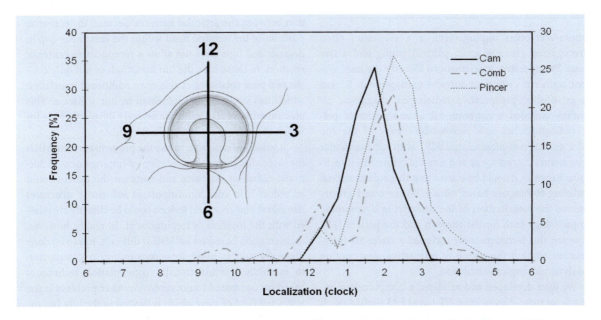

■ **Fig. 58.8.** Distribution of the sum of impingement points for the three different impingement subgroups described in the established clock-wise manner. This theoretical distribution matches perfectly the intra-operative observation of labral and chondral lesions independently from the type of impingement [8, 15]

Effect of Surgical Intervention for FAI on the Resulting ROM

The effect of surgical treatment on the resulting ROM was determined for virtual acetabular rim trimming and femoral offset creation only and for a combined treatment. In order to have comparable values for all the patients, we trimmed consistently 3 mm of the acetabular rim of the individually displayed impingement zone independent from severity of impingement and individual preoperative ROM. Accordingly, the femoral head-neck offset was improved by 3 mm for each patient with a cam or combined pathology.

As a result, there was a statistically significant increase of ROM after virtual joint reshaping for internal rotation in 90 degrees of flexion and for pure flexion.

The mean improvement of internal rotation (in 90 degrees of flexion) after segmental rim trimming/femoral head neck offset creation was 5.6 degrees for pincer hips and 8.8 degrees for cam hips, respectively. For hips with a mixed impingement and a combined treatment, the mean ROM was increased by 14 degrees (8.1 degrees after acetabular rim trimming and 5.9 degrees after additional femoral head reshaping).

Discussion

Femoro-acetabular impingement is a common, often unrecognized cause of groin pain in young and active adults. Pre-operative assessment to identify the impingement source is critical to surgical management. So far, the established preoperative radiological diagnostic algorithm included a conventional antero-posterior pelvic radiograph, an axial »crosstable« view of the hip and a special two-dimensional MRI with intra-articular gadolinium contrast agent and a radial reformation technique. Recently, it could be shown that three-dimensional rendering techniques based on a CT-scan could greatly improve the visualization of the underlying dysmorphic hip pathology both for the surgeon and the patient [15]. However, this technique only included a static 3D interpretation without the option of interactive joint motion and dynamic surgical simulation.

We have developed and validated a computerized approach for three-dimensional CT-based FAI simulation. It could be shown that our software »HipMotion« represents an accurate and reliable tool for simulation of individual hip ROM, the location of the acetabular and/or femoral area of impingement and surgical simulation of the necessary osteoplasties. All measurements and surgical indicators are related to strict anatomical references, including a pelvic and a femoral coordinate system for angle calculation and a clockwise system of the acetabulum for intraoperative comparison and implementation of the planned osteoplasties. Our preliminary results of the pilot study show for the first time that – after elimination of individual tilt and rotation – hips with FAI have a significantly decreased flexion, abduction and internal rotation in 90 degrees of flexion when referred to anatomical landmarks. In addition, the benefit of isolated rim trimming, normal offset contour creation of the femoral head or a combined treatment on the resulting ROM was detected.

When comparing the location of impingement points detected in patients with FAI with HipMotion, a similar distribution to the previously reported and intra-operatively observed distribution of labral and chondral lesions was found. Therefore, the hypothesis that FAI creates joint damage at the specific location of impingement can be supported by our findings.

HipMotion is not applicable to all hips. Severely altered hips with advanced osteoarthritis cannot be analyzed reliably due to two reasons. First, a correct segmentation of the femoral head and the acetabulum is not possible since the loss of joint space hampers a reliable determination between the articular surfaces. Second, the eccentric position of the femoral head within the acetabular cup in degenerated hips does not allow a reproducible center of rotation. In these hips the hip motion does not only consist of a pure rotation but also of an additional translation which has not been implemented in our software. This phenomenon is also valid for severely dysplastic hips for which the software is not applicable either.

It would be desirable to use the proposed arthro-MRIs for three-dimensional simulation of impingement. Additional radiation exposure and costs for the patient could be reduced. In addition, important soft-tissue structures like labral and chondral lesions could be directly correlated with the location of impingement. In reality, however, segmentation based on an MRI is difficult, has to be done manually and is more time-consuming in comparison to established semiautomatic segmentation techniques based on computed tomography. Another problem is the restricted field of view which is limited to the hip. Important anatomical landmarks (particularly the distal femoral or the contra-lateral reference points) cannot be digitized in this data volume.

In summary, this computer-assisted non-invasive method represents a novel approach to a pathoanatomical mechanical problem of the hip that has not been studied extensively so far with sophisticated computer programs. It will help the surgeon to quantify the severity of impingement and guide him in decision making of the appropriate treatment option. For the patient, a more logical visualization of their pathomorphology will improve the understanding resulting in a better compliance. HipMotion represents the basis for future steps where navigated instruments will allow intra-operatively executing the previously planned osteoplasties. This could be combined with less invasive techniques such as hip arthoscopy or smaller incisions without full surgical dislocation of the hip.

Acknowledgements. Part of this work was funded by a fellowship for prospective researchers of the Swiss National Science Foundation (SNF), the NCCR »Computer-Aided and Image Guide Guided Medical Interventions« of the SNF, a Research Fellowship Award of the New England Baptist Hospital, Boston, MA, and the International Society for Computer Assisted Orthopaedic Surgery (CAOS-International).

References

1. Nolte LP, Langlotz F (2004) Basics of Computer-Assisted Orthopaedic Surgery (CAOS). In: Stiehl JB, Konermann WH, Haaker RG (eds) Navigation and robotics in total joint and spine surgery. Springer, Berlin Heidelberg New York, pp 3–9

2. Tannast M, Langlotz U, Siebenrock KA, Wiese M, Bernsmann K, Langlotz F (2005) Anatomic referencing of cup orientation in total hip arthroplasty. Clin Orthop 436: 144–150

3. Ganz R, Parvizi J, Beck M, Leunig M, Nötzli H, Siebenrock KA (2003) Femoroacetabular Impingement: A cause for osteoarthritis of the hip. Clin Orthop 417: 1–9

4. Wagner S, Hofstetter W, Chiquet M, Mainil-Varlet P, Stauffer E, Ganz R, Siebenrock KA (2003) Early osteoartritic changes of human femoral head cartilage subsequent to femoro-acetabular impingement. Osteoarthritis Cartilage 11: 508–518

5. Murphy SB, Ganz R, Müller ME (1995) The prognosis in untreated dysplasia of the hip. J Bone Joint Surg Am 77: 985–989

6. Lavigne M, Parvizi J, Beck M, Siebenrock KA, Ganz R, Leunig M (2004) Anterior femoroacetabular impingement. Part I: Techniques of joint preserving surgery. Clin Orthop 418: 61–66

7. Ganz R, Gill TJ, Gautier E, Krügel N, Berlemann U (2001) Surgical dislocation of the adult hip. J Bone Joint Surg Br 83: 1119–1124

8. Siebenrock KA, Schöniger R, Ganz R (2003) Anterior femoro-acetabular impingement due to acetabular retroversion and its treatment by periacetabular osteotomy. J Bone Joint Surg Am 85: 278–286

9. Kubiak-Langer M, Tannast M, Langlotz F, Ganz R, Siebenrock KA (2004) A CT based system to calculate range of motion of the hip joint and to simulate the femoroacetabular reshaping. In: Langlotz F, Davies BL, Stulberg SD (eds) Computer Assisted Orthopedic Surgery, Proceedings of the 4th Annual Meeting of CAOS-International 2004, pp 143–145.

10. DiGioia AM, Jaramaz B, Blackwell M et al. (1998) The Otto Aufranc Award: Image guided navigation system to measure intraoperatively acetabular implant alignment. Clin Orthop 355: 8–22

11. Murphy SB, Simon SR, Kijewski PK, Wilkinson RH, Griscom T (1987) Femoral anteversion. J Bone Joint Surg Am 69: 1169–1176

12. Hu Q, Langlotz U, Lawrence J, Langlotz F, Nolte LP (2001) A fast impingement algorithm for computer-aided orthopedic surgery. Comput Aided Surg 6: 104–110

13. Tannast M, Kubiak-Langer M, Langlotz F, Ganz R, Siebenrock KA, Murphy SB (2005) Prediction of individual hip joint motion and impingement: A validation study using surgical navigation. In: Langlotz F, Davies BL, Stulberg SD (eds) Computer Assisted Orthopaedic Surgery, 5th Annual Meeting of CAOS-International Proceedings, Helsinki, Finland, pp 457–459

14. Kubiak-Langer M, Tannast M, Murphy SB, Siebenrock KA, Langlotz F (2005) Reliability study of the CT based system for range of motion calculation within the native hip joint. In: Langlotz F, Davies BL, Schlenzka D (eds) Computer Assisted Orthopaedic Surgery, pp 261–263

15. Beaulé PE, Zaragoza E, Motamedi K, Copelan N, Dorey FJ (2005) Three-dimensional computed tomography of the hip in the assessment of femoroacetabular impingement. J Orthop Res 23: 1286–1292

Imageless Navigated Posterior Minimally Invasive Total Hip Replacement with the Orthosoft Navitrack System

A. Malik, Z. Wan, L.D. Dorr

Introduction

Historically, the acetabulum has been positioned by the judgment and experience of the surgeon without intra-operative knowledge of the true relationship of the acetabulum to the pelvic position, nor its relationship to femoral anteversion. The consequence of clinical judgment alone has been the risk of component mal-position with impingement which can cause dislocation, pain, accelerated wear and loosening [1–8]. The ideal cup position, when mated with the femur, allows coverage and stability of the prosthetic femoral head, provides good contact areas for the articulation surface, and prevents impingement in multiple body positions.

Clinical studies pioneered by DiGioia et al. [9] showed that navigation was definitely possible for total hip replacement with the benefit of controlling the highly variable pelvic orientation between patients [9–12]. Image based navigation with computed tomography hip software was validated on cadavers to have a precision of 1 to 3 degrees [13]. Clinically, DiGioia et al. observed with computed tomography based navigation that the acetabular cup alignment was within 5 degrees of the preoperatively planned position of 45 degrees abduction and 20 degrees flexion [9].

The problem of verification of true cup position was demonstrated by Murray et al. [14]. DiGioia et al. [9] found a discrepancy of 0–20 degrees between measurements for anteversion obtained by computer-assisted navigation versus radiographs and attributed this to intra-operative pelvic motion.

Our interest was to work on imageless navigation technology because the preoperatively CT based programs did not account for the imprecision associated with reaming or cup placement during surgery [9]. Imageless technology allows real-time intra-operative knowledge of the quantitative direction and depth of reaming; adjustment during reaming for variations in the bony anatomy to allow for correct cup coverage with optimal inclination; and allows adjustment of the anteversion of a cup to a desired combined anteversion through knowledge of the fixed femoral anteversion. In this study we determined the accuracy of, and reproducibility of, measurements of inclination, anteversion, and reproduction of the correct center of rotation of the acetabulum using the Orthosoft navigation program. Pelvic tilt was used to adjust the inclination and anteversion. Radiographs do not reflect the accuracy of the computer. The computer allows accurate real-time control of the placement of the acetabular components. If the femoral preparation is done first, so that the anteversion of the femoral component is known, the acetabulum can be customized for each patient to achieve a combined prosthetic mean anteversion of 35 +/– 5 degrees. The computer improved the skill of the surgeon to correctly and reproducibly implant the components.

Methods

After obtaining Institutional Review Board approval and proper informed consent for prospective review of data, 90 consecutive patients with 102 hips were included in the study using the Navitrack Imageless Computer Hip System (ORTHOsoft, Montreal, Canada) between July 2004 and March 2005. The patients had computer navigation data

☐ **Table 59.1.** Demographics	
Patients:	**88**
Hips Navigated	100
Age	62.4± 12.7 years
Sex	40 men (45%), 48 women
Height	1.7 ± 0.1 meters
BMI	27.2 ± 4.7
Weight	79.3±18.2 kg

collected during total hip replacement. Two hips in two patients had failure of the collection technique during the operation and the computer navigation was not used for component placement. Therefore, 100 hips in eighty-eight patients are included in this report. The demographics are listed in ☐ Table 59.1. The diagnosis was osteoarthritis in eighty-eight hips (88%), dysplasia in seven, avascular necrosis in four, and rheumatoid arthritis in one. The Hips were classified in four different categories according to our classification method as published [15].

Additional Measurements of Tilt

Pelvic tilt has been shown to have a profound effect on the visualization of the acetabulum and has been shown to vary during the different stages of surgery [15, 17]. When Murray [14] published his sets of equations for comparison of the anatomic, intra-operative and radiographic planes of inclination and anteversion, an assumption was made that the pelvis was neutral in the supine position. However, this is not true all the time. Computer navigation provides us with the capacity to incorporate a patient's pelvic tilt during cup positioning and thus obtain adjusted inclination and anteversion values. We routinely use tilt and adjusted anteversion and inclination for component control during surgery.

Computer Measurements of Inclination and Anteversion

Murray [14] defined cup position relative to anatomical, intra-operative (as directed by mechanical guides) and

radiographic variables for inclination and anteversion. Computer systems base their angle calculations against the anterior plane of the pelvis (the anatomical inclination and anteversion described by Murray). Classically, surgeons are accustomed to visualizing the cup in radiographic planes, which are calculated on the supine plane (radiographic inclination and anteversion described by Murray). Because it makes more intuitive clinical sense to the surgeon when all values for inclination and anteversion on the computer are displayed as converted from the anatomical plane (anterior pelvic plane) to the radiographic plane, the anatomical values were converted directly by the software program to values of adjusted anteversion and inclination that were visualized on the computer screen. These are equivalent to values of the radiographic plane, compatible with the classic training of surgeons.

Surgical Technique

The approach used in all cases was the posterior mini-incision [15, 16]. The type of incision does not compromise the use of computer navigation, and navigation can be used with either anterior or posterior incisions. The technique of imageless navigation for THR has been described by us [15, 17].

Instruments for computer navigation were calibrated by the operating room technicians while the patient was being brought to the room. For registration we used baseplates which were secured on the pelvis and femur with three threaded 1/8" pins to bone. An optical tracker was attached to the baseplate. The anterior pelvic plane was registered by percutaneous digitization of both anterosuperior iliac spines and the pubis near the tubercles. For pubis registration, because of the thickness of the mons pubis fat, the skin was punctured by the sharp tip of the digitizer and the tip advanced until firm bone contact. The patient was then moved to the lateral position and secured with two pelvic supports and two chest supports (Sunmed, Redding, CA). The femoral baseplate was attached to the anterior lateral femur 8 cm cephalad from the superior pole of the patella and anterior to the anterior edge of the iliotibial band. The pins were drilled through the anterior lateral cortex into, but not through, the medial cortex.

The longitudinal axis of the body was measured by touching the two posterior supports in the shape of a triangle (□ Fig. 59.1). The software computed the angle of the anterior pelvic plane relative to the long axis of the body and this was termed pelvic tilt.

Femoral Preparation

In our surgical technique the preparation of the femur was performed first so that the anteversion of the femur was known prior to the preparation and implantation of the acetabulum. When the first incision is made to the level of the trochanter, the leg is registered for leg length and offset measurement. After femoral preparation of reaming and broaching, the intra-medullary canal of the femur was registered with a dedicated instrument by touching 5 points within the femoral canal. The software computed the anteversion as the broach (and subsequently the stem) was impacted into the bone (□ Fig. 59.2).

Acetabular Preparation

After exposure of the acetabulum, different parameters were registered for real time referencing while reaming and placing the trial and cup (□ Fig. 59.3):

1. Center of rotation and diameter of the bony acetabulum. The acetabulum was digitized sixteen times in order to obtain these values.
2. Mosaic of the peripheral and medial walls obtained by digitizing these surfaces.
3. Inclination and anteversion of the bony acetabulum by touching the bone six times. This was adjusted by the software for the tilt of the pelvis to obtain the adjusted values.

Reaming

The reamer has a tracking device attached to it so that the position of the reamer in relation to the bony acetabulum was seen on the computer screen (□ Fig. 59.4). The computer quantifies exactly where the reamer is in relation to the bony center of rotation so that the surgeon can be aware of the measurement change in the center of rotation (in mm) for cephalo-caudal (CC), medio-lateral (ML) and antero-posterior (AP) directions. Our aim on reaming was to achieve the necessary depth medially and superiorly to permit correct cup

coverage while maintaining the center of rotation as close to correct as possible. Correct coverage meant that the antero-superior edge of the cup was flush with bone and the inferior-medial edge was inside the transverse acetabular ligament.

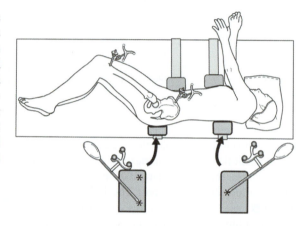

□ **Fig. 59.1.** The patient is in the lateral position for the operation and supported by two pelvic and two chest supports. The triangle is formed using the posterior supports of the pelvis and the chest to register the longitudinal axis of the body. This is illustrated with two points on the pelvic support and one on the chest support

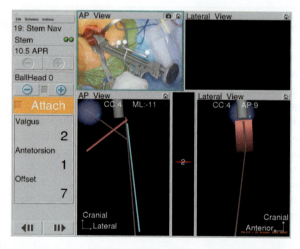

□ **Fig. 59.2.** As the broach is inserted into the femur the light emitting diode (LED) on the broach handle allows the computer to recognize the broaches position in the intra-medullary canal. The broach is in 2 degrees of valgus to the intra-medullary canal and in 1 degree of anteversion; the offset of the femur from the center of rotation of the cup is 7 mm

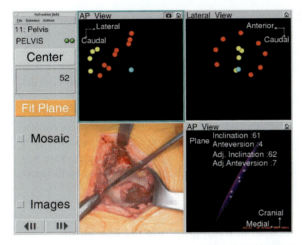

Fig. 59.3. The acetabular bone is touched by the pointer guide as seen in the *lower left-hand quadrant*. The mosaic of the bony acetabulum is shown on the computer screen in the two planes. The *red dots* outline the periphery of the acetabulum and the *yellow dots* outline the medial wall. The *blue dot* is the center of rotation of the bony acetabulum. The *lower right quadrant* shows the inclination and anteversion of the native acetabulum as determined by the fit plane

Cup Placement

We always implant a trial cup before the definite cup, and for both the holder has a tracking device to obtain readings for inclination and anteversion (❑ Fig. 59.5). With the trial cup we can judge for pressfit size and stability. The real cup was implanted with qualitative visualization of its position which is displayed on the computer screen, and the quantitative change of its center of rotation relative to the bony center of rotation. The position of the cup could be manipulated into the desired inclination and anteversion by viewing the numbers as the cup was implanted. The numbers for center of rotation of the cup represent the center of rotation with the polyethylene liner in place, which is known data *a priori* in the software.

In order to measure any change in cup position caused by the installation of the liner, 6 points were digitized on the edge of the liner (termed the cup plane) to register the inclination and anteversion of the cup (❑ Fig. 59.6). The difference in the cup plane measurement compared to that with the cup holder was considered the variability

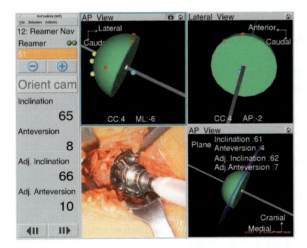

Fig. 59.4. The reamer in the acetabulum is shown in the lower left hand quadrant. The position of the reamer relative to the acetabular peripheral bone and medial wall is shown in the upper two quadrants. The CC number shows the position of the reamer superior to the center of rotation of the osseous acetabulum (negative numbers mean inferior displacement); ML is medio-lateral displacement from the center of rotation by the reaming (negative number means medial displacement); AP is the antero-posterior position of the reamer (negative number means posterior displacement). The numbers on the left give the angular position of the reamer in the acetabulum both by inclination and anteversion, which is also adjusted

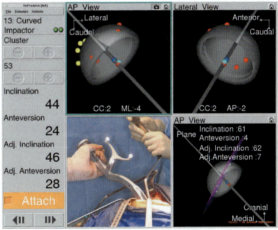

Fig. 59.5. The trial cup implantation is shown in the lower left quadrant. The upper quadrant shows the position of the cup relative to the acetabulum including the medial wall. The CC, ML and AP numbers provide the center of rotation superior displacement (CC), medialization (ML) and AP displacement (AP). The numbers on the left give the numerical inclination and anteversion, and adjusted inclination and anteversion. The lower right quadrant gives the native acetabulum values, and the gray lines show what portion of the cup would be uncovered

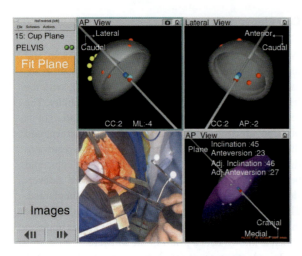

■ **Fig. 59.6.** The fit plane of the cup is measured by touching the edge of the metal shell in six places with the pointer guide. The fit plane registers the inclination and anteversion of the cup. The fit plane is repeated once the plastic liner has been inserted as in the picture by touching the cup six times again. In our experience, insertion of the liner changes the inclination/anteversion numbers for up to 3 degrees. This however is of no clinical significance, especially with a margin of error of 2 degrees

of motion of the cup in the bone. Motion greater than 5 degrees, (that occurred when the liner was malleted into place) was considered an unstable cup and the cup required screw fixation.

The combined anteversion of cup and stem were targeted at 35 +/– 5 degrees. In 68 hips we assessed impingement of the greater trochanter on the pelvis, the lesser trochanter to the ischium, and metal neck impingement against the edge of the cup and compared it to inclination and the combined anteversion.

Data Obtained from Radiographic Measurements

Pre-operative, immediate post-operative, and six week post-operative antero-posterior pelvis radiographs with the beam centered over the symphysis pubis were used for measurements. Measurements from post-operative radiographs included:

1. Cup Coverage. Correct cup coverage was defined as the inferior edge being ±10 mm of the transteardrop line with no more than 5 mm uncovered at the superolateral edge of the acetabulum.

2. Inclination of the cup was measured by the method of Callaghan et al. [18]. In this study a correction factor of –2 degrees was used for inclination measured with the beam centered over the symphysis pubis (so as to simulate the level of the center of rotation of the hip).

3. Anteversion of the Cup was measured with a method previously described [19, 20]. In this study, a correction factor of 4 degrees was added to the anteversion measurement on the postoperative antero-posterior pelvic radiograph with the beam centered on the symphysis pubis.

Precision of Radiographs to the Computer Navigation System

Precision was measured by comparing the adjusted computer inclination and anteversion with the postoperative radiographic values. If the computer navigation value for inclination and/or anteversion was not within ±5 degrees of the radiographic value, the radiograph was considered an outlier to the standard of the computer.

Accuracy of the Computer Navigation System

The accuracy of computer navigation was measured by comparing the adjusted inclination and anteversion with a post-operative computed tomography scan taken according to known protocols [12].

Statistics

The statistical analysis was performed with SPSS software (SPSS Inc., Chicago, IL). The Kolmogorov-Smirnov test for normal distribution was used before further statistical analysis was conducted. For analysis of measurements, the means and standard deviations were calculated. One-way Anova was used to determine statistical difference in measurements between antero-posterior pelvic tilt. Discriminate analysis was used to identify the influence of numerous variables on the impingement. A Chi Square test was used to determine if there was a difference in sex distribution, and head size distribution between hips with impingement and without. A Student's unpaired t test was used to determine the difference of medialization, computer inclination and the combined anteversion between hips with impingement and without. The repeatability between femoral anteversion of computer navigation and computed tomography scans were calculated using Intraclass Correlation Coefficient by the reliability analysis. The bias and precision were calculated according to the American Society for Testing and Materials (ASTM) definitions. A p value of less than or equal to 0.05 was considered to be statistically significant.

Results

The accuracy of computer measurements for adjusted inclination and adjusted anteversion were validated by postoperative CT scans (◘ Table 59.2). The bias for inclination was 0.53 degrees and for anteversion was 1.6 degrees. The bias reflects the accuracy which is therefore 0.53 degrees for inclination, and 1.6 degrees for anteversion.

The precision of computer measurements to radiographic measurements was statistically compared. Comparison of computer navigation of adjusted inclination and adjusted anteversion to radiographic values in 100 hips are displayed in ◘ Table 59.3. The precision of radiographic results to the computer results for inclination was 7.8 degrees with a bias of -0.002 degrees; for anteversion the precision of the radiographs was 7.2 degrees with a bias of 1.1 degrees.

Post-operative CT scan verification of femoral anteversion was done in nine patients (◘ Table 59.4). The mean femoral anteversion was 7 +/- 4.3 degrees (range 0 to 19 degrees, precision equals 6.2 degrees). Femoral

◘ **Table 59.2.** Accuracy of Computer Navigation for acetabulum

	CT Inclination	Navitrack Inclination	CT Anteversion	Navitrack Anteversion
N hips	23	23	23	23
Mean Value	41.8 ± 4.6	41.2 ± 4.7	24.4 ± 6.3	22.8 ± 8.9
t-Test	P > 0.05 NS		P > 0.05 NS	
Mean of Differences (bias)	0.53		1.6	
95% CI of Differences	-0.67 to 1.73		-1.24 to 4.34	
ICC	0.9		0.79	

N hips is the number of hips studied. *Mean value* is in degrees. *95% CI* is confidence interval. *ICC* is intraclass correlation coefficent.

◘ **Table 59.3.** Computer measurements compared to radiographic measurements

Computer measurement	Inclination	Anteversion
Bony Acetabular Anatomy	54.4 + 7.4 (39–71)	11 + 7.0 (0–28)
Cup unadjusted	41.6 + 5.0 (31–51)	26.3 + 6.6 (9–45)
Cup adjusted	41.5 + 4.1 (32–50)	27.1 + 2.7 (19–37)
Cup plane adjusted	41.5 + 5.7 (31–49)	26.8 + 3.4 (20–45)
Liner plane adjusted	42.0 + 4.4 (28–51)	26.9 + 2.6 (20–34)
Radiographic	41.5 + 4.3 (28–51)	26.1 + 2.9 (15–32)

Numbers are in degrees. Unadjusted numbers are not adjusted for tilt while adjusted numbers are. Radiographic measurements are included to compare to computer numbers.

■ Table 59.4. Accuracy of computer navigation for femoral anteversion

Statistics	CT inclination	Navitrack inclination
N hips	9	9
Mean value	9 ± 6.2	6.8 ± 4.5
t-Test	p = 0.07 NS	
Mean of Differences (bias)	2.2	
95% CI of Differences	-0.23 to 4.67	
ICC	0.906	

N hips is the number of hips studied. *Mean value* is in degrees. *95% CI* is confidence interval. *ICC* is intraclass correlation coefficent.

anteversion for men was a mean 5.0 +/– 3.0 degrees while for women was 8.8 +/– 4.5 degrees (p=0.024).

The mean combined anteversion for both men and women was 34.3 +/– 4.5 degrees (range 25 to 49 degrees).

With our definition for correct coverage we found that 66 hips had less than 5 mm superior-lateral cup uncovered, 25 hips had 5.1 to 10 mm cup uncovered, and 9 hips had over 10 mm of cup uncovered. Eighty-one cups were within 10 mm of Kohler's line and 19 not within 10 mm.

Pelvic Tilt

Influence of tilt on inclination and anteversion is shown in ■ Table 59.5 which has a comparison of the adjusted and unadjusted measurements. Unadjusted measurements are statistically related to pelvic tilt, whereas when the anteversion is adjusted for the tilt the values are the same, no matter the tilt.

Impingement

Twenty-two of 68 hips (32%) had impingement. Women were found to have statistically more impingement with 19 of 41 compared to 3 of 24 men having impingement (p=0.002). Women had an increased incidence of impingement because they have smaller bones and require a smaller femoral head which resulted in a worse head-neck ratio.

A second statistical variable for impingement was acetabular inclination. Hips with impingement had a mean inclination of 39.5 +/– 3.9 degrees and those without had a

mean of 42.3 +/– 5.1 degrees (p=0.03). The third statistical variable was medialization of the cup with impingement having a mean 3.2 +/– 3.5 mm medialization versus 5.8 +/– 4.9 mm in those hips without (p=0.03). A fourth variable statistically related to impingement was combined anteversion of the hip. Hips with impingement had combined anteversion of 36.8 +/– 4.8 degrees (femoral anteversion of 9.1 +/– 4.1 degrees) whereas in hips without impingement it was 33.9 +/– 4.1 degrees (femoral anteversion 6.6 +/– 4.3 degrees) (p=0.03). This increased combined anteversion with impingement was in women who had greater femoral anteversion, but smaller head/neck ratios.

On analyzing statistically cup coverage and impingement we found no relation between supero-lateral uncoverage and impingement, nor between the lower edge to transverse tear drop line distance and impingement.

Discussion

An important goal of this study was to verify that imageless computer navigation provided accurate information »in vivo« during surgery [17]. This is vital if orthopedic surgeons are going to be able to trust this technology as a sophisticated and better instrumentation. The reproducibility of acetabular component placement accuracy was validated by postoperative CT scans to be 0.53 degrees for inclination and 1.6 degrees for anteversion.

Precision measurements showed that radiographs are not as accurate as the computer. The lack of complete agreement between radiographs and computer values have been previously confirmed by others [9, 12, 13]. The im-

□ Table 59.5. Influence of anterior-posterior pelvic tilt on inclination and anteversion

Computer measurement	Posterior tilt 10–20 degrees	Posterior tilt 1–9 degrees	Anterior tilt 0–9 degrees	Anterior tilt 10–20 degrees	P value
Computer inclination*	40.4 + 4.4	38.7 + 3.5	42.0 + 4.5	49.2 + 4.2	0.001
Computer adjusted inclination	41.7 + 4.5	41.7 + 3.6	40.6 + 4.0	43.1 + 4.0	0.38
Computer anteversion*	24.2 + 3.7	17.3 + 5.9	29.5 + 3.4	36.7 + 3.9	0.001
Computed adjusted anteversion	27.3 + 3.2	26.8 + 3.4	27.2 + 2.2	27.2 + 2.0	0.93

Numbers in degrees for inclination and anteversion. The anteroposterior tilt of the pelvis is divided into four categories according to the number of degrees of tilt. The effect of adjustment by pelvic tilt is shown by the difference in unadjusted computer inclination and anteversion values compared to the similarity of adjusted inclination and adjusted anteversion values.
*The number of degrees of anterior-posterior pelvic tilt is statistically related to these measurements.

precision of 7 to 8 degrees is consistent with the difference of radiographic and navigation measurements which has been reported to occur because of variable flexion of the pelvis on the X-ray table, the rotation of radiographs, and variations from the direction of the X-ray beams [9, 12].

One of the critical factors for achieving accuracy was the knowledge of pelvic tilt. The computer corrects for tilt and the software then considers the position of the acetabulum relative to the pelvis during cup implantation [10]. The data in □ Table 59.5 clearly show the importance of knowledge of the pelvic tilt. This knowledge is a defining difference from conventional mechanical hip guide systems which do not reference the patient's pelvic position, but work off the patient's body axis for cup placement. With mechanical guides the true alignment of the pelvis (tilt), and the changes that occur to the pelvis during surgery, are not taken into consideration and therefore outliers of component position are frequent.

In this study we learned that femoral component anteversion is not the 10 to 15 degrees that laboratory studies have used [2, 5]. With non-cemented components the mean femoral anteversion was 7 degrees and was greater by 4 degrees in women than men, which confirmed the cadaver study of Maruyama et al. [21]. Furthermore, the anteversion of the non-cemented femoral component was fixed and therefore not a variable that the surgeon could control. This fact makes it important to customize the cup for each patient which requires a paradigm shift in the performance of the total hip replacement operation. To customize the cup, rather than use target numbers, requires femoral preparation prior to acetabular preparation. This paradigm shift permits acetabular anteversion

to be controlled to provide a combined anteversion of 35 +/- 5 degrees. Customizing the implant position for the patient's anatomy can only be done using navigation systems with this paradigm shift of preparation.

We also learned that the computer navigator was a useful tool in reducing impingement. We could achieve inclination between 40 and 45 degrees with coverage of the cup by knowledge of the medialization and superior displacement of the center of rotation. If the anatomic bony inclination was 55 to 65 degrees, the cup must be medialized more by reaming to achieve a covered cup with 40 degrees inclination than if the bony inclination was 45 to 50 degrees. The computer measurements provide the data for knowledge of the anatomic bony acetabulum, the number of mm of reamed depth and the cup inclination and anteversion. Bony coverage can be observed by the surgeon. This technique prevents lateralization of the cup which is the primary cause of impingement of the metal neck on the metal shell. We learned the technique of medialization to prevent lateralization of the cup and yet have inclination of 40 degrees during the course of this study. Therefore, we had one-third of cups which were excessively uncovered superior-lateral in these hips. Navigation is a great source of data for evaluating component positioning and correlating this with impingement. This knowledge should lead to better results for hip replacement in the short and long term [9, 13, 22, 23]. We hypothesize that even in the short term the patient should benefit from correct component position which avoids impingement.

Computer navigation provides accurate knowledge during reaming to maintain the center of rotation. With the advent of minimally invasive surgery [15, 16, 22], computer navigation can reduce errors in cup placement and help restore the center of rotation despite the decreased vision associated with the smaller incision. The computer software allows the surgeon to visualize the change in the center of rotation in all directions as well as the adjusted for tilt positions of cup inclination and anteversion. It has not always been common knowledge that the center of rotation of the cup is related to the longevity of a THR [23]. With computer navigation the change in center of rotation is known, even if it is necessary to superiorly displace the center of rotation for adequate cup fixation. Because of deformity of the acetabulum it is not always possible to ideally restore the center of rotation. In these patients, the mean superior displacement of the center of rotation was 1.56 +/− 3.3 mm and medialization was -5.19 +/− 5.4 mm which is well within accepted limits of reconstruction of the center of rotation [23].

Over 25 years have passed since Lewennik et al. [24] described the safe zone for acetabular component positioning as 30 to 50 degrees for inclination and 5 to 25 degrees for anteversion. Until recently, the ability to reproducibly position a cup to any target numbers had depended greatly on a surgeon's experience and intuition. However, even the accuracy of experienced surgeons varies at different surgeries, and it is impossible to say that at every surgery the desired cup position can be obtained [9, 13, 25, 26]. Furthermore, with these computer studies we found the safe zone for inclination to be only 40 +/- 5 degrees and for anteversion to be 20 to 30 degrees. The computer is needed to reproducibly obtain these positions. The intra-operative knowledge provided by the computer is helpful for an experienced surgeon [25], but it is even more important for the less experienced or low volume surgeon in their efforts to achieve consistent results. The classic tutored learning procedure for a surgeon through trial and error may be modified with this new system.

Objections to navigation systems are that they are expensive, generate additional radiation exposure in image based systems, are time consuming and require special intra-operative planning procedures [26]. However, when considering these inconveniences, the cost generated by revisions associated with dislocation, early component wear due to mal-position and impingement, decreased range of motion, and long term wear are very important factors which may be reduced by use of the computer. The time added to surgery with navigation should be weighed against the knowledge of correct component position

and biomechanical reconstruction, which replaces several minutes of decision making when the surgeon is using conventional methods [17].

This clinical study of the efficacy, accuracy, and precision of computer navigation for total hip replacement provides valuable knowledge to the utility of this technology. The imageless program eliminates the need for pre-operative CT scans, intra-operative fluoroscopy and is accurate within 0.5 to 1.5 degrees for cup position. The center of rotation can be controlled during cup preparation, and when combined with known inclination and anteversion, impingement can be reduced. The best use of the computer requires a paradigm shift in performance of THR because femoral preparation must precede acetabular preparation as only the acetabular cup position can be varied. This technologically sophisticated instrumentation will accelerate the technical performance of inexperienced and low volume surgeons by providing the same intra-operative information that experienced surgeons had learned by trial and error through time.

References

1. Charnley J, Cupic Z (1973) The 9 and 10 year results of the low-friction arthroplasty of the hip. Clin Orthop 95: 9–25
2. Barrack RL, Lavernia C, Ries M, Thornberry R, Tozakoglou E (2001) Virtual reality computer animation of the effect of component position and design on stability after total hip arthroplasty. Orthop Clin North Am 32: 569–577
3. Scifert CF, Brown TD, Pedersen DR, Callaghan JJ (1998) A finite element analysis of factors influencing total hip dislocation. Clin Orthop 355: 152–162
4. Shon, WY, Baldini T, Peterson MG, Wright TM, Salvati EA (2005) Impingement in total hip arthroplasty: A study of retrieved acetabular components. J Arthroplasty 20: 426–435
5. D'Lima DD, Urquhart AC, Buehler KO, Walker RH, Cowell CW (2000) The effect of the orientation of the acetabular and femoral components on the range of motion of the hip at different head-neck ratios. J Bone Joint Surg 82-A: 315–321
6. Yamaguchi M, Akisue T, Bauer TW, Hashimoto Y (2000) The spatial location of impingement in total hip arthroplasty. J Arthroplasty 15: 305–312
7. Barrack RL, Butler RA, Laster DR, Andrew P (2001) Stem design and dislocation after revision total hip arthroplasty: Clinical results and computer modeling. J Arthroplasty 16 (Suppl 1): 8–12
8. Patil S, Bergula A, Chen PC, Cowell CC, D'Lima DD (2003) Polyethylene wear and acetabular component orientation. J Bone Joint Surg 85-A (Suppl 4): 56–63
9. DiGioia AM, Jaramaz B, Blackwell M et al. (1998) The Otto AuFranc Award. Image guided navigation system to measure intraoperatively acetabular implant alignment. Clin Orthop 355: 8–22

10. DiGioia AM 3rd, Jaramaz B, Plakseychuk AY, Moody Je Jr, Nikou C, Labarca RS, Levison TJ, Picard F (2002) Comparison of a mechanical acetabular alignment guide with component placement of the socket. J Arthroplasty 17: 359–364
11. DiGioia AM, Plakseychuk AY, Levison TJ, Jaramz B (2003) Mini-incision technique for total hip arthroplasty with navigation. J Arthroplasty 18: 123–128
12. Jaramaz B, DiGioia AM, Blackwell M, Nikou C (1998) Computer assisted measurement of cup placement in total hip replacement. Clin Orthop 354: 70–81
13. Amiot LP, Poulin F (2004) Computed tomography-based navigation for hip, knee, and spine surgery. Clin Orthop 421: 77–86
14. Murray DW (1993) The definition and measurement of acetabular orientation: J Bone Joint Surg 75-B: 228–232
15. Dorr L (2006) Hip arthroplasty minimally invasive techniques and computer navigation. Saunders Elsevier, pp 16–28, 167–177
16. Berry DJ, Berger RA, Callaghan JJ, Dorr LD, Duwelius RJ, Hartzband MA, Lieberman JR, Mears DC (2003) Minimally invasive total hip arthroplasty. Development, early results and a critical analysis. J Bone Joint Surg 85-A(11): 2235–2246
17. Dorr LD, Hishiki Y, Wan Z, Newton D, Yun A (2005) Development of imageless computer navigation for acetabular component position in total hip replacement. Iowa Orthop Journal 25: 1–9
18. Callaghan JJ, Salvati EA, Pellicci PM, Wilson PD Jr, Ranawat CS (1985) Results of revision for mechanical failure after cemented total hip replacement 1979 to 1982. A two to five-year followup. J Bone Joint Surg 67-A: 1074–1085
19. Wan Z, Dorr LDD (1996) Natural history of femoral focal osteolysis with proximal ingrowth smooth stem implant. J Arthroplasty 11: 718–725
20. Ackland MK, Bourne WB, Uhthoff HK (1986) Anteversion of the acetabular cup. J Bone Joint Surg 68-B: 409–413
21. Maruyama M, Feinberg JR, Capello WN, D'Antonio JA (2001) Morphologic features of the acetabulum and femur: anteversion angle and implant positioning. Clin Orthop 393: 52–65
22. Inaba Y, Dorr L, Wan Z, Sirianni L, Boutary M (2005) Operative and patient care techniques for posterior mini-incision total hip arthroplasty. Clin Orthop 441: 104–114
23. Karachalios T, Hartofilakidis A, Zacharakis N, Tsekoura M (1993) A 12–18 year radiographic followup study of Charnley low friction arthroplasty. The role of the center of rotation. Clin Orthop 296: 140–147
24. Lewinnek GE, Lewis JL, Tarr R, Compere CL, Zimmerman JR (1978) Dislocations after total hip-replacement arthroplasties. J Bone Joint Surg 60A: 217–220
25. Leenders T, Vandevelde D, Mahieu G, Nuyts R (2002) Reduction in variability of acetabular cup abduction using computer assisted surgery: A prospective randomized study. Comp Aided Surg 7: 99–106
26. Jolles BM, Genoud P, Hoffmeyer P (2004) Computer-assisted cup placement techniques in total hip arthroplasty improves accuracy in placement. Clin Orth 426: 174–179

Navigating The Two-Incision Total Hip Arthroplasty

M.A. Hartzband, G.R. Klein

Introduction

Minimally-invasive techniques have gained popularity over the past few years and are changing the practice of orthopedic surgery today. The objectives of minimally-invasive total hip replacement are to minimize surgical dissection and, as a result, potentially decrease postoperative pain, shorten hospital stay, and accelerate recovery [1–4]. However, it is critical that the present long term success, reliability and safety of total hip arthroplasty is maintained. The two-incision total hip arthroplasty [5, 6] which takes advantage of a tissue-sparing approach offers the potential for a marked decrease in morbidity with a dramatically more rapid recovery.

Computer-assisted surgery offers the potential of more accurate component orientation without complete visualization of the bony landmarks [7]. Thus, navigation is a natural complement to accurately performing a truly minimally-invasive surgical procedure. Navigation has been shown to increase the accuracy of component positioning, while decreasing variability of component placement [8, 9]. This technology provides real time measurements of acetabular position such as cup abduction angle and anteversion, which should result in a significant reduction in technical errors and complications related to mal-positioning of the components [10]. Navigation also allows the surgeon to accurately measure leg-lengths and hip offset intra-operatively. It is important to remember that leg-length discrepancy and patient dissatisfaction represent one of the most common reasons for litigation against the orthopedic community [11], and hopefully with naviga-

tion, this risk can be minimized or eliminated. In addition, navigation may be used as a teaching tool in the early stages of surgeon education so as to limit the admittedly steep learning curve of complex minimally-invasive surgical procedures such as two-incision total hip arthroplasty. Image-guided surgery utilizes high-speed computers coupled with advanced tracking devices to enable more accurate and precise surgery [12]. Navigation technology can be loosely classified as image-guided or imageless technology. Image guided navigation includes CT based, fluoroscopic based, and ultrasonic based technology in which there has been some early work. Although CT-guided imaging is accurate and reliable, it is expensive and requires significant patient registration and preoperative planning. Currently it is less popular for joint arthroplasty applications at this time than either fluoroscopically-based or imageless systems. Fluoroscopy is available in any operating room and the vast majority of orthopedic surgeons are familiar with the use of image intensification. In addition, fluoroscopic systems allow intra-operative planning and are relatively inexpensive with the exception of technician time. Fluoroscopy based systems provide the surgeon with a real-time instrument tracking in a multiplanar setting, and provides the surgeon with data in both the AP and lateral planes. Fluoroscopic based navigation is an ideal match for two-incision incision hip arthroplasty because the two-incision total hip arthroplasty is a procedure that currently requires five to 30 seconds of fluoroscopy, depending on the individual surgeon's preference and experience. By utilizing the fluoroscopy-based navigation system, the need for live intra-operative fluoroscopy is eliminated. With only three static fluoroscopic images, the surgeon can plan, visualize intra-operatively and gain valuable real-time information specific to each patient. The navigation system can aid the surgeon in identifying critical points such as proper incision location, neck osteotomy location and angle, cup abduction and anteversion, femoral component version and seating, as well as leg length and offset measurements. By using these simple few static images taken pre-operatively, x-ray exposure to the surgeon, operating room staff, and patient is minimized.

Technique

This technique uses a Medtronic image guidance system (Memphis, TN) which is a combination of specialized surgical hardware and image-guidance software that enables a surgeon to track the position of a surgical instrument in the operating room and continuously update this position within one or more still-frame fluoroscopic images acquired pre-operatively from a C-arm.

There are three basic phases of navigated two-incision total hip arthroplasty 1) »off-the-clock« navigation, 2) »on-the-clock« acetabular navigation, and 3) »on-the-clock« femoral navigation. The first is the so-called »off-the-clock« navigated portion. As with any navigated procedure it is necessary to integrate the surgical world and computer world. »Off-the-clock« begins with acquiring the empty image which involves placing a calibration grid on the fluoroscopy unit and allowing the computer to communicate with the grid. Following this the surgeon follows the computer prompts to select the operative side and enter relevant data. The final phase of »off-the-clock« navigation is instrument verification. This is a portion of the procedure that requires no additional surgical time as it is performed by a scrub technician while the »on-the-clock« navigation portion of the procedure begins. Instrument verification involves orienting the computer, via passive arrays, to the orientation and position of each instrument.

The »on-the-clock« acetabular navigation includes the actual surgical process. There are eight separate phases to »on-the-clock« acetabular navigation: (1) frame placement, (2) image acquisition, (3) establishment of pelvic and femoral checkpoints, (4) establishment of pelvic and femoral landmarks, (5) locate anterior incision, (6) navigate neck osteotomy, (7) ream acetabulum, and (8) navigate acetabular component insertion.

The patient is placed in a supine position on the operating table; a bolster which can be inflated or deflated during the procedure is placed under the ipsilateral hemipelvis. The acetabular exposure is performed with the bolster inflated so as to elevate the operative side of the patient's pelvis 20 degrees with respect to the non-operative side. This facilitates acetabular exposure and reaming. The pillow will be taken down at the conclusion of this phase of the procedure and prior to definitive cup insertion.

Once the patient has been prepped and draped with the pillow deflated, the reference frames are placed. The reference frame is of a set of optical markers mounted on a metal frame that can be rigidly attached with respect to the patient anatomy.

While the surgeon is placing the reference frames, the surgical technician can register and calibrate all instruments with the navigation system. A stab wound is made at the crest of the ilium approximately two to three finger-breadths posterior to the antero-superior iliac spine. A threaded pin is drilled far enough into the ilium in order to obtain good fixation, the fixator clamp is slid over this pin and the second pin location is drilled using the fixator frame as a drill guide. The screws of the fixation clamp are tightened gently and the reference frame is set to a desirable position in the line of site of the camera. It is important to place the construct in a position that will always be seen by the camera. Once visibility has been assured, the fixation device and reference frame are definitively tightened.

The femoral reference frame is using a similar technique at the antero-lateral aspect of the junction of middle and distal thirds of the femur. The knee should be flexed during this portion of the procedure to avoid tethering the quadriceps mechanism and the pin should be drilled starting just anterior to the palpable longitudinal defect of the fascia lata and intermuscular septum Bicortical fixation is recommended to enhance stability. A passive array is affixed to the femoral pin cluster (◘ Fig. 60.1). The frame should be only provisionally tightened until appropriate line of site with the camera is confirmed in multiple anticipated leg positions. It is important to keep in mind that the femoral component most commonly used with a two-incision procedure is a fully-coated stem, 160 mm in length. This requires straight reaming of the proximal femoral canal, and it is critical to ensure that the femoral reference frame be located distal to the area of anticipated intra-medullary femoral reaming.

The next step is to acquire the necessary images. A minimum of three images is required to perform this

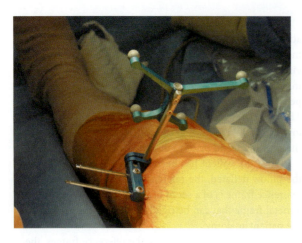

■ Fig. 60.1. Femoral reference frame placed in the antero-lateral aspect of the femur

procedure: (1) an antero-posterior (AP) image of the affected hip joint; this image will be used to navigate the anterior incision, the femoral osteotomy, the acetabular reamers, and the acetabular implant in the AP plain. (2) an AP image of proximal femur; this image will be used to navigate the femoral awl, the straight femoral reamers and femoral broaches in an AP plain. (3) a lateral image of the proximal femur; this view is used to navigate the femoral awl, straight reamers, femoral broaches, and the femoral stem from a lateral view.

Although only a minimum of three images is required to perform the procedure, additional images are recommended to obtain different views of the patient's anatomy and theoretically improve the accuracy of the navigation. Additional images may include: (1) a pelvic inlet and outlet image which would be necessary only if the physical landmark of the pubic symphysis is inaccessible to the pointer probe. For example a distorted pelvis or an obese patient. The pelvic inlet and outlet views allow the surgeon to landmark, via cross correlation, in which points are chosen on two image plains displayed on a computer screen rather than on the patient himself. (2) Oblique-affected cup. This image provides an additional view of the acetabulum to further increase the procedure's accuracy.

After acquisition of images and labeling of the images on the computer screen, the next phase is to identify landmarks on the patient. Traditional arthroplasty instruments such as cup holders and reamers orient the cup with respect to an overall impression of body position and

do not take into account subtle changes in pelvic orientation. With navigation, however, the patient's pelvis can be accurately tracked in real-time in a three-dimensional space. Therefore, accurate pelvic position is independent of how that patient is positioned and how the surgical field is affected by retractors or leg manipulation. In order to track the pelvis in a three-dimensional space, three specific landmarks (the ipsilateral anterosuperior iliac spine (ASIS), contra-lateral ASIS, and pubis symphysis) must be captured on the pelvis. Femoral tracking uses two landmarks on the femur and two on the tibia. This landmarking is done by one of two methods. Landmarks may be either directly palpated with the computer assisted pointer probe or in some circumstances such as obese patients or patients with substantial deformity the landmarks are inaccessible to the pointer probe. In these instances, landmarks may be chosen by selecting the same point in two orthogonal images on a navigation screen; for example, a landmark in the center of the femoral shaft can be identified by choosing the center of the femoral shaft in both the AP and lateral images. The three pelvic landmarks are typically directly palpated with the navigated pointer probe. These three landmarks create the anterior pelvic plane or the coronal plane of the pelvis. The line that connects the affected or non-affected AS iliac spines describes the medio-lateral (ML) axis of the pelvis. The line that passes through the pubic symphysis perpendicular to the ML axis describes the supero-inferior (SI) axis of the pelvis. The antero-posterior (AP) axis is perpendicular to both the ML and SI axes. The plane created by the SI and AP axes is the sagittal plane of the pelvis. The plane created by the ML and AP axes is the transverse plane of the pelvis. The cup anteversion and abduction values reported by the computer software are directly related to the orientation of the surgical instrument with respect to the planes created by these landmarks (■ Fig. 60.2).

Landmarks for femoral navigation include: (1) proximal and distal ends of the intra-medullary canal of the femur, and (2) proximal and distal end of the tibial midline. These landmarks help define the anatomic axis of the proximal femur along which the femoral implant will align. The AP and ML axes of the femur will determine the basis for femoral rotation (version). One cannot overly stress the importance of accurate landmarking. If landmarks are incorrect, all data generated by the computer, particularly acetabular version, will be subject to error.

Once landmarking is complete, the surgeon may begin the formal surgical procedure [2]. Localizing the anterior incision can be a difficult step during the learning curve of this procedure. The anterior incision is oriented parallel to the long axis of the femoral neck. By using a navigated pointer probe on the skin at the anticipated incision site, the surgeon can see, in real-time, this pointer superimposed on a static fluoroscopic image (AP of the hip joint) on the computer screen (□ Fig. 60.3). This procedure helps locate the ideal location for the anterior incision. Without navigation, this portion of the operation can consume significant time and radiation exposure.

Prior to making the incision, the previously-placed bolster is inflated in order to elevate the operative hemipelvis 20 degrees with respect to the contra-lateral pelvis. This effectively lateralizes the incision and helps to avoid injury to the lateral femoral cutaneous nerve (LFCN). Dissection is carried down through the subcutaneous tissue and the tensor fascia lata and sartorius muscles are identified. A longitudinal incision is made in the fascia of the tensor fascia lata (TFL) approximately one centimeter lateral to the true Smith-Peterson interval. Locating the fascial incision in the fascia of the TFL further protects the LFCN from injury. Digital dissection will easily separate the sartorius from the tensor fascia lata to expose peri-capsular fat and the direct head of the rectus femoris. A Cobb elevator is utilized to elevate the rectus femoris off the hip capsule and the peri-capsular fat is similarly elevated to expose the hip capsule. The anterior femoral circumflex vessels are usually found at the inferior pole of the incision. These vessels are often of significant size and must be isolated and electrocoagulated prior to proceeding. A longitudinal capsular incision is then made extending from the acetabular rim to the base of the femoral neck. With experience, there is no need to extend this incision in a T or H fashion, and specially designed self-illuminated retractors are then placed intra-capsularly on the superior and inferior surface of the femoral neck.

After the femoral neck has been exposed, the software will prompt the surgeon to navigate the osteotomy guide. The osteotomy guide is placed through the anterior incision into a position on the anterior surface of the femoral neck. This guide is rendered on-screen and the osteotomy line is generated over the static fluoroscopic image of the femoral neck. Once the guide is positioned into the correct osteotomy angle at the appropriate preoperatively templated level, the bone is marked and the osteotomy is made with a fine oscillating saw blade. A vertical osteotomy is made just at the articular margin of the lateral border of the femoral head. A second vertical osteotomy

θ_1 = Anteversion
θ_2 = Abduction

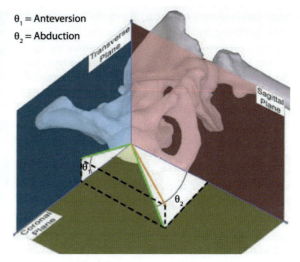

□ **Fig. 60.2.**Schematic of the transverse, sagittal and coronal reference planes the navigation system uses to aid in pelvic preparation and component placement

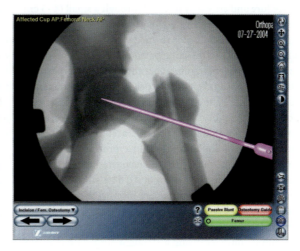

□ **Fig. 60.3.** Navigation-assisted anterior incisions placement

is made lateral to this point just at the medial border of the greater trochanter, and this intercalary segment of lateral femoral neck is removed with a Kocher clamp or rongeur. With slight traction and external rotation placed on the limb, the femoral neck and head fragment can be easily elevated anteriorly and exposed. A special cork screw with rotational tines, which is part of the two-incision set, is then malleted into the cut cancellous surface of the femoral head and neck fragment up into the femoral neck thereby obtaining purchase. The cork screw is tightened and then the assembly is twisted so as to rupture the ligamentum. The head and neck are then delivered from the wound. The osteotomy guide should now be reinserted along the cut surface of the femoral neck to verify the angle and height of femoral neck cut. The information is archived by the computer and will assist the surgeon in avoiding over-impaction of the femoral component during stem placement. The acetabular labrum is excised and the fovea is débrided. A retractor is placed antero-inferiorly just anterior to the transverse acetabular ligament. A second retractor is placed at 180 degrees to this on the postero-superior acetabular wall. A third retractor is placed anteriorly between these two. Care must be taken, particularly with this third retractor's placement, to avoid injury to the femoral nerve or vessels. Placement of this retractor should be performed only by the operating surgeon and cavalier extra-capsular placement should be avoided. The reamers are then inserted. Hemisphere plus, side-cut acetabular reamers are typically used with this procedure and are easily inserted through a small (4–5 cm anterior) incision regardless of templated acetabular diameter. The acetabulum is reamed starting with a reamer 2 mm smaller than the anticipated acetabular component size. It is important to remember that the pelvis is elevated 20 degrees on a bolster. This pelvic tilt is automatically accounted for by the computer, thereby simplifying this portion of the procedure as compared to the use of standard mechanical guides. Once the acetabulum has been reamed to the desired position and appropriate host-bone contact has been generated, the navigated cup inserter is used to insert the cup (■ Fig. 60.4). The surgeon selects, on-screen, the size of the cup and inserts the cup with the navigated inserter in view of the camera. Once desired parameters for abduction and version have been obtained, the cup is impacted using a standard surgical technique. The acetabular liner is then introduced and locked into position.

Femoral component insertion is also aided by the use of navigation. Navigating the femur allows an accurate real-time location of the posterior incision. The limb is adducted approximately 25–30 degrees and the tibia held roughly vertical by a first assistant on the non-operative side of the table. The navigated pointer probe is placed at the anticipated incision site and a real-time representation of the probe in relation to actual femoral anatomy is displayed on-screen. A starting point for the femoral incision

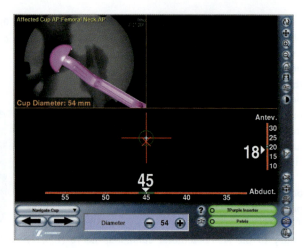

■ **Fig. 60.4.** Navigated cup insertion

is created by identifying a coaxial point of the probe on the patient's proximal femoral anatomy. Once the desired incision location has been identified, the skin is marked and the incision is made. Fat and subcutaneous tissues are divided with electrocautery. The risk of an inappropriate starting point and resultant abductor damage can be significantly diminished.

Once the posterior incision has been made, a tapered awl with a passive array attached is inserted into the femoral canal. The corresponding image on the navigation screen displays a virtual extension of the awl on both the AP and lateral femoral images (■ Fig. 60.5). This allows the insertion of the awl at an appropriate angle, position and depth.

A side cutting reamer with a passive array attached is then inserted in 2 mm increments and the femoral neck is laterally reamed with confirmation of position by the reamer. A straight reamer approximately 2 mm smaller than that pre-operatively templated can be inserted in the femoral canal through the posterior incision, and the surgeon can follow the path of this reamer in real time on the computer screen to ensure that it is being inserted at the appropriate angle and depth. In a similar fashion, progressive femoral rasps attached to passive arrays are inserted. The software allows for optimal placement of the stem by quantifying the degree of version of the implant. The navigated stem inserter is utilized to seat the stem. The computer will provide information to confirm ap-

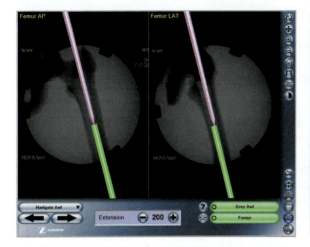

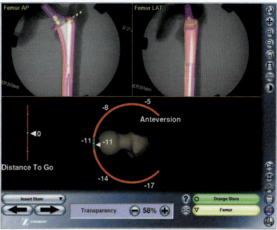

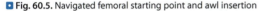

Fig. 60.5. Navigated femoral starting point and awl insertion

Fig. 60.6. Navigated femoral stem insertion

propriate seating and version of the specific implant with relation to the specific patient's anatomy (◘ Fig. 60.6). The previously-archived osteotomy line is utilized to avoid stem over-impaction or under-impaction. Optimal implant positioning may reduce the likelihood of dislocation [13] and impingement [14] and may result in an increase in the life of the arthroplasty.

In the navigated two-incision hip procedure, verification of leg length and offset is performed during the trial reduction phase of the surgery. After the trial head is inserted, the limb is reduced and placed in the same position that preoperative leg-length measurement was recorded. The ability of the system to locate both referenced frames is confirmed, and the navigation screen provides data (◘ Fig. 60.7) to allow the surgeon to make necessary adjustments in terms of neck lengths (and potentially acetabular polyethylene offsets) to minimize any discrepancy in postoperative leg length or offset. Both wounds are then irrigated copiously.

The actual femoral head is impacted with an offset head impactor and the hip is reduced. The capsule is easily repaired with this approach with 1–3 interrupted #1 Vicryl sutures, and the wound is closed over a small drain anteriorly that is removed approximately six hours postoperatively, prior to patient discharge from the hospital. The patients are typically ambulated within three hours of the procedure and are almost invariably discharged home within 24 hours of the procedure.

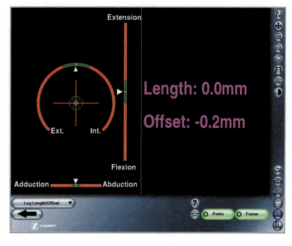

Fig. 60.7. Navigated leg-length and offset parameters

Results

A review of our initial 15 cases of fluoroscopically-navigated, two-incision total hip arthroplasties revealed a total fluoroscopy time of 21 seconds (high 30 seconds and a low 17 seconds). Between 4 and 7 seconds of this 21-second average was used to recheck and confirm component position at the conclusion of the procedure.

This additional time has not been required with further experience and confidence. An average of 20.5 minutes was added to the total surgical time. Of the 20.5 min, 5 min represented time for insertion of the pelvic reference frame (range 3–8 min), 4.7 min represented time for insertion of the femoral reference frame (range 2.5 to 6 min). The acquisition of images averaged 7 min with a range of 5–8 min, and landmarking of the patient averaged 3.8 min with a range of 3–4 min, initial incision to close averaged 67.3 min with a range of 54–78 min. Of this initial group, there have been no dislocations, no leg-length discrepancy of more than 2 mm, no component subsidence, infection, or revision for any reason.

Conclusion

There are many advantages of computer assisted navigation of the two-incision hip arthroplasty. Navigation facilitates both the acetabular and femoral incision placement without use of additional fluoroscopy and enhanced visibility of the osteotomy positions to avoid over-impaction during stem placement. Acetabular and femoral position may be improved and component placement may be more reproducible. Leg length and offset are also displayed in real time thereby allowing the surgeon to maximize the quality and accuracy of the arthroplasty. In addition, patient data and component type and position are archived.

Similar to any new technology or procedure concerns do exist. Bicortical fixation of the tracking pins is required, which takes additional time, although the time burden becomes minimal with experience. The risk of fracture remains a real concern, although none have occurred during the senior author's experience with fluoroscopic-based navigation and there are no reports of fracture related to navigation pins in the literature.

One of the greatest concerns of navigation is the consequences of inaccurate landmarking. The commonly-used expression »garbage in = garbage out« is particularly appropriate to this technology in that inaccurate landmarking will lead to inaccurate navigation data and inaccurate component position. Bone-tracking errors are also a significant concern in any navigation system requiring the placement of fixation pins. Loosening or movement of these pins or trackers relative to the bone can create navigation inaccuracies. These inaccuracies may be unknown to the surgeon, potentially resulting in an error.

The use of »checkpoints« can be used to identify these errors, but require slight additional time during the setup of the procedure.

An additional concern is that of over reliance of computer-generated data by the less-experienced surgeon. It is important that the surgeon understand software applications and the basis of computer-generated calculations so as to landmark as accurately as possible and appropriately evaluate data generated by the computer. Longer operative times are not only a potential risk to the patient in terms of infection and blood loss, but will significantly impact surgeon acceptance of this technology if times become too prolonged. Navigation should be used to aid to the surgeon and should only be used as another instrument or tool in the surgeon's armamentarium. This technology should not replace the surgeon's experience, training and intuition.

In conclusion, minimally-invasive techniques and computer-assisted surgical techniques are an obvious combination. Minimally-invasive techniques are difficult to teach and difficult to learn. They are often more tactile and differing surgeons have varying abilities to adapt to these techniques. Computer-assisted surgery is time-consuming and may be of limited value when applied to conventional surgical procedures. If computer-assisted techniques can be successfully applied to minimally-invasive surgical techniques, surgeons will be able to learn these techniques more easily and avoid technical errors.

References

1. Berger RA (2004) Mini-incision total hip replacement using an anterolateral approach: technique and results. Orthop Clin North Am 35: 143–151
2. Berger RA (2004) The technique of minimally invasive total hip arthroplasty using the two-incision approach. Instr Course Lect 53: 149–155
3. Sculco TP (2004) Minimally invasive total hip arthroplasty: in the affirmative. J Arthroplasty 19: 78–80
4. Sculco TP, Jordan LC, Walter WL (2004) Minimally invasive total hip arthroplasty: the Hospital for Special Surgery experience. Orthop Clin North Am 35: 137–142
5. Berger RA, Duwelius PJ (2004) The two-incision minimally invasive total hip arthroplasty: technique and results. Orthop Clin North Am 35: 163–172
6. Berry DJ, Berger RA, Callaghan JJ, Dorr LD, Duwelius PJ, Hartzband MA, Lieberman JR, Mears DC (2003) Minimally invasive total hip arthroplasty. Development, early results, and a critical analysis. Presented at the Annual Meeting of the American Orthopaedic

Association, Charleston, South Carolina, USA, June 14, 2003. J Bone Joint Surg Am 85-A: 2235–2246

7. DiGioia AM, Jaramaz B, Blackwell M et al. (1998) The Otto Aufranc Award. Image guided navigation system to measure intraoperatively acetabular implant alignment. Clin Orthop Relat Res:8–22

8. Wixson RL, MacDonald MA (2005) Total hip arthroplasty through a minimal posterior approach using imageless computer-assisted hip navigation. J Arthroplasty 20: 51–56

9. Nogler M, Kessler O, Prassl A, Donnelly B, Streicher R, Sledge JB, Krismer M (2004) Reduced variability of acetabular cup positioning with use of an imageless navigation system. Clin Orthop Relat Res:159–163

10. Kennedy JG, Rogers WB, Soffe KE, Sullivan RJ, Griffen DG, Sheehan LJ (1998) Effect of acetabular component orientation on recurrent dislocation, pelvic osteolysis, polyethylene wear, and component migration. J Arthroplasty 13: 530–534

11. Murray DW (1993) The definition and measurement of acetabular orientation. J Bone Joint Surg Br 75: 228–232

12. Leenders T, Vandevelde D, Mahieu G, Nuyts R (2002) Reduction in variability of acetabular cup abduction using computer assisted surgery: a prospective and randomized study. Comput Aided Surg 7: 99–106

13. Lewinnek GE, Lewis JL, Tarr R, Compere CL, Zimmerman JR (1978) Dislocations after total hip-replacement arthroplasties. J Bone Joint Surg Am 60: 217–220

14. Yamaguchi M, Akisue T, Bauer TW, Hashimoto Y (2000) The spatial location of impingement in total hip arthroplasty. J Arthroplasty 15: 305–313

Part V　Reconstruction and Trauma Surgery

High Tibial Osteotomy with a Kinematic Navigation System

M. Prymka, J. Hassenpflug

Introduction

In the last years, joint saving operations were thrusted into the background, compared to joint arthroplasty. High tibial osteotomies too are more and more displaced by unicondylar knee prostheses.

This seems to be unjustified, when looking to two long term studies of our hospital about each 200 patients after high tibial osteotomy. In 96% and 75%, an implantation of a knee endoprosthesis could be avoided until 10 years postoperative. The complication rate all in all was low, but wrong sawing directions, incomplete osteotomies, and over- or undercorrections could be detected.

With the help of the navigation-system OrthoPilot (Aesculap, Tuttlingen) we developed further the traditional operative technique. With this technical support we hope to improve the intra-operative realization of the preoperative planning, and to standardize the quality of the operation.

When using a navigation system, the data from the conventionally done preoperative planning were put into the computer. Intra-operative reference markers (so-called rigid bodies) were fixed to the tibia and femur with a screw. These rigid body are located optoelectronically as well as further reference points at the bone. By this way, the Navigation system is able to detect the exact position of the leg. The technology could be used for closing wedge and opening wedge operations.

In the closing wedge procedure, after preparation of the bone a cutting jig and the saw itself could be positioned exactly with the help of the navigation. In this way the first, horizontal osteotomy and the second osteotomy could be performed. During the sawing procedure the surgeon is informed about the sawing angle and the distance between tip of the saw and the medial cortical bone on the monitor. In the opening wedge procedure the leg axis changes are detected simultaneously. Therfore the opening procedure can be performed until the planned correction angle is reached with the help of the navigation system.

We have now use this system for 3 years and have positive experiences. Post-operative X-rays showed, that we always got the exact correction angle compared to the pre-operative planning. We could not detect any complications caused by the navigation system.

Methods

In Patients suffering from gonarthrosis, which is limited to the medial aspect of the knee joint, high tibial valgisation osteotomy appears to be an appropriate alternative to knee-arthroplasty [7, 10]. In 1958, Jackson described this procedure for axis correction of the proximal tibia [9] for the first time. This operation was modified in 1965 by Coventry [3]. At first it was used mainly for correction of valgus deformities. According to the knee base-line in valgus deformity, distal femur osteotomy may be recommended [1, 8]. For a long time the indication for high tibial osteotomy was not subject to discussion [2]. Within the last years high tibial osteotomy was performed more seldom and seemed to be replaced by uni- or bicondulary knee-arthroplasty. Taking into account the biomechanical basics and the very positive long term results, which were achieved by the traditional osteotomy technique this change of treatment does not seem to be warranted.

The aims of a high tibial osteotomy are:
- correction of the joint deformity to release the loading of the medial joint compartment,
- pain-reduction and improvement of the joint-function,
- possibility of a biological joint healing with additional intra-articular procedures to enhance regeneration of the joint-surface.

With correction of the deformity weight-bearing of the affected medial part of the joint could be reduced significantly. Even partial regeneration of the cartilage is possible [4, 11]. With an additional intra-articular cartilage reconstruction, the biological joint-resurfacing could be significantly improved, so that perhaps one day we can speak of a »bio-prosthesis«, which could allow preservation of function and reduction of pain for a longer time. In total, high tibial valgisation osteotomy for varus gonarthrosis still is frequently performed at our hospital. Long time follow-up studies have demonstrated positive outcome. Follow-ups between 5 and 17 years of several authors presented an improvement of pain and joint function in more than ¾ of the operated patients [12, 13]. In our first long term study we reported on 177 patients [6], which were operated between 1974 and 1983. In the 10-year follow-up of 74% of the patients subjectively were very satisfied. During the follow-up period the presumption that the patients who needed knee arthroplasty was less than 5%. The complication rate was very low. In an unpublished study 226 high tibial osteotomies done between 1984 and 1993 were evaluated and there were similarly good clinical results as compared to the first study. Parallel with the first study, the complication-rate revealed only a few cases of the peroneus nerve palsy, but we saw more cases of disturbed healing of bone. In 8 cases this could be treated by plaster-cast, further 8 patients had to be treated with an external fixator. Also loosenings of the Coventry staples in 7 cases less than 4 weeks after the operation were found. In 3 patients we observed an overcorrection, which had to be revised. One fracture of the tibial plateau and one deep and six skin-near infections could be documented.

Surgical Technique and Results

The principle of the high tibial osteotomy seems to be easy, but for this operation precise planning and an exact intra-operative transformation of the planning is required. Therefore, this operation is not an operation for beginners although the technical procedure itself seems to be easy. The failure analysis leads to the assumption, that the results of high tibial osteotomies could be improved by means of a navigation-system, moreover the use of a navigation-system could decrease major and minor failures of the operation. In cooperation with Aesculap (Tuttlingen, Germany) we developed a software-program to perform high tibial osteotomies with the help of a navigation-system (»Ortho-Pilot«) computer-assisted. Now the software-package is commercially available. By means of this system the conventional pre-operative planning, using x-ray templates, could be transformed intra-operatively with precision and without intra-operative X-ray control. The positioning of the saw-jigs was also performed with the help of the navigation-system as was the size and position of the osteotomy wedge. The navigation-system is used for the orientation of the saw-jigs and to navigate the sawing-procedure itself. For the development of the system and the intra-operative transformation several pre-requisitions have to be fulfilled:
- *stable fixing of the saw-jig:* After the navigated positioning of the jig it must not be moved. The stability of the jigs could be improved with the help of specially designed self-cutting spongious screws.
- *rigidly stable saw-blade:* The saw-blade is not allowed to flex during the cutting procedure, because the calibration relatively to the rigid body at the corpus of the saw would not remain exact and therefore a control during the cutting-procedure would not be possible. This problem could be solved with the help of specially designed saw-blades. Therefore visual control of the cutting procedure is possible.
- *Intra-operative control of the leg axis:* It is necessary to mark the position of the upper leg. This is possible with the help of a 2nd reference marker at the distal femur and additional definition of the hip centre.

The navigation system is possible to differ between opening wedge- and closing wedge technique.

Closing Wedge Technique

Before the procedure, the planning data, which were achieved by X-ray, are loaded into the computer into the Orthopilot system. The correction angle is required as well as the exact width and depth of the tibial plateau. Therefore planning X-rays must be performed with a

61

reference scale. The operation starts in a classical style after exposure of the peroneal nerve with a shortening osteotomy of the fibula. Then the lateral tibial metaphysis is preparated for the osteotomy and the first reference marker (rigid body) is fixed 10 cm below the joint space

(◙ Fig. 61.1a). This marker has to be stably fixed such that it does not move during the whole operation. An additional marker is fixated at the distal femur. By moving of hip, knee and ankle-joint the joint centers and the leg-axis is determined exactly by the system (◙ Fig. 61.2). After

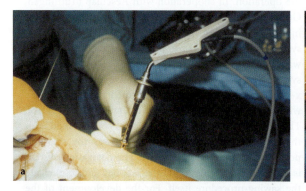 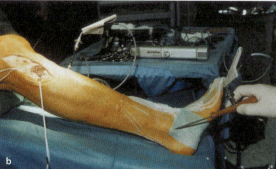

◙ **Fig. 61.1a,b.** Fixing of the rigid body in the tibiae (**a**), referencation, palpation of the lower leg, here of the lateral malleolus (**b**)

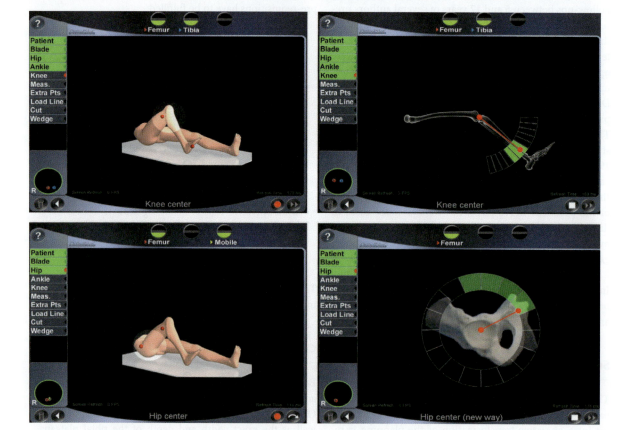

◙ **Fig. 61.2.** Monitor view when moving hip and knee joint (kinematic referencation)

that the geometry of the lower leg is calibrated with the system by palpating exact defined points at the lower leg (◘ Fig. 61.1b). For this palpation we use a special measurement tool with opto-electronical reference.

By means of the navigation-system the saw-jig for the first, horizontal osteotomy can be positioned exactly according to the preoperative planning (◘ Fig. 61.3). The surgeon can control this positioning on the system monitor with the help of two virtual horizons for the a.p. and sagittal view. Now the cutting procedure is performed. During the cutting procedure the positioning of the saw-blade and the distance between the tip of the saw-blade and the medial cortex of the tibia can be controlled on the monitor (◘ Fig. 61.4). The exact cutting angle of the saw blade is also documented on the monitor in real time. With a check-blade, where also reference markers are fixed, the osteotomy surface can be checked on the monitor. At this stage the pivoting point of the osteotomy is determined. After fixing of the 2nd saw-jig, which is pivoted with the help of the navigation system around the check blade (◘ Fig. 61.5) the 2nd osteotomy can be performed. Again the saw blade is leaded by the navigation system (◘ Fig. 61.6). The system gives visual feedback about the distance between the tip the saw blade and the pivoting point. After removal of the lateral based bone-wedge the osteosynthesis can be performed with Coventry staples (◘ Fig. 61.7) or a bone plate as an angle-stable device for higher primary stability. ◘ Figure 61.8 showes the pre- and post-operative X-rays of a 20-year old female athlete, who was operated because of a painful varus knee deformity.

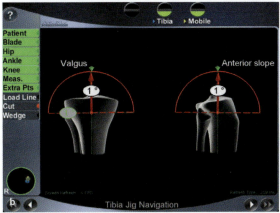

◘ **Fig. 61.3a,b.** Jig for the first osteotomy (**a**), picture of the monitor (**b**)

Opening Wedge Technique

Similar to the closing wedge technique the planning data of the patient have to be loaded to the navigation system. Similar to the procedure described above, rigid bodies are fixed fix at the distal femora and the proximal tibia. Then the leg axis can be measured. We now present a surgical technique, that is modified form the technique published by Galla and Lobenhoffer 2004 [5]. After measuring the leg axis, the operation can performed.

The 5–8 cm long skin incision runs from a point anterior to the insertion of the pes anserinus in a postero-cranial direction. The incision ends over the postero-medial corner of the medial tibial plateau. After division of the subcutaneous tissues and the fascia, the pes anserinus tendons are retracted posteriely with a hook.

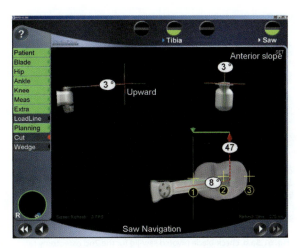

◘ **Fig. 61.4.** Monitor view of the first osteotomy (cutting procedure)

61

A Hohmann retractor is inserted behind the tibia. At the anterior edge of the incision the insertion of the patellar tendon into the tibial tuberosity and the medial border of the patellar tendon are exposed. The cranial end of the patellar tendon must be clearly visualized to allow a later determination of the endpoint of the anteriorly ascending osteotomy. The extended knee is now viewed in the exact AP plane showing the joint space. Under image intensification two K-wires are inserted into the tibial plateau and they mark the direction of the osteotomy. Care has to be taken that the thickness of the tibia plateau cranial to the planned osteotomy site leaves sufficient space for the placement of two locking screws for fixing the plate. The wires are aimed at the caudal third of the tibio-fibular joint. The wires end 0,7 cm inside the lateral tibial cortex.

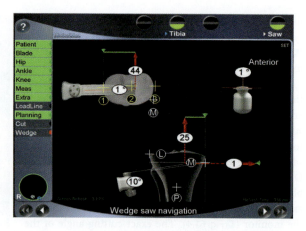

■ **Fig. 61.6.** cutting procedure of the second osteotomy (monitor view)

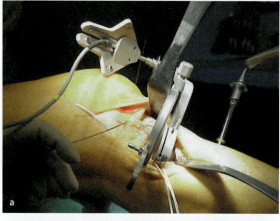

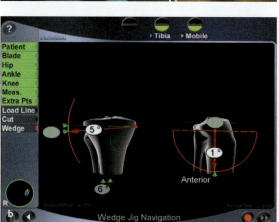

■ **Fig. 61.5a,b.** check-blade pivoted saw-jig for the 2nd osteotomy (a), monitor view (b)

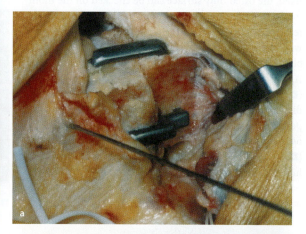

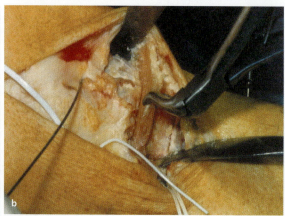

■ **Fig. 61.7a,b.** removal of the bone-wedge (a); closing ot the osteotomy, osteosynthesis with Coventry-clamps (b)

The first wire is placed posteriorly at the cranial border of the pes. The second wire is inserted 2 cm exactly anterior (with help of X-ray control) to the first wire. As both wires end at the ending point of the first osteotomy, the depth of the osteotomy can be measured by positioning a third wire in contact with the medial tibial cortex along the first wire and measuring against the overall length of the third wire and subtracting this from the length of the first two wires. The depth is marked on the saw blade. The anterior ascending osteotomy is marked with an electrocautery, leaving 15–20 mm of intact bone on the side of the tuberosity. The osteotomy is made just distal and parallel to the wires with an oscillating saw. Both wires help to guide the proper direction. While osteotomizing the hard posterior tibial cortex, it is important to protect the posteriorly lying structures with a Hohmann retractor. Sawing must be done carefully and slowly with little pressure. Loss of resistance is felt when the posterior cortex has been traversed. Constant irrigation during sawing is mandatory. Only the posterior two thirds of the tibia are cut leaving about 1.5 cm intact tibial bone in the front. Having achieved the planned depth of cutting, the anteriorly ascending cut (135°) is done with the narrower blade. This osteotomy lying in the frontal plane must cross the cortex also at the lateral side. The lateral bony bridge allows the preservation of a sufficient bony contact. The anterior osteotomy guarantees stability in the sagittal plane. Insertion of a broad flat chisel into the transverse osteotomy is done up to the lateral bony bridge. The maximal depth of insertion corresponds to the depth of cutting; it should be marked on the chisel. A second chisel is then carefully hammered in between the first chisel and the guide wires; its depth of insertion should be 5 mm less than that of the first chisel. During the insertion of the chisels care has to be taken not to enter the bony bridge or to brake it; increase of resistance is felt when contacting the bridge. The osteotomy gap opens slowly now (Fig. 61.9).

Further flat chisels are placed between the two chisels already in place; each additional chisel should be advanced to a lesser depth. During this procedure one always has the control of the navigation system, how much correction angle already has been reached. Chisels are added until the exact correction angle has been reached according to the navigation system (Fig. 61.10).

It is very important, that the gap is opened slowly over several minutes allowing a plastic deformation of the lateral bony bridge and avoiding breaking this bridge. The two guide wires are left in place during the spreading; they increase the rigidity of the cranial fragment thus preventing a fracture into the articular surface. The medial collateral ligament tends to inhibit posterior opening of the osteotomy and, consequently, can increase the posterior slope of the tibial articular surface. To counteract this, it is important to sufficiently detach the superficial fibers of this ligament and to check the opening of the posterior

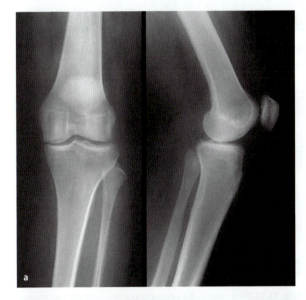

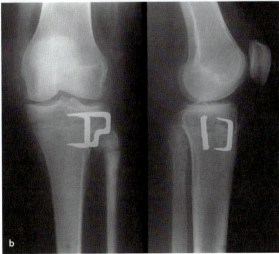

 Fig. 61.8a,b. Case: female 28 y., preoperative (a); 7 weeks postoperative (b)

61

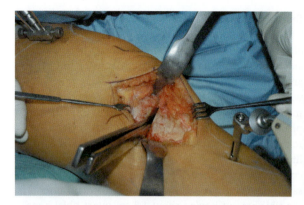

Fig. 61.9. After biplanal sawing two chisles open the osteotomy

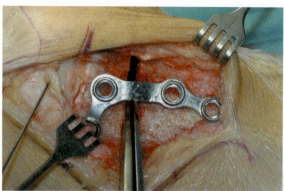

Fig. 61.11. Positioning of the L-Form plate while chisles are still inside the osteotomy

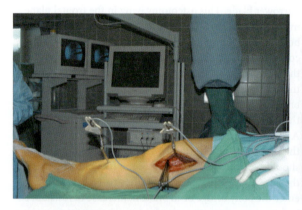

Fig. 61.10. Intraoperative Situation while checking the correcting angle during chiseling

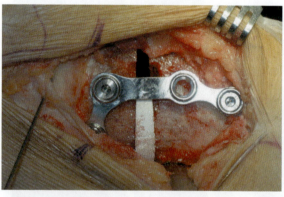

Fig. 61.12. Placement of the interlocking screws and the caciumtriphosphat wedge

part of the osteotomy gap. Therefore, it is necessary to place the chisels sufficiently towards the postero-medial corner of the gap.

While the chisels hold the osteotomy in corrected position, an L-form angular-stable plate is placed at the medial tibia (Fig. 61.11). With four screws and interlocking screws the plate can be fixated to the proximal tibia with angular stability. The exact correction angle can be controlled via the navigation system. The chisels are removed and a special calcium triphosphat wedge is pushed press-fit into the osteotomy gap (Fig. 61.12). After 6 weeks of only 10–20 kg weight bearing under the use of crutches, and a X-ray control, full weight bearing is allowed. Figure 61.13 shows the example of an severe varus deformity, 6 weeks after correction osteotomy in opening technique.

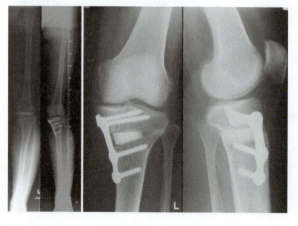

Fig. 61.13. Case Female, 24 Y, preoperative and 6 weeks postoperatively

Use of a navigation system in high tibial osteotomy ensures exact intra-operative orientation without X-ray-control. The size of the wedge and its position can be chosen optimally. Smoother osteotomy surfaces could lead to enhanced healing and rehabilitation. We expect to decrease of the operative complication rate. The described system is used at the Orthopaedic Department of the University of Kiel and is now developed for commercial use. We have used this system for 3 years and have excellent experience. Post-operative X-rays have shown that the navigated ostetomies achieve exact correction angle compared to the pre-operative planning. We could found detect any complications utilizing this technique.

We prefer the opening wedge technique with angular stable osteosynthesis because the degree of correction may be visualized by the navigation system simultaneously during the procedure.

References

1. Blauth W, Schuchardt E (1986) Orthopädisch-chirurgische Operationen am Knie. Thieme, Stuttgart New York
2. Blauth W, Stünitz B, Hassenpflug J (1993) Die interligamentäre valgisierende Tibiakopfosteotomie bei Varusgonarthrose. Operative Orthopädie und Traumatologie 5: 1–15
3. Coventry M (1965) Osteotomy of the upper portion of the for degenerative arthritis of the knee. J Bone Joint Surg 47A: 984–990
4. Coventry M (1985) Upper tibial osteotomy for osteoarthritis. J Bone Joint Surg 67A: 1136–1140
5. Galla M, Lobenhoffer P (2004) High tibial open wedge valgus osteotomy stabilized with the Tomofix plate fixator. Operat Orthop Traumatol 16: 397–417
6. Hassenpflug J, Haugwitz V, Hahne A (1998) Langfristige Ergebnisse nach Tibiakopfosteotomie. Z Orthop 136: 154–161
7. Hassenpflug J, Plötz GMJ (2000) Alternativen zur Endoprothetik. In: Eulert J, Hassenpflug J (Hrsg) Praxis der Knieendoprothetik. Springer, Berlin Heidelberg New York Tokio, S 7–18
8. Healy WL, Anglen JO, Wasilewski SA, Krackow KA (1988) Distal femoral varus osteotomy. J Bone Joint Surg 70A: 102
9. Jackson JP (1958) Osteotomy for osteoarthritis of the knee. J Bone Joint Surg 40B: 826
10. Jerosch J, Heisel J (1999) Knieendoprothetik. Springer Berlin Heidelberg New York Tokio, S 38–41
11. Maquet PGJ (1984) Biomechanics of the knee. Springer, Berlin Heidelberg New York Tokyo, pp 9–74
12. Naudie D, Bourne RB, RorabeckCH, Bourne TJ (1999) Survivorship of high tibial valgus osteotomy – a 10 to 22 year follow up study. Clin Orthop 367: 18–27
13. Rinonapoli E, Mancini GB, Corvaglia A, Musiello S (1998) Tibial osteotomy for varus gonarthrosis. Clin Orthop 353: 185–193

Principles of Computer-Aided Surgery in Trauma Surgery

Y. Weil, R. Mosheiff, L. Joskowicz, M. Liebergall

Introduction

Computer-Aided Surgery (CAS) has started to have a significant impact on the practice of orthopaedic surgery [1]. Together with concurrent surgical and technological trends, such as minimal invasiveness and improved digital imaging, it has the potential to improve results, shorten operative time, reduce morbidity, and reduce variability in a number of common surgical orthopaedic procedures.

Despite a slow beginning, in the last five years CAS has made inroads in orthopaedic trauma by providing support for the planning and execution of surgical procedures. Preoperative planning consists, among others, of digital two and three-dimensional implant templating with properly scaled digital X-ray and CT images, accurate measurements of anatomical angles and axes, and osteotomy planning. Intra-operative execution consists of fluoroscopy and CT-based navigation of surgical instruments and implants, and in some cases, mechatronics and robotic devices.

Navigation systems are by far the most commonly used in orthopaedic trauma and hence our discussion is focused on them. First, we describe the types of navigation systems currently used in orthopaedic trauma. Next, we discuss the clinical considerations for fluoroscopy-based navigated trauma surgery and describe the clinical procedures in which it is used. We conclude with perspectives and our view of future developments.

Navigation Systems for Trauma

There are four types of navigation systems currently in use in orthopaedics: 1) CT-based; 2) two-dimensional (conventional) fluoroscopy-based; 3) three-dimensional (volumetric) fluoroscopy-based; and 4) imageless (kinematics). All of them rely on optical tracking technology.

CT-Based Navigation

Introduced in the early 1990s, CT-based navigation systems were the first-image guidance systems used in orthopaedics. They were designed to assist surgeons in pedicle screw insertion and in acetabular component placement during total hip arthroplasty. Preoperative planning consists of determining the location and diameter of the pedicle screw pilot holes; the implant and/or acetabular cup type and size; and location on a preoperative CT. Intra-operatively, a dynamic reference frame is rigidly attached on or near the site of interest to a bony structure and the CT images are aligned (registered) to the patient's anatomy. The plan, together with a graphical template of the surgical tools in their real-time location are then superimposed on the CT images and shown on a computer screen.

The first CT-based systems in trauma appeared in the late 1990's for percutaneous iliosacral screw insertion and for intra-medullary nailing of femoral shaft fractures [2]. The two main advantages of CT-based systems over conventional fluoroscopy are: 1) they provide axial and spatial, real-time multi-image visualization of bony anatomy and surgical tools and 2) they significantly reduce the use of fluoroscopy.

Despite the above, the current use of CT-based systems in orthopaedic trauma is very limited. First, preoperative CT images of long bone fractures are not always indicated and might delay definitive fracture care and increase the burden on the health care system. Second, even when indicated and available (e.g. pelvic fractures), a registration process, which can be cumbersome, error-prone, and time consuming is required. Third, unstable fractures cause bone displacement that alters the registration, introducing errors that invalidate image-based navigation. Although useful, most trauma applications have moved away from CT-based navigation.

Intra-operative CT or MRI-based navigation systems overcome some of these drawbacks but are cumbersome, costly, and can lengthen the operative time. Furthermore, their availability is very restricted [3–5].

Two-Dimensional Fluoroscopy-Based Navigation

Conventional two dimensional C-arm fluoroscopy-based navigation systems are the most commonly used navigation systems in current orthopaedic surgery [6]. Their main advantage is that they are the closest to conventional fluoroscopy, the »work horse« of orthopaedic trauma. In these systems, a tracking and calibration cage is attached to the C-arm image intensifier and sterilized or draped. Once the patient is prepared on the operating table, the surgeon attaches a dynamic reference frame on or near the bony structure of interest and acquires a set of fluoroscopic images. The images are stored and shown on a computer screen with the actual surgical instruments' location superimposed on them, in effect creating augmented, multiplanar real-time virtual fluoroscopy. Additional fluoroscopic images can be acquired during the procedure, both for validation and for navigation.

There are many advantages to fluoroscopy-based navigation. First, it enables surgeons to better plan and execute surgical actions without the need to perform actual additional fluoroscopy. For example, surgeons can plan and correct the direction of straight implants such as percutaneous screws or intra-medullary nails, or plan the extraction of foreign bodies, by simultaneously following the implant and surgical instruments' positions on all augmented fluoroscopic images. This is a significant improvement over the conventional method, in which implants are positioned by repeatedly adjusting the implant location in each plane (typically coronal and sagittal), and acquir-

ing a control image for each step of the procedure. This results in better implant placements, shorter time, and significantly less radiation to the patient and surgical staff [6]. Unlike CT-based systems, no intraoperative registration is necessary. However, the line of sight between the position sensor (camera) and the trackers must be maintained at all times, and the dynamic reference frame must remain rigidly attached throughout the procedure. Unlike CT-based navigation systems, no axial or spatial views are available.

Three-Dimensional Fluoroscopy-Based Navigation

A recent addition to the orthopaedic intra-operative imaging arsenal is intra-operative CT-like imaging with an isocentric 3D fluoroscope (e.g. the Siremobil IsoC-3D, Siemens, Germany). This new type of fluoroscope is a motorized C-arm unit that captures up to 100 two-dimensional fluoroscopic images in sequence by rotating the C-arm by 180° around the anatomical region of interest. It produces axial CT-like slices with 25–50% less radiation than that required by a conventional high-resolution CT scanner [7]. Despite the lower image quality, the resulting images show sufficient detail of bony anatomy and are adequate for most trauma applications [7, 8].

Navigation with three-dimensional fluoroscopy proceeds as with conventional fluoroscopy. However, the field of interest changes along the course of the surgical instrument, thus the image is updated according to the precise spatial location of the tool (◻ Fig. 62.4). A set of three-dimensional fluoroscopic images are acquired after C-arm draping and reference frame attachment. The actual axial views and the computed sagittal, coronal, oblique, and spatial images can be viewed simultaneously with the tracked surgical instruments superimposed on them. Additional two- and three-dimensional fluoroscopic images can be acquired during the procedure.

The advantages of three-dimensional fluoroscopy are that they provide intra-operative CT-like images without additional registration. However, the field of view is currently small (9" in current fluoroscopes, unsuitable for long trajectories), image quality is limited (e.g. in the thoracic region and in obese patients), and radiation dosage is significant. To date, it has been successfully used for inserting pedicular screws [9] and for retrograde drilling of osteochondral talar lesions in treating foot and ankle lesions [10].

Imageless Navigation

A recent addition to computer-aided orthopaedic navigation is imageless navigation. Today, it is predominantly used in total hip and total knee arthroplasties. In imageless navigation, a dynamic reference frame is attached to at least two bone sites (e.g. femur and tibia). The extremities are then moved and the kinematic and joint axis data is acquired. The relative angular data, such as hip inclination and anteversion are updated in real time. For total knee arthroplasty, the surface of the tibial plateau can be sampled with a pointer to reconstruct its shape and plan the cuts.

The advantage of imageless navigation is that it provides kinematic and joint motion data that is difficult or impossible to obtain with images. While this technique is effective in joint reconstruction and can be useful for fracture reduction, no use of it has to date been reported in orthopaedic trauma. Still, it may have a role in post traumatic reconstructions such as corrective osteotomies.

Clinical Considerations for Navigated Fluoroscopy-Based Trauma Surgery

Fluoroscopy-based navigation is by far the most commonly used type of navigation in orthopaedic trauma. Common important issues include indications, hardware and setup, attachment of the reference frame, fluoroscopic image capture, and radiation reduction.

Indications. Fluoroscopy-based navigation relies on previously acquired images. Thus, a constant and stable fracture reduction is a prerequisite for navigation. Nondisplaced or provisionally reduced fractures by means of traction, external fixators and Kirschner wires are examples of appropriate indications.

Hardware and Setup. Fluoroscopy-based navigation requires the following equipment: 1) a pre-calibrated custom surgical instrument or a standard one fitted with a tracker rigidly attached to it; 2) a calibration and tracking cage attached to the C-arm image intensifier; 3) a reference frame rigidly attached to the bony anatomy and; 4) a position sensor (usually an optical tracker camera) positioned in the operating room so as to maintain at all times a line of sight with the C-arm, the dynamic reference frame, and the tracked surgical instrument. The additional navigation setup time and effort is minimal once the surgeon has understood the navigation requirements and has become familiar with them.

Attachment of the Reference Frame. Fluoroscopy-based navigation requires rigidly attaching a reference frame on or near the anatomy of the operated site to compensate for its motions. The actual attachment location is determined by anatomical, procedural, and technical requirements. For example, the greater trochanter is the usual site for navigated femoral intra-medullary nailing. When the reference frame is too close to the surgical site, possibly interfering with surgical instruments, it should be moved out of the way. However, the further the reference frame is from the tracked instrument, the lower is the tracking accuracy, as angular and translational errors increase. A distance of up to 20 cm between the tracked instrument and the reference frame yields acceptable results in terms of accuracy with current optical tracking technology. In a recent study of cannulated screw fixation of the hip [11], the reference frame was alternatively placed on the ipsilateral iliac crest and on the fracture table, with the patient tightly secured to it, instead of on the greater trochater. The errors were 1.5 mm and 1° in translation, which is acceptable for this procedure.

Fluoroscopic Image Capture. The type of views and number of fluoroscopic images to be used in navigation is procedure-dependent. For example, the insertion of a percutaneous iliosacral screw for posterior pelvic ring disruptions requires 2–4 views of the pelvis (inlet, outlet, lateral and roll over) [12]. The percutaneous insertion of cannulated screws for hip fractures requires a single AP and lateral images of the hip.

Radiation Reduction. An advantage of fluoroscopy-based navigation is the reduction of radiation to both the patient and the surgical team. One minute of intra-operative fluoroscopy of the pelvis is equivalent to about 40 mSv of radiation, 250 radiographs of the chest, or one pelvic CT scan [6, 13]. Thus, the maximum allowable amount of radiation to the hands and eyes is reached after 50 cases [13]. A prospective randomized study of navigated versus standard distal locking of intra-medullary nails showed significant radiation reduction when using navigation [14].

Clinical Applications of Navigated Fluoroscopy-Based Trauma Surgery

We now describe the clinical applications of fluoroscopy-based navigation in four types of surgical procedures. The first three support fracture fixation: 1) trajectory navigation with two-dimensional fluoroscopy; 2) navigation with three-dimensional fluoroscopy; and 3) navigation of complex-shaped instruments and implants. The fourth supports fracture reduction of long bone fractures.

Trajectory Navigation with Two-Dimensional Fluoroscopy

Insertion of straight surgical fixation implants such as screws, nails, or wires is an everyday task in orthopaedic traumatolgy. Often times, such procedures are performed percutaneously or through small incisions, without actual visualization of the target organ. Usually, fluoroscopic imaging is used to monitor the direction of the implant in the target bone using multiple projection, typically a minimum of two orthogonal images (such as anteroposterior and lateral). Significant skill, practice, and time are required to perform this hand/eye coordination task involving the mental reconstruction of a dynamic spatial situation from a sequence of static images.

Navigated two-dimensional fluoroscopy provides a natural computerized enhancement for this surgical action. By simultaneously following the real-time position of both the actual surgical instrument tip and axis, and its projected straight-line trajectory on one or more images, the surgeon can aim and continuously correct the position and orientation of the surgical instrument with respect to a target. This improved surgeon's hand/eye coordination results in more accurate placements in shorter time, with less radiation.

A tracked, pre-calibrated drill guide is used in most applications (❏ Fig. 62.1). The drill guide is a cannula with interchangeable internal sleeves of various diameters through which drill bits and guide wires are introduced. The computer extrapolates the trajectory of the planned implant and superimposes it on the previously acquired fluoroscopic images. For visualization, the trajectory line diameter and extension can be chosen as appropriate (see ❏ Fig. 62.1, bottom). To place a screw, the surgeon brings the tracked drill guide tip to the entry point and orients it according to the augmented images until the axis coincides with the desired target direction. Since these adjustments are done before the actual drilling takes place, drilling attempts and »false routes« are avoided [15].

Most commercial systems allow for attaching trackers to long straight surgical instruments such as awls, taps, drill bits, and graspers and for calibrating them intra-

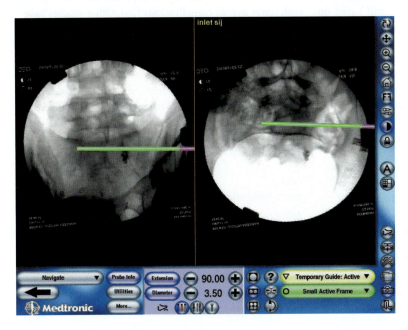

❏ **Fig. 62.1.** Insertion of a percutaneous ilio-sacral screw using two-dimensional fluoroscopy-based navigation. The pink line shows the actual drill guide axis and tip; the green one its predicted trajectory. The diameter and extension of the trajectory line are shown at the center bottom of the screen.

62

operatively. This allows for tracking instrument progress into the bone after insertion and to correct its position accordingly. However, the surgeon must watch for bending and deflection of long instruments, since this may result in inaccurate results [15].

It is important to once again emphasize that any actual change in anatomy, such as fracture displacement or motion of the reference frame will cause a mismatch between the displayed image and the trajectory shown on the screen. If any suspicion arises, additional fluoroscopic images should be acquired for confirmation.

We next describe four routine clinical surgical applications for trajectory navigation: 1) percutaneous pelvic ring and acetabular fractures fixation with a cannulated screw; 2) screw removal; 3) hip fracture pinning; and 4) intramedullary nailing.

Percutaneous Pelvic Ring and Acetabular Fractures

Percutaneous iliosacral screw insertion is a demanding procedure: the »safe zone« for screw placement is narrow due to the presence of nearby nerve structures [16]. Routt [17] has shown that the screws can be safely inserted by adjusting the drill bit trajectory based on alternate pelvic inlet, outlet and lateral fluoroscopic images. While CT-based navigation has also been used to place the screws, the most practical method is navigated two-dimensional fluoroscopy. The desired trajectory is planned based on a pair of pelvic inlet and outlet views, and the drill guide trajectory is adjusted to be on the center of the safe zone in all images. A single drill attempt is performed, with a very high probability of being inside the safe zone. Operative time is thus reduced to a few minutes per screw, and radiation dosage is similarly reduced [12, 18]. Note, that multiple screws can be placed using the same images, and therefore stronger constructs can be installed to increase stability [19].

Other screws for the fixation of pelvic and acetabular disruptions can be placed percutaneously in a similar fashion, and these in turn may assist in minimizing the surgical dissection associated with formal approaches. A classical example is the placement of an anterior column screw for the transverse component of an acetabular fracture via a posterior approach. While these screws are not placed percutaneously, their placement requires repeated use of intra-operative fluoroscopy, which can be totally avoided with navigation [12, 20].

Screw and Hardware Removal

The removal of pelvic fixation screws and other hardware is indicated in some cases, such as for women of child bearing age. This task may be challenging since these implants are deeply seated and extensive soft tissue dissection cannot be avoided. Fluoroscopy-based navigation can be used to direct the surgeon towards the implants, thus reducing the risk of damage to soft tissues and decreasing the radiation to the pelvis [21]. The technique is identical to that of pelvic screw insertion, with the difference being that the surgeon reaches for the head of the screw with the navigated screwdriver. Other applications include the removal of broken screws, missiles or other foreign bodies using pre-calibrated special drills and instruments, such as a hollow mill or a cement grabber.

Hip Fracture Pinning

Cannulated screw fixation of hip fractures is a common undertaking with conventional fluoroscopy. Recent studies [22–25] show that particular screw spreads and configurations are preferred in order to prevent complications such as collapse and subtrochanteric fractures. Navigation can be used to achieve the desired spread. A study comparing the accuracy of navigated cannulated screw insertion with fluoroscopy-based navigation versus conventional fluoroscopy, demonstrated superior formation of the screws with respect to parallelism and spread, with fewer overall complications [26]. Other studies have also demonstrated increased accuracy in the pinning of slipped capital femoral epiphysis in adolescents [27, 28].

The surgical technique for placing these screws is similar to the one presented above. First, the fracture is reduced and the reference frame is attached to the involved side iliac crest. Next, a pair of AP and lateral images of the involved hip are acquired and used for insertion of all three screws. A verification X-ray image is shot after all guide wires are in place and screws are inserted in the standard fashion.

Intra-Medullary Nailing

Although routinely performed, intra-medullary nailing is not devoid of complications. Two issues are starting point selection and screw locking. Accurately placing the starting point can prevent complications such as avascular necrosis of the femoral head, unnecessary cartilage damage (especially in the knee and shoulder), fractures, and risk to neurovascular structures. Locking screw insertion requires repeated trial and error, usually with heavy use of fluoroscopy.

Trajectory navigation with fluoroscopy is indicated for both starting point selection and screw locking [29]. The starting point can be determined with a tracked cannulated drill guide by choosing an entry point and ob-

serving the planned trajectory on the screen (◘ Fig. 62.2). Once the fracture has been reduced and the nail inserted, freehand navigated screw locking can be performed with the »perfect circle« technique (◘ Fig. 62.3). First, the reference frame is fixed to the bony anatomy near the locking screws' location. Then, an AP view in which the nail holes

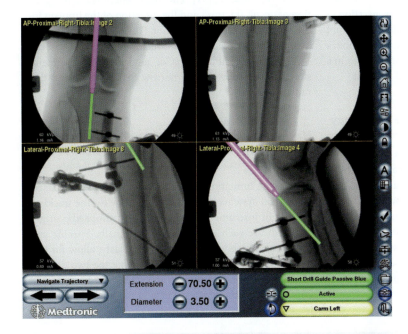

◘ **Fig. 62.2.** Computerized assisted nailing of a tibial shaft fracture: determination of the entry point.

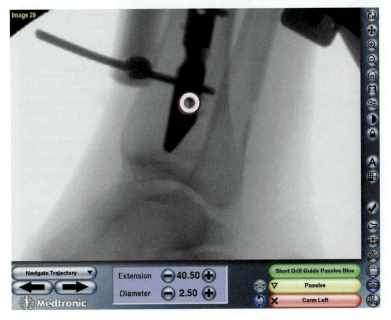

◘ **Fig. 62.3.** Computer screen showing lateral view of distal locking. The concentric circles show the position and orientation of the drill.

appear as circles is acquired. An additional lateral view may be taken to determine screw length measurement. The tracked drill guide is then drawn towards the locking screw area and is navigated until a circle within the hole appears on the computer screen. This is followed by drilling through the tracked drill guide and inserting the locking screw. Sometimes, such as in the case of the tibial nail, the same AP and lateral views can be used for insertion of two or three adjacent locking screws. A single drill attempt usually suffices for the locking screw. In a similar fashion, a blocking or »poller« screw for stabilizing narrow nails in a wide metaphyseal bone can be planned and inserted.

Navigation with Three-Dimensional Fluoroscopy

Three-dimensional fluoroscopy by itself is useful in the reduction of articular fractures such as calcaneal, tibial plateau or plafond, acetabular, distal radius, etc. It may provide data regarding articular surface congruency, implant position and intra-articular fragments or hardware and may change the course of a case [10, 30].

Coupled with navigation, three-dimensional fluoroscopy provides the main advantage of CT-based navigation; axial and spatial views, without the need for registration: The indications for the use of this modality are currently evolving and they already include pedicle screw insertion [18] and percutaneous fixation of non-displaced or provisionally reduced fractures in which the field of view is relatively narrow (e.g., acetabular, calcaneal, talar, proximal and distal tibia). A preliminary report of three-dimensional fluoroscopic navigation in talar osteochondral lesions is promising [31]. The main benefit is the recognition of occult fractures and the direction of the implant in the optimal direction for fixation (◘ Fig. 62.4), which may be unachievable with conventional fluoroscopy.

The current limitations of navigated three-dimensional fluoroscopy are the narrow field of view and the radiation dosage.

Navigation with Complex-Shaped Instruments and Implants

One of the limitations of commercial fluoroscopy-based navigation systems is that they only allow for the tracking of straight instruments. This excludes orthopaedic surgical hardware such as plates and most nails. Specific applications, notably in total hip arthroplasty, allow for the navigation of rasps and cups by showing the two dimensional projection of both cup and stem in order to assess component placement, especially in the axial plane [32].

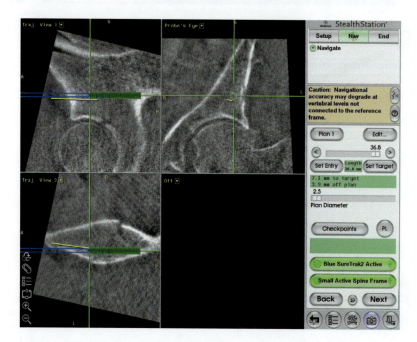

◘ **Fig. 62.4.** An acetabular fracture treated by navigated percutaneous fixation using three-dimensional fluoroscopy.

Navigating complex-shaped, non-straight instruments and implants in orthopaedic trauma is still in its infancy. Two examples include a preliminary trial with a Less Invasive Stabilisation System (LISS) plate [33] and a design for the Gottfried Percutaneous Compression Plating (PCCP) plate (■ Fig. 62.5). To navigate these instruments, a precise description of their geometry must be made available to the navigation system, along with their custom calibration specifications. The navigation system then computes the silhouette of the instruments and superimposes them on the fluoroscopic images. The main advantage is that the actual implant profile and position are simultaneously shown in the fluoroscopic images, facilitating its final positioning and thereby saving operative and radiation time.

Navigation in Fracture Reduction

Long bone fracture reduction, especially of the femoral shaft, is considered to be the key step in the treatment of skeletal injuries. Currently, the reduction requires extensive use of fluoroscopy, with inevitable exposure to the surgeon's hands. Inaccurate results, especially in peri-axial rotation, are not uncommon and may result in long term complications [34, 35].

Fluoroscopy-based navigation for long bone fracture reduction is obviously appealing, although to date only a couple of commercial systems support it. The first obstacle is technical, as earlier systems did not support tracking of two bony segments with a reference frame attached to each. Traditionally, the navigation systems track only a surgical instrument and a reference frame. An elegant solution is to insert a tracked intra-medullary device in one bone fragment and tracking the other fragment with the bone tracker for fracture reduction [36]. Systems that allow tracking and alignment of two fragments are now available. Further research and clinical experience are still needed to prove their efficacy (■ Fig. 62.6).

Perspectives and Conclusions

Wider availability of navigation systems and their routine clinical use, along with support for more procedures and instruments are the most immediate issues that will contribute to the advancement of CAS in orthopaedic trauma.

In addition, computer-aided navigation can support surgery planning in the operating room, shortly before or even during surgery. The navigation system can be used as an intra-operative measuring device, thus providing valuable data that blurs the distinction between preoperative

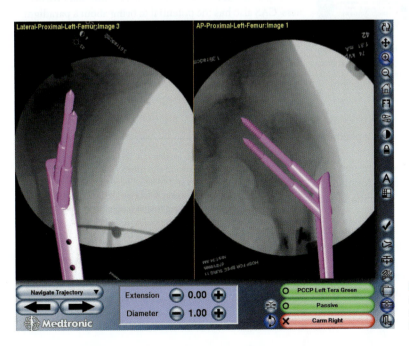

■ **Fig. 62.5.** Navigation of a complex-shaped implant – and experimental model of the Gotfried PerCutaneous Compression Plate (PCCP).

62

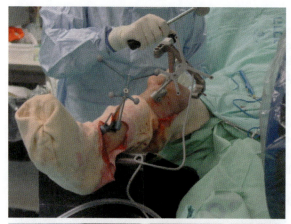

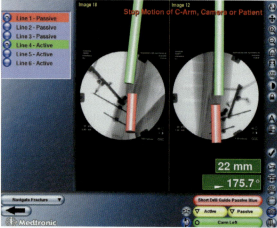

■ **Fig. 62.6.** Fracture reduction. Top: photograph showing the location of the trackers. Bottom: computer screen showing the proximal (top, green line) and the distal (bottom, red line) fragment axes.

4. planning the trajectory and length of a fixation device, such as a screw or an intramedullary nail, thereby avoiding inappropriate or misplaced hardware; and

5. planning the restoration of normal limb alignment, such as planning the poller (blocking) screw position in intra-medullary nailing of metaphyseal fractures. To avoid coronal or sagittal deviation of the limb axis due to narrow nail diameter, a metaphyseal screw can be implanted outside the nail to reduce the volume available for the nail and to assist in fracture reduction.

Fracture reduction is a topic that elicits much interest and for which planning and navigation modules are being developed. When available, the anatomy of the healthy side can be used as a guide for the reduction. This comparative method has been successfully used with CT-based systems in total knee and total hip arthroplasty. CT-based planning enables the matching of both surface anatomy and peri-axial rotation based on the relation of the femoral neck anteversion to the posterior condylar line with respect to the healthy side [37].

In trauma, a fluoroscopy-based method is more desirable. The main issues are: 1) the definition of fragment boundaries; 2) coronal, sagittal, and axial alignment; and 3) ease of use of the system.

Together with other trends, such as minimal invasiveness, CAS also has the potential to bring about a paradigm shift in the treatment of trauma. Besides its current main use in intra-operative planning and support, CAS technology serves as the basis for basic and clinical research, quality control, and surgeon training.

and intra-operative planning. Examples of such planning include:

1. performing accurate measurements on the post reduction fracture for the assessment of restoration of normal anatomy thus helping in the planning of the reduction;

2. determining an implant position after fracture reduction by positioning an implant template on post reduction fluoroscopic images;

3. planning a fracture reduction by identifying the axes of each fragment in multiple planes or by graphically outlining the fracture fragments on the fluoroscopic images and then aligning them;

References

1. Liebergall M, Mosheiff R, Joskowicz L (2006) Computer-aided orthopaedic surgery. Rockwood and Green's Fractures in Adults, 6th edn. Lippincott, Williams and Wilkins, Philadelphia

2. Joskowicz L, Milgrom C, Simkin A, Tockus L, Yaniv Z (1999) FRACAS: A system for computer-aided image-guided long bone fracture surgery. Computer-Aided Surgery 3(6): 271–288

3. Ebmeier K, Giest K, Kalff R (2003) Intraoperative computerized tomography for improved accuracy of spinal navigation in pedicle screw placement of the thoracic spine. Acta Neurochir (Suppl) 85: 105–108

4. Haberland N, Ebmeier K, Grunewald JP, Hliscs R, Kalff RL (2000) Incorporation of intraoperative computerized tomography in a newly developed spinal navigation technique. Computer Aided Surgery 5(1): 18–27

5. Hoffmann J, Dammann F, Reinert S (2002) Initial experience with intraoperative computed tomography in maxillofacial surgery. Biomedical Technology 47 (Suppl 1) Pt 1: 470–473

6. Kahler DM (2004) Image guidance: fluoroscopic navigation. Clin Orthop 421: 70–76

7. Wieners G, Pech M, Beck A, König B, Erdmenger U, Stöckle U, Wust P, Felix R, Schröder RJ (2005) Comparison of radiation dose and image quality of Siremobil-IsoC(3D) with a 16-slice spiral CT for diagnosis and intervention in the human pelvic bone. Rofo 177(2): 258–264

8. Konig B, Erdmenger U, Schroder RJ, Wienas G, Schaefer J, Pech M, Stockle U (2005) Evaluation of image quality of the Iso C3D image processor in comparison to computer tomography. Use in the pelvic area. Unfallchirurg 108(5): 378–385

9. Briem D, Linhart W, Lehmann W, Begemann PG, Adam G, Schumacher U, Cullinane DM, Rueger JM, Windolf J (2006) Computer-assisted screw insertion into the first sacral vertebra using a three-dimensional image intensifier: results of a controlled experimental investigation. Eur Spine J, 15(6):757–63

10. Richter M, Geerling J, Zech S, Goesling T, Krettek C (2005) Intraoperative three-dimensional imaging with a motorized mobile C-arm in foot and ankle trauma care: a preliminary report. J Orthop Trauma 19(4): 259–266

11. Ilsar I, Weil Y, Joskowicz L, Mosheiff R, Liebergall M (2005) Table-mounted vs. bone-mounted reference frame attachment in computer-assisted orthopaedic surgery – an assessment of accuracy. Proc. CAOS-Int. Annual Meeting, Helsinki

12. Mosheiff R, Khoury A, Weil Y, Liebergall M (2004) First generation of fluoroscopic navigation in percutaneous pelvic surgery. J Orthop Trauma 18(2): 106–111

13. Mehlman CT, DiPasquale TG (1997) Radiation exposure to the orthopaedic surgical team during fluoroscopy: »how far away is far enough?« J Orthop Trauma 11(6): 392–398

14. Suhm N. Messmer P, Zuna I, Jacob LA, Regazzoni P (2004) Fluoroscopic guidance versus surgical navigation for distal locking of intramedullary implants. A prospective, controlled clinical study. Injury 35(6): 567–574

15. Mayman D, Vasaehelyi EM, Long W, Ellis RE, Rudan J, Pichora D (2005) Computer-assisted guidewire insertion for hip fracture fixation. J Orthop Trauma 19(9): 610–615

16. Matta JM, Saucedo T (1989) Internal fixation of pelvic ring fractures. Clin Orthop 242: 83–97

17. Routt Jr MLC, Simonian PT (1996) Closed reduction and percutaneous skeletal fixation of sacral fractures. Clin Orthop 329: 121–128

18. Collinge C, Coons D, Tornetta P, Aschenbrenner J (2005) Standard multiplanar fluoroscopy versus a fluoroscopically based navigation system for the percutaneous insertion of iliosacral screws: a cadaver model. J Orthop Trauma 19: 254–258

19. Yinger K, Scalise J, Olson SA, Bay BK, Finkemeier CG (2003) Biomechanical comparison of posterior pelvic ring fixation. J Orthop Trauma 17(7): 481–487

20. Crowl AC, Kahler DM (2002) Closed reduction and percutaneous fixation of anterior column acetabular fractures. Comput Aided Surg 7(3): 169–178

21. Weil Y, Liebergall M, Khoury A, Mosheiff R (2004) The use of computerized fluoroscopic navigation for removal of pelvic screws. Am J Orthop 33(8): 384–385

22. Gurusamy K, Parker MJ, Rowlands TK (2005) The complications of displaced intracapsular fractures of the hip: the effect of screw positioning and angulation on fracture healing. J Bone Joint Surg (Br) 87-B: 632–634

23. Booth KC, Donaldson KJ, Dai QG (1998) Femoral neck fracture fixation: a biomechanical study of two cannulated screw placement techniques. Orthopedics 21: 1173

24. Kloen P, Rubel IF, Lyden JP, Helfet DL (2003) Subtrocanteric fractures after cannulated screw fixation of femoral neck fractures: a report of four cases. J Orthop Trauma 17: 225–229

25. Maurer SG, Wright KE, Kummer FJ, Zuckerman JD, Koval KJ (2003) Two or three screws fixation of femoral neck fractures? Am J Orthop 32: 438–442

26. Liebergall M, Ben David D, Weil Y, Peyser A, Mosheiff R (2006) Computerized navigation for the internal fixation of femoral neck fractures. J Bone Joint Surg (A) 88(8):1748–54

27. Weil Y, Pearle A, Simanovsky N, Porat S, Mosheiff R (2006) Computerized Navigation for treatment of Slipped Femoral Capital Epiphysis. HSSY, in press

28. Perlick L, Tingart M, Wiech O, Beckmann J, Bathis H (2005) Computer-assisted cannulated screw fixation for slipped capital femoral epiphysis. J Pediatr Orthop 25(2): 167–170

29. Hazan E, Joskowicz L (2003) Computer-assisted image-guided intramedullary nailing of femoral shaft fractures. Tech Orthop 18(2): 130–140

30. Atesok K, Kallur A, Peleg E, Weil Y, Liebergall M, Mosheiff R (2005) Intraoperative 3-dimensional imaging Iso-C(3D) in trauma surgery, 25th Annual Meeting of the Israeli Orthopaedic Association, Tel Aviv, Israel

31. Kendoff D, Geerling J, Mahlke L, Citak M, Kfuri M Jr, Hufner T, Krettek C (2003) Navigated Iso-C(3D)-based drilling of a osteochondral lesion of the talus, Unfallchirurg 106(11): 963–967

32. Weil Y, Mattan Y, Kandel L, Eisenberg O, Liebergall M (2006) Navigation-assisted MIS 2-incision total hip arthoplasty – Surgical technique and primary results. Orthopaedics 29(3):200–206

33. Grutzner PA, Langlotz F, Zheng G, Recum JV, Keil C, Nolte LP, Wentzensen A, Wendl K (2005) Computer-assisted LISS plate osteosynthesis of proximal tibia fractures: Feasibility study and first clinical results. Comput Aided Surg 10(3): 141–149

34. Gugenheim JJ, Probe RA, Brinker MR (2004) The effects of femoral shaft malrotation on lower extremity anatomy. J Orthop Trauma 18(10): 658–664

35. Jaarsma RL, Pakvis DF, Verdonschot N, Biert J, van Kampen A (2004) Rotational malalignment after intramedullary nailing of femoral fractures. J Orthop Trauma 18(7): 403–409

36. Mosheiff R, Weil Y, Peleg E, Liebergall M (2004) Computerized navigation for closed reduction during femoral intramedullary nailing. Injury 36: 866–870

37. Ron O, Joskowicz L, Milgrom C, Simkin A (2002) Computer-based periaxial rotation measurement for aligning fractured femur fragments from CT: a feasibility study. Comput Aided Surg 7(6): 332–341

Integration of Computer-Based Systems in Foot and Ankle Surgery

M. Richter, J. Geerling, S. Zech, T. Hüfner, M. Citak

Introduction

Foot and ankle surgery at the end of the 20th century was characterized by the use of sophisticated computerized preoperative and postoperative diagnostic and planning procedures [1, 9]. However, intra-operative computerized tools that assist the surgeon during his or her struggle for the planned optimal operative result are missing. This results in an intra-operative »black box« without optimal visualization, guidance and biomechanical assessment [9]. The future will be characterized by breaking up this intra-operative »black box«. We will have more intra-operative tools to achieve the planned result [9]. Intra-operative three-dimensional imaging (ISO-C-3D), Computer Assisted Surgery (CAS) and Intra-operative Pedography (IP) are three possible innovations to realize the planned procedure intra-operatively [9]. These devices might be especially helpful for minimally invasive surgery.

These novel methods are in clinical use at our institution for further development. This chapter especially analyzes the feasibility and potential clinical benefit of navigation for foot and ankle surgery. Since the intra-operative three-dimensional imaging (ISO-C-3D) and intra-operative pedography (IP) are two other innovations that are closely connected to navigation, these two methods are also described.

Intra-Operative Three-Dimensional Imaging (ISO-C-3D)

In foot and ankle trauma care, mal-position of extraosseous or intra-articular screws and gaps or steps in joint lines frequently remain undiscovered when using intra-operative fluoroscopy, and are only recognized on postoperative computed tomography (CT) scans [3]. Earlier preclinical studies showed that evaluation of reduction and implant position with a new C-arm based three-dimensional imaging device (ISO-C-3D) is better than with plain films or C-arm alone and comparable to CT scans [3].

Study Results

A prospective consecutive clinical study was performed in a level one trauma center [9]. The hypothesis was that the ISO-C-3D could detect failures of reduction or implant position that had not been detected with a conventional C-arm in a considerable percentage.

Patients with foot and ankle trauma or reconstruction surgery that were treated in the Trauma Department of the Hannover Medical School between July 1, 2003 and June 30, 2005 were considered for inclusion in the study. Before the use of the device, the reduction and implant position had to judged to be correct by the surgeon using a conventional C-arm. The patients were either placed on a special metal-free carbon table or on a standard table. Time spent, changes after use of the ISO-C-3D and surgeons' ratings (visual analogue scale, VAS, 0–10 points) were recorded. The surgeons' ratings for image quality for the carbon table and the standard table were compared (t-test, significance level 0.05). The surgeons' ratings for image quality for the carbon table and the standard table were compared (t-test, significance level 0.05).

101 patients/cases (no bilateral ISO-C-3D use) were included (Fractures: pilon, n=15; Weber-C ankles, n=12;

isolated dorsal Volkmann, n=3; talus, n=7; calcaneus, n=32; navicular, n=2; cuboid, n=2; Lisfranc-fracture-dislocation, n=8; ankle/hindfoot arthrodesis with or without correction, n=4/16). Carbon table was use in 80 (79%) cases and a standard table in 21 (21%). The operation was interrupted for 430 seconds on average (range, 300–700); 100 seconds on average for preparation, 120 seconds on average for the ISO-C-3D-scan and 210 seconds on average for evaluation of the images by the surgeon. In 39% (39 of 101) of the cases, the reduction (n=16, 16%) and/or implant position (n=30, 30%) was corrected after ISO-C-3D-scan during the same procedure. The ratings of the eight surgeons involved were 9.2 (5.2–10) for feasibility, 9.5 (6.1–10) for accuracy and 8.2 (4.5–10) for clinical benefit. The image quality was rated 9.1 (8.0–10) for the carbon tables, and 8.7 (7.0–10) for the standard tables (difference rating carbon table versus standard table, t-test, p>0.05). The image quality was rated 9.1 (8.0–10) for the carbon tables, and 8.7 (7.0–10) for the standard tables (difference rating carbon table versus standard table, t-test, n.s.). ◘ Figure 63.1 shows a clinical example.

In this study, in almost 40% of cases, reduction and/or implant position was corrected after ISO-C-3D-scan at the same procedure. The radiation contamination is comparable to a standard CT scan and corresponds to 39 seconds fluoroscopy time with a modern digital C-arm. The image quality with a carbon table is not better than with a standard table. Consequently, the use of a carbon table is not necessary for ISO-C-3D-scan at the foot region.

In conclusion, the intra-operative three-dimensional visualization with the ISO-C-3D can provide important information in foot and ankle trauma care that cannot be obtained from plain films or C-arm alone [12]. The use is not considerably time consuming. The ISO-C-3D is extremely useful in evaluating reduction and/or implant position intra-operatively and can replace a postoperative CT scan.

Computer-Assisted Surgery (CAS)

CT-Based CAS

The accuracy of the reduction in hind- and midfoot fractures and fracture-dislocations correlates with the clinical result [14, 20]. The same is true for the correction of hind- and midfoot [16, 17, 19]. However, an accurate correction or reduction with the conventional C-arm based procedure is challenging [19]. CT-based Computer Assisted Surgery (CAS) has become a valuable tool for the correction and reduction in other body regions [2, 5, 6]. Especially a more exact reduction could be achieved [5–7].

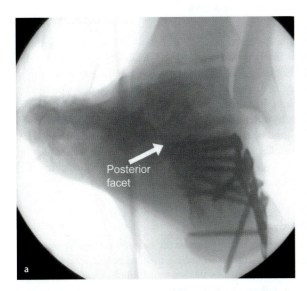

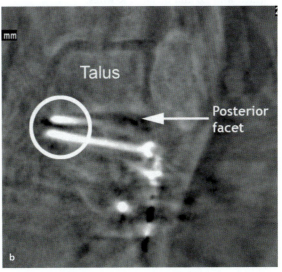

◘ **Fig. 63.1a,b.** Intra-operative three-dimensional imaging (ISO-C-3D). Calcaneus fracture after open reduction and internal fixation with plate and screws. After evaluation with C-arm including Broden´s view (**a**), a cor-

rect reduction and implant position was confirmed by the surgeon. The ISO-C-3D-scan showed a screw penetrating the posterior facet medially (**b**), and the screw position was corrected during the same procedure

CT-based CAS may also be useful for the correction of hind- and midfoot deformities and for the reduction in hind- or midfoot fractures and fracture-dislocations.

Study Results

The purpose of an experimental study at our institution was to compare CT based CAS assisted correction of hind- and midfoot deformities with C-arm based correction [8].

Sawbone™ (Pacific Research Laboratories, Vashon, WA, USA) specimen models »Large Left Foot/Ankle«, »Large Left Foot/Ankle With Equinus Deformity«, »Large Left Foot/Ankle With Calcaneus Malunion«, »Large Left Foot/Ankle With Equinovarus Deformity« were used. A CT-scan of each deformity specimen model (n=3) was performed. The goal of the correction was to transform the shape of the pathology specimen models into the shape of the normal specimen model. Two methods were used for the correction, a, conventional C-arm based correction, and, b, CAS (CT based, Surgigate™, Medivision, Oberdorf, Switzerland & Northern Digital Inc., Waterloo, Ontario, Canada) based correction. Five specimens of each deformity model were corrected with each method. The surgeon's direct view to the specimens was disabled by drapes. During the correction procedure, the visualization of the specimen was exclusively provided by the image of the C-arm or the CAS device. Retention was performed with 1.8 mm titanium K-wires.

The shape was graded normal in all specimens (n=15) in the CAS group, and in eight of the specimens in the C-arm group (other grades in C-arm group: nearly normal, n=6, abnormal, n=1, Chi^2-test, p=0.05). The time needed for the procedure was longer in the CAS group, and the fluoroscopy time was shorter in the CAS group than in the C-arm group (mean values and range shown, t-test utilized):

- time entire procedure, CAS, 782 (450–1020) s, C-arm, 410 (210–600) s, p<0.001;
- fluoroscopy time, CAS, 0s, C-arm, 11 (8–19) s, p<0.001.

The measurement *differences* between the corrected specimens and the normal specimen model were as follows (mean values and standard deviation shown, t-test utilized): foot length, CAS, -1.7 +/- 1.9 mm, C-arm, –4.1 +/- 3.8 mm, p=0.03; length of longitudinal arch, CAS, –0.9 +/- 0.9 mm, C-arm, –5.6 +/- 4.9 mm, p=0.001; height of longitudinal arch, CAS, –0.1 +/- 0.5 mm, C-arm, 1.7 +/–

4.3 mm, p=0.14; calcaneus inclination, CAS, 0.1 +/– 1.4°, C-arm, 2.7 +/– 4.8°, p=0.05; calcaneus length, CAS, –0.5 +/- 0.4 mm, C-arm, –2.8 +/- 1.3 mm, p=0.005; Boehler's angle, CAS, 0.4 +/– 1.1°, C-arm, 4.1 +/– 8.6°, p=0.37.

In conclusion, in an experimental setting, CT based CAS provided higher accuracy for the correction of hind- and midfoot deformities than C-arm based correction [8].

The reasons for the double time needed with CT-based CAS in comparison with the C-arm based method are the requirements of the data transfer of the DICOM-data of the pre-operative CT scan to the CAS device and especially the very time consuming matching process during the registration procedure. The main problems with the matching are based on the difficult bony architecture of the foot with 28 bones and more than 30 joints. Due to these anatomic conditions, the foot does not regularly maintain its complete integrity and position during the pre-operative CT and the registration. This makes the registration in the foot much more difficult than in other body regions like the spine or the pelvis with lesser and bigger bones and joints [2, 5, 6]. Fortunately, during this experimental study was planned and performed, two CAS methods without registration were intended: the C-arm based CAS and the ISO-3-D based CAS. These CAS methods without registration are especially interesting for the foot region.

ISO-C-3D-Based CAS

In our institution ISO-C-3D based CAS was co-developed and firstly used for retrograde drillings in osteochondral defects of the talus [9]. CT-based Computer Assisted Surgery (CAS) guided retrograde drilling of osteochondral lesions had been previously described with promising results as a new technique [4]. In addition to the current method of arthroscopic evaluation and treatment and CT based CAS, we also introduce an alternative technique of using lSO-C-3D based CAS guided retrograde drilling of the lesion.

Study Results

All patients with symptomatic osteochondrosis dissecans stadium I and II according to Berndt and Harty of the talus between June 1st, 2003 and July 31st were included in a follow-up study (Fig. 63.2a). The patients were treated with ISO-C-3D based navigated retrograde drilling. Time spent, accuracy, problems, surgeons' rating (Visual Analogue Scale [VAS], 0–10 points) were recorded and analyzed. The accuracy of the drillings were assessed by the intra-operative three-dimensional imaging device (ISO-C-3D™) Follow-up were performed clinical and radiological using following scores: Visual Analogue Scale Foot and Ankle (VAS FA) and SF 36 (standardized on a possible 100 point maximum for better comparison with the VAS FA).

Technical Background. An ISO-C-3D description above, see ▪ Fig. 63.1) was connected to a navigation system (Surgigate™, Medivision, Oberdorf, Switzerland & Northern Digital Inc., Waterloo, Ontario, Canada). After fixation of a Dynamic Reference Basis (DRB) to the bone, an ISO-C-3D scan follows (▪ Fig. 63.2b). The data are transferred to the navigation system. The starting- and end-point, direction and length of the drilling is planned on the screen of the navigation system using the standard software. A trajectory for the following drilling is placed in the virtual bone on the screen. The drilling is performed with a modified navigated electrical power drilling machine (Powerdrive™, Synthes Inc., Bochum, Germany, ▪ Fig. 63.3). The direction and length of the drilling is shown on the monitor of the navigation device. Standard fluoroscopy is not needed during the entire procedure.

Ten patients (n=6 at lateral talar shoulder; n=4 at medial talar shoulder) were treated with ISO-C 3D based CAS guided retrograde drilling. Time needed for preparation, including the placement of the DRB, scanning time and preparation of the trajectories was 580 s (500–750). All drillings were in correct position (deviation from planned position less than 2° and 2 mm). No surgery related com-

plication, especially no infection occurs. The surgeons' ratings were: feasibility, VAS 9 (7.3–10); accuracy 8.5 (5.8–10); clinical benefit 8.5 (5.7–10). Time of follow-up was 18 (12–28) month. Nine patients could be included in the follow-up study. One patient required OATS after initial clinical improvement. This patient had to be excluded. The VAS FA was 92 (86–98), the SF 36 89 (79–97). The different score categories averaged as follows:

- Pain: VAS FA 85 (69–100), SF36 87 (80–100);
- Function: VAS FA 94 (88–99), SF36 96 (83–100);
- Other complains: VAS FA 96 (87–99), SF36 85 (67–93).

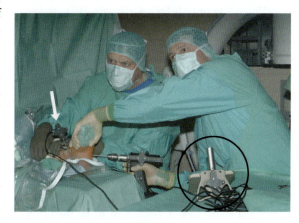

▪ **Fig. 63.3.** ISO-C-3D-based Computer Assisted Surgery (CAS). ISO-C-3D-based CAS guided retrograde drilling in osteochondrosis dissecans tali. Retrograde drilling with starting point at the lateral talar process and visualization on the screen of the CAS device in real time [*white arrow*, Dynamic Reference Base (DRB) fixed to the talar neck through a stab incision; black arrow, drilling machine equipped with DRB; circle, device for drill calibration]

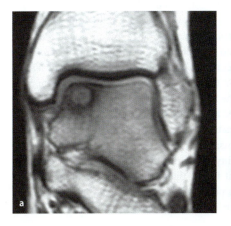
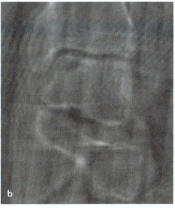

▪ **Fig. 63.2a,b.** ISO-C-3D-based Computer Assisted Surgery (CAS). ISO-C-3D-based CAS guided retrograde drilling in osteochondrosis dissecans tali. MRI image (**a**) and ISO-C-3D image from data transferred to navigation system (**b**) of an osteochondrosis dissecans tali (Berndt & Harty stadium II)

The introduced system was reliable and in frequent use at our department for surgical procedures in different body regions. The advantages of the introduced technique are an actual and almost real-time intra-operative three-dimensional imaging for the use of navigation without the need for anatomical registration and an immediate intra-operative control of surgical treatment [9]. Our results reveal that ISO-C-3D-based Computer Assisted Surgery (CAS) guided retrograde drilling is an alternative to arthroscopically guided or open drilling for osteochondral lesions of the talus. To date we use the same ISO-C-3D but a different navigation device which is easier to use (VectorVision™, BrainLAB Inc., Kirchheim-Heimstetten, Germany; descripition see below). The tremendous device costs for the ISO-C-3D based CAS will prevent standard use for retrograde drilling in osteochondral lesions of the talus alone despite the advantages. However, the ISO-C-3D based CAS is also useful for other body regions like spine and pelvis (see other chapters). Furthermore, the ISO-C-3D alone is a valuable tool for intra-operative three-dimensional visualization as described above.

C-arm Based CAS

As described above CAS is considered to be useful for the correction of hind- and midfoot deformities and for the reduction in hind- or midfoot fractures and fracture-dislocations [8]. CT based CAS provided high accuracy in an experimental setting but the very cumbersome obligatory registration process prevented the clinical use [8]. A registration free C-arm based CAS guided correction was fortunately developed and studied at our institution.

Study Results

Patients with posttraumatic deformities of the ankle or subtalar joint with deformity (mal-alignment) were included in a prospective clinical follow-up study. C-arm based CAS guided arthrodeses with correction of the deformity were performed. Time spent, accuracy, problems, surgeons' rating (Visual Analogue Scale [VAS], 0–10 points) and follow-up (Visual-Analogue-Scale Foot and Ankle (VAS FA), American Orthopaedic Foot and Ankle Society Hindfoot Score (AOFAS), SF36) were analyzed. The accuracy of the corrections was assessed by a new C-arm based three-dimensional imaging device (ISO-C-3D).

Technical Background. A navigation system with wireless Dynamic Reference Bases (DRB) was used (VectorVision™, BrainLAB Inc., Kirchheim-Heimstetten, Germany). The system was connected with a modified C-arm (Exposcope™, Instrumentarium Imaging Ziehm Inc., Nuernberg, Germany, ◘ Fig. 63.4a). One DRB was fixed to each of the two bones or fragments that had been planned for correction in relation to each other. With the C-arm, anteroposterior and lateral digital radiographic images were obtained, and the data were transferred to the navigation device. Then the correction was performed. During the correction, the angle motion and translational motion between the bones or fragments in all degrees of freedom were displayed on the screen of the navigation system (◘ Fig. 63.4b). Furthermore, virtual radiographs with the moving bones or fragments were displayed on the screen. C-arm use was not used during the correction process. After correction, retention was performed with 2.0 mm K-wires. Then the accuracy of the correction was checked with C-arm and intra-operative three-dimensional imaging with ISO-C-3D (Siemens Inc., Germany). Finally screw fixation followed. The insertion of the screws was also C-arm based CAS guided (data not shown).

12 patients were included (ankle correction arthrodesis, n=3; subtalar correction arthrodesis, n=6; combined ankle/subtalar joint correction arthrodesis, n=2; Lisfranc correction arthrodesis, n=1). Time needed for preparation, scanning time and preparation on the screen for the correction was 500 s (400 – 900). The correction process took 45 s (30–60). All planned angles and translations were exactly achieved as planned before (deviation from planned correction less than ±2° for angles or ±2 mm for translations). Three surgeons were involved. Feasibility, VAS 9.5 (9–10); accuracy 9.8 (9.5–10); clinical benefit 9 (8–10). 10 (83%) patients completed follow-up after 14 (6–27) months. All arthrodeses were fused at follow-up. The corrected angles and translations at follow-up (analyzed on radiographs) did not differ significantly from those measured intra-operatively (see above; t-test, p>.05). The VAS FA averaged 47 (25–81), the AOFAS Hindfoot Score 57 (40–64), and the SF36 54 (34–80). The different score categories averaged as follows: pain: VAS FA 47 (14–85), SF36 46 (11–93); function: VAS FA 41 (14–85), SF36 45 (8–85); other complaints: VAS FA 52 (19–83), SF36 70 (55–84).

The feasibility of the introduced method was favorable. The time spent is less than 10 minutes for preparation. The correction process is very fast and extreme accurate, especially regarding the problems with the conventional

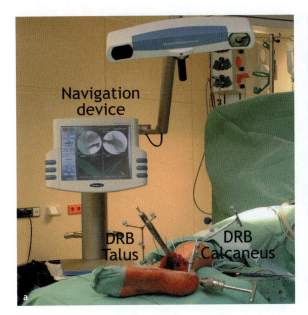

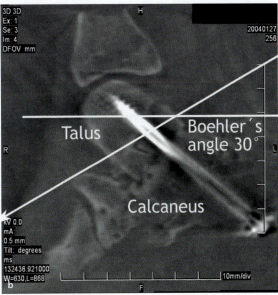

Fig. 63.4a,b. C-arm based Computer Assisted Surgery (CAS). C-arm based CAS guided correction of hindfoot deformity after mal-united calcaneus fracture. Fixation of a wireless Dynamic Reference Base (DRB) to the talar neck and the tuber calcanei. Image acquisition with a modified digital C-arm (**a**). Antero-posterior and lateral digital radiographic images were obtained, and the data were transferred to the navigation device. During the correction, the angle motion and translational motion between the bones or fragments in all degrees of freedom were displayed on the screen of the navigation system (**b**). Furthermore, virtual radiographs with the moving bones or fragments were displayed on the screen

C-arm based correction. In our experience, the correction without CAS guidance needs more time because the necessary frequent C-arm controlling. Furthermore, it is much more difficult, not only because of the difficult visualization but also because the very demanding correction process with three-dimensional motion of two different fragments in relation to each other.

In conclusion C-arm based CAS guided correction of posttraumatic deformities of the ankle and hindfoot region is feasible and provides very high accuracy and a faster correction process [11]. The significance of the introduced method is high in those cases, because the improved accuracy may lead to an improved clinical outcome [16, 17, 19].

Intraoperative Pedography (IP)

For any kind of reduction or correction at the foot and ankle an immediate biomechanical assessment of the

reduction result would be desirable [16, 17, 19]. This is especially true for a CAS-guided reduction or correction, that is supposed to be more accurate than a conventional reduction [13]. The reduction or correction control is normally performed with a C-arm or an ISO-C-3D if available [8, 12]. Analyzing the position of the bones radiographically allows conclusions about the biomechanics of the foot [19]. However, pedography is considered to be more effective for the analysis of the biomechanics of the foot [15]. So far, pedography for biomechanical assessment was only available during clinical follow-up [9]. An intra-operative pedography (IP) would be useful for immediate intraoperative biomechanical assessment [9].

Study Results

A new device was developed to perform IP. A feasibility study was first performed. Then a study for validation followed to compare introduced method with standard dynamic pedography [10]. Finally, a prospective consecutive randomized multi-center study is in progress to analyze the clinical benefit of IP

For an intra-operative introduction of standardized forces to the foot sole, a device named Kraftsimulator Intraoperative Pedographie (KIOP, manufactured by the Workshop of the Hannover Medical School, Hannover, Germany; Registered Design No. 20 2004 007 755.8 by the German Patent Office, Munich, Germany) was developed (◘ Fig. 63.5). The pedographic measurement is performed with a custom-made mat with capacitive sensors (PLIANCE™, Novel Inc., Munich, Germany). The system allows real-time pedography and comparison to the contra-lateral side. The measurements were performed in neutral ankle position. In this neutral ankle position, the influence of the missing muscle action in the anaesthetized patient is considered to be minimal since the EMG in awake standing individuals with comparable ankle position is silent [18].

Validation Study. The validation was performed in two steps:

- Step 1: Comparison of standard dynamic pedography (three trials, walking, third step, three trials, mid stance force pattern), static in standing position (three trials) and pedography with KIOP in healthy volunteers (three trials, total force 400 N). For dynamic pedography and pedography in standing position, a standard platform (EMED™, Novel Inc., Munich, Germany) was used.
- Step 2: Comparison of pedography in standing position, pedography with KIOP in non-anaesthetized and anaesthetized patients (three trials, total force 400 N). Patients with operative procedures performed at the knee or distal to the knee were excluded. Only patients with general or spinal anesthesia were included.

Additionally, a qualitative analysis was performed for both steps (◘ Fig. 63.6). The analysis was focused on the force distribution and not on the force values. The relation of the forces of different regions as hindfoot, midfoot, forefoot (1st metatarsal, 2nd-4th metatarsal, 5th metatarsal), and medial versus lateral were compared. The different measurement and qualitative analyses were compared (t-test, Oneway ANOVA).

The results of the validation process were as follows.

Step 1: 30 individuals were included (age, 26.1±8.6 years; gender, male: female = 24: 6). Step 2: 30 individuals

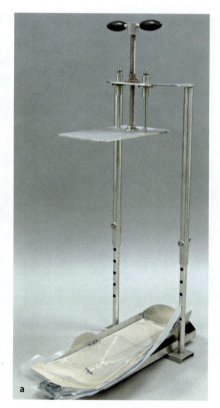

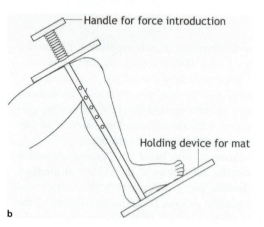

Handle for force introduction

Holding device for mat

b

◘ **Fig. 63.5a,b.** Intra-operative Pedography (IP). The newly developed device for intra-operative force introduction (Kraftsimulator Intraoperative Pedographie® (KIOP®), registered design no. 202004007755.8, German Patent Institute, Munich, Germany & St. Paul, MN, USA, **a**). The custom made mat for force registration (pliance®, Novel, Munich, Germany & St. Paul, MN, USA) is covered intra-operatively with a sterile plastic bag and is placed on the KIOP® as also shown in Fig. 64.4. The size of the mat is 16×32 cm. The mat includes 32×32 sensors with a sensor size of 0.5×1 cm. **b** A scheme of the modus for intra-operative pedography (IP)

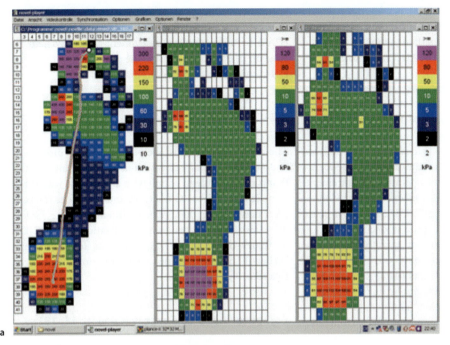

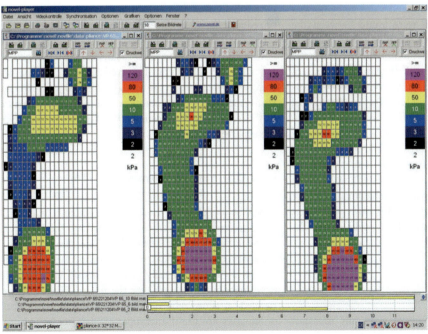

☐ **Fig. 63.6a,b.** Intra-operative pedography (IP). Images from the qualitative analysis of the validation process of IP. **a** Step 1; awake volunteer; *left*, pedography with KIOP; *middle*, static pedography in standing position; *right*, standard dynamic pedography. For dynamic pedography and pedography in standing position, a standard platform (EMED™, Novel Inc., Munich, Germany) was used. **b** Step 2; non-anesthetized/anesthetized patient; *left*, pedography in standing position; *middle*, pedography with KIOP in non-anaesthetized individual; *right*, IP in anesthetized individual

were included (age, 55.3±30.3 years; gender, male: female = 24: 6). No statistical significant differences were found in both steps between the methods, and between the methods of step 1 and 2 (t-test & ANOVA, p>0.05).

Clinical Prospective Study. Sixteen patients were included until March 15, 2006 (ankle correction arthrodesis, n=2; subtalar joint correction arthrodesis, n=4; correction arthrodesis midfoot, n=4, correction forefoot, 4; Lisfranc-fracture-dislocation). Nine patients were randomized for the use of intra-operative pedography, whereas four had no intra-operative measurement. The mean preoperative scores were as follows: AOFAS: 51.6±22.6; VAS FA: 45.2±14.4; SF36: 47.3±21.4. No score differences between the two groups occurred (t-test, p>0.05). The mean interruption of operative procedure for the intra-operative pedography was 323±32 seconds. In four of the nine patients (44%) changes were made after intra-operative pedography during the same operative procedure (correction modified, n=3; screw tightened, n=1). The follow-up has not been completed so far.

In conclusion, IP is feasible and valid since no statistical significant differences were found between the measurements of the introduced method for IP in anaesthetized individuals and the standard dynamic and static pedography. In the future dynamic IP with registration of the entire foot sole is planned for an even more sophisticated biomechanical assessment [10]. During the clinical use, in 50% of the cases a modification of the surgical correction were made after intra-operative pedography in the same surgical procedure. A follow-up of these patients has to be completed to show if these changes improve the clinical outcome. In any case, IP was be able to detect Insufficient biomechanical behavior of the foot and may lead to modifications in the same procedure, and not after pedography in the office weeks or months later [10].

What Do We Need When?

The perfect surgeon who does not make any mistakes without any guidance does not need any of the introduced systems. However, the surgical staff involved in foot and ankle surgery consists of experienced surgeons as well as interns, residents and fellows in training. In times of increasing legal pressure regarding working hours, the

acquisition of surgical experience is harder. Tools for improved intra-operative imaging (ISO-C-3D), guidance (CAS) or biomechanical assessment (IP) may help the surgeon in training to achieve the planned result with less experience [9].

ISO-C-3D [12]

The ISO-C-3D is most helpful in closed procedures and/or when axial reformations provide information that is not possible to obtain with a C-arm or with direct visualization. Weber-C fractures and calcaneus fractures are examples for these special situations. The ISO-C-3D is less helpful when easy visualization with a C-arm or under direct vision is possible as for example in Weber-B fractures during open reduction and internal fixation.

Computer-Assisted Surgery (CAS) [8, 11, 13]

CAS is helpful in complex three-dimensional corrections or reduction, and in closed placement of drillings and/or screw positioning [8]. The significance of the introduced CAS-methods is high in those cases, because the improved accuracy may lead to an improved clinical outcome like complex corrections in the hind- and midfoot deformities [16, 17, 19]. CAS is too complex and time consuming for all those cases that are accurately and easily performed by the experienced surgeon.

Intra-Operative Pedography (IP) [10]

IP will be useful for all those cases in which biomechanical assessment may lead to an immediate improvement of the achieved surgical result [9]. The same cases that are analyzed with clinical pre- or postoperative pedography so far, will potentially profit from IP. The surgeons experience is also crucial for the use of IP, since experienced surgeons who do not use pedography in their office, may not use it intra-operatively also. IP as introduced was made possible by the newly developed device for intra-operative force introduction (Kraftsimulator Intraoperative Pedographie (KIOP), registered design no. 202004007755.8, German Patent Institute, Munich, Germany).

Integrated Computer System for Operative Procedures (ICOP)

For the future, the integration of the different computerized systems will improve the handling and clinical feasibility. An integration of preoperative pedography, planning software, CAS, ISO-C-3D and IP in one Integrated Computer System for Operative Procedures (ICOP) will be favorable. Within this kind of ICOP, the preoperative computerized planning will be able to include preoperative radiographic, CT, MRI and pedography data. The preoperative computerized planning result will be transferred to the CAS device. An intra-operative two-dimensional (C-arm) or three-dimensional (ISO-C-3D) imaging will allow registration-free CAS and will be matched with preoperative CT and or MRI images. The CAS-system will be guided by biomechanical assessment with IP that allows not only morphological but also biomechanical based CAS. The intra-operative three-dimensional imaging (ISO-C-3D) data and the IP-data will be matched with the data from the planning software to allow immediate improvements of reduction, correction and or drilling/implant position in the same procedure [9].

In conclusion, in the future computerized methods for improved intra-operative imaging, guidance and biomechanical assessment will help to realize the planned operative result [9].

References

1. Dahlen C, Zwipp H (2001) Computer-assisted surgical planning. 3-D software for the PC. Unfallchirurg 104(6): 466–479
2. DiGioia AM, III, Jaramaz B, Plakseychuk AY, Moody JE, Jr., Nikou C, Labarca RS, Levison TJ, Picard F (2002) Comparison of a mechanical acetabular alignment guide with computer placement of the socket. J Arthroplasty 17(3): 359–364
3. Euler E, Wirth S, Linsenmaier U, Mutschler W, Pfeifer KJ, Hebecker A (2001) Comparative study of the quality of C-arm based 3D imaging of the talus. Unfallchirurg 104(9): 839–846
4. Fink C, Rosenberger RE, Bale RJ, Rieger M, Hackl W, Benedetto KP, Kunzel KH, Hoser C (2001) Computer-assisted retrograde drilling of osteochondral lesions of the talus. Orthopade 30(1): 59–65
5. Langlotz F, Bachler R, Berlemann U, Nolte LP, Ganz R (1998) Computer assistance for pelvic osteotomies. Clin Orthop (354): 92–102
6. Merloz P, Tonetti J, Pittet L, Coulomb M, Lavallee S, Troccaz J, Cinquin P, Sautot P (1998) Computer-assisted spine surgery. Comput Aided Surg 3(6): 297–305
7. Radermacher K, Portheine F, Anton M, Zimolong A, Kaspers G, Rau G, Staudte HW (1998) Computer assisted orthopaedic surgery with image based individual templates. Clin Orthop (354): 28–38
8. Richter M (2003) Experimental Comparison Between Computer Assisted Surgery (CAS) based and C-Arm Based Correction of Hind- and Midfoot Deformities. Osteo Trauma Care 1129–1134
9. Richter M (2006) Computer Based Systems in Foot and Ankle Surgery at the Beginning of the 21st Century. Fuss Sprungg 4(1): 59–71
10. Richter M, Frink M, Zech S, Vanin N, Geerling J, Droste P, Krettek C (2006) Intraoperative pedography – a new validated method for intraoperative biomechanical assessment. Foot Ankle Int (in press)
11. Richter M, Geerling J, Frink M, Zech S, Knobloch K, Dammann F, Hankemeier S, Krettek C (2006) Computer Assisted Surgery Based (CAS) based correction of posttraumatic ankle and hindfoot deformities – Preliminary results. Foot Ankle Surg 12: 113–119
12. Richter M, Geerling J, Zech S, Goesling T, Krettek C (2005) Intraoperative three-dimensional imaging with a motorized mobile C-arm (SIREMOBIL ISO-C-3D) in foot and ankle trauma care: a preliminary report. J Orthop Trauma 19(4): 259–266
13. Richter M, Geerling J, Zech S, Krettek C (2005) ISO-C-3D based Computer Assisted Surgery (CAS) guided retrograde drilling in a osteochondrosis dissecans of the talus: a case report. Foot 15(2): 107–113
14. Richter M, Wippermann B, Krettek C, Schratt E, Hufner T, Thermann H (2001) Fractures and Fracture Dislocations of the Midfoot – Occurence, Causes and Long-Term Results. Foot Ankle Int 22(5): 392–398
15. Rosenbaum D, Becker HP, Sterk J, Gerngross H, Claes L (1997) Functional evaluation of the 10-year outcome after modified Evans repair for chronic ankle instability. Foot Ankle Int 18(12): 765–771
16. Sammarco GJ, Conti SF (1998) Surgical treatment of neuroarthropathic foot deformity. Foot Ankle Int 19(2): 102–109
17. Stephens HM, Walling AK, Solmen JD, Tankson CJ (1999) Subtalar repositional arthrodesis for adult acquired flatfoot. Clin Orthop (365): 69–73
18. Trepman E, Gellman RE, Solomon R, Murthy KR, Micheli LJ, De Luca CJ (1994) Electromyographic analysis of standing posture and demi-plie in ballet and modern dancers. Med Sci Sports Exerc 26(6): 771–782
19. Zwipp, H. (1994) Chirurgie des Fußes. Springer, Berlin Heidelberg New York Tokio
20. Zwipp H, Dahlen C, Randt T, Gavlik JM (1997) Komplextrauma des Fusses. Orthopäde 26(12): 1046–1056

New CAS Techniques in Trauma Surgery

G. Zheng, X. Zhang, X. Dong, S. Sagbo, P.A. Grützner, F. Langlotz

Introduction

There is a trend towards less invasive and percutaneous treatment in trauma surgery that aims for shorter hospital stays, faster recovery and better cosmetic results. However, such a treatment is also a technically demanding procedure. Toray's less invasive procedures that show great advantages in healing and therapy often do not allow controlling instruments through direct sight, because muscles and skin left in place hide the surgical target. The surgeon has to rely on intra-operative imaging means such as fluoroscopy or ultrasound. Techniques like the placement of guide-wires prior to the ultimate intervention are used to monitor an intended trajectory with the use of fluoroscopy and subsequently enable safe guidance of the surgical instrument. Preoperatively acquired images such as radiograph, CT, and MRI may also be referred to obtain more detailed information with high image quality. The surgeon is responsible for bringing the information gained from different imaging modalities into spatial relationship within the situation on the operating table.

The introduction of computer-assisted surgery (CAS) technique in more than a decade ago overcomes certain difficulties in less invasive treatment and brings following potential advantages: improving accuracy, reducing invasiveness, facilitating planning and simulation, and reducing X-ray radiation for both patent and surgical team. This chapter aims for reviewing recently and currently developed CAS techniques in trauma surgery including: (1) registration-free CT-based navigation; (2) zero-dose fluoroscopy-based close reduction and osteosynthesis of diaphyseal fracture of long bone; (3) virtual implant management; and (4) robot-assisted trauma surgery.

Registration-Free CT-Based Navigation

CT-based surgical navigation made it possible to achieve a link between the pre-operatively acquired three-dimensional (3D) image data and the intra-operative instrument position. The surgeon sees his instrument in a virtual medical image in real time. This is achieved by fitting the instrument with infrared light-emitting diodes (active markers) or reflective spheres (passive markers) and by tracking it with a positional locator. Conceptually, CT-based navigation systems can be compared with global positioning systems (GPS), e.g. those frequently used in cars [1]. The positional locator placed in the operating room takes the role of the GPS satellite. It remotely measures the position of the surgical instruments with respect to a reference coordinate system established on the operated anatomy by means of a so-called dynamic reference base (DRB) [2]. The associated coordinates are then transformed into the frame of reference of the image data through an intra-operative registration process and allow visualization of the instruments, just like a car-mounted GPS receiver indicates its position on a map. Although in a variety of pro- and retrospective clinical trials these systems have proven to be superior to conventional surgical techniques, particularly in anatomically complex situations [3, 4], these system did not become widely available for trauma surgery due to the challenging and often time-consuming intra-operative registration process as well as the limitation imposed by the assumption that the bone morphology can be represented by a rigid body throughout the complete surgical action.

Recent developments in registration-free navigation [5] or modality-based navigation [6] revitalize the application of CT-based navigation in trauma surgery. The principle of registration-free navigation can be summarized by two key steps: (1) offline calibration step, and (2) intra-operative navigation step. In the first step, the correlation between the 3D image volume and a device reference coordinate system affixed to the imaging modality is determined through a paired-point matching process. This device reference coordinate system is permanently established by calibrating the active or passive markers attached to the imaging modality. After this step, the position and orientation of the image volume in this device reference coordinate system is known. This calibration process is procedure-unrelated and typically carried out through an offline process at regular time intervals. Intra-operatively, as soon as the image volume of the patient is acquired, the navigation system knows immediately its position and orientation in the patient reference coordinate system due to the offline calibration measurement. No intra-operative registration is required anymore. Registration-free navigation has been successfully applied in treatments to various fractures including articular fractures [5], spine fractures[7] and pelvic fractures [8].

Zero-Dose Fluoroscopy-Based Reduction and Osteosynthesis of Diaphyseal Fracture of Long Bone

Diaphyseal fracture of long bone belongs to one of the most common injuries encountered in clinical routine trauma surgery. Most of them are displaced and need to be surgically reduced. The past 15 years witnessed the shift from direct reduction and rigid fixation to biological internal fixation using indirect reduction techniques with correct alignment of axes, rotation, and correct reconstruction of bone length without open surgical exposition of the fracture sites [9]. While in the past, fractures used to be exposed considerably to allow the surgeon direct view of the fracture site and stabilized with accordingly sized plates, it is now generally agreed that the technique of minimally invasive osteosynthesis yields superior results. Minimization of the skin incision and reduction of the induced soft tissue damage results in a number of advantages

for the patient including both the cosmetic results as well as improvement in function and healing time [10].

One of the difficulties with minimally invasive techniques in long bone fracture treatment is caused by the absence of direct visual contact to fracture reduction and implant positioning. As a consequence, the fluoroscope, also known as C-arm, is used more intensively during modern surgical techniques for visualizing underlying bone, implant, and surgical tool positions. The disadvantages of fluoroscope include two-dimensional (2D) projection image from single view, limited field view, distorted images, and last but not least, high radiations to both the patient and the surgical team [11]. The integration of conventional fluoroscopes into computer assisted navigation systems has been established as one means to overcome certain of these drawbacks [12–21].

Fluoroscopy-based navigation systems try to intrinsically and extrinsically calibrate fluoroscopes to compensate for their distortions and to create a virtual fluoroscopy, which provides the missing link between intra-operative imaging information of the surgical reality with the surgical action for different surgical applications [17]. The one specific application area is long bone fractures, especially femoral diaphyseal fracture reduction. In [13] static fluoroscopic images was replaced with a virtual display of 3D long bone models created from pre-operative Computed Tomography (CT) and tracked intra-operatively in real time. Fluoroscopic images were used to register the bone models to the intra-operative situation. In [15] a computer-assisted fluoroscopy-based navigation system for reduction of femoral fracture and antetorsion correction was developed. In this system, the bone fragments were represented by their individual axes and alignment of bone fragments during fracture reduction was monitored through real-time visualization of line graphics. Bi-planar landmark reconstruction was proposed to contactlessly determine the coordinates of deep-seated landmarks. A patient-specific coordinate system was then established based on these reconstructed landmarks for measuring changes of leg length and antetorsion. Recently we have proposed to enhance this system using a 3D cylindrical model representation of each bone fragments, which is interactively reconstructed from the acquired fluoroscopic images [18].

Although a number of authors reported excellent experiences in restoration of leg lengths and antetorsion for femoral diaphyseal fracture reduction with currently existing systems for virtual fluoroscopy [18–20], two disadvantages of these devices can be identified during routine clinical use: (1) the bone fragments were represented either by simple 3D models (lines or cylinders) interactively reconstructed from the acquired fluoroscopic images or by complex surface models constructed from pre-operative CT data. The former represents the surgical reality in a rather abstract way and the latter requires a pre-operative CT data, which adds financial burden and radiation to the patient; (2) changes in the bony anatomy due to fracture reduction can only be analyzed by the re-acquisition of C-arm images causing additional radiation to patient and surgical staff and requiring cumbersome re-positioning of the fluoroscope at the patient during surgery.

To address these issues, a novel technique has been developed to create a computed fluoroscopy for computer-assisted close reduction and osteosynthesis of long bone fractures [21], as shown by ▪ Fig. 64.1. With this novel technique, repositioning of bone fragments during fracture reduction will lead to image updates in each acquired imaging plane, which is equivalent to using several fluoroscopes simultaneously from different directions but without any X-ray radiation. This novel technique is achieved with a two-step procedure: (1) *data preparation,* which is done be-

fore fracture reduction and osteosynthesis but after image acquisition, automatically estimates the size and the pose of the diaphyseal fragments through three-dimensional morphable model fitting using a parameteric cylinder model. The projection boundary of each estimated cylinder, a quadrilateral, is then fed to a region information based active contour model [22] to extract the fragment contours from the input fluoroscopic images. After that, each point on the contour is interpolated relative to the four vertices of the corresponding quadrilateral, which resulted in four interpolation coefficients per point. The second step, *image updates,* repositions the fragment projection on each acquired image during close reduction and osteosynthesis using a computerized method. It starts with interpolation of the new position of each point on the fragment contour using the interpolation coefficients calculated in the first step and the new position of the corresponding quadrilateral. The position of the quadrilateral is updated in real time according to the positional changes of the associated bone fragments, as determined by the navigation system during fracture reduction. The newly calculated image coordinates of the fragment contour are then fed to a OpenGL® based

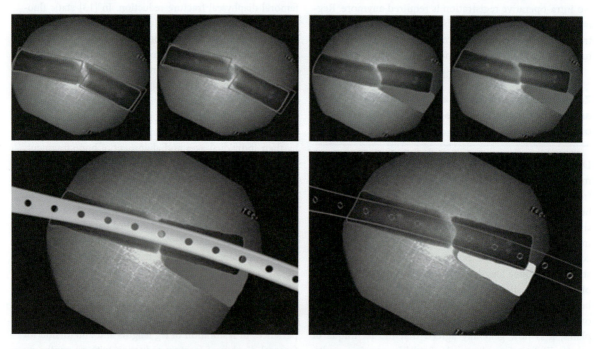

▪ **Fig. 64.1.** *Top left:* Fragment identification and projection contour extraction; *top right:* image dynamization for close fracture reduction; *bottom left:* photorealistic rendering of osteosynthesis plate where the

anatomical structures are occluded by the virtual plate; *bottom right:* non-photorealistic rendering of osteosynthesis plate texture warping pipeline to achieve a real-time image updates. This novel technique has been successful applied to close reduction and osteosynthesis of proximal tibia fractures and demonstrated very promising results [23].

Virtual Implant Management

A wide variety of different plates, screws, and nails are used in trauma surgery [24]. However, the scaled visualization and tracking of these devices and tracking of these devices and their corresponding surgical instrument is currently only possible using fluoroscopy, which implies a risk of high irradiation.

Computer-assisted surgery has made tremendous progress over the past 10 years. Navigation systems have been recognized as important tools that help trauma surgeons, and various such systems have been developed for trauma surgery. A disadvantage of these systems is that each system uses its own proprietary technique to manage implants. As a result, there is no standardized concept for implant and tool management or data formats to store information of implants for use in planning and navigation.

A novel concept has recently been developed to provide this functionality [25]. The concept centers around a virtual implant database [26] that contains both geometrical and calibration information for trauma implants and instruments. This should enable realistic navigation of various implants through a common interface, and could be used with any navigation application. This database contains various virtual representations of osteosynthesis implants and anchoring devices for fracture reduction and fixation. It can be browsed for details of any stored virtual implant. Currently it supports the planning and navigation parameters of LISS and LC-DCP plates (Synthes AG, Chur, Switzerland), as well as searching functionalities based on implant size, manufacturer, bone part, or implant type. The system has been successfully tested for several computer-assisted trauma surgery applications [26–27]. A management tool aiming for automating the process from implant CAD files to a standardized XML-based implant database has also been developed [28].

Robot-Assisted Trauma Surgery

Robot-assisted trauma surgery is an emerging field where the robot is directed and manipulated by the trauma surgeons in order to enhance and complement their free-hand abilities. Although computer-assisted surgery has made tremendous progress in trauma surgery by the beginning of 21st century, the use of robots in trauma surgery was only explored in laboratory settings at the same period [29]. This may be attributable to the difficulty and invasiveness of registration and immobilization of robot in a fracture treatment.

This situation is changing by a recently introduced miniature robot [30] with a parallel architecture that can be directly mounted on the bone with a minimally invasive attachment jig. A surgical instrument or tool guide is attached to the moving platform of this robot so that it can be precisely positioned and oriented by the robot controller to a desire location close to the mounting site The application of such a robot in trauma surgery can be summarized by four steps: (1) *pre-operative planning*, where the entry point and the trajectory are planned by the surgeons based on preoperatively acquired X-ray, CT, or MRI images; (2) *intra-operative robot fixation*, in which the miniature robot together with the targeting guide is rigidly attached to the bony structure close to the surgical site with a minimally invasive way; (3) *registration*, where a rigid transformations between the coordinate systems of the robot, the target anatomy, and the preoperative plan are established; and (4) *execution of surgical plan*, in which the robot controller aligns the targeting guide with the preoperatively planned trajectory to allow the surgeon to execute the surgical action precisely. Such a device is currently available for spine fusion and distal locking in intra-medullary nailing [30].

Conclusions

It has been identified that a potential impact area for the relatively new field of computer-assisted surgery should be orthopaedic trauma [31], where surgeons frequently must perform delicate surgery without the benefit of a firsthand look at what they will be operating on. Fracture orientation can be difficult to conceptualize, especially in the acetabulum or spine. Anatomic reduction and stable fixation remain a challenge and have required long incisions with wide exposure, sometimes with increased postoperative morbidity. The introduction of CAS technology into trauma surgery provides a new tool for accurate and safe implant placement in percutaneous applications about the pelvis, spine, and long bones. Recently and currently developed new CAS techniques now allow this technology to be applied to routine fracture care, with the potential to improve accuracy, while reducing invasiveness and decreasing radiation exposure to the patient and the surgical team.

References

1. Langlotz F (2002) State-of-the-art in orthopaedic surgical navigation with a focus on medical image modalities. J Visualization Comput Animat 23: 77–83
2. Nolte LP, Zamorano LJ, Visarius H, Berlemann U, Langlotz F, Arm E, Schwarzenbach O (1995) Clinical evaluation of a system for precision enhancement in spine surgery. Clinical Biomechanics 10: 293–303
3. Laine T, Lund T, Ylikoski M, Lohikoski J, Schlenzka D (2000) Accuracy of pedicle screw insertion with and without computer assistance: a randomised controlled clinical study in 100 consecutive patients. Eur Spine J 9(3): 235–240
4. Digioia AM 3rd, Jaramaz B, Plakseychuk AY, Moody JE Jr, Nikou C, Labarca RS, Levison TJ, Picard F (2002) Comparison of a mechanical acetabular alignment guide with computer placement of the socket. J Arthroplasty 17(3): 359–364
5. Grutzner PA, Hebecker A, Waelti H, Vock B, Nolte L-P, Wentzensen A (2003) Clinical study for registration-free 3D-navigation with the SIREMOBIL Iso-C3D Mobile C-arm. Electromedica 71 (Suppl 1): 7–16
6. Messmer P, Gross T, Suhm N, Regazzoni P, Jacob AL, Huegli RW (2004) Modality-based navigation. Injury 35 SA-24–SA-29
7. Wendl K, von Recum J, Wentzensen A, Grutzner PA (2003) Iso-C3D-assisted navigated implanation of pedicle screws in thoracic lumbar vertebrae. Unfallchirurg 106(11): 907–913
8. Huegli RW, Staedele H, Messmer P, Regazzoni P Steinbrich W, Gross T (2004) Displaced anterior olumn acetabular fracture: closed reduction and percutaneous CT-navigated fixation. Acta Radiologica 6: 618–621
9. Leunig M, Hertel R, Siebenrock KA et al. (2000) The evolution of indirect reduction techniques in the treatment of fractures. Clin Orthop 375: 7–14
10. Krettek C, Gerich T, Miclau T (2001) A minimally invasive medial approach for proximal tibial fractures. Injury SA4–SA13
11. Yampersaud YR, Foley KT, Shen AC, Williams S, Solomito M (2000) Radiation exposure to the spine surgeon during fluoroscopically assisted pedicle screw insertion. Spine 2637–2645
12. Hofstetter R, Slomczykowski M, Bourquin I, Nolte L-P (1997) Fluoroscopy based surgical navigation – concept and clinical applications. Proceedings of the 11th International Symposium on Computer Assisted Radiology and Surgery, pp 956–960
13. Joskowicz L, Milgrom C, Simkin A et al. (1998) FRACAS: a system for computer-aided image-guided long bone fracture surgery. Comp Aid Surg 277–288
14. Hofstetter R, Slomczykowski M, Sati M, Note L-P (1999) Fluoroscopy as an image means for computer-assisted surgical navigation. Comp Aid Surg 65–76
15. Hofstette R, Slomczykowski M, Krettek C et al. (2000) Computer-assisted fluoroscopy-based reduction of femoral fractures and ante-tortion correction. Comp Aid Surg 311–325
16. Nolte L-P, Slomczykowski M, Berlemann U, Matthias MJ, Hofstetter R, Schlenzka D, Laine T, Lund T (2000) A new approach to computer-aided spine surgery: fluoroscopy-based surgical navigation. Eur Spine J S78–S88
17. Foley K, Simon D, Rampersaud YR (2001) Virtual fluoroscopy: Computer-assisted fluoroscopic navigation. Spine 347–351
18. Grutzner PA, Zheng G, Vock B, Keil C, Nolte L-P, Wentzensen A (2004) Computer-assisted osteosynthesis of long bone fracture. In: Stiehl JB, Konermann W, Haaker R (eds) Navigation and robotics in total joint and spine surgery. Springer, Berlin Heidelberg New York Tokio, pp 449–454
19. Suhm N, Jacob AL, Nolte L-P, Regazzoni P, Messmer P (2000) Surgical navigation based on fluoroscopy – clinical application for computer-assisted distal locking of intramedullary implants. Comp Aid Surg 391–400
20. Slomczykowski M, Hofstetter R, Sati M, Krettek C, Nolte L-P (2001) Novel computer-assisted fluoroscopy system for intraoperative guidance: feasibility study for distal locking of femoral nails. J Orthop Trauma 122–131
21. Zheng G, Dong X, Langlotz F, Gruetzner PA (2005) Zero-dose fluoroscopy-based close reduction and osteosynthesis of diaphyseal fracture of femurs. Stud Health Technol Inform 119: 592–594
22. Ronfard R (1994) Region-based strategies for active contour models. Int J Comput Vision 13(2): 229–251
23. Grutzner PA, Langlotz F, Zheng G, von Recum J, Keil C, Nolte LP, Wentzensen A, Wendl K (2005) Computer-assisted LISS plate osteosynthesis of proximal tibia fractures: feasibility study and first clinical results. Comp Aid Surg 141–149
24. Suhm N (2004) Long bone trauma. In: DiGioia AM, Jaramaz B, Picard F, Nolte LP,(eds). Computer and robotic assisted knee and hip surgery. Oxford University Press, Oxford, pp 297–306
25. Zheng G (2002) Advancements of fluoroscopy-based navigation for less invasive orthopaedic interventions. Ph.D. thesis, MEM Institute for Surgical Technology and Biomechanics, University of Bern, Bern, Switzerland
26. Sagbo S, Zheng G, Vangenot C, Moumni J, Nolte LP (2004) Virtual implants database for computer assisted surgery: a new unified implant access interface for surgical planning, navigation and simulation. Proceedings of MICCAI 2004/DiDaMIC-2004 Workshop on Distributed Databases and Processing in Medical Image Computing, St Malo/Rennes, France, pp 26–35
27. Anderegg C, Langlotz F (2004) The planning of fracture treatment using digital templates. Proceedings of 4th Annual Meeting of the International Society for Computer Assisted Orthopaedic Surgery (CAOS 2004), Chicago, IL. pp 115–117
28. Sagbo S, Blochaou F, Langlotz F, Vangenot C, Nolte L-P, Zheng G (2005) New orthpaedic implant management tool for computer-assisted planning, navigation, and simulation: from implant CAD files to a standarized XML-based implant database. Comp Aid Surg 311–319
29. Fuchtmeier B, Egerdoerfer S, Mai R, Hente R, Dragoi D, Monkman G, Neilich M (2004) Reduction of femoral shaft fractures in vitro by a new developed reduction robot system 'RepoRobo'. Injury SA-113–SA-119
30. Shoham M, Burman M, Zehavi E, Joskowicz L, Batkilin E, Kunicher Y (2003) Bone-mounted miniature robot for surgical procedures: concept and clinical applications. IEEE T Robotics and Automation 19(5): 893–901
31. Kahler DM (2004) Image guidance – fluoroscopic navigation. Clin Orthop 421: 70–76

Navigated High Tibial Osteotomy with Vector Vision System

K.-W. Cheung, W.-P. Yau, K.-H. Chiu, K.-Y. Chiu

Introduction

High tibial osteotomy (HTO) was first introduced in the 1960's for the treatment of symptomatic osteoarthritis of the knee with varus deformity [1–2]. It has been proven to be successful in terms of pain relief and restoration of function [3–16]. Despite the fact that the number of HTO being performed is declining in the recent years [17], it is still a useful operation for a well selected group of patients.

In patients suffering from knee osteoarthritis, the varus or valgus deformity leads to an abnormal distribution of the stress at the joint during weight bearing, and subsequently accelerates degenerative changes in the compartment with increased load. For a knee with varus deformity, the stress is concentrated over the medial compartment of the tibial-femoral joint. The principle of HTO is to correct the varus mal-alignment of the lower limb so that the medial compartment of the tibial-femoral joint is unloaded, and the stress is shifted to the healthy lateral side. Coventry described the closing wedge osteotomy over the proximal tibia in 1965 [2]. Good results were reproduced by many other surgeons [3–16]. Other techniques, such as dome osteotomy and medial opening wedge osteotomy, were later described [16, 18, 19].

Careful selection of the patient is critical to obtain good results. The ideal candidates to receive HTO are active young individuals with isolated medial tibial-femoral osteoarthritis of the knee. The patients should be (1) younger than 60 years old, (2) have a pre-operative alignment of less than varus 10°, (3) pre-operative knee flexion contracture of less than 10° and (4) pre-operative knee flexion of more than 90°.

The initial success of HTO deteriorates with time. It is usually due to the progression of the osteoarthritis and the recurrence of the deformity and pain. Using conversion to total knee arthroplasty (TKA) as the end-point, the survivorship of HTO ranged from 73% to 97% at 5 years, 51% to 96% at 10 years and 39% to 87% at 15 years after the index operation [5, 14–15]. Risk factors of failure included the amount of valgus correction, age, severity of osteoarthritis at presentation, the presence of a lateral tibial thrust, pre-operative knee alignment, pre-operative flexion arc, ligamentous instability, body mass and non-union at osteotomy site.

The most common cause of early failure is perhaps the under-correction of the deformity in the frontal plane. The symptomatic improvement in the early post-operative period was less satisfactory [3, 7, 16]. There was an increased chance of early recurrence of the varus deformity, and a corresponding increase in the patient's pain [5, 15, 16]. Coventry recommended an additional over-correction of 3° to 5° on top of the normal anatomical alignment. On the other hand, excessive over-correction may lead to poor results [3, 8, 16] because of over-loading of the lateral compartment and subsequent pre-mature progression of the osteoarthritis. Other potential complications of HTO include intra-articular fracture during the osteotomy [8, 14–16] and hardware penetration into the joint. These usually occurred when the osteotomy site was made too close to the articular surface. In order to avoid these complications, many surgeons perform the operation under fluoroscopic control.

Beside the correction in the alignment of the lower limb in the frontal plane, it is increasingly recognized in recent years that HTO can result in unintentional change in the tibial slope in the sagittal plane [20–23]. This leads to an alteration in the tension of the anterior and posterior cruciate ligaments. The effect is not yet fully understood, but this will definitely result in an altered biomechanical environment inside the knee joint. On the other hand, some surgeons combined the anterior cruciate ligament reconstruction with HTO in patients suffering from concomitant chronic anterior cruciate ligament insufficiency and mild osteoarthritis of the medial compartment of the tibial-femoral joint. They deliberately changed the tibial slope to optimize the tension in the cruciate ligaments [24, 25].

In the operating room, it is very difficult to know the exact limb alignment even with fluoroscopic guidance. Grid plate is an additional tool to help aligning the limb but the view of the fluoroscopy is still very limited. The slope of proximal tibia, level of osteotomy, size of the wedge and the Fujisawa point determination [26] are very difficult to be determined. Fujisawa considered the ideal point of joint correction as 62% intersection measuring from medial to lateral border of tibial plateau, in order for the ulcerated cartilage over the medial tibial plateau to repair by themselves. In addition, the use of fluoroscopy increases the radiological hazard to the medical personnel involved in the procedure. Because of these issues, we began to explore the use of navigated HTO in 2003.

Keppler et al. first reported on computer assisted medial open wedge HTO in 2004 [27]. They studied techniques on saw bone models and then on cadavers. It was found that the mechanical axis passed through the Fujisawa point in 80% of the subjects. Kendoff et al. in 2004 [28] and Hüfner et al. [29] in 2005 reported that navigated HTO was more accurate than conventional technique. However, these studies were performed without arthroscopic assistance. The anatomy and landmarks of proximal tibia were not fully utilized in generating the navigation model. We think that with the use of arthroscopy during the procedure, the proximal tibia anatomy can be fully appreciated. It may help to provide a more accurate determination of the final limb frontal plane alignment and also the tibial slope.

Techniques

The navigation system we use is the BrainLAB Vector Version 1.0 system (◻ Fig. 65.1). It is an imageless navigation system. It can use either cutting block guided without K wire, or image-guided placement of K wire (with or without athroscopic assistance) to navigate the bone cut. The arthroscopic assisted, image-guided placement K wire method is used by the authors.

4.0 mm tracker anchoring pins are inserted into the distal femur and proximal tibia. Two pins are needed on each side, and the pins are inserted through both cortices. The tracker anchoring clamps are then fixed securely to the pins. The lower limb is moved from extension to full flexion to test the receiving filed of the detection camera. The trackers are passive ones and reflect the infra-red light generated from the camera.

The registration of the hip center is first performed through rotation of the hip. About 100 points were obtained throughout the hip movements. The movements

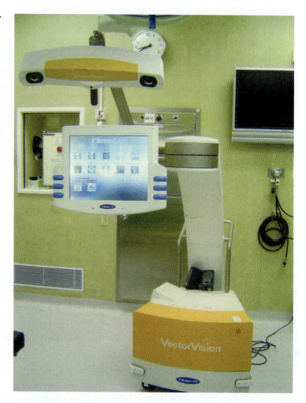

◻ **Fig. 65.1.** BrainLAB Vector Version system

have to be gentle, and the assistant has to stabilize the pelvis by pressing firmly onto the anterior superior iliac spines. This will prevent the pelvis from lifting off the operating table, and causes pelvic rotation instead of hip rotation. The computer will calculate the accuracy of the hip centre determination. If the latter is more than 3 mm, there will be 1° of deviation of the mechanical axis. The most prominent points of the medial and lateral malleoli are then registered. Theses two landmarks help to determine the centre of the ankle point. The medial and lateral borders of tibial plateau are registered for the computer to calculate the width of the tibial plateau. The latter provides the system with the definition of the medial proximal tibial axis, which along with the mechanical axis determines the medial-proximal tibial angle (MPTA). The tibial antero-posterior direction is registered with the computer. The information is used for determining the direction of the tibial slope. The medial and lateral femoral epicondyles are registered percutaneously. They are the references for the relative femoral rotation.

The intra-articular landmarks are registered with arthroscopy (◘ Fig. 65.2). Standard antero-lateral and antero-medial arthroscopic portals were used. The distal point of the mechanical axis of femur is registered. It is about 10 mm anterior to the femoral insertion of posterior cruciate ligament. The proximal point of the mechanical axis of tibia is also registered. It is over the tibial insertion of anterior cruciate ligament. These data are used to define the long leg mechanical axis, and thus the varus/valgus and the flexion/extension alignment of the femur/tibia as well as the tibial posterior slope. The anatomies of the medial and lateral tibial plateaus are then registered. About 30 points are collected on each plateau. This step is for registering the natural tibial slope. The anatomy around the tibial tuberosity is then registered. This guides the surgeon in determining the level of the osteotomy, which is above the tibial tubercle.

The computer will then generate a pre-cut model of the limb. These include the pre-cut deformity and the range of movement before the osteotomy. The computer will calculate the ideal alignment if the mechanical axis is to pass through the Fujisawa point (◘ Fig. 65.3). The surgeon then determines the plane of the osteotomy. The start and end points of the osteotomy are first defined. These two points will determine the initial center of rotation point on the tibia (hinge of the open wedge). The start point (medial) can be determined through the antero-medial longitudinal incision and the end point (lateral) can be determined percutaneously with fluoroscopic guide. The computer can provide information on how far the entry and exit points are from medial and lateral joint line respectively. The surgeon can use this as a guide and compare it with the pre-operative plan. The computer will generate a pre-planned osteotomy plane.

The next step is to determine the actual plane of the osteotomy. This can be done by the insertion of two guide pins. The first guide pin will determine the level and direction of the osteotomy. The second guide pin will determine the slope of the osteotomy. The computer can help to navigate these two guide pins and help the surgeon

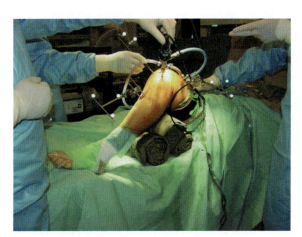

◘ **Fig. 65.2.** Intra-articular registrations through arthroscopy

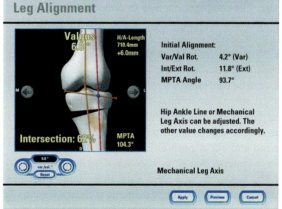

◘ **Fig. 65.3.** Computer calculation of the ideal alignment before the osteotomy was made

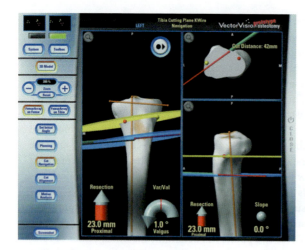

Fig. 65.4. Planning of the osteotomy

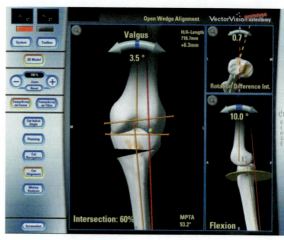

Fig. 65.5. Final alignment of the lower limb

to determine the level and direction of osteotomy and also the slope of the osteotomy (Fig. 65.4). We do not want to change the tibial slope as much as possible.

After all the registrations and guide pins insertion, the osteotomy is performed. The surgeon will make the osteotomy with reference to the guide pins and with the help of fluoroscopy. The completeness of osteotomy has to be determined by the surgeon's experience and also with the help of fluoroscopy. If the osteotomy is opened too early, it may result in intra-articular fracture of tibial plateau. The ideal osteotomy is to leave behind a hinge at the proximal tibial-fibular joint.

The next step is to determine the extent of the opening wedge. The computer can help to decide the limb axis as the surgeon start to open the wedge. The computer can also provide information on how far the limb axis is from the Fujisawa point, and whether the tibial slope changes when the surgeon opens the wedge (Fig. 65.5). The positions can be confirmed with fluoroscopy. In the past when navigation system was unavailable, the author used a long straight rod to check the limb alignment after osteotomy. The long straight rod was positioned over the centers of the hip and ankle, position check with fluoroscopy and then the intersection at the knee was determined.

The wedge is then filled with either bone graft or hydroxyapatite wedge. The osteotomy is fixed with internal fixation device. The computer can also navigate the direction of the drill and thus minimize the risk of intra-articular penetration by screws.

Results

From 2004 to 2005, arthroscopic assisted medial open wedge HTO was performed in six patients. All patients had isolated medial tibial-femoral osteoarthritis. The average age at the time of operation was 50 years old (range 47 to 53). All patients had arthroscopy at the same time of HTO to assess the cartilage status of all three knee compartments. Patients with Outerbridge grade IV degeneration received microfracture at the same time, and partial meniscectomy was performed when there was degenerative tear of the meniscus. The average tourniquet time of the operation was about 30 min more than the conventional HTO.

The average post-operative coronal plane alignment of the lower limb (mechanical axis) was 2.5° valgus. All patients had valgus alignment in the post-operative radiographs (Fig. 65.6). On average, the post-operative radiographic alignment showed 0.8° deviations from the computer output in the operating room. Four cases with post-operative radiographs showed less valgus alignment than the computer output, the other two cases showed more valgus alignment than the computer output.

The average intersection of the mechanical axis of the lower limb over the tibial plateau was 57%. There was an average deviation of 2.8% from the computer. The mechanical axis in the post-operative radiographs tended to be closer to the Fujisawa point than the computer outputs. This might be due to the rotation of the

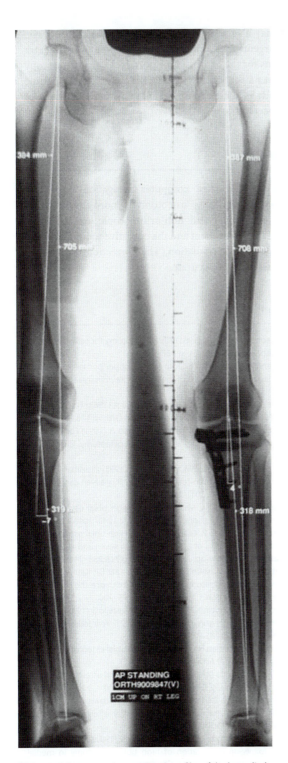

Fig. 65.6. Post-operative standing long film of the lower limb

limb in the operating room that affected the intersections shown on the computer screens. If the limb was in an externally rotated position, the intersection tended to be increased compared with if the limb was in the neutral position.

The average post-operative tibial slope was 7.5°. Compared with the pre-operative radiographs, the tibial slope changed by an average of 0.75° (range, 1° less to 5° more). The tibial slope was not navigated throughout the operation because it needed placement of tracker pins into the proximal tibial osteotomy fragment. The latter was only 3 cm in width, and the tracker pins could hinder the placement of the fixation device.

There was no complication. There was no loss of alignment of the limb at one year follow up.

Discussion

Navigated HTO performed without arthroscopic assistance has been reported by several authors in the past two years. Kendoff et al reported that the correction of MPTA with a fluoroscopy based navigation technique was better than conventional technique [28]. Hüfner et al performed a cadaveric study comparing conventional and navigated HTO, and the navigated HTO was significantly more accurate than conventional HTO [29]. The variability of the corrections was significantly lower in the navigated group. In the multicenter study reported by Wang et al [30], the mean error was 0.9° and the maximum error was 2° in medial open wedge HTO using CT-free navigation. Gebhard et al used an imageless navigation system and alignments were verified with fluoroscopy in the operating room [31]. There was ±2° difference between post-operative radiographs with pre-operative planning. There was also ±2° difference between post-operative radiographs with intra-operative displayed values. Maurer et al reported the use of a CT-free navigation system and found the post-operative leg axis was 3° ± 1° valgus and related exactly to intra-operative measure provided by the navigation system [32]. Wiehe et al. reported good correlation between radiographic data and intra-operative data provided by the computer, there was an average 1.6° of deviation in the coronal plane [33]. Our results obtained with arthroscopic assisted navigated HTO are comparable in this regard.

One advantage of using arthroscopy for the navigated HTO is that the registration of the tibial plateau anatomy enables the surgeon to gather information on the pre-op-erative tibial slope. The latter helps to avoid unintentional change in the tibial slope after the osteotomy. This is impossible for navigated HTO done without arthroscopy. Because of this, the studies mentioned in the above para-graph only addressed alignment in the coronal plane, and did not compare changes in tibial slope between navigated and non-navigated HTO. In the present study, the post-operative tibial slope deviated from the pre-operative sta-tus by an average of 0.75° (range, 1° less to 5° more). The tibial slope determination in this setting may be affected by the problems during the registration process. The surgeon may find it difficult to determine which point is the optimal direction for registration of the tibial antero-posterior axis. To register the most posterior point of the tibial plateau during the arthroscopy may also be difficult. An easy identifiable landmark, e.g. posterior horn of medial of lateral meniscus, may be used for registration. In addition, the deviation in the tibial slope may be due to the cutting error made by the surgeon. Moreover, the placement of the wedge may also affect the posterior tibial slope. If the wedge is placed too anterior, the posterior tibial slope will increase and vice versa.

Arthroscopy at the same time of the navigated HTO offers other advantages. Without arthroscopy, a medial proximal tibial osteophyte may shift the intersection of tibial mechanical axis towards the medial plateau and thus causes under correction of the deformity. With arthrosco-py, the intra-articular anatomic landmarks are visually se-lected, and the accuracy and precision of the mechanical axes formulated can be increased. The appreciation of the tibial plateau anatomy provides invaluable information in helping surgeons to plan the osteotomy and the inser-tion of hardware. Intra-articular fracture and hardware penetration into the joint can thus be minimized even without intra-operative fluoroscopy. In addition, arthros-copy permits concomitant intra-articular procedures to be carried out.

A few downsides exist for arthroscopic assisted navi-gated HTO. It is technically demanding and takes more time than conventional HTO for registration. Registra-tion through arthroscopic portals is not easy. The intact cartilage of the tibial plateau makes it very slippery and it is quite difficult to perform the pivoting action at the start of the registration. If there is any »air point« (reg-istration without actual touching the anatomical land-mark) collected during the registration process, it may affect the overall alignment. The registration process

itself may also scratch and damage the intact cartilage. The surgeon must inform the patients about the extra incisions for the arthroscopic portals. Using arthroscopy to assist navigation in HTO will increase operative time especially in the learning period. This may add costs to the procedure.

Conclusion

Arthroscopic assisted computer navigation in medial open wedge high tibial osteotomy is more advantageous than conventional and non-arthroscopic assisted navi-gated HTO. The patient and the operative room personnel are pone to less irradiation. The correction of the limb alignment is more accurate.

References

1. Jackson JP, Waugh W (1961) Tibial Osteotomy for osteoarthritis of the Knee. J Bone Joint Surg 43B: 746–751
2. Coventry MB (1965) Osteotomy of the upper portion of the tibia for degenerative arthritis of the knee: a preliminary report. J Bone Joint Surg 47A: 984–990
3. Aglietti P, Rinonapoli E, Stringa G, Taviani A (1983) Tibial osteoto-my for the varus osteoarthritic knee. Clin Orthop 176: 239–251
4. Berman AT, Bosacco SJ, Kirshner S, Avolio A (1991) Factors influ-encing long-term results in high tibial osteotomy. Clin Orthop 272: 192–198
5. Coventry MB, Illstrup DM, Wallrichs SL (1993) Proximal tibial os-teotomy: A critical long-term study of eighty-seven cases. J Bone Joint Surg 75A: 196–201
6. Insall JN, Joseph DM, Msika C (1984) High tibial osteotomy for varus gonarthrosis. J Bone Joint Surg 66A: 1040–1048
7. Ivarsson I, Myrnerts R, Gillquist J (1990) High tibial osteotomy for medial osteoarthritis of the knee: A five to seven and an eleven to thirteen year follow-up. J Bone Joint Surg 72B:238–244
8. Matthews LS, Goldstein SA, Malvitz TA, Katz BP, Kaufer H (1988) Proximal tibial osteotomy: Factors that influence the duration of satisfactory function. Clin Orthop 229: 193–200
9. Rinonapoli E, Mancini GB, Corvaglia A, Musiello S (1998) Tibial os-teotomy for varus gonarthrosis. A 10- to 21- Year follow-up study. Clin Orthop 353: 185–193
10. Ritter MA, Fechtman RA (1988) Proximal tibial osteotomy: A survi-vorship analysis. J Arthroplasty 3: 309–311
11. Rudan JF, Simurda MA (1991) Valgus high tibial osteotomy: A long-term follo-up study. Clin Orthop 268: 157–160
12. Stuart MJ, Grace JN, Ilstrup DM, Kelly CM, Adams RA, Morrey BF (1990) Late recurrence of varus deformity after proximal tibial osteotomy. Clin Orthop 260: 61–65
13. Yasuda K, Majima T, Tsuchida T, Kaneda K (1992) A ten to fifteen year follow-up observation of high tibial osteotomy in medial compartment osteoarthritis. Clin Orthop 282: 186–195

14. Koshino T, Yoshida T, Yuki A, Saito I, Saito T (2004) Fifteen to twenty-eight years' follow-up of high tibial valgus osteotomy for osteoarthritic knee. Knee 11: 439–444

15. Naudie D, Bourne RB, Rorabeck CH, Bourne TJ (1999) Survivorship of the high tibial valgus osteotomy. A 10- to 22- Year Follow-up Study. Clin Orthop 367: 18–27

16. Hernigou PH, Medevielle D, Debeyre J, Goutallier D (1987) Proximal tibial osteotomy for osteoarthritis with varus deformity. J Bone Joint Surg 69A: 332–353

17. Wright J, Heck D, Hawker G et al. (1995) Rates of tibial osteotomies in Canada and the United States. Clin Orthop 319: 266–275

18. Maquet P (1976) Valgus osteotomy for osteoarthritis of the knee. Clin Orthop 120: 143–148

19. Sundaram NA, Hallet JP, Sullivan MF (1986) Dome osteotomy of the tibia for osteoarthritis of the knee. J Bone Joint Surg 68B: 782–786

20. Billings A, Scott DF, Camargo MP, Hofmann AA (2000) High tibial osteotomy with a calibrated osteotomy guide, rigid internal fixation, and early motion. J Bone Joint Surg 82A: 70–79

21. Kaper BP, Bourne RB, Rorabeck CH, MacDonald SJ (2001) Patella infera after high tibial osteotomy. J Arthroplasty 16: 168–173

22. Cullu E, Aydogdu S, Alparslan B, Sur H (2005) Tibial slope changes following dome-type high tibial osteotomy. Knee Surg Sports Traumatol Arthrosc 13: 38–43

23. Brouwer RW, Bierma-Zeinstra SMA, Koeveringe AJV, Verhaar JAN (2005) Patellar height and the inclination of the tibial plateau after high tibial osteotomy. The open versus the closed-wedge technique. J Bone Joint Surg 87B: 1227–1232

24. Bonin N, Ait Si Selmi T, Donell ST, Dejour H, Neyret P (2004) Anterior Cruciate reconstruction combined with valgus upper tibial osteotomy: 12 years follow-up. Knee 11: 431–437

25. Noyes FR, Barber SD, Simon R (1993) High tibial osteotomy and ligament reconstruction in varus angulated, anterior cruciate ligament-deficient knees. A two- to seven-year follow-up study. Am J Sports Med 21: 2–12

26. Fujisawa Y, Masuhara K, Shiomi S (1979) The effect of high tibial osteotomy on osteoarthritis of the knee. An arthroscopic study of 54 knee joints. Orthop Clin North Am 10(3): 585–608

27. Keppler P, Gebhard F, Grutzner PA, Wang G, Zheng G, Hufner T, Hankemeier S, Nolte LP (2004) Computer aided high tibial open osteotomy. Injury 35S: A68-A78

28. Kendoff D, Hankemeier S, Wang G, Zheng G, Geerling J, Hüfner T, Notle L, Krettek C (2004) Navigated high tibial osteotomy – experimental comparison to the conventional technique. 4th Annual Meeting of Computer Assisted Orthopaedic Surgery – International Proceedings, pp 44–45

29. Hüfner TM, Hankemeier S, Kendoff D, Wang G, Zheng G, Krettek C (2005) Navigated open wedge high tibia osteotomy – advantages and disadvantages in comparison to the conventional technique in a cadaver study. 5th Annual Meeting of Computer Assisted Orthopaedic Surgery – International Proceedings, pp 168–169

30. Wang G, Zheng G, Grützner PA, Müller-Alsbach UW, Staubli AE, Nolte LP (2004) A generic CT-free intra-operative planning and navigation system for high tibial osteotomy. 4th Annual Meeting of Computer Assisted Orthopaedic Surgery – International Proceedings, pp 42–43

31. Gebhard F, Keppler P, Kuzik J, Maier G (2005) Computer assisted high tibial osteotomy. 5th Annual Meeting of Computer Assisted Orthopaedic Surgery – International Proceedings, pp 106–107

32. Maurer F, Wassmer G (2005) Navigation guided high tibial osteotomy (HTO) – Is it worth the effort? 5th Annual Meeting of Computer Assisted Orthopaedic Surgery – International Proceedings, pp 312–313

33. Wiehe R, Becker U, Bauer G (2005) Does computer-assisted navigation increase the precision of the high tibial osteotomy? 5th Annual Meeting of Computer Assisted Orthopaedic Surgery – International Proceedings, pp 502–504

Navigated Correction Operation of the Pelvis

T. Hüfner, J. Geerling, D. Kendoff, M. Citak, T. Pohlemann, T. Gösling, C. Krettek

Introduction

Non unions or clinical relevant posttraumatic mal-unions of the pelvis are rare entities due to the application of standardized treatment protocols. However, these problems may occur also with an optimal primary treatment [17, 19]. After instable pelvic ring fractures type B and C Tile gives an estimation of about five percent post traumatically mal unions of the pelvis [22]. Other authors report 55 to 75% non unions and mal unions after non operative treatment of pelvic C type fractures [4, 6, 18].

Pain, instabilities and persistent and relevant problems during daily activities are the indication for a correction operation of the pelvis.

Pain is the most frequent symptom, which is related to the instability or the displacement within the sarco-iliacal region [21]. After a correction operation of a mal united pelvic fracture the pain within the posterior pelvic ring can be reduced significantly (16). The clinical diagnosis of a pelvic ring fracture may be quite visible in severe instabilities; the diagnosis of a non union is very difficult with clinical examination only.

Instability with compression can not be provoked frequently by the examiner of the pelvic ring. Weight bearing radiographs with left or right leg standing may be helpful in documentation instability.

In our own experience a fluoroscopy controlled infiltration of painful regions of the pelvic ring with local anesthesia may help also for a more precise diagnosis.

Limping or sitting incongruence are other typical symptoms. Frequently cranial or posterior displacements rota-

tional displacements are to be seen according to the initial pelvic ring fracture (16). With the initial clinical examination these displacements can be diagnosed. Another typical symptom is sitting incongruence as the patient complains about having pain while sitting or lying on the back. An internal rotation of one hemipelvis leading to external rotation of the spina iliaca posterior superior becoming more prominent is the reason therefore is. The sacrum or coccygeum might be prominent as well if one hemipelvis is shifted cranially and may lead to pain while sitting.

Limping is due to a cranial displacement of the hemi pelvis, which leads to functional shortening of the leg. 3 to 6 cm have been described in the literature due to leg differences (16). Internal or external displacements may lead to limping, too.

AP, inlet and outlet views and with acetabular involvements the Judet views as well are the standard radiological examination. These conventional radiographs allow an initial quantitative analysis of the displacement. The cranial displacement is visible in the AP-view and posterior displacements are diagnosed best with the inlet view.

For further thorough analysis the spiral computer tomography is the most important examination. The three dimensional views provide the surgeon with an excellent whole overview of the problem. The reformations in axial sagittal and coronar planes allow an excellent analysis in all planes. The software allows measurements of angles and distances within one millimeter. A model of the pelvis (»rapid prototyping«) may be helpful in special cases.

A thorough neurological examination is essential to exclude other problems according to fresh pelvic ring injuries. Huittinen found 50% neurological lesions with instable pelvic fractures (3). The nerval routes L5 and S1 are most frequently damaged. The other sacral roots may be involved, too. Further neurophysiologic examinations as EMG and ENG may be necessary.

Operation

An extended planning for correction operations of the pelvis is required. After the above mentioned examinations have been done further examinations are necessary. There is the need of knowledge of previous operations (operation report), prior incisions and possible infections (antibiogram).

The operation itself must be planned preoperatively in detail. To achieve a high correction potential Letournell reports three steps of the operation [15]. According to the displacement the patient is first in prone and then in spine and after this again in prone position, changed according to the displacement.

The osteotomy of pelvic or liberating of a non union is the first operation step. After this the mobilization of the hemipelvis and the reduction are done. The definitive stabilization is performed in a third part.

Osteotomies should be done within the old fracture line. Dissection of a sacro-tuberal and sacroiliac ligaments must be done first in case of cranial displacement of a hemipelvis since this is necessary to mobilize the hemipelvis.

Navigated Pelvic Correction Operations

The intra-operative visualization is limited in conventional pelvic correction operations contrary to the pre-operative excellent visualization. The direct visualization is limited with extended approaches and the intra-operative fluoroscopy does not reflect the complex three dimensional displacements.

The advantages and limitations of a navigated correction operation of a mal healed pelvic fracture are discussed in the following case report.

Case Report

Using an ilioinguinal approach an isolated transiliac pelvic ring fracture type C 1 21 was operated in an outside institution [18] and an incomplete reduction was per-

formed using a plate osteosynthesis. 4 months after the motor cycle accident the 22 year old women presented with pain while walking. She required a crutch for walking with full weight-bearing. Mal positioning and partial non union were shown in conventional radiographs and CT. A partial lesion of the ischiadic nerve was found in neurological examination. The operation was planned to be done with navigation. The Surgigate System, (Medivision, Oberdorf, Switzerland) were used with the CT dataset of the pelvis using the spine modul. The operation was performed within three steps. In prone position the dissection of the sacro-tuberal ligaments for mobilization of the right hemipelvis were performed. Suturing was done immediately. Patient was placed in prone position. Using the Kocher–Langenbeck approach a neurolysis of the ischiadic nerve was performed. A partial osteotomy within the primary fracture line was done using navigation (Medivision, Oberdorf, Switzerland). The spine module and navigated chisels from the PAO module were used. After wound closing patient was placed again in supine position. Two dynamic reference bases (DRB) were fixed to the pelvis and the later fragment. Registration was performed after the ilio-inguinal approach was completed. The module developed for periacetabular osteotomies was used [9]. The osteotomy, again navigated, was completed from anterior after implants were removed. Afterwards the navigated reduction was performed. In real-time on the monitor screen the reduction maneuver was controlled. Unfortunately, the DRB placed nearby the symphysis was loosening at the end of the reduction maneuver. Another registration was not possible due to a changed situation compared to the initial CT dataset. The operation was completed in conventional manner.

Discussion

Correction operations of the pelvic ring are rare, usually last long and are patient-loading operations. The intra-operative control of the reduction is done through the approaches supported by fluoroscopy control. Fluoroscopy control should be performed after each reduction at least within three planes (AP, in- and outlet) for three dimensional analysis. The radiation exposure for the patient as well as for the surgeon has to be mentioned. Furthermore, this procedure is time consuming. Implants or retractors can be a limiting factor using intra-operative fluoroscopy as well.

The morbidity for the patient is much higher using extended approaches for better visualization. A prospective study of the pelvis study group of the German Traumatology Society revealed an increased blood loss of 1392 (700–3000 ml) using extended approaches compared to 680 (200–7600 ml) using simple approaches (ilio-inguinal, Kocher-Langenbeck).

Navigation could be the solution for improved results of these operations. It is based on CT datasets providing excellent images. The accuracy is excellent if the registration procedure is performed correct. The surgeon has the three dimensional images displayed on the monitor screen during the critical steps, as osteotomy and reduction. Virtual instruments are displayed in relationship to the patient's anatomy additionally.

This is crucial for perfect cuts and improved reduction and reduced radiation exposure.

The osteotomy is planned on the *intact* pelvis using the PAO module. Within this software there are still some limitations. Cuts can be done only on the three-dimensional model and not using reformations (axial, sagittal and coronar plane). The chisels are not displayed in relationship to the planned cuts during operation. The surgeon must perform the cuts according to the preoperative planning, because an intra-operative deviation of the osteotomy can not be registered by this system.

A potential pitfall might be loosing of the DRB during the reduction maneuver is. The information displayed on the monitor is not correct if this problem is not recognized.

Conclusion and Future Developments

For pelvic correction operations navigation is very helpful. The preoperative planning increases the three-dimensional knowledge of the surgeon. Intra-operatively the increased visualization improves the quality of the cuts and the reduction.

But even with rapidly growing number of clinically available software modules for CT-based navigation systems, available applications are restricted to navigation within a solid bony structure. The accurate reduction is essential in fracture surgery and can influence the immediate course of an operation. The long-term out- come is directly affected by the quality of reduction. This has been reported in several series for pelvic ring and acetabular fractures.

Therefore, an experimental study was performed evaluating the use of a conventional CT-based navigation system (Surgigate™, Medivision, Oberdorf, Switzerland) enhanced by a newly developed software package. The system enables real-time tracking of two fragments for navigated reduction. This alpha-version was developed in cooperation with the Maurice Müller Institute of Biomechanics in Berne, Switzerland. The system to work with volumetric datasets (Voxel graphic) extracted from conventional CT datasets and surface models (vector graphics) due to combination of this software. Automated generated surface models from voxel data enables real-time bone fragment tracking.

For experimental set-up, two models were used: at one plastic model and one anatomic specimen following injury types were created: (a) A combined symphysis and sacroiliac joint disruption, classified as Type 61 C 1.2 according to the AO classification [18] and (b) a combined symphysis disruption and transforaminal sacral fracture, classified as Type 61 C 1.3. [18]

With both objects same experiments were performed. CT data were acquired from each object with the Spiral CT Somatom Plus4 (Siemens, Erlangen, Germany) (140 kV; 171 mA; slice thickness, 2 mm; reconstruction index, 2 mm; pitch, 1 mm). After segmentation and surface generation a dynamic reference base was attached to each fragment. Due to currently only pair-point registration the landmarks were marked with titanium fiducials (diameter, 2 mm) for better reproducibility. Four points per fragment located close to the fracture line are required. Verification was done using a navigated pointing device at the following points: superior and inferior iliac spine, the pubic tubercle, and two specific fiducials at the fracture site. Registration was repeated if one of both, the calculated system error (root mean square error) or verification, was greater than 1 mm. The fragments were fixed to modified three-dimensional holders allowing three-dimensional manipulation and easy fixation. For measurement of the accuracy of the reduction an electromagnetic touchless three-dimensional tracking system (Polhemus, Colchester, VT) was attached to the fragments. The accuracy of the system was 0.1 mm in the translational axes (x, y, and z axes) and 0.1 mm in rotational angles. The Polhemus motion sensor was attached to each fragment and connected to the motion tracking system. Before testing, the fracture plane was defined. With a calibration tool the x and y axes were defined with the fracture reduced (sacroiliac joint, transforaminal sacrum. The z axis was calculated by the tracking system.

Reduction was defied as complete fragment apposition without any step-off. This position was used to calibrate the motion sensor to the start-up position with all axes and angles reset to zero. Without limitation of time using visual controlled reduction with full direct sight and tactile information for definition of the ideal results (control) or solely navigated reduction (monitor sight) with the examiner blinded to the object and manipulating the fragments the reduction was performed only with the three-dimensional arms. During reduction the display on the screen could be manipulated using zooming function or turning the objects to obtain different views – inlet, outlet). The reduction maneuver was performed 20 times. The starting position for reduction was the position of maximum displacement which was equivalent in all trials ($p > 0.05$). The position judged by the examiner as the position of anatomic reduction was defied as the end point of the experiment, only based on the information from the navigation screen. The three-dimensional arms were fixed rigidly preserving the end point position with no additional movement. Data frames were captured continuously during the displacement and reduction maneuver. At the position of maximal displacement and anatomic reduction the position was held for 10 seconds to acquire the data at 1 Hz. The residual displacement was measured in the axes (mm) and angles (degrees). Using Euclidean geometry the resulting reduction accuracy was calculated. The Euclid distance (translation) and the residual rotations were compared with the start-up (zero) position. Statistical analysis using commercially available statistical software (SPSS, SPSS Inc, Chicago, IL) included the Levene test and non-paired t test. The significance level was set at $p < 0.05$.

Within the C 1.2 injury, residual translation was increased for navigated reduction compared to visually controlled reduction in both, foam model or anatomic specimen. ($p < 0.01$). Mean deviation was 1.1 mm for the navigation group. The visual controlled reduction led to significantly lower residual rotation compared with reduction control by navigation ($p < 0.05$).

Residual rotation of the pelvis specimen was lower than the foam models for visual and navigated reduction ($p < 0.05$).

For the C1.3 injury residual translation increased with navigated reduction compared with visual control with an average difference of 0.7 mm.

The residual rotation of the foam models was not increased ($p > 0.05$) using reduction control with navigation., navigated reduction led to increased angles ($p < 0.05$) in pelvic specimen compared with visual controlled reduction. Generally, the specimen models had lower residual rotation when compared with the foam models ($p < 0.05$).

A high intra-operative precision are required for several standard procedures. Navigation systems have been included this precision in the available software including pedicle screw insertion, pelvic osteotomy, and cup and stem implantation of hip prostheses.(7,10–14) The registration procedure required for each bone fragment is one of the limitations of image-guided surgery. Tracking one or several fragments requires tracker fixation to each fragment and independent registration. Some authors reported CT-based navigation for pelvic fracture surgery as fixation of pelvic ring fractures or pelvic non-union. However, in this situations no additional fracture reduction or movement was necessary [5, 23].

A new software for computer-assisted peri-acetabular osteotomy was introduced by Langlotz [11] allowing independent tracking of a second fragment after the osteotomy. The primary registration is limited to the intact pelvis and the second fragment can be generated only virtually in contrast to the presented software prototype. This software has been used successfully for osteotomies and reduction control in late reconstructions of malunited pelvic ring fractures as described above. One main problem is an alteration of the dynamic reference base during these usually long-lasting operations due to repeated manipulations. There is no possibility of an update to the actual situation. By using independent and repetitive registration for each fragment and real-time movement tracking the software version introduced in the current study overcomes these limitations. Currently, only paired-point registration is available. Furthermore these points must be close to the fracture line limiting the setup to experimental design only.

However, in the experimental setup an accurate reduction control was seen. The segmentation algorithm and generation of the surface models were reliable for foam models and specimens. The focus of the study was on clinically relevant issue of residual displacement after pelvic ring reduction. The reduction was monitored and controlled by visual and tactile information or visual control with the navigation system alone. Although the latter provided three-dimensional models, it is a two-dimensional view in contrast to the visual control with real three-dimensional information. This might be one of the reasons why the results differed. Further development of the software may allow axial, sagittal, and coronal planes for preoperative planning and intra-operative performance.

Differences between visual and navigated reduction control were found. However, both groups remained within a range of pelvic reduction which generally is accepted as an anatomic result. Surgeon's observation is limited due to the surgical approach and in minimal techniques by the two dimensional fluoroscopic images. Furthermore bowel gas and obesity can impair observation in closed techniques especially of the posterior pelvic ring, with the risk of increased complication rates. An intra-operative CT scan has been suggested but requires repeated CT data acquisition during a reduction maneuver. These problems could overcome with the proposed reduction module. In the experimental setup used in the current study one disadvantage is the absence of a soft tissue envelope. This may alter the quality of a closed reduction, however, due to intact ligamentotaxis, a more precise outcome is possible. Additional experiments are planned with a more realistic set-up. The smaller residual rotation displacement seen in the specimen when compared with foam models seems to be attributable to a better fit of the fragments after reduction was done. Additional development of the software prototype with integration of surface registration, enhanced surface model generation, and the display of reformatted CT views may lead to improved handling and facilitated multifragment tracking. Use in the clinical setting seems possible in the near future.

References

1. Bosch U, Pohlemann T, Haas N, Tscherne H (1992) Klassifikation und Management des komplexen Beckentraumas. Unfallchirurg 95: 189–196
2. Hüfner T, Pohlemann T, Gänsslen A et al. (1999) Computer assisted surgery for correction of a malhealed pelvic ring fracture in a young female patient. Comput Aided Surg 4: 154
3. Huittinen V, Slätis, P (1972) Nerve injury in double vertical pelvic fractures. Acta Chir Scand 138: 571–575
4. Hundley J (1966) Ununited unstable fractures of the pelvis. J Bone Joint Surg 48-A: 1025
5. Kahler DM, Zura RD, Mallik K (2000) Computer Guided Placement of Iliosacral Screws Compared to Standard Fluoroscopic Technique. In: Nolte LP (ed). Fifth International Symposion on Computer Assisted Orthopedic Surgery. Davis, Switzerland
6. Kellam J (1989) The role of external fixation in pelvic disruptions. Clin Orthop 241: 66–82
7. Laine T, Lund T, Ylikoski M, Lohikoski J, Schlenzka D (2000) Accuracy of pedicle screw insertion with and without computer

8. Laine T, Makitalo K, Schlenzka D et al. (1997) Accuracy of pedicle screw insertion: a prospective CT study in 30 low back patients. Eur Spine J 6(6): 402–405
9. Langlotz F, Bächler R, Berlemann U, Nolte LP, Ganz R (1998) Computer assistance for pelvic osteotomies. Clin Orthop 354: 92–102
10. Langlotz F, Bächler R, Berlemann U, Nolte LP, Ganz R (1998) Computer assistance for pelvic osteotomies. Clin Orthop 354: 92–102
11. Langlotz F, Stucki M, Bächler R, Ganz R, Nolte LP (2000) A novel system for complete THR planning and intraoperative free-hand navigation. In: Nolte LP (ed) Fifth International Symposium on Computer Assisted Orthopedic Surgery. Davis, Switzerland
12. Langlotz U, Langlotz F, Hiogne D, Rohrer U, Nolte LP (2000) A novel system for complete THR planning and intraoperative free-hand navigation. In: Nolte LP (ed) Fifth International Symposium on Computer Assisted Orthopedic Surgery. Davos, Switzerland
13. Lavallée S, Sautot P, Troccaz J, Cinquin P, Merloz P (1995) Computer-assisted spine surgery: A technique for accurate transpedicular screw.xation using CT data and a 3-D optical localizer. J Image Guid Surg 1: 65–73
14. Lavallée S, Troccaz J, Sautot P et al. (1996) Computer-assisted spine surgery using anatomy-based registration. In: Taylor R, Lavallée S, Burdea G, Moesges R (eds) Computer-integrated surgery. MIT Press, Cambridge, pp 77–97
15. Letournel E (1993) Open reduction internal fixation of acetabular fractures: long term results and analysis of 1040 cases. 1st International Symposium on surgical treatment of acetabular fractures, May 10–11, Paris, 1993
16. Matta J, Dickson K, Markovich G (1996) Surgical treatment of pelvic nonunions and malunions. Clin Orthop 329: 199–206
17. Matta J, Saucedo T (1989) Internal fixation of pelvic ring fractures. Clin Orthop 242: 83–97
18. Orthopedic Trauma Association Committee for coding and classification (1996) Fracture and dislocation compendium. J Orthop Trauma 10 (Suppl 1): V–IX
19. Pennal G, Massiah K (1980) Nonunion and delayed union of fractures of the pelvis. Clin Orthop 151: 124–129
20. Routt Jr ML, Simonian PT, Mills WJ (1997) Iliosacral screw fixation: Early complications of the percutaneous technique. J Orthop Trauma 11: 584-589
21. Semba R, Yasukawa K, Gustillo R (1983) Critical analysis of results 53 Malgaigne fractures of the pelvis. J Trauma 23(6): 535–537
22. Tile M (1988) Pelvic ring fractures: should they be fixed? J Bone Joint Surg 70-B: 1–12
23. Zura RD, Kahler DM (2000) A transverse acetabular nonunion treated with computer-assisted percutaneous internal fixation: A computer-assisted surgery report. J Bone Joint Surg 82A: 219–224

Computer-Assisted Osteosynthesis of Long Bone Fractures

P.A. Grützner, G. Zheng, C. Keil, L.P. Nolte, A. Wentzensen, J. von Recum, F. Langlotz, N. Suhm

Introduction

The fluoroscope, also know as C-arm, is the most important and most commonly used imaging modality in traumatology and orthopaedic surgery. It is an important instrument for intra-operative diagnostics, for the precise visualization of an achieved fracture reduction, for the position checking of surgical instruments such as drill bits, and for the verification of the correct placement of osteosynthesis material or joint replacement.

In recent decades traumatological techniques underwent considerable modifications. While in the past, fractures used to be exposed considerably and stabilized with accordingly sized plates, it is now commonly agreed that the technique of minimally invasive osteosynthesis is superior. The concept includes the closed fracture reduction with correct alignment of axes, the rotation and correct reconstruction of length whereas the former goal of anatomical reconstruction has been abandoned except for articular fractures. Minimization of the skin incision and reduction of the induced soft tissue damage result in a number of considerable advantages for the patient including the cosmetic result as well as improvements regarding function and time of healing.

One of the difficulties related to minimally invasive techniques in fracture treatment is caused by the absence of direct visual contact to the implant inside the bone and to the currently achieved reduction. As a consequence, the fluoroscope is used more intensively during modern surgical techniques. For that reason, both, patient and surgical staff are exposed to high radiation doses [5, 8]. In addition, C-arm imaging suffers from certain restrictions. Each image is a two-dimensional projective representation. Moreover, only one fluoroscope is usually available. i.e., only one projection may be visualized at a time, requiring permanent repositioning of the C-arm. The surgeon must position the implant in one view, and then obtain additional images in other planes for trial and error placement of the implant. During image acquisition, the device must be placed in the operation field, potentially hindering surgical treatment.

The integration of conventional fluoroscopes into computer-assisted navigation systems has been established as one means to overcome certain of these drawbacks and to establish solutions or elements of solutions to the describe problems [1, 3, 4, 6].

Although a number of authors report excellent experiences with currently existing systems for virtual fluoroscopy, two disadvantages of these devices can be identified during routine clinical usage. The purely linear, two-dimensional representation of surgical tools represents the tracked objects only in a rather abstract way. Moreover, changes in the bony anatomy due to fracture reduction or osteotomies can be respected only by the re-acquisition of C-arm images which imposes additional radiation to patient and surgical staff and requires re-positioning of the fluoroscope with respect to the patient.

Materials and Method

Intra-Operative Guidance by Virtual Fluoroscopy for Distal Interlocking

In one clinical application we applied intra-operative guidance by virtual fluoroscopy for drilling the distal locking holes during intra-medullary nailing osteosynthesis.

Though locked nailing is a standard surgical technique in the operative treatment of diaphyseal fractures, insertion of distal interlocking bolts remains technically demanding. Mechanical or fluoroscopic guidance are commonly applied to pass the drill through the interlocking hole. For mechanical guidance methods, the precision of bolt placement is typically problematic; for fluoroscopic guidance methods, the fluoroscopic time is the issue. Applying virtual fluoroscopy to drill the holes for distal locking suggests improvements in these two points [7].

The intra-operative setup as position of the computer cart, tracking device, C-arm fluoroscope and nail reference base varied with the fracture to be treated and with the type of implant used. Principally the computer cart should be placed opposite to the surgeon in order to guarantee direct sight on the computer screen. The tracking unit should be localized behind the surgeon to secure visibility of all reference bases during image acquisition and drilling the interlocking holes. Guidance is required in a single plane for distal interlocking and the nail is the object to target at.

Computer-assisted distal locking of intra-medullary implants was performed in two steps: First, computer controlled precision alignment of the fluoroscope. Proper alignment of the fluoroscope prior to image acquisition is an essential prerequisite for successful distal locking: after implantation into the medullary canal of the long bone the implants locking holes must be imaged as perfect circles. To perform computer controlled precision alignment of the fluoroscope, the nail reference base was rigidly connected with the nail insertion handle prior to implantation. The C-arm fluoroscope was positioned until the interlocking holes were imaged as perfect circles. A single fluoroscopic shot was transferred to the SurgiGATE system.

The drill-bit was calibrated for the actual position within the referenced driver. When the referenced driver approached the interlocking holes, it's actual position is projected into the fluoroscopic image that was displayed on the workstation screen.

The drill bit was moved along the surface of the bone until the simulated drill tip was projected into the center of the distal interlocking hole. The entrance point was fixed by impression of the drill's tip into the bone. Next, the longitudinal axis of the drill was aligned parallel to the axis of the interlocking hole and the length measuring algorithm was initiated. After penetration the bone's second cortex, the length measuring algorithm was stopped and the distance passed by the drill was displayed. This allowed determination the correct length of the interlocking bolt.

Clinical evaluation included recording precision of the interlocking procedure, fluoroscopy time and procedure time needed for computer assisted distal locking. Problems with technical equipment during the procedure were reported [9].

Virtual Fluoroscopy for Guide-Wire Placement

In a second application, intra-operative guidance by virtual fluoroscopy was applied for guidewire placement during DHS implantation to stabilize pertrochanteric femoral fractures and during screw fixation of femoral neck fractures. In these applications simultaneous guidance in multiple views is required and the proximal femoral bone is the referenced object to target at.

The principle is to perform fracture reduction and temporary fracture fixation with Kirschner wires. Next, the DRB is fixed to a Schanz screw that is inserted into the proximal femoral bone through a stab wound. Anterior-posterior and axial fluoroscopic shots of the proximal femoral bone are acquired, transferred to the navigation system and the C-arm fluoroscope is removed from the patient.

The entrance point and axis of the guide-wire is simulated and thus can be corrected simultaneously in both fluoroscopic image planes. Correct guide-wire placement was verified fluoroscopically prior to implant insertion.

Reality Enhancement

For the integration of the three-dimensional geometry of navigated instruments and implants into the navigation process, it was hypothesized, that by this approach more complex objects such as osteosynthesis plates or nails could be visualized within C-arm images in a more realistic way. For this purpose, three-dimensional computer aided design (CAD) drawings served as input. To avoid the re-acquisition of images after bony manipulations, the simultaneous dynamization of conventional fluoroscopic images in different projection planes was developed. Dynamization denotes the segmentation of bony objects within individual images and the independent referencing and tracking of the associated fragments. It was assumed that this technique would enable a more realistic visualization of the three-dimensional fracture reduction process in navigated C-arm images.

The interactive segmentation of the images uses a concept of »virtual cylinders« that benefits from the cylindrical shape of long bones. In a first step, at least two two-dimensional projections of each fragment are framed by a three-dimensional cylinder. The cylinder is created semi automatically by drawing the contour of the bones in the registered images in different planes. Then the cylinder is used to separate the fragment that it encapsulates from the background of the X-ray image. Spatial changes in position of the associated bone object (as determined by the independent tracking) can then be reflected by synchronously moving the segmented image section over the static background (◻ Fig. 67.1).

It is therefore possible to control the reduction process in real-time in a radiation-free manner. A further step towards enhanced reality in virtual fluoroscopy is the aforementioned three-dimensional visualization of tools in two-dimensional images. Using the known locations of the X-ray source and intensifier unit during image acquisition as well as two projected images, a three-dimensional space is reconstructed in which the operated bony structures and all navigated tools are placed in relation to each other [2]. Correct proportions of the implant and the bone are being adapted automatically (◻ Fig. 67.2).

The Less Invasive Stabilization System LISS® (Stratec-Medical, Oberdorf, Switzerland) is an osteosynthesis system allowing minimally invasive fixation of problematic metaphyseal fractures with angular stabilization. In a sense it is comparable to an internal fixator. However, its implantation is challenging and usually does not forgive any errors. The usual »reduction against the plate« known from conventional fracture treatment is inapplicable. Instead the implant has to fit the convexity of the bone precisely. After successful laboratory evaluation the newly developed module was integrated into the existing navigation system. This technology was then applied during osteosynthesis supported by LISS for the first time in our clinic. We performed a consecutive case study of three patients with four fractures of the proximal tibia between June and August 2001. All patients were primary fixed with an external fixator or unreamed tibia nailing

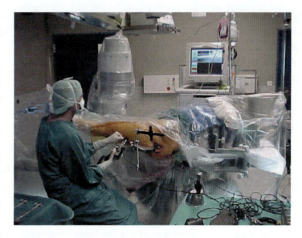

◻ **Fig. 67.1.** Computer assisted distal locking of a PFN® implant. The cross-shaped nail DRB is attached to the insertion handle. The referenced drill is moved along the bone surface. The actual drills position is projected into the stored fluoroscopic images on the computer screen in front of the surgeon. The C-arm fluoroscope is removed from the patient

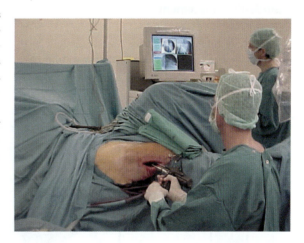

◻ **Fig. 67.2.** Guide-wire placement with biplane virtual fluoroscopic guidance. The bone reference and the referenced driver are visible for the tracking unit (not visible). The C-arm fluoroscope is removed from the patient

and secondary stabilized with the LISS. In two patients a proximal tibia fractures in combination with severe soft tissue damage (3°) due to the accident were present. In the primary treatment the fractures were stabilized by external fixation. The soft tissue damage was treated by local flaps or skin transplantation. After healing of the soft tissue the treatment was changed from external fixation to internal stabilization. One patient was treated with an unreamed tibia nail in another hospital with a proximal tibia fracture and 2° soft-tissue damage. In this patient a severe instability was remaining. All patients were in follow-up for 18 months.

Intra-operatively OR time, blood loss, and X-ray duration were recorded. The sequence of the navigation part of the OR was as followed described.

First, DRBs were fixed to the proximal and distal main fragments. Fluoroscopic images were acquired in two different planes both, proximally and distally of the fractures as well as at the levels of the fractures. Subsequently, the fractures were reduced and fixated. With the help of virtual cylinders three-dimensional structures were created from the image pairs that represented the bone volumes.

Results

Pilot Study with Virtual Fluoroscopy Applied for Guide-Wire Placement

In a pilot study computer guidance was successfully applied for guidewire placement in 11 patients with proximal femoral fractures. In seven patients the guidewire for a Dynamic Hip Screw (DHS, Stratec, Oberdorf, Switzerland) could be placed exactly within the femoral neck during osteosynthesis of pertrochanteric femoral fractures (◘ Fig. 67.3). In four patients guide-wires were placed for fixation of femoral neck fractures with cannulated screws. No intra-operative problems have been observed within these early clinical applications.

Controlled Prospective Clinical Study on Guidance Methods for Distal Interlocking

Computer-assisted distal locking was evaluated in a controlled clinical study with two branches. Patients in both branches were divided into control group and study group. For patients diagnosed with pertrochanteric femoral fractures (study branch 1) distal locking was performed with mechanical guidance in the control group and with virtual fluoroscopy in the study group. For patients diagnosed with diaphyseal fractures of the lower extremity (study branch 2) distal locking was performed with fluoroscopic guidance in the control group and with virtual fluoroscopy in the study group (◘ Table 67.1).

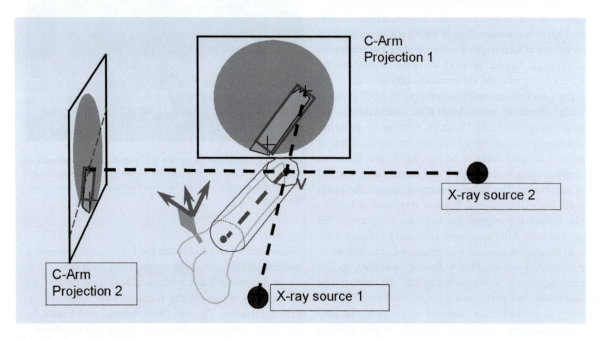

◘ **Fig. 67.3.** Virtual three-dimensional space created from two-dimensional X-ray projections

◩ **Table 67.1.** Results of the controlled prospective clinical study for distal locking. In study branch 1 (grey) virtual fluoroscopy was compared with mechanical guidance. In study branch 2 virtual fluoroscopy was compared with fluoroscopic guidance. The accuracy achieved while drilling the interlocking holes was rated as misplaced interlocking hole/drilling the hole with contact to the implant/ drilling the hole without contact to the implant

Guidance method	Virtual fluoroscopy	Mechanical	Virtual fluoroscopy	Fluoroscopy
Patients (n)	26	24	25	19
Procedure time (min)	38	6.5	17	12.5
Fluoroscopy time (s)	6	6	6	107
Intra-operative Problems	4	2	3	1
Accuracy	(2/8/35)	(1/13/31)	(2/11/28)	(1/9/31)

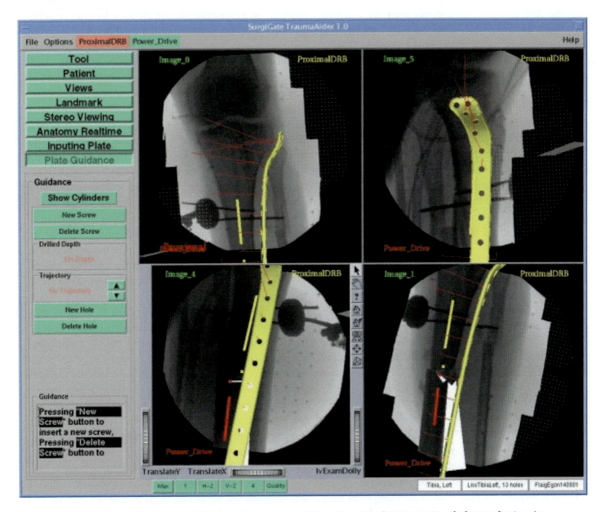

◩ **Fig. 67.4.** User interface with visualization of X-ray dynaminization and three-dimensional representation of a fracture fixation plate

Virtual fluoroscopy required significantly shorter fluoroscopy time than fluoroscopic guidance (p<0.0001) but in both branches caused a significant increase of the procedure time (virtual fluoroscopy versus mechanical guidance (p<0.0001); virtual fluoroscopy versus fluoroscopic guidance (p=0.029)) and in the number of intraoperative problems compared with the standard guidance techniques.

Reality Enhancement

As a result, the acquired images could dynamized, and the entire reduction procedure could be carried out without additional fluoroscopic checking. In real-time the LISS plates, the drill and the screw driver with the attached screws were visualized three-dimensionally and in their correct spatial relation to the acquired images. The introduction of the plates as well as the subsequent fixation procedure could be navigated including drilling, depth measurement, and screw insertion. For verification purposes, the acquisition of two C-arm images of the fracture area completed the procedure. These final images were acquired from different directions with both DRBs as well as the LISS marker shield still in place. As a consequence the resulting images could be re-loaded into the navigation system and the matching between the X-ray shadow of the implanted plate and its overlaid graphical model could be verified.

It turned out to be possible to carry out the entire reduction and fixation procedure under navigational guidance without the need for additional image updates and associated radiation exposure. During all four surgeries correct fracture reduction and plate placement was achieved at first trial. Disadvantageous were the uncomfortable interface of this prototype software and the necessity to have an additional person control the application. Compared to the conventional approach, the additional need of OR time to be about 15 min (range from 10 to 20).

Discussion and Conclusion

The goal of virtual fluoroscopy is to supply an adequate means for intra-operative guidance in order to improve efficiency of image guided orthopedic procedures.

There is no need for preoperative planning steps such as image processing or interactive definition of anatomical landmarks. The system does not require the intra-operative registration of preoperative image data (matching) as it is mandatory for CT based navigation. Another advantage of virtual fluoroscopy is the ability to update the navigational image data at any time, which may appear necessary after changes to the anatomical situation due to fracture reduction maneuvers or osteotomies.

Our controlled clinical study on computer guidance by virtual fluoroscopy for distal locking demonstrated the capability of such system to provide online guidance with significantly reduced fluoroscopy times. As distal locking of intra-medullary implants requires guidance in a single plane, this clinical model is not able to demonstrate all the advantages offered by virtual fluoroscopy such as simultaneous multiplanar guidance. Virtual fluoroscopy applied for guide-wire placement in a laboratory setup demonstrated the potential of the method to reduce procedure times.

The proposed virtual cylinder concept, combined with the virtual fluoroscopy, provides the surgeon with 3D virtual models of the fractured fragments, and includes several advantages. It allows disposing simultaneously several views of the fractured, bone during reduction. It is possible to visualize the fracture from any viewpoint. With this reality augmented navigation system, a close, indirect reduction in the real word has been turned into an open, direct reduction in the virtual world. It allows controlling instruments through direct insight in the virtual world. Furthermore, it also facilitates the effective extraction of the contour of the fragment projection image. The further development leads to an algorithm that for the first time allows the radiation free updates of fluoroscopic images, which decreases considerably the radiation exposure of the surgical team.

A universal concept is also proposed to navigate various implants into various surgical guidance systems. It allows not only realistic visualization of virtual implants but also provides the surgeon with additional navigation information and functional parameters for a specific implant. A generic database structure, combined with two generic operations defined on it, allows easy extension with any newly developed implants on the one hand, and flexible integration with any navigation system on the other hand. Our preliminary work on integrating LISS plate for fracture reduction and fixation has verified these points.

The proposed non-photorealistic rendering methods for visualization of virtual surgical instruments or implants not only allow the surgeon to interpret the associated 3D structures but also keep the image details from occlusion for a better understanding the positional relationship between surgical instruments or implants and underlying anatomies, taking the acquired image as the projection background.

However, there are several advantages observed in this preliminary clinical trial. The fracture reduction could be achieved and monitored for the whole surgical procedure without acquiring new fluoroscopic images. This would have required the use of four C-arms operating in constant mode from different viewing angle. The visualization of fracture reduction and the implant placement could be achieved simultaneously. This paves the way for less invasive fracture reduction and fixation. In our clinical cases, no implant misplacement or replacement intra-operatively due to the direct visual feedback provided by the reality augmented virtual system was observed. All implants could be optimally placed in the first try. There was very low radiation time observed compared to the conventional procedure.

Navigation systems are quickly spreading through operating rooms in traumatology and orthopedics. This technology does not turn novices into experts, but should be seen as a useful tool for the experienced surgeon that helps improving the quality of the process and the outcome while decreasing variability. Our experiences indicate that only the consequent application of navigation even during standard cases leads to acceptance by the surgical staff and ultimately to trust and safety when using the system. Future will show if only the individual patient can directly benefit from this technology or if it also has positive socio-economic effects by reducing the intra-operative complication rate.

Navigation systems, and in particular the utilized software programs, undergo constant improvements including better user interfaces, easier interaction, and last but not least reduced costs. As a consequence their broader application can be foreseen.

Future advancements of our system aim at the simplification of the intra-operative setup, the improvement of image quality, and the adaptation of new instruments. Although the virtual cylinder concept that we presented in the thesis allows effective bone extraction from fluoroscopic images, it can only provide a rough approximation of real reality. More development needs to be done to transfer the simplified augmented reality approaches towards a full 3D virtual surgical scene. Three-dimensional model reconstruction based on a limited number of

registered projections should be investigated. The reconstructed model could be used to provide a more precise representation of the associated anatomy.

The preliminary implementation of the proposed concept for navigating various implants could be further expanded. The solutions realized so far are focused on a particular type of implant and do not define a common data format to store these information for usage for various planning and navigation applications.

The potential of the technique appears tremendous. Advantages that can be identified already now include the reduction of intra-operative radiation doses to the patient and surgical staff, as well as the improved operative precision providing more safety to the patient.

Navigated osteosynthesis can overcome the disadvantages of the minimally invasive procedure by visualizing reduction, implant placement, and fixation.

References

1. Foley KT, Simon DA, Rampersaud YR (2001) Virtual fluoroscopy: computer-assisted fluoroscopic navigation. Spine 26: 347–351
2. Grützner PA, Vock B, Zheng G, Kowal J, Nolte L, Wentzensen A (2001) Minimal invasive, computerassistierte Plattenosteosynthese bei Frakturen langer Röhrenknochen. Hefte zu: Der Unfallchirurg 283: 160
3. Hofstetter R, Slomczykowski M, Sati M, Nolte LP (1999) Fluoroscopy as an imaging means for computer-assisted surgical navigation. Comput Aided Surg 4: 65–76
4. Nolte LP, Slomczykowski MA, Berlemann U et al. (2000) A new approach to computer-aided spine surgery: fluoroscopy-based surgical navigation. Eur Spine J 9 (Suppl 1): S78–S88
5. Rampersaud YR, Foley KT, Shen AC, Williams S, Solomito M (2000) Radiation exposure to the spine surgeon during fluoroscopically assisted pedicle screw insertion. Spine 25: 2637–2645
6. Slomczykowski MA, Hofstetter R, Sati M, Krettek C, Nolte LP (2001) Novel computer-assisted fluoroscopy system for intraoperative guidance: feasibility study for distal locking of femoral nails. J Orthop Trauma 15: 122–131
7. Suhm N (2001) Intraoperative accuracy evaluation of virtual fluoroscopy-A method for application in computer-assisted distal locking. Comput Aided Surg 6: 221–224
8. Suhm N, Jacob AL, Zuna I, Roser HW, Regazzoni P, Messmer P (2001) Radiation exposure of the patient by intraoperative imaging of intramedullary osteosyntheses. Radiologe 41: 91–94
9. Suhm N, Jacob AL, Zuna I, Regazzoni P, Messmer P (2003) Fluoroskopiebasierte chirurgische Navigation versus mechanisches Zielsystem für perkutane Eingriffe. Unfallchirurg 106: 921–928

Navigated Screw Placement in Sacro-Iliac Trauma

D.M. Kahler

Introduction

The modern trauma surgeon makes heavy use of intraoperative radiographic imaging in the form of c-arm fluoroscopy. Most orthopaedic surgeons are very proficient in the use of this standard technique for minimally invasive implant placement. Unfortunately, the decreased invasiveness that is facilitated by image-intensification comes at the expense of significant radiation exposure for both the patient and the surgeon. There is also a risk of inadvertent damage to important structures during the first pass of the drill or guide wire, as conventional imaging is available in only one plane at a time. The risk of iatrogenic injury increases when working around the complicated anatomy of the pelvis.

Complete disruptions of the posterior pelvic ring are severe injuries that usually require surgical stabilization. The initial goals of surgical management focus on pelvic ring reduction and fixation to control bleeding, promote safe mobilization, and decrease the chance of further morbidity [1, 2]. Initial stabilization of the pelvic ring with an external fixator can promote tamponade of bleeding sites. Definitive management of these injuries using anterior external fixation alone is often associated with loss of reduction and unacceptable shortening of the extremity [3]. For definitive management of the unstable posterior pelvis, internal fixation has been shown to be superior to both external fixation and non-operative treatment, especially for posterior disruptions involving the sacroiliac joint alone [4, 5].

The high complication rates reported with formal open exposure of the pelvis and acetabulum have led to increased interest in the use of percutaneous procedures. Less invasive techniques have the potential to minimize the morbidity associated with treatment of these fractures. When combined with appropriate anterior pelvic ring fixation, percutaneous placement of iliosacral screws using fluoroscopic guidance has been shown to provide stable fixation and eliminates the wound complications associated with open surgical approaches [6, 7]. Accurate screw placement, however, requires excellent image intensification in the operating room, as well as an appreciation of the appropriate pelvic radiographic landmarks [8]. The use of fluoroscopy is technically demanding in terms of positioning of the unit and patient, the requirement for frequent and repeated imaging, and alternating between the various views necessary for visualization of implant placement. Intra-operative radiographic visualization may be limited due to patient obesity, excessive bowel gas, or the presence of radiographic contrast media in the bowel. There is significant risk of injury to the L5 or S1 nerve roots, cauda equina, or major vessels if pertinent radiographic landmarks are not adequately visualized [9]. The safe target zone for screw placement in some cases measures less than one centimeter in its minor diameter [2]. Nonetheless, ilio-sacral screw placement using intra-operative fluoroscopy has been shown to be effective for percutaneous fixation of posterior pelvic ring disruptions, and remains the most popular conventional technique [2, 6, 7].

Another concern is radiation exposure to the patient and surgeon, as percutaneous techniques typically require heavy reliance on intra-operative fluoroscopic imaging. It has recently been demonstrated that the radiation safety guidelines established by the Occupational Safety and Health Administration (OSHA) are probably routinely exceeded by practicing orthopaedic surgeons during their careers, and possibly even during residency [10]. Current radiation safety guidelines abandon strict limits for radiation exposure in favor of »ALARA« (As Low As Reasonably Attainable), meaning that any option that decreases radiation exposure should be routinely employed. It should always be remembered that the patient, rather than the surgeon, absorbs most of the ionizing radiation used during C-arm based minimally invasive surgery.

The quest for decreased invasiveness, improved accuracy, and decreased radiation exposure has recently led to increased interest in computer-assisted orthopaedic surgery (CAOS). In general, computer-guided techniques utilize a stored patient-specific imaging data to provide intra-operative guidance, rather than relying on continuous updating of a fluoroscopic image in the operating room. This technology is often referred to as image-guided surgery (IGS), or surgical navigation, and has recently been applied to the treatment of traumatic injuries to the pelvis [11–13]. Although this technology has been used successfully in other fields, such as neurosurgery and otolaryngology, it has been relatively slow to gain traction in the orthopaedic community.

The development of computer-assisted surgical navigation has made it possible to accurately place cannulated screws in the pelvis using percutaneous technique, using stored radiographic images rather than real-time radiographic guidance. There are currently two basic types of image guided surgery techniques for trauma: 3D-CT technique, and fluoroscopic navigation.

The 3D-CT technology was adapted for use in orthopaedic trauma in 1997. This technique relies on a pre-operatively obtained CT scan that is then loaded onto an IGS system. Using a CT-derived virtual model on a computer workstation, the surgeon may pre-operatively plan an optimal trajectory for screw placement. Optically tracked surgical instruments are then used to precisely execute the surgical plan in the operating room. Unfortunately, the reliance on the preoperative CT for guidance limits the utility of this technique in trauma cases where a reduction is necessary, as any manipulation of the fracture corrupts the stored 3D model, making it unsuitable for use in navigation. This limited the use of the 3D-CT technique to fractures in which a reduction was not necessary,

or in which a closed reduction could be obtained with an external fixator prior to CT imaging.

A newer technology, fluoroscopic navigation, allows intra-operative harvesting and storage of multiple images following fracture reduction. These stored images are then used during implant placement. Fluoroscopic navigation systems became available for clinical use in 1999, and are now marketed by several manufacturers. This technology provides multiplanar guidance during implant placement without the need for repeated fluoroscopic imaging, and has essentially replaced 3D-CT technique in the authors practice. The chief advantage of fluoroscopic navigation over 3D-CT technique is that the surgeon may easily obtain additional images for navigation following a reduction maneuver or implant placement. This advantage makes fluoroscopic navigation more versatile in fracture management, and greatly expands the indications for the use of IGS in routine fracture care.

In this study, early surgical experience with computer-assisted technique is compared to conventional fluoroscopic technique in order to determine its relative merit with regard to accuracy, operative time, and radiation exposure to both the patient and the surgeon. The study group consists of patients with posterior pelvic ring disruptions treated between 1997 and 2003 using computer-assisted technique. Surgical experience in this group is compared to a series of patients treated in the prior two years using conventional percutaneous fluoroscopic technique.

Methods and Surgical Technique

3D-CT Technique

An existing system for pedicle screw placement (Stealth-Station, Sofamor-Danek, Memphis, TN) was modified for use in pelvic trauma in 1996, by increasing the field of view and incorporating a paired point registration system using an external fixator. Based on the favorable results of a cadaver feasibility study [2], approval was granted to proceed with clinical use of the integrated computer guidance system. The orthopaedic software package was granted a Food and Drug Administration exemption in February, 1997.

Patients undergoing computer-assisted internal fixation for posterior pelvic ring disruption were typically provisionally stabilized by the application of an anterior

68

pelvic external fixator. A fiducial array with four aluminum spherical fiducials was attached to the patient's anterior iliac crest on the contralateral side of the disruption using standard external fixator components, or to the anterior frame itself. Each patient received a preoperative CT scan to allow segmentation of the pelvis and fiducials. The digitized CT scans were downloaded to the integrated computer workstation. An array of three CCD digital cameras attached to a boom positioned over the operative field provides optical tracking of the surgical instruments and patient. A dynamic reference frame with four light emitting diodes (LEDs) was clamped to the threaded end of the fiducial array on the external fixator in order to allow optical tracking of the pelvis as a rigid body. This safety feature allows continuous tracking of the pelvis in the operating room in case of camera or patient movement during the operative procedure.

A volumetric three-dimensional reconstruction of the pelvis and fiducials was built as a virtual model on the workstation. Each fiducial was registered on the virtual pelvis model by centering cross hairs on each aluminum sphere in three planes. During surgery, proper orientation was provided by sequentially registering each actual fiducial on the external fixator, using a concave hemisphere-tipped probe equipped with LED's to allow optical tracking.

The registration process essentially shows the computer the location of the patient's pelvis in the operating room. The pelvis is then continually tracked during the procedure by the dynamic reference frame in the event of any patient or camera movement, preventing the need for repeated registration. Limited fluoroscopy is then used to identify bony landmarks and validate the accuracy of registration prior to proceeding. Using this paired-point registration scheme, mean fiducial registration error of less than 0.5 mm was routinely obtained.

A surgical plan was created pre-operatively by selecting appropriate entry and exit points on the three-dimensional model on the workstation. The path of fixation is represented in two perpendicular navigation views along the intended path of the screw. The workstation calculates the path length of the surgical plan, thereby accurately determining the length of the screw required. A stop is placed on the guide wire to prevent drilling beyond the end of the surgical plan.

In most cases, acceptable reduction of the sacral fracture or sacroiliac disruption was obtained at the time of initial external fixation, and the pelvis was then internally fixed in situ. Using a calibrated LED-equipped drill guide with a power drill, a 2.8-mm guide wire was drilled into the safe zone of the S1 body as determined by the surgical plan. The workstation produces real time feedback of the drill guide trajectory on the two orthogonal projections of the surgical plan, while also displaying the planned path of fixation. The goal was to precisely match the planned trajectory when passing the guide wire (🞏 Fig. 68.1).

After placing the guide wire to the appropriate depth, final fluoroscopic radiographic images were taken to confirm accurate guide wire placement. The appropriate 7.3 mm screw (Synthes, West Chester, PA) was then passed over the guide wire. The only radiation requirements intra-operatively were the few seconds of fluoroscopy required for validation of accuracy of registration and screw placement.

During the three years following approval of the system for clinical use, computer assisted fixation was performed in 21 cases of posterior pelvic ring disruption in 17 patients. Operative time and fluoroscopy time was recorded for the 27 screws placed using 3D-CT computer assisted technique.

Fluoroscopic Navigation

Fluoroscopic navigation became available for clinical use in 1999. This technology relies on retrofitting of a standard C-arm fluoroscopy unit with a calibration target. The target may then be tracked by the IGS system while fluoroscopic images are being obtained. The images are then warped by the IGS system to eliminate distortion and make them suitable for navigation. As with 3D-CT technique, a reference frame is attached to the patient's pelvis, allowing tracking of the patient during imaging and insertion of the guide wire. Fluoroscopic images are then obtained and stored on the IGS workstation (VectorVision, BrainLAB AG, Munich; or iON/FluoroNav, Medtronic, Memphis, TN). Up to four images may be simultaneously displayed on the workstation. Pelvic inlet, outlet, AP, and oblique lateral views are typically obtained for navigation during iliosacral screw insertion. An optically tracked drill guide is brought into the surgical field, and recognized by the IGS system. The position of the drill guide can then be displayed relative to the stored fluoroscopic images. The surgeon may choose to plan appropriate screw trajectory on the stored images, or simply use the real-time feedback of the navigation system dur-

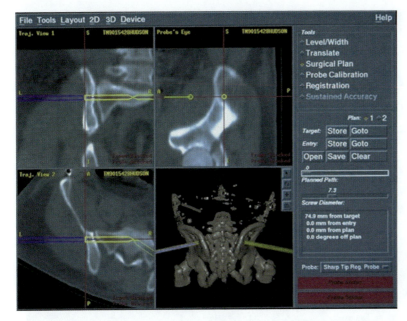

■ **Fig. 68.1.** This is the screen output during 3D-CT guided insertion of ilio-sacral screws for a bilateral posterior pelvic ring disruption. The surgical plan for insertion of the screw into the right hemipelvis is seen in *yellow*, while the drill guide is seen in *blue*

ing guide wire placement. Fluoroscopic navigation eliminates the need for a preoperative CT and the sometimes time-consuming registration step necessary with 3D-CT technique. The technique is self-registering, as the position of the instrument is simply superimposed onto the stored images.

The main advantage of fluoroscopic navigation over 3D-CT technique is that the stored images may be easily updated intra-operatively following fracture reduction. In the earlier technique, reliance on a pre-operative CT limited its use to cases in which an intra-operative reduction was not required. For this reason, fluoroscopic navigation has essentially replaced the 3D-CT technique in actual practice. The CT-based technique is now reserved for cases in which c-arm imaging is limited by retained bowel gas or contrast material, or for the very obese patient.

During treatment of displaced fractures, a two pin external fixator is usually placed to maintain fracture reduction while applying longitudinal traction on a Judet table. Following reduction, the starting point for skin incision and screw trajectory was determined with a trajectory extension feature in the software. The soft tissues are dilated along the path of screw insertion. The optically-tracked drill guide is then placed down to bone along the precisely defined trajectory for screw placement. A 2.8-mm guide wire is then passed along the proposed trajectory. Depth

of drilling is controlled by placing a stop on the guide wire based on the trajectory length as determined by the guidance system (■ Fig. 68.2). A 7.3-mm cannulated screw of appropriate length is then placed over the guide wire. Accurate reduction and screw placement is confirmed with additional inlet and outlet images. The external fixator is then removed, and the wounds irrigated and closed with one or two simple interrupted nylon sutures.

Between September, 1999 and January, 2003, 44 posterior pelvic ring disruptions in 35 patients were stabilized with one or two 7.3 mm cannulated screws using fluoroscopic navigation. A total of 55 screws were placed, and fluoroscopic time and operative time were prospectively recorded.

Control Group

Charts were obtained of 25 patients that underwent surgical repair of a sacral fracture or ilio-sacral disruption from 1995 to 1997. The author in this study had already attained proficiency in ilio-sacral screw placement, and performed all of the procedures in the control group and the experimental groups. Patients eventually requiring an open procedure were eliminated from the study, leaving 15 patients with 17 posterior pelvic ring disruptions

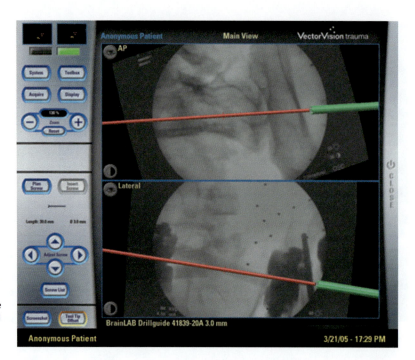

Fig. 68.2. Screen output during insertion of a left-sided ilio-sacral screw using fluoroscopic navigation. The representation of the drill guided is seen in *green* on the inlet and outlet views, while the trajectory ahead of the drill guide is seen in *red*

who had undergone percutaneous internal fixation using fluoroscopic guidance. These records were retrospectively reviewed.

For all groups, blood loss, fluoroscopic time, and procedure time (end of surgical prep/drape to skin closure) were recorded in the surgical record; this was done prospectively for the image-guided groups. All patients were mobilized with protected weight bearing on the affected extremity and begun on early range of motion exercises. All patients were given prophylaxis against deep venous thrombosis with warfarin or low molecular weight heparin unless there were contraindications to anticoagulation. Accuracy of screw placement was evaluated using post-operative inlet and outlet radiographs. Post-operative CT was not performed unless there was concern regarding accuracy of screw placement, or other indications for repeat pelvic imaging.

Results

Accurate screw placement was possible using all three techniques. Although postoperative CT was not obtained in every case, inlet and outlet views of the pelvis failed to

reveal any radiographic evidence of screw mal-position in either of the two computer assisted series. One patient in the historical control group had late symptoms and CT evidence of violation of the S1 foramen with the threads of one screw, and required hardware removal after her pelvis had healed.

Using 3D-CT computer-assisted technique, a total of 27 screws were successfully placed into the S1 or S2 body in 21 cases. The mean total operative time per screw was 25 minutes with a range from 11 to 43 minutes. The mean fluoroscopy time required for validation of screw placement was 13 seconds, with a range from 11 to 26 seconds per screw.

Using virtual fluoroscopy, a total of 55 screws were placed in 44 cases. The mean total operative time per screw was 35 min, with a range from 24 to 68 min. Fluoroscopy time per screw averaged 29 s, with a range from 16 to 46 s. Operative and fluoroscopic times included both fracture reduction and screw placement in this group. Longer surgical times were related to cases with more difficult reductions.

Traditional fluoroscopic ilio-sacral screw placement was performed in 17 cases in the control group. Mean operative time was 34 minutes per screw with range from

□ Table 68.1. Operating time and radiation exposure during ilio-acral screw placement using three different techniques

Technique	Cases (number of screws)	Operative time (range)	Fluoroscopy time (range)
Standard technique	17 (17)	34 min (23–61)	76 s (63–104)
3D-CT technique	21 (27)	25 min (11–43)	13 s (11–26)
Fluoroscopic navigation	44 (55)	35 min (24–68)	29 s (16–46)

23 to 61 min per screw, and the mean fluoroscopy time required was 76 s per screw, with a range from 63 to 104 s per screw.

Computer-assisted technique required significantly less operative time in the 3D-CT group, similar operative time in the fluoroscopic navigation group, and significantly less fluoroscopic time in both groups (□ Table 68.1).

Discussion

Surgical navigation and computer-assisted techniques have recently been applied to several orthopaedic subspecialties. A major concern regarding this new technology has been that it invariably increases operative time during joint replacement and spine surgery. When used in trauma applications, however, the minimal setup time is easily offset by improved first-pass accuracy of implants. Neither computer-assisted group required significantly more operative time than standard fluoroscopic technique. Both computer-assisted groups used significantly less fluoroscopic time than standard technique.

In the treatment of posterior pelvic ring disruptions in this study, the use of computer assisted surgical navigation decreased intra-operative radiation exposure to both the patient and the surgeon, without significantly increasing operative time. The IGS techniques completely eliminate radiation exposure to the surgeon's hands. Although accurate screw placement was possible using all techniques, there were no clinically significant screw mal-positions in either of the IGS groups.

Fluoroscopic navigation required more operative time than 3D-CT technique. It is important to note, however, that the 3D-CT group had already undergone placement of the external fixator and closed reduction prior to obtaining the CT scan and prior to the navigation procedure. The actual navigated screw insertion in the fluo-

roscopic group required little operative time; most of the time was consumed by fracture reduction and harvesting of images.

New technology employing isocentric C-arm imaging provides the capability of obtaining a 3D dataset in the operating room, allowing imaging and navigation similar to the 3D-CT technique without a preoperative CT. Unfortunately, image quality and a small field of view have limited the utility of the Iso-C 3D technique in pelvic applications. A recent study showed that the best accuracy during placement of iliosacral screws was obtained using a fluoroscopic navigation interface [14].

The best indicator of the radiation risk to a patient or surgeon from a diagnostic radiological procedure comes from using both the skin radiation exposure and the organ radiation exposure. At our institution, a PA chest radiograph exposes the patient to between 10 and 15 mRads, and a lateral chest radiograph results in 20–30 mRads. A CT of the pelvis exposes the patient to between 3 and 5 Rads. The ionizing radiation exposure of portable operative fluoroscopy about the pelvis is 4 Rads (40 mSv)/min [15]. The patient absorbs most of this radiation, although some may be reflected by the patient to the surgeon, or intercepted by the hands of the careless surgeon. In this study, the fluoroscopic time saved was approximately 55 s per screw in the 3D-CT group, thus sparing the patient approximately 4 Rads (40 mSv)/screw, or the equivalent of 250 routine chest radiographs. Fluoroscopic navigation reduced radiation exposure to the patient by over 60%, and eliminated radiation exposure to the surgeon's hands.

Reduction in exposure to radiation is becoming an important concern for orthopaedic surgeons. It is clear that low doses of occupational radiation exposure may have measurable health effects. One minute of fluoroscopy time about the pelvis is equivalent to 40 mSv of radiation, which is the equivalent of about 250 chest radiographs.

Career high-altitude airline pilots receive an average of 3–6 mSv of radiation over environmental background exposure per year; this is equivalent to only a few seconds of fluoroscopy exposure in the operating suite. Despite this low level of increased radiation exposure, pilots are subject to a five-fold increase in myeloid malignancies and three-fold increase in skin cancers when compared to the general population [16]. Although the excess skin cancer risk is believed to be due to sun exposure, radiation exposure is the only risk factor identified for the myeloid malignancies. We believe that reduction of radiation exposure to both the patient and the surgeon should be a goal for all surgeons performing percutaneous surgery.

Conclusion

Image-guided surgery techniques have the potential to improve the accuracy of implant placement, while decreasing operative time and eliminating radiation exposure to the surgeon. Fluoroscopic navigation in particular appears to have broad potential applications in orthopaedic trauma. The surgeon using these techniques must have the diligence to obtain good images prior to proceeding with implant placement, as well as the discipline to abandon the procedure if imaging is inadequate. These procedures should be attempted only by experienced fracture surgeons, in the event that reversion to a formal open procedure is necessary.

References

1. Olsen SA, Pollak A (1996) Assessment of pelvic ring stability after injury. Clin Orthop Relat Res 329: 15–27
2. Routt, ML Jr, Simonian PT (1996) Closed reduction and percutaneous skeletal fixation of sacral fractures. Clin Orthop Relat Res 329: 121–128
3. Webb LX, Caldwell K (1988) Disruption of the posterior pelvic ring caused by vertical shear. South Med J 81: 1217–1221
4. Matta JM, Tornetta P (1996) Internal fixation of unstable pelvic ring injuries. Clin Orthop Relat Res 329: 129–140
5. Moed B (1996) Techniques for reduction and fixation of pelvic ring disruptions through the posterior approach. Clin Orthop Relat Res 329: 102–114
6. Keating JF, Werier J, Blachut P, Broekhuyse H, Meek RN, O'Brien PJ (1999) Early fixation of the vertically unstable pelvis. J Orthop Trauma 13(2): 107–113
7. Routt MLC, Kregor P, Simonian PT, Mayo KA (1995) Early results of percutaneous iliosacral screwsplaced with the patient in the supine position. J Orthop Trauma 9: 207–214
8. Routt ML Jr., Simonian PT, Agnew SG, Mann FA (1996) Radiographic recognition of the sacral alar slope for optimal placement of iliosacral screws: a cadaveric and clinical study. J Orthop Trauma 10: 171–177
9. Mostafavi HR, Tornetta P (1996) Radiologic evaluation of the pelvis« Clin Orthop Relat Res 329: 6–14
10. Mehlman CT, DiPasquale TG (1997) Radiation exposure to the orthopaedic surgical team during fluoroscopy: »How far away is far enough?« J Orthop Trauma 11(6): 392–398
11. Kahler DM (2004) Image Guidance: Fluoroscopic Navigation. Clin Orthop Relat Res 421: 70–76
12. Hinsche AF, Giannoudis PV, Smith RM (2002) Fluoroscopy-based multiplanar image guidance for insertion of sacroiliac screws. Clin Orthop Relat Res 395: 135–144
13. Stöckle U, König B, Schaser K, Melcher I, Haas NP (2003) CT and fluoroscopy based navigation in pelvic surgery. Unfallchirurg 106 (11): 914–920
14. Smith HE, Yuan PS, Sasso R, Papadopoulos S, Vaccaro AR (2006) An evaluation of image-guided technologies in the placement of percutaneous iliosacral screws. Spine 31(2):234–238
15. Agarwal SK (1999) Ionizing Radiation Exposure at the University of Virginia. Unpublished data
16. Gundestrup M, Sturm HH (1999) Radiation-induced acute myeloid leukaemia and other cancers in commercial jet cockpit crew: a population-based cohort study. Lancet 354: 2029–2031

68

Computer-Assisted Surgery for Correction of Skeletal Deformities

M.A. Hafez, E.H. Schemitsch, M. Fadel, G. Hosny

Introduction

The term »orthopaedics« was originated from the Greek words ortho and »paideia« and has been traditionally used to describe the branch of medicine concerned with the correction or prevention of skeletal deformities. The burden of bone and joint deformities in developing countries is huge due to the prevalence of congenital, post-traumatic, metabolic (rickets), neurological (poliomyelitis) and other underlying conditions. Verma [1] reported that in India, a very large number of infants with genetic disorders are born every year, almost half a million with malformations and 21,000 with Down syndrome. In developed countries, skeletal deformities may have a different distribution and etiology but the burden on health care is still significant. Deformities secondary to Paget's disease and inflammatory arthropathy are relatively more common in developed countries.

There is a common association between skeletal deformities and arthritis and in some cases, surgeons may debate which is the cause or the result. In arthritic joints, the location of deformities could be around the joint or in the shafts of long bones. There are different trends for treating arthritis that are associated with deformities particularly, those around the joint. In developing countries, there is a trend to treat osteoarthritis and correct deformities by osteotomies. In developed countries, the trend is to treat arthritis by joint replacement and correct the deformities according to their location. In addition to the location of deformities, there are other factors such as age that can influence the choice of treatment options. Whatever the type of treatment, accu-racy and reproducibility are important factors for successful outcome of procedures such as knee replacement [2, 3] or osteotomy [4, 5]. Accuracy and precision are required for pre-operative planning and surgical implementation.

Computer-assisted surgery (CAS) is an enabling technology that has the potential to improve accuracy and reproducibility and overcome drawbacks of conventional techniques. Literature is now abundant with reports comparing navigation against conventional techniques, particularly for total knee replacement (TKR). Several randomized trials [6–12] showed superior accuracy of navigation techniques. Other comparative trials [13–18] showed more precise placement of implants with navigation techniques. The elimination of IM rods reduces the risk of blood loss and fat embolism [7, 19]. CAS systems can act as training tools and can measure operative performance and surgical outcome, thus supporting research and documentation. Deformity correction is also well suited for CAS, as corrective procedures require accurate planning and precise performance. CAS systems can also provide real time intra-operative guidance similar to fluoroscopic images and subsequently reduce the screening time and radiation exposure, which is on the rise [20]. There are reports of different CAS techniques used for deformity correction such as robotics, navigation and planning software.

The authors present their experience in using different CAS techniques for deformity correction, namely navigation, patient-specific templates and planning software (Taylor Spatial Frame). This chapter also reflects the different CAS approaches applied in both developed and developing countries.

Navigation for Deformity Correction

At St Michael Hospital, University of Toronto, an image-free navigation system has been used routinely for total knee arthroplasty (Stryker navigation) and other procedures such as hip resurfacing (VectorVision, BrainLab & Smith and Nephew). Many of the navigated TKR procedures involved the correction of deformities around the knee such as varus, valgus and flexion contracture that are frequently associated with osteoarthritis and inflammatory arthritis. The image-free navigation normally incorporates the kinematic and morphologic data that are intra-operatively collected from the patient to compute the mechanical axis and to guide the surgeon in achieving the required alignment for TKR during bone cutting. This automatically corrects associated bone deformities. The navigation system also guides the surgeon to correct joint deformities and imbalances by measuring the soft tissue tension and by providing a real time feedback to the surgeon during soft tissue release. The initial results of navigated TKR in our institute are encouraging but formal outcome assessment has not been published yet. In this section, we (EHS & MAH) present the use of an image-free navigation system for a complex case of lower limb deformity associated with an ipsilateral failed total knee arthroplasty that required revision (Fig. 69.1). The patient was an 85-year-old woman who had a left total knee replacement performed in 1995 and did well for about 10 years until she had a fall a year ago and then developed valgus instability of the left knee with limited mobility. She had a right hip replacement in 1987 and coronary artery bypass grafting in the past. She was overweight with valgus mal-alignment and subluxation of the left knee. Her x-rays confirmed the diagnosis of lateral subluxation of the prosthesis with deformity in the femur. The deformity was found to be secondary to rickets.

Treatment options including revision arthroplasty and a femoral osteotomy were discussed with the patient who decided to have a left total knee arthroplasty revision. A decision was made to use a navigation system, partly because of the deformed femur that precluded the use of intra-medullary guides and also to accurately restore the mechanical axis. Routine steps were performed for revision TKR and also for the use of the image-free navigation system. After removal of old implants and cement, the femoral cut was navigated to be at 0° for both coronal and sagittal alignment. Because of the femoral bowing and deformity, the femoral implant was positioned more laterally

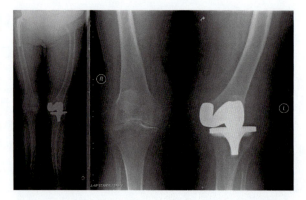

 Fig. 69.1. Pre-operative radiographs show a failed left TKR and a deformity secondary to rickets. A right total hip replacement is also shown

and an 80-mm stem was inserted with an offset of 8 mm. The proximal end of the stem was very close to the medial cortex. A distal augment of 10 mm was used on the lateral and medial sides. The tibial cut was navigated aiming at 0° for both coronal and sagittal alignment. A tibial component with a stem that had an offset of 8 mm was used. A 10-mm augment was inserted under the tibial component and a 14-mm tibial insert was applied. A constrained condylar prosthesis (TS Scorpio, Stryker) was finally implanted and the knee was stable with good range of motion. Surgery was performed without any complications and the postoperative course was uneventful. Postoperative radiographs showed satisfactory position of the implants and acceptable alignment of the lower limb (Fig. 69.2).

There is controversy with regard to the treatment of osteoarthritis (OA) of the knee or failed TKR in the presence of a considerable deformity of the femoral or tibial shafts. The first option is to correct the deformity by an osteotomy at the deformity level and to perform TKR after the healing of the osteotomy. The disadvantages of this approach are the need for two surgical procedures and the consequences of two sessions of anesthesia, preoperative preparation, longer hospital stay and longer rehabilitation time. There is a risk of delayed or nonunion of the osteotomy and higher risk of failure of TKR after osteotomy procedures.

The second option is to perform the corrective osteotomy at the level of the deformity at the same sitting as the TKR. In this situation, prostheses with long stems are used possibly with locking screws beyond the osteotomy level. The disadvantages of this approach are the conse-

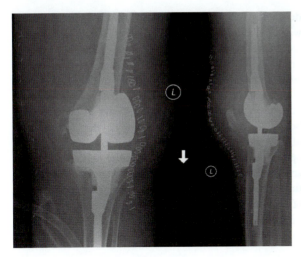

quences of a major and a lengthy procedure that may lead to higher risk of intra-operative and postoperative complications. There is a risk of nonunion of the osteotomy, implant failure and longer rehabilitation time.

The third option is to perform TKR and indirectly correct the deformity at the level of the knee joint. The disadvantages of this approach are the technical demand and the risk of ligamentous damage at the level of the knee joint. In addition, the use of intra-medullary guides in such cases is not possible and may lead to complications. A literature review showed no comparative studies for the application and the outcome of the above three options.

In our case, the capabilities of the navigation system have made the third option more attractive. By restoring the mechanical axis while planning the alignment and bone cutting for TKR, it was possible to indirectly correct shaft deformities by adjusting the inclination of bone cuts at the level of the knee. Using this technique, it was possible to plan bone cuts without compromising collateral ligaments, the patellar tendon or the level of the joint line. Using conventional techniques, it would have been difficult to insert the IM rod and its insertion may have lead to alignment errors and complications. At present, we are conducting an experimental investigation using the treatment options mentioned above with comparison between navigation and conventional techniques. The experiment involves 3 surgeons operating on 24 plastic knee specimens that have femoral or tibial shaft deformities.

Patient Specific Templating

MAH previously reported [21, 22] the use of a novel CAS technique called »patient specific templating« (PST). This technique is currently confined to TKR and it aims at providing patient-specific templates (PST) or custom cutting guides that can completely replace conventional instruments (CI) for TKR (☐ Fig. 69.3). Computed tomography based preoperative planning was used for sizing, alignment and bone cutting and then the designing of two virtual templates. Using rapid prototyping technology, virtual templates were transferred into physical templates (cutting blocks) with surfaces that matched the distal femur and proximal tibia. The technique was used in 45 experimental TKR procedures (16 cadaveric and 29 plastic knees) and showed that it was possible to perform TKR without CI systems, medullary guides, tracking or registration. The mean time for bone cutting was 9 minutes (15 minutes for CI systems), when the surgeon had an assistant and 11 minutes (30 minutes for CI systems), when the surgeon was unassisted. Postoperative CT scans from 6 randomly selected cadaveric specimens showed mean errors of 1.7° and 0.8 mm (maximum 2.3° and 1.2 mm) for alignment and bone resection respectively. The technique was tested by multiple new users and showed significant intra-observer and inter-observer agreement for 5 observers with a mean alignment error of 0.67° (maximum 2.5°) and a mean bone resection error of 0.32 mm (maximum 1 mm). The PST technique showed several advantages over conventional instrumentation and proved to be a simple, less expensive alternative to navigation and robotic techniques for TKR. This technique is described in more detail in Chapter 24 in this book.

In addition, the advantage of providing a CT-based 3-D pre-operative planning and the elimination of medullary guides make the PST an attractive technique for TKR in patients with complex multiplane deformities. The PST technique was tried on 4 plastic knee specimens that had complex femoral or tibial deformities (unpublished study) (☐ Fig. 69.4). Each case had a CT scan with segmentation and 3-D reconstruction of images. The degree of the deformity was calculated in 3-D and the mechanical axis was established. Pre-operative planning for TKR was performed including sizing of implants, alignment and bone cutting. Routine steps for the PST technique mentioned above were implemented.

The experiment proved that it was possible to plan TKR and the correction of the shaft deformity at the level of the knee joint and then perform the surgery using patient specific templates without resorting to conventional instruments. By restoring the mechanical axis while planning for TKR, it was possible to indirectly correct shaft deformities by adjusting the inclination of bone cuts at the level of the knee. The amount of bone cutting at the distal femur and proximal tibia was variable depending on the location and direction of the deformity. For example, while dealing with varus deformity at the mid shaft tibia, the lateral tibial plateau was cut at 10 mm as per standard techniques for TKR but the medial tibial plateau, was

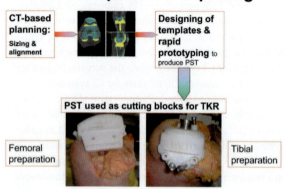

Fig. 69.3. Technical steps for patient specific templating technique

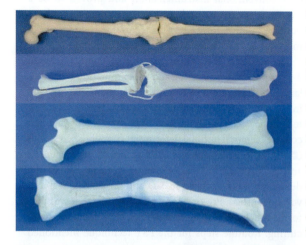

Fig. 69.4. Plastic specimens (Foam Cortical shell, Sawbones, Sweden) with deformities around the knee joint and in the tibial or femoral shafts

deficient below the level of the cut. Metal augmentation was considered for treating bone deficiency. Using this technique, it was possible to plan bone cuts without compromising collateral ligaments, the patellar tendon or the level of the joint line.

The accurate planning of CAS has opened a new horizon in managing complex TKR with deformed long bones. The correction of the deformity in the same setting of TKR and at the level of the knee joint is an attractive option for patients since it obviates the need for further anesthetics, another procedure and longer rehabilitation time. The elimination of IM guides may reduce the risk of bleeding, fat embolism, infection and fractures. More importantly, the accurate pre-operative planning may lead to better performance and survival of TKR implants.

Planning Software (Taylor Spatial Frame)

We (MF and GH) present our experience in using a simple form of CAS that is better suited in countries, where skeletal deformities are relatively more common while other CAS systems such as robotics and navigation are currently less practical. Osteotomy, acute correction, and internal or external fixation are possible in one plane but it is difficult with combined angular and translational deformities. In such cases, gradual correction with an Ilizarov frame is preferable. In Egypt, the Ilizarov external fixator (IEF) is commonly used and has been a useful surgical tool for many orthopaedic surgeons, particularly for the treatment of lower limb deformities, bone loss and non-union of fractures [23, 24]. Ilizarov techniques require sequential correction for multiplane deformities and may involve the use of hinges with independent lengthening, translation and rotation that could be time consuming [25]. A circular external fixator, the Taylor spatial frame (TSF) (Fig. 69.5) that relies on the use of a computer software program was developed [26]. Using TSF, surgeons can simultaneously manage multiple angles and translations while correcting limb deformities. The computer program encompasses a six-axis deformity analysis and provides a print-out schedule for turning and adjusting the controls on the struts. Full correction of the deformity will be achieved when the struts are restored to their pre-calculated length.

Several authors reported the use of TSF [27–30]. We conducted a community-based assessment for the usefulness of TSF in lower limb lengthening and deformity correction [31]. Between 1999 and 2001, we treated 22 patients using the TSF. There were 14 females and eight males, and their mean age was 16.5 (range: 6–42) years. The etiology was four cases of tibia vara, two cases of valgus knee, three congenital short femurs, two equinus feet, five short tibiae, five short and deformed tibiae following trauma, and one posttraumatic short femur. Measurements were made both clinically and from antero-posterior and lateral standing radiographs using Paley's technique [32]. We measured five of the six deformity parameters using radiographs. The sixth deformity parameter and the three frame parameters were measured by clinical examination. We also recorded four mounting parameters. These 13 parameters were loaded into the Chronic Deformity Correction Program, which then returns six specific strut lengths, which allows adjustment of the fixator to exactly mimic the deformity. Patients were reviewed weekly for 1 month, then every 2 weeks, and radiographs were taken at appropriate intervals. The frame was removed when »tricortical« consolidation was seen on antero-posterior and lateral radiographs. If deformity remained after the

proximal and distal rings were parallel, a further program of correction was started using a second »print out«.

The mean number of operations before the application of the spatial frame was 2.6 (range 1–6). The operative time ranged from 1.5 to 3 hours, and the period in the spatial frame was between 2 to 9 (average 5.27) months. The mean follow-up was 3.2 (range 2.5–4.5) years. The treatment objectives were lengthening in eight patients, correction of deformities in eight, and both in six. A multifactor objective grading system was developed using a modification of that devised by Tucker [33]. Our results were 18 excellent, two good, and two fair. One patient was unable to complete the entire procedure. Mean lengthening was 5 (range 3.5–8) cm. Mean healing index was 42 (range 33–48) days/cm. Bifocal lengthening was performed in two patients.

Pin tract inflammation occurred in all our patients, and 12 of these infections required antibiotics. There was loosening of three frames that had been treated by debridement, addition or replacement of wires. Fracture of the regenerated bone occurred in two patients due to

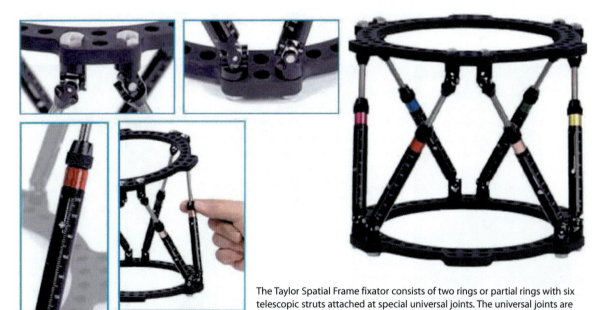

The Taylor Spatial Frame fixator consists of two rings or partial rings with six telescopic struts attached at special universal joints. The universal joints are passive and do not require clamping. Strut lengths are changed by rotating an adjustment knob. These strut lengths may be read directly off each strut. From an initial 'neutral' position struts may be lengthened or shortened as necessary.

◻ **Fig. 69.5.** Taylor Spatial Frame (With permission from JC Taylor)

premature frame removal. One patient developed deep vein thrombosis and two patients required a second attempt, which failed in one.

Traditional Ilizarov techniques use distraction rods with hinges and include other mechanical joints in order to permit gradual reciprocal angulation or rotation of the rings [34]. These hinges and translation mechanisms are specifically oriented for each deformity, and this means that the surgeon must design a new frame for the treatment of each patient, which requires time and expertise. Using TSF, this drawback is markedly reduced. Correction of residual deformity is difficult using the Ilizarov system, as it is necessary to make further adjustments after the oblique plane angular deformity has been corrected. This leads to an undesirable sequential correction of the deformity. We used the residual program successfully in two patients and our results are in agreement with Feldman et al. [35]. We used TSF in cases of genu valgus and equinus foot and we achieved successful correction. One knee of a patient with bilateral genu valgus was completely corrected and was rated as good (Fig. 69.6).

There is a steep learning curve associated with the use of the Ilizarov system in the management of multiaxial deformity [36]. However, Feldman et al. [35] were able to correct multiaxial deformities using the TSF with relative ease. The relatively high cost and the steep learning curve limit the broad based application of the TSF technique. However, our results are encouraging and we consider the TSF as a useful method for treatment of lower limb deformities in our community. The recent introduction of a web-based software program and the universal struts will facilitate the determination of the amount and direction of strut correction.

References

1. Verma I (2001) Burden of genetic disorders in India. Indian J Pediatr. 2000;67-893-898. Erratum in: Indian J Pediatr 68(1): 25
2. Fehring TK, Odum S, Griffin WL, Mason JB, Nadaud M (2001) Early failure in total knee arthroplasty. Clin Orthop Relat Res 392: 315–318
3. Sharkey PF, Hozack WJ, Rothman RH, Shastri S, Jacoby SM (2002) Insall Award paper. Why are knee replacements failing today? Clin Orthop Relat Res 404: 7–13
4. Chillag KJ, Nichollas PJ (1984) High tibial osteotomy: A retrospective analysis of 30 cases. Orthopaedics 7: 1821
5. Coventry MB, Ilstrup DM, Wallrichs SL (1993) Proximal tibial osteotomy. A critical long-term study of eighty-seven cases. J Bone Joint Surg 75-A-2: 196–201
6. Sparmann M, Wolke B, Czupalla H, Banzer D, Zink A (2003) Positioning of total knee arthroplasty with and without navigation

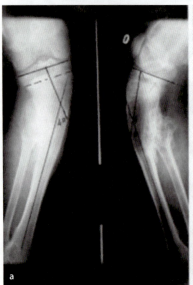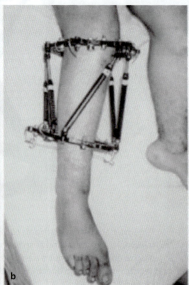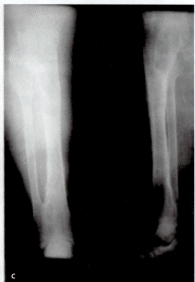

 Fig. 69.6. AP and LAT radiograph of the right leg of an 18-year-old male patient with bilateral genu valgus; **b** during treatment; **c** radiograph after frame removal [31]

support. A prospective, randomised study. J Bone Joint Surg Br 85: 830–835

7. Chauhan SK, Scott RG, Breidahl W, Beaver RJ (2004) Computer-assisted knee arthroplasty versus a conventional jig-based technique. A randomised, prospective trial. J Bone Joint Surg Br 86-3: 372–377

8. Saragaglia D, Picard F, Chaussard E, Montbarbon F, Leitner F, Cinquin P (2001) Computer assisted total knee arthroplasty: comparison with a conventional procedure. Results of a 50 case prospective randomized study. First Annual Meeting of Computer Assisted Orthopedic Surgery. Davos, Switzerland

9. Chin PL, Yang KY, Yeo SJ, Lo NN (2005) Randomized control trial comparing radiographic total knee arthroplasty implant placement using computer navigation versus conventional technique. J Arthroplasty 20: 618–626

10. Decking R, Markmann Y, Fuchs J, Puhl W, Scharf HP (2005) Leg axis after computer-navigated total knee arthroplasty: a prospective randomized trial comparing computer-navigated and manual implantation. J Arthroplasty 20: 282–288

11. Victor J, Hoste D (2004) Image-based computer-assisted total knee arthroplasty leads to lower variability in coronal alignment. Clin Orthop Relat Res 428: 131–139

12. Stockl B, Nogler M, Rosiek R, Fischer M, Krismer M, Kessler O (2004) Navigation improves accuracy of rotational alignment in total knee arthroplasty. Clin Orthop Relat Res 426: 180–186

13. Nabeyama R, Matsuda S, Miura H, Mawatari T, Kawano T, Iwamoto Y (2003) The accuracy of image guided knee replacement based on computed tomography. J Bone Joint Surg Br 86: 366–371

14. Perlick L, Bathis H, Tingart M et al. (2004) Navigation in total-knee arthroplasty: CT-based implantation compared with the conventional technique. Acta Orthrop Scand 75: 464–470

15. Bolognesi M, Hoffman A (2005) Computer navigation versus standard instrumentation for TKA: a single-surgeon experience. Clin Orthop Relat Res 440: 162–169

16. Anderson KC, Buehler KC, Markel DC (2005) Computer assisted navigation in total knee arthroplasty: comparison with conventional methods. J Arthroplasty 20 (Suppl 7): 132–138

17. Kim SJ, MacDonald M, Hernandez J, Wixson RL (2005) Computer assisted navigation in total knee arthroplasty: improved coronal alignment. J Arthroplasty 20 (Suppl 3): 123–131

18. Haaker RG, Stockheim M, Kamp M, Proff G, Breitenfelder J, Ottersbach A (2005) Computer-assisted navigation increases precision of component placement in total knee arthroplasty. Clin Orthop Relat Res 433: 152–159

19. Kalairajah Y SD, Cossey AJ, Verral GM, Spriggins AJ (2005) Blood loss after total knee replacement: Effects of computer-assisted surgery. J Bone Joint Surg Br 87: 1480–1482

20. Hafez M, Smith R, Matthews S, Kalap N, Sherman K (2005) Radiation exposure to the hands of orthopaedic surgeons: Are we underestimating the risk? Arch Orthop Trauma Surg 125: 330–335

21. Hafez MA, Chelule K, Seedhom BB, Sherman KP (2006) Computer-assisted total knee arthroplasty using patient-specific templating. Clin Orthop Relat Res 444: 184–192

22. Hafez MA, Jaramaz B, Di Gioia A III (2006) Computer Assisted Surgery of the Knee: An overview. In: Insall JN, Scott N (eds) Surgery of the Knee, 4th edn, vol. 2. Churchill Livingston, Philadelphia, pp 1655–1674

23. Hosny G (2005) Treatment of tibial hemimelia without amputation: preliminary report. J Pediatr Orthop B 14: 250–255

24. Hosny G, Fadel M (2003) Ilizarov external fixator for open fractures of the tibial shaft. Int Orthop 27: 303–306

25. Taylor J (2002) Six-axis deformity analysis and correction. In: Paley D (ed) Principles of Deformity Correction. Springer, Berlin Heidelberg New York, pp 411–436

26. Taylor JC (2005) The correction of general deformities with the taylor spatial frame fixator,« http://www.jcharlestaylor.com

27. Rodl R LB, Bohm A, Winkelmann W (2003) Correction of deformities with conventional and hexapod frames--comparison of methods. Z Orthop Ihre Grenzgeb 141: 92–98

28. Rozbruch SR HD, Blyakher A (2002) Distraction of hypertrophic non-union of tibia with deformity using Ilizarov/Taylor Spatial Frame: reportof two cases. Arch Orthop Trauma Surg 122: 295–298

29. Seide K WD, Kortmann HR (1999) Fracture reduction and deformity correction with hexapod Ilizarov fixator. Clin Orthop Relat Res 363: 186–195

30. Sluga M PM, Kotz R, Nehrer S (2003) Lower limb deformities in children: two-stage correction using the Taylor spatial frame. J Pediatr Orthop B 12: 123–128

31. Fadel M, Hosny G (2005) The Taylor spatial frame for deformity correction in the lower limbs. Int Orthop 29: 125–129

32. Paley D (2002) Radiographic assessment of lower limb deformities. In: In: Paley D, ed. Principles of Deformity Correction. Springer, Berlin Heidelberg New York, pp 31–60

33. Tucker HKJ, Kinnebrew TE (1992) Management of unstable open and closed tibial fractures using the Ilizarov method. Clin Orthop Relat Res 280: 125–135

34. Ilizarov G (1992) Transosseous osteosynthesis. Springer, Berlin Heidelberg New York, pp 287–543

35. Feldman DS, Madan S, Koval KJ (2003) Correction of tibial malunion and nonunion with six-axis analysis deformity correction using the Taylor Spatial Frame. J Orthop Trauma 17: 549–554

36. Tetsworth KD, Paley D (1994) Accuracy of correction of complex lower extremity deformities by the Ilizarov method. Clin Orthop Relat Res301: 102–110

Part VI   Spinal Surgery

Navigation in Cervical Spine Surgery

A. Weidner

Introduction

In general there is no difference in stabilization techniques of the cervical spine compared with the lumbar spine: screws are inserted into the spine and connected with rods (posterior) and a plate (anterior) to achieve primary stability. Transarticular screw fixation is introduced by Magerl for C1/C2. Judet described another fixation technique for fracture of the pars interarticularis of C2 in which a screw bridges the both fracture parts.

Landmarks in the operating field include facet joints and transverse processes, which serve for identification of the screw's entry point. Because drilling direction and screw length is difficult to judge precisely, intraoperative fluoroscopic examination is required. The main difference between lumbar and cervical spine is the different size of anatomical structures. Therefore, manual feed back while drilling into a pedicle is less helpful in the cervical spine, where additionally important structures are nearby and thus at risk: vertebral artery, spinal nerve, or spinal cord. Cervical spine surgery has a lower frequency as compared with lumbar spinal surgery, a fact that leads to a limited amount of relevant clinical studies.

Intraoperative navigation promises preoperative planning of screw alignment and intraoperative transfer of these data for optimal screw positioning. Due to the fact that cervical anatomy is more complex higher precision standards and reliability are demanded for surgical navigation tools.

Cervical Spine Navigation: Intraoperative Techniques

Two different navigation techniques are available, which differ in the type of digital data sets loaded into the work station: CT scan data provide three-dimensional reconstruction in comparison with intraoperative fluoroscopy, which delivers two-dimensional images only.

CT-Based Navigation

CT-based navigation requires a special CT protocol preoperatively. Consecutive axial images of 1.5 mm thickness are mandatory for precise screw placement planning. Screw entry point and screw direction are calculated preoperatively by navigational software in order to minimize potential risks of damaging vital structures including spinal cord, spinal nerve and vertebral artery. Also screw length and diameter are determined preoperatively.

Preoperative planning is transferred intraoperatively into the surgical field, provided that the virtual anatomy can be matched with intraoperative land-marks, a process referred to as »registration«. Surgical instruments equipped with light emitting diodes (LEDs) are linked with the navigation system via an optoelectrical camera tracing them in a three-dimensional space, thus identifying the location of the instruments in the virtual field. The surgeon can use this virtual field as a reference for precise positioning of all instruments. The reference frame, also equipped with LEDs linked by the camera to the work station, traces also excursion of the thorax caused by breathing or manipulation by the surgeon from the surgical to the virtual field. The surgeon identifies spinal landmarks touching and digitizing them. All acquired data are matched with the digitized CT scan. The entry points of screws are identified and matched with the virtual image on the screen for optimal placement.

Fluoroscopy-Based Navigation

With this technique the computer is loaded intraoperatively with a number of two-dimensional fluoroscopic views of the cervical spine. The image intensifier is equipped with LEDs feeding continuously information to the navigation computer. When fluoroscopic views are taken, the position of the image intensifier is known, so matching of virtual and surgical field is not necessary. LED-equipped tools are calculated into the two-dimensional fluorographs. However, the third dimension (depth) has to be added by the imagination and experience of the surgeon.

Cervical Spine Applications

Transarticular Screw Fixation C1/C2 (Magerl Technique)

A 1.5 mm CT scan is required for this technique. Dorsal flexion of the neck during scanning provides reduction of the altlantodental subluxation. This set of data is transferred into the computer for optimal screw alignment planning (■ Fig. 70.1). First the centerpoint in the interarticular part of C2 has to be identified where the vertebral artery has the closest contact to C2. With a diameter of less than 6 mm a safe transarticular screw placement is impossible. From this centerpoint the cranial direction of the screw is determined: On the sagittal plane the screw must cross the C1/C2 joint at the dorsal or middle third of the joint and should be anchored at least 10 mm into the lateral mass of C1. On the coronal plane the screw should be placed in the middle third of C1/C2 (see ■ Fig. 70.1 and ■ Fig. 70.2b).

The screw tip will not be monitored correctly in the virtual field because C1 is not matched with the surgical field. Position of C1 must be evaluated via the fluorographs after positioning of the patient. Intraoperative atlantodental distance should be nearly similar to the distance during data acquisition of the CT, so that conclu-

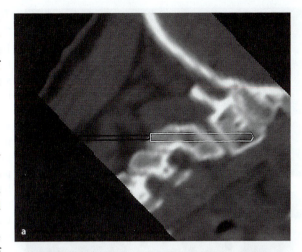

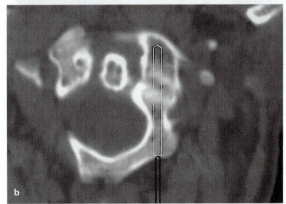

■ **Fig. 70.1a,b.** Preoperative planning CT scan for C1/C2 transarticular screw fixation. **a** Sagittal, **b** axial screw direction

sions can be drawn from this virtual surgical field with regards to screw placement within the first vertebra. The screws were inserted according to preoperative planning. In our own reported series of 115 patients (108 suffering from rheumatoid arthritis) transarticular screw fixation was performed because of atlantodental subluxation [10]. In 37 cases the screws were inserted utilizing CT-based navigation, in a control group of 78 cases the conventional technique based on anatomical landmarks and intraoperative fluoroscopy was utilized.

Out of 230 theoretical screw placements 228 screws could actually be implanted. In two patients one screw could not be inserted. There were no infections or injuries of the dura or neurological structures. One female patient from the control group died in consequence of a vertebral

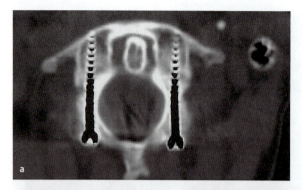

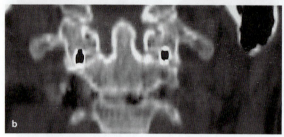

□ Fig. 70.2a,b. Postoperative CT follow up of transarticular screw fixation of C1/C2. **a** The axial, and **b** coronal view, are perpendicular to the screw direction at the level of the C1/C2 joints

artery injury by a screw; the screw was biomechanically placed correctly, yet the vertebral artery showed an anatomical variation, which was not detected prior to surgery.

Screw placement was evaluated by the classification of Madawi [6]: Correct screw position includes a more than 5 mm screw insertion into C1, protrusion of the screw tip over the anterior arch of C1 of less than 5 mm on the lateral radiograph (see □ Fig. 70.1a). Furthermore, the screw tip should be projected in the middle third of the C1/C2 joint seen on an anteroposterior radiograph (□ Fig. 70.1b, □ Fig. 70.2b). Deviation exists, if the screw is not placed in this middle third, but still within the interarticular part of C2. The screw is malpositioned if medially and laterally outside of the interarticular part of C2.

Lateral deviation was most commonly observed. In the navigation group four screws only were deviating into the lateral third. Lateral deviation was significantly higher in the control group, where 23 screws deviated. There were no screws malpositioned in the navigation group compared to eight screws in the control group, without any clinical consequences. That number was too little for drawing statistically significant conclusions.

Transpedicular C2 Screw Fixation

In Hangman's fractures (fracture of pars interarticularis of C2) direct screw fixation of both fragments can prevent spinal fusion and therefore neck mobility is not impaired by surgery. Arand et al. [1] reported two cases that were treated with such a technique (Judet's fixation) performed with the aid of CT-based navigation. All screws could be inserted through the fracture cleft fully covered by bone inside of the interarticular part of C2. We were able to perform this technique in four patients with a minimally invasive approach by stab incision guided by CT-based navigation. Postoperative follow-up revealed correct position of all screws.

Navigation in Anterior Cervical Spine Surgery

CT-based navigation of anterior cervical spine surgery is possible, but identification of anatomical landmarks in this area is unequally more difficult for matching than at the dorsal aspect of the craniovertebral junction. Bolger et al. [2] reported 40 surgeries in which the navigation could not be executed in the first seven because of landmark identification problems. The following five had considerably prolonged surgery time; however, in the final 28 a precision of 0.74 mm ± 0.4 mm could be achieved without delay. We performed this technology in few cases of tumors only. Often a conventional radiograph is sufficient for intraoperative orientation. For anterior cervical spine osteosynthesis, computer-navigation technique has no major advantage over conventional technique, because the screw entry point is clearly visible and modern screw design allows monocortical purchase. Neither two-dimensional conventional fluoroscopy (because of accuracy of the fluorograph) nor three-dimensional CT-based navigation technology (because after inserting a bone graft the position of the vertebral body is changed compared to the preoperative image) is currently capable of imaging the posterior cortex of the vertebral body.

Navigation in Posterior Cervical Spine Surgery

During a posterior approach in cervical spine surgery screws are inserted either into the lateral mass or into the pedicle. Nerve root or vertebral artery injuries are reported. Richter et al. [8] found that in 92% of all pedicle screws inserted with navigation a perforation of the pedicle wall did not occur. In another study, in 36 cases the pedicle screw was reportedly inserted correctly [4]. Lateral mass screws, however, can be inserted safely without navigation in cervical spine surgery. The direction of the screw is parallel to the facet joint plane and the screw is directed 20 degrees anterolaterally. This procedure is monitored easily by direct observation.

Discussion

Intraoperative navigation in spine surgery increases precision. This has been demonstrated to be true for the lumbar spine in a randomized prospective clinical study [5]. However, no clinical advantage could be established so far [9]. Few studies are published for cervical spine surgery. We were able to show a significantly improved screw position with the use of navigation, however, this does not directly indicate a decreased incidence of vertebral artery injuries [10].

The most important factor of a new technology has to include clinical improvement and outcome: This would be a decreased incidence of pseudarthrosis in this group of patients. However, there are no data currently available supporting this to be the result of navigation. Developing pseudarthrosis is multifactorial and therefore it is difficult to apply a reduced rate of pseudarthrosis to navigation alone, particularly in a disease where radiographic findings and clinical symptoms do not necessarily correlate.

Therefore, CT-based navigation at present should not be considered as standard and always superior to conventional techniques. This would be the case, if prospective randomized and controlled studies would demonstrate significantly improved outcomes. Additional radiation (CT scan) is another issue of concern, particularly taking the fact into account that only few patients' first CT scans are precise enough for making it relevant for navigation. Only improved clinical results would justify the costs of this technology.

However, navigation may be indicated in complex anatomical situations, such as malformations, or in revision surgeries. CT navigation makes sense for screw fixation of C1/C2 instability and for C2 fractures (Hangman's), as well as for surgeries where it is difficult to obtain intra-operative images, e.g. the craniocervical and cervicothoracic regions. The latter is not routinely performed in most centers due to difficult registration.

For insertion of multiple cervical pedicle screws at several levels, each vertebra would have to be registered and matched individually – a procedure that is time consuming and impossible after laminectomies, because no reference frame can be attached. Insertion of lateral mass screws can be safely monitored by the surgeon.

Matching of preoperative CT scan and intraoperative radiographs will certainly open new ways for minimally invasive methods in cervical spine surgery, but this should be associated with the development of entirely new surgical techniques to get more benefits from the advantages of navigation.

References

1. Arand M, Hartwig E, Kinzl L, Gebhard F (2001) Spinal navigation in cervical fractures – a preliminary clinical study on Judet-osteosynthesis of the axis. Comput Aided Surg 6: 170–175
2. Bolger C, Wigfield C, Melkent T, Smith K (1999) Frameless stereotaxy and anterior cervical surgery. Comput Aided Surg 4: 322–327
3. Foley K, Smith M (1996) Image-guided spine surgery. Neurosurg Clin N Am 7: 171–186
4. Kamimura M, Ebara S, Itoh H, Tateiwa Y, Kinoshita T, Takaoka K (2000) Cervical pedicle screw insertion: assessment of safety and accuracy with computer-assisted image guidance. J Spinal Disord 13: 218–224
5. Laine T, Lund T, Ylikoski M, Lohikoski J, Schlenzka D (2000) Accuracy of pedicle screw insertion with and without computer assistance: a randomised controlled clinical study in 100 consecutive patients. Eur Spine J 9: 235–40; discussion 241
6. Madawi AA, Casey AT, Solanki GA, Tuite G, Veres R, Crockard HA (1997) Radiological and anatomical evaluation of the atlantoaxial transarticular screw fixation technique. J Neurosurg 86: 961–968
7. Nolte LP, Zamorano L, Visarius H, Berlemann U, Langlotz F, Arm E, Schwarzenbach O (1995) Clinical evaluation of a system for precision enhancement in spine surgery. Clin Biomech 10: 293–303
8. Richter M, Amiot LP, Neller S, Kluger P, Puhl W (2000) Computer-assisted surgery in posterior instrumentation of the cervical spine: an in-vitro feasibility study. Eur Spine J 9 [Suppl 1]: S65–70
9. Schulze CJ, Munzinger E, Weber U (1998) Clinical relevance of accuracy of pedicle screw placement – a computed tomographic-supported analysis. Spine 23(20): 2215–2221
10. Weidner A, Wahler M, Chiu ST, Ullrich CG (2000) Modification of C1-C2 transarticular screw fixation by image-guided surgery. Spine 25: 2668–2673; discussion 2674

Navigated Pedicle Screw Placement in Lumbar Spine Fusion Surgery

J. Geerling, D. Kendoff, M. Citak, A. Gösling, T. Gösling, C. Krettek, T. Hüfner

Introduction

For the treatment of spinal instabilities arising from injuries, tumors and deformities devices with the use of transpedicular screws has become a routine procedure since the introduction by Roy-Camille [25]. However, due to the small diameter and its relation to neural structures and the screws are directed to major vessels, these technique may lead to serious complications due to misplacement of these screws [6].

Most surgeons use fluoroscopy for localizing the pedicle. But with this conventional technique the cortical perforation rate is high. Within the lumbar spine the misplacement rate is up to 30 [9, 27]. Within the thoracic spine the pedicle placement is more difficult because of the smaller diameter of the pedicle and the closeness of the spinal cord. In the literature cortical perforations of the pedicle are described up to 55 percent [29]. The incidence of neurological complications arising of such misplacements is described up to 5% [6, 9, 18]. In some cases even a placement through the cauda equina is described [5].

But also from the biomechanical point of view it is useful to hit the pedicle as precise as possible. The better the screw fills the pedicle, the higher is the fixation strength [2]. This effect is higher with a screw as long as possible.

CT-Based Navigation

To decrease the misplacement rate computer assisted spinal navigation systems has been developed in the nineties as first application in orthopaedic surgery. In the beginning these systems were CT based. The advantage of these technique is the three dimensional visualization of the pedicle in axial, sagittal and coronal planes allowing the observation of the placement in relationship to the anatomy structures and the possibility of a pre-operative planning of the pedicle screw. The disadvantages are the image acquisition pre-operatively with the possibility of motion of the vertebra during the interim between the scan and the operation itself [4]. Furthermore, there is the need of the so-called registration meaning the correlation of the patient's anatomy and the data on the computer.

The registration, also called »matching« is the most important step in CT-based navigation. There are two different kinds of procedures.

— *Pair-point-registration:* At least three, due to own experience up to five points, not on a straight line, are identified on the surface as well as on the therapeutical as on the virtual object. Preoperatively these points are marked on the virtual object at the navigation system. These points should have an as large distance as possible and should be on different levels. Intra-operatively the corresponding points are localized on the therapeutical object. These points are digitalized with an instrument recognized by the navigation system, the so called »pointer«. Due to the pairs of the corresponding points the computer can calculate the position of both coordinate systems, the virtual and the real one, and overly both.

— *Surface registration:* Using this registration technique, a three dimensional model of the bony surface of the CT-dataset is calculated pre-operatively. Intra-operatively a cloud of several points is digitalized on the real bony surface. The computer calculates these points to the surface of the model. These points should be as symmetric as possible on the posterior cortex of the vertebra, including the posterior process.

Most navigation systems use both registration forms to increase the accuracy. Each vertebra should be registrated on its own due to the flexibility of the spine. The CT-scan is performed on the back, operation in prone position. This can change the position and relationship between the segments, as well as intra-operative movements. The single vertebra itself is a rigid body. Therefore the registration for each vertebra can be performed independent from the positioning of the spine. The DRB has to be placed to each vertebra that is operated on at the posterior process.

Several authors [17, 26] reported a longer insertion time per screw, however the total operation time was not reported to be significantly longer [17, 28]. Despite to these limitations with the use of computer assisted spine surgery the misplacement rate could be decreased to 4.5 to 10% [1, 17, 19, 20, 28]. Furthermore, no neurological complications were described in the actual literature placing pedicle screws with computer assistance.

However, there are several pitfalls to avoid during CT based spinal navigation. While calculating the surface of the vertebra the surface might not be calculated correctly due to an osteoporotic bone or other artifacts like pointing with still soft tissue on the bone. With an incorrect surface calculation the position of the vertebra might be calculated incorrect leading to the mistake that the pedicle screw is displayed on the correct position on the monitor screen but is wrong in reality.

Fluoroscopy-Based Navigation

The limitations of the CT-based navigation is absent in fluoroscopy based navigation. Within this navigation technique the registration process is automated and there is the possibility of updating the dataset due to new acquisition of fluoroscopic images at any time during surgery. The limitation is the two dimensional image information and the decreased image quality within the thoracic spine.

A definite improvement of the navigation systems within the last past years is the implementation of intra-operative fluoroscopy and to use these images for the navigation (modality based navigation). These actual images can be used multimodal for navigation (spine, pelvis, extremities). The images can be actualized after reduction or an additional plane can be integrated. Furthermore the orthopedic surgeon is familiar with the intra-operative use of a fluoroscope.

The principle of fluoroscopy based navigation in the spine is: The DRB is placed to the posterior process in the known manner. With the fluoroscope an a. p. and a lateral view is taken. With small rotation of the fluoroscope out of the a.p. it is possible to perform oblique views of the vertebra as well. The images are placed into a »library« at the navigation system. If the image quality is good, the fluoroscope can be removed from the operation situs. The surgeon can choose the images to navigate in. There is a maximum of four views displayable simultaneously. Without a paired-point or surface registration it is possible to navigate the instruments within these images. The images will be stay static on the monitor and the instruments are displayed in real time. Beneath the advantages of multiplanar visualization in real time a reduction of the radiation exposure is possible.

The accuracy of Fluoroscopy spinal navigation is quite as precise as CT-based navigation

Choi [3] performed an experimental study using cadaver specimens from T1 to S1 comparing the accuracy of a CT-based navigation system vs. a fluoroscopy based robot system. In his study he found 12.7% perforations within the CT-navigated group vs. 17.9% misplacements in the fluoroscopy based group.

Fritsch used fluoroscopy based navigation for pedicle screw placement in 30 patients within a clinical evaluation. Within a postoperative CT-scan the evaluation of the placement was performed. 5.6% of the screws showed misplacement, divided in 9% in the thoracic spine and 3.8% in the lumbar spine.

In a recently published study Rampersaud [21] found an overall pedicle wall breach of 15.3% within a clinical study. The pedicle screw placement was performed between T2 and S1. Evaluating the misplacement in thoracic and lumbar spine the rate within thoracic spine was significantly higher with 31.6% vs. 10.6% in the lumbar spine. Due to an associated error of 1–2 mm due to metal artefacts [22, 30] he rated misplaced screws of below 2 mm as clinically acceptable resulting in a misplacement rate of 5.1% in the thoracic and 1.4% in lumbar spine.

Iso-C-3D-Based Navigation

The newly developed Iso-C-3D (Siemens, Erlangen, Germany) allows directly intra-operative three dimensional imaging in multiplanar views due to multiple fluoroscopic images around an isocenter [15, 24]. The scanned volume is 12 cm^3. The scan itself takes 120 seconds with a fluoroscopy radiation time of 20 seconds. This new intra-operative three dimensional method correlates accurate with imaging with computer tomography [7, 16, 23].

In alliance with a computer-assisted surgery system the combination of this three dimensional dataset with the advantages of the fluoroscopy based navigation is given. No anatomy based registration is necessary due to an automated registration process during the scan. Furthermore data update is possible at any time during surgery with a new scan.

There are only a few reports for Iso-C-based navigation for pedicle screw placement. Grützner [10] reported in a clinical study with 302 pedicle screws implanted with Iso-C-3D navigation of a misplacement rate of more than 2 mm in 1.7%. In an earlier paper of the same group Wendel [28] reported of 0.7% misplacements in 141 screws. In his paper he compared the misplacement rate with CT- and fluoroscopy based navigation within the same hospital. In the »historical« comparison group 4.5% of the CT based and 2.8% of the fluoroscopy based navigated pedicle screws were misplaced. The misplacements with Iso-C-based navigation occurred in the thoracic spine.

Hott evaluated the clinical screw placement in 86 placements from cervical to lumbar spine. He reported of 4% misplacements in cervical, 6% in thoracic and non in lumbar spine [12].

Holly [11] performed a laboratory evaluation of the Iso-C navigation using three fresh-frozen intact human torsos. For this study he placed a reference to a spinous process and performed the navigated screw placement at this level and one above and below. Pedicles of T1 down to L5 were instrumented. For image-guided drill placement a small skin incision was made therefore. Of 102 pedicle screws 94.7% were placed correctly, 100% in lumbar and 92% in thoracic spine.

Within the thoracic spine the misplacement rate was higher than in the lumbar spine. This overall misplacement rate is smaller compared with the pedicle perforation rate using CT or fluoroscopy based navigation. However, there is the question of the reason for this rate.

Within the reported clinical cases no reason for this small inaccuracy was reported, neither a movement of the reference base or other reasons like the influence of freehand placement.

Pitfalls

One mistake during navigation with one of the above mentioned modalities is the right definition of the vertebra to operate on. The correct localization must be defined by the surgeon. Within the lumbar spine most time this is easy, but it is still necessary to use a fluoroscope to verify the correct high. Within the thoracic spine a fluoroscope is essential to localize the right posterior process of the navigated vertebra.

Precision Analysis of CT and ISO-C Navigation

The purpose of an own study was to evaluate the basic accuracy of the CT and Iso-C-based navigation due to the above-mentioned difference in precision. Therefore, an experimental study was performed using a plastic model of a whole spine with the help of the »reversed verification« described by Hüfner et al. [14].

Methods

The Surgigate™ navigation system (Medivision, Oberdorf, Switzerland), either the spine module, version 3.1 or the Iso-C module, version 1.0 was used.

An intact foam model of the entire spine (Synbone™, Malans, Switzerland) from C1 to sacrum was marked with titanium markers, 1.6 mm in diameter and 8 mm length at level Th4, Th8, Th12, L2, and L4. These markers were placed at the five vertebras at the lateral side of the pedicle, the lateral side of the vertebra, and ventral at the inferior and superior edge of the vertebra.

A CT scan of this spine in supine position was performed using the volume zoom scanner (Siemens, Erlangen, Germany) with the following protocol: 120 kV, 150 mAs, Thick slices 1.25 mm, table feed 5.5 mm, reconstruction interval 0.6 mm. The marked vertebra, one above and two below were scanned. The reason for scanning two vertebras below was the overlapping anatomy of the spinal process within the thoracic spine [8].

For CT-based navigation the matching was performed using five defined landmarks: tip of the spinous process and superior and inferior facet on both sides. This procedure was performed at each vertebra marked with the titanium marker. The reference base was placed to the spinous process and the registration was performed. Once the matching has been calculated, a number, witch reflects the quality of the registration is displayed. The matching result is the root-mean-square of the distances between the digitized points projected into the CT images and their corresponding points in the image. Using the Calculate/Skip worst button the system enables a new calculation with one pair less, the worst one. The new matching result is then displayed.

If this matching result is larger than 1 the pair point matching was repeated.

Surface matching was performed afterwards when the given result of the calculation was good. It was performed with 12 points symmetrically at the dorsal aspect of the vertebra including the spinal process. Again, if the matching result was larger than 1 the surface matching was repeated.

For Iso-C navigation the reference base was also placed rigidly to the marked vertebra. The isocenter was defined with an ap and a lateral fluoroscopic image placing the vertebra centrally. Therefore the whole spine was placed into special holders at both ends of the spinous model to verify that no other metal is in the x-ray beam. Both holders were placed upon a radiolucent table, also (◘ Fig. 71.1).

With two different setups the accuracy analysis was performed:

Point Accuracy

The accuracy at the placed markers were analyzed. Within the verification mode the pointer has to be placed to a selected point and this position should be compared with the displayed point within the dataset. According to Hüfner [14], we also used the »reversed verification«.

Therefore, the pointer was placed after the registration procedure in a special holder. This holder allows a three-dimensional movement of the pointer until the tip of the virtual displayed pointer hit a marker on the navigation system (◘ Fig. 71.2). Fixing the holder rigidly the distance in reality between the marker and the tip of

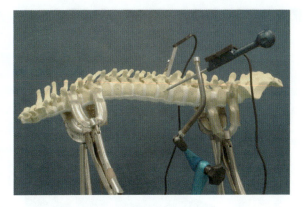

◘ **Fig. 71.1.** »Reversed Verification«: At the navigated vertebra the reference base is placed at the spinous process. In a special three-dimensional holding device the pointer is fixed allowing free movement of the pointer in space. The device can be fixed when achieved the correct position of the pointer

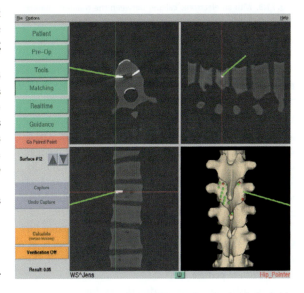

◘ **Fig. 71.2.** Monitor screenshot: The pointer was fixed with the holding device when hitting the titanium markers displayed on the monitor screen

the pointer was measured. An electronically calliper (CD-15CP, Mitutoyo, Inc., Aurora, IL) was used (◘ Fig. 71.3). The accuracy of the calliper was 0.1 mm, according to the manufacturer. All six titanium markers at each marked vertebra were selected as reference points for this reversed verification.

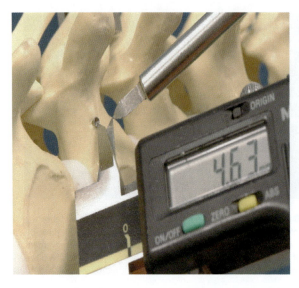

Fig. 71.3. With an electronic calliper between the titanium marker and the tip of the pointer the deviation in reality was measured

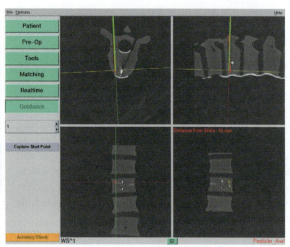

Fig. 71.4. Monitor screenshot: In the prepared holes a trajectory (*red*) was planned and the navigated pedicle awl was placed into the drill hole. The deviation of the angle and the deviation of the entrance point was measured on the screenshot

Pedicle Accuracy

The accuracy for pedicle screw placement was analyzed placing drill-holes for a pedicle screw at Th4, Th8, Th12, L2, and L4 with the navigated pedicle awl of the navigation system. The placement was performed manually without navigation. A CT scan with the same protocol mentioned above was performed of each instrumented vertebra with one vertebra above and two below.

A trajectory was exactly planned within the canal for the pedicle screw witch was visible within the dataset. The diameter of the trajectory was planned as 4 mm, the diameter of the pedicle awl.

For registration same landmarks as for pair-point-matching and surface registration as mentioned above was used. The reference base was placed at the prepared vertebra.

After registration the pedicle awl was placed to the prepared drill hole exactly fit the hole without any motion due to preparing with the same instrument. The navigated awl was displayed on the navigation monitor in green as a line. A screenshot of the monitor was performed and transferred to a commercial laptop. Using CorelDraw 7 (Corel Corperation, Otawa, ON), the screenshots were analyzed measuring the deviation of the planned trajec-

tory and the displayed pedicle awl. The maximum difference between both lines and the angular deviation in each direction was measured (Fig. 71.4).

The analysis at each vertebra was performed three times at all markers or at the left and right pedicle with a new registration, either CT based or with a new Iso-C scan, in between.

Results

Point Accuracy

The mean deviation using CT-based navigation was 1 mm including all markers at one vertebra at the whole spine and 0.5 mm with Iso-C navigation. However, the difference was not significant.

The highest deviation with the CT-based navigation was 2.8 mm, with Iso-C-based navigation 1.88 mm. In almost fifty percent of the measurements a correct imaging, e.g. no difference in reality, was registered with Iso-C navigation. This was just in 25% with CT-based navigation the result. A deviation of more than 2 mm was not registered with Iso-C navigation, in 12% of the CT-based procedure (Fig. 71.5).

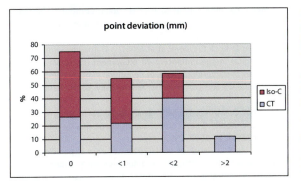

Fig. 71.5. Iso-C-based navigation showed a higher point accuracy. However, between both modalities there was no statistical difference

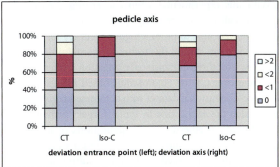

Fig. 71.6. *On the left side* the deviation at the entrance point of both navigation modalities is shown in mm. *On the right side* the deviation of the pedicle axis is shown. Between both navigation modules there is no statistical significance

Pedicle Accuracy

The mean deviation in CT-based navigation was 0.78 mm with a maximum deviation of 4 mm. Iso-C-3D-based navigation showed a maximum deviation of 1.5 mm with a mean deviation of 0.23 mm. Over 75% of the measurements showed no deviation at the entrance point with Iso-C-3D based navigation in contrast to 43% with CT based navigation. No deviation higher than 2 mm occurred with Iso-c-3D based but in 6.6% in CT based navigation (Fig. 71.6).

Almost 80% of the pedicle axis of the inserted pedicle awls hit the defined trajectories correct with Iso-C-3D navigation. In less than 5% an angle of 1 to 2 degree and no deviation greater than 2° occurred. In CT based navigation two third of the inserted pedicle awls showed no deviation. However, a deviation of more than 2° occurs in 6.6%.

The mean deviation in Iso-C-based navigation was 0.2 degree with a maximum deviation of 1.9°. CT-based navigation showed a mean deviation of 0.6 degree with a maximum of 4.5° (see Fig. 71.6).

Discussion and Conclusion

During CT-based navigation, pPossible errors and inaccurate point registration and therefore miscalculations of the dataset can be achieved. The planned landmarks have to be reproduced accurately for CT-based navigation.

The time-consuming step of registration is automated in Iso-C-based navigation. This special point might be the reason for higher accuracy using Iso-C-based navigation for pedicle screw placement.

Within this experimental study, the accuracy compared to CT-based navigation was not significant different. However, comparing the measured accuracy in point as well as in pedicle accuracy the Iso-C-based navigation is more accurate. Furthermore with Iso-C-based navigation no special CT has to be prepared preoperative. an update of the dataset is always possible performing a new Iso-C scan if an anatomic change occurs intra-operatively.

The disadvantage of decreased image quality in osteopenic or obese patients as described by Hott [11, 13] has to be mentioned but was not present in the experimental setup, of course. However, this point has to be considered during Iso-C-based navigation especially in thoracic spine.

The overall accuracy of both three dimensional navigation tools is accurate. In the literature the misplacement rate for pedicle screw placement is slightly higher using CT-based navigation compared to Iso-C-based navigation. However, the amount of literature concerning CT-based spinal procedures is higher than of the most recent technological advantage in navigation using a combination with the Iso-C. The question to answer was if the recently published studies evaluating the Iso-C are concurrence good due to a small number of patients or if the Iso-C-based navigation provides a higher accuracy than CT based navigation.

With this experimental setup concerning the overall image to reality accuracy using a »reversed verification« model, we were able to proof a higher accuracy for Iso-C-based navigation. Within this technique combining a »fluoroscope« with three dimensional navigation it offers some advantages over CT- or Fluoroscopic based navigation. A true three-dimensional dataset with automated registration will broaden the application in spinal surgery providing a high accuracy. Furthermore the applications of minimal invasive techniques in spinal surgery seem possible.

Due to the performed study and resulting accuracy results we will still advice using intra-operative fluoroscopy for intra-operative control of the displayed accuracy of both modalities.

References

1. Arand M, Hartwig E, Kinzl L et al. (2001) Spinal navigation in cervical fractures--a preliminary clinical study on Judet-osteosynthesis of the axis. Comput Aided Surg 6: 170–175
2. Brantley AG, Mayfield JK, Koeneman JB et al. (1994) The effects of pedicle screw fit. An in vitro study. Spine 19: 1752–1758
3. Choi WW, Green BA, Levi AD (2000) Computer-assisted fluoroscopic targeting system for pedicle screw insertion. Neurosurgery 47: 872–878
4. Delorme S, Labelle H, Poitras B et al. (2000) Pre-, intra-, and postoperative three-dimensional evaluation of adolescent idiopathic scoliosis. J Spinal Disord 13: 93–101
5. Donovan DJ, Polly DW Jr, Ondra SL (1996) The removal of a transdural pedicle screw placed for thoracolumbar spine fracture. Spine 21: 2495–2498; discussion 9
6. Esses SI, Sachs BL, Dreyzin V (1993) Complications associated with the technique of pedicle screw fixation. A selected survey of ABS members. Spine 18: 2231–2238; discussion 8–9
7. Euler E, Wirth S, Linsenmaier U et al. (2001) Comparative study of the quality of C-arm based 3D imaging of the talus. Unfallchirurg 104: 839–846
8. Gebhard F, Kinzl L, Arand M (2000) Limits of CT-based computer navigation in spinal surgery. Unfallchirurg 103: 696–701
9. Gertzbein SD, Robbins SE (1990) Accuracy of pedicular screw placement in vivo. Spine 15: 11–14
10. Grutzner PA, Beutler T, Wendl K et al. (2004) Intraoperative three-dimensional navigation for pedicle screw placement. Chirurg 75: 967–975
11. Holly LT, Foley KT (2003) Three-dimensional fluoroscopy-guided percutaneous thoracolumbar pedicle screw placement. Technical note. J Neurosurg 99: 324–329
12. Hott JS, Deshmukh VR, Klopfenstein JD et al. (2004) Intraoperative Iso-C C-arm navigation in craniospinal surgery: the first 60 cases. Neurosurgery 54: 1131–1136; discussion 6–7
13. Hott JS, Papadopoulos SM, Theodore N et al. (2004) Intraoperative Iso-C C-arm navigation in cervical spinal surgery: review of the first 52 cases. Spine 29: 2856–2860
14. Hufner T, Geerling J, Kfuri M Jr et al. (2003) Computer assisted pelvic surgery: registration based on a modified external fixator. Comput Aided Surg 8: 192–197
15. Kotsianos D, Rock C, Euler E et al. (2001) 3-D imaging with a mobile surgical image enhancement equipment (ISO-C-3D). Initial examples of fracture diagnosis of peripheral joints in comparison with spiral CT and conventional radiography. Unfallchirurg 104: 834–838
16. Kotsianos D, Wirth S, Fischer T et al. (2004) 3D imaging with an isocentric mobile C-arm comparison of image quality with spiral CT. Eur Radiol 14: 1590–1595
17. Laine T, Lund T, Ylikoski M et al. (2000) Accuracy of pedicle screw insertion with and without computer assistance: a randomised controlled clinical study in 100 consecutive patients. Eur Spine J 9: 235–240
18. Lonstein JE, Denis F, Perra JH et al. (1999) Complications associated with pedicle screws. J Bone Joint Surg Am 81: 1519–1528
19. Merloz P, Tonetti J, Pittet L et al. (1998) Pedicle screw placement using image guided techniques. Clin Orthop Relat Res 39-48
20. Merloz P, Tonetti J, Pittet L et al. (1998) Computer-assisted spine surgery. Comput Aided Surg 3: 297–305
21. Rampersaud YR, Pik JH, Salonen D et al. (2005) Clinical accuracy of fluoroscopic computer-assisted pedicle screw fixation: a CT analysis. Spine 30: E183–190
22. Rao G, Brodke DS, Rondina M et al. (2002) Comparison of computerized tomography and direct visualization in thoracic pedicle screw placement. J Neurosurg 97: 223–226
23. Rock C, Kotsianos D, Linsenmaier U et al. (2002) Studies on image quality, high contrast resolution and dose for the axial skeleton and limbs with a new, dedicated CT system (ISO-C-3 D). Rofo 174: 170–176
24. Rock C, Linsenmaier U, Brandl R et al. (2001) Introduction of a new mobile C-arm/CT combination equipment (ISO-C-3D). Initial results of 3-D sectional imaging. Unfallchirurg 104: 827–833
25. Roy-Camille R, Saillant G, Berteaux D et al. (1979) Vertebral osteosynthesis using metal plates. Its different uses (author's transl). Chirurgie 105: 597–603
26. Schlenzka D, Laine T, Lund T (2000) Computer-assisted spine surgery. Eur Spine J 9 (Suppl) 1: S57–64
27. Weinstein JN, Spratt KF, Spengler D et al. (1988) Spinal pedicle fixation: reliability and validity of roentgenogram-based assessment and surgical factors on successful screw placement. Spine 13: 1012–1018
28. Wendl K, von Recum J, Wentzensen A et al. (2003) Iso-C(3D0-assisted) navigated implantation of pedicle screws in thoracic lumbar vertebrae. Unfallchirurg 106: 907–913
29. Xu R, Ebraheim NA, Ou Y et al. (1998) Anatomic considerations of pedicle screw placement in the thoracic spine. Roy-Camille technique versus open-lamina technique. Spine 23: 1065–1068
30. Yoo JU, Ghanayem A, Petersilge C et al. (1997) Accuracy of using computed tomography to identify pedicle screw placement in cadaveric human lumbar spine. Spine 22: 2668–2671

Navigation in Spinal Surgery using Fluoroscopy

E.W. Fritsch

Introduction

Since popularized by Roy Camille [22], pedicle screws are widely used in combination with rods or plates (internal fixator) for spinal fixation in different conditions because of the biomechanical superiority of this construct [15, 27]. Furthermore, higher fusion rates are reported with the use of an internal fixator [3, 28].

The main problem with transpedicular screws is the proximity of the spinal cord in the thoracic area [26] and the proximity to the nerve roots at the lumbar spine [4] with the possibility of neurological complications as a consequence of screw mal-placement especially medial-screw mal-placement.

It is reported that between >2 mm [10, 26] and >6 mm [11, 24] medial mal-placement beyond the pedicle cortex a neurological deficiency becomes predictable. As a consequence, the rate of neurological problems due to screw mal-placement using conventional screw-insertion techniques is up to 7% [5].

With the background of up to 39.9% screw mal-placement overall and a 28.5% rate of medial mal-placement [11] using conventional pedicle screw-insertion techniques, it seems understandable that the first attempt of computer-aided orthopedic surgery (CAOS) or image-guided surgery (IGS) was to improve the accuracy of pedicle screw placement [16, 22] which is meanwhile proven in prospective randomized trials at the thoracic and lumbar spine [2, 14] for CT-based IGS.

But CT-based navigation still has limits for everyday routine use.

According to Gebhard et al. [9] the limitations are:

- The limited calculation capacity of the computers used limits the number of available projections and the number of CT-scan slices that are processable.
- The pre-operative planning is influenced by superposing scan protocols and artifacts.
- The CT scan used for navigation reflects the preoperative status of the anatomy-making navigation suitable only with intact vertebral bodies.
- Despite a correct registration process failures in navigation can occur due to mathematical tilting of a vertebral body which is detectable only with intraoperative fluoroscopy.
- The alteration of the preoperative dataset by intraoperative changes of the anatomical situations due to reposition maneuvers are not addressable.

Furthermore, the radiation dose applied with the preoperative CT scan is higher than the radiation dose by intraoperative fluoroscopic control [25] which is of importance especially in scoliosis surgery.

Because of the limitation of CT-based image-guided surgery and with the aim to reduce the radiation dose using the fluoroscope to control every single step during pedicle-screw insertion, fluoroscopic-based navigation [17] (»virtual fluoroscopy« [7,8]) was developed.

Acknowlegements: I want to thank Dr. Iris Grunwald and Prof. Dr. med Wolfgang Reith, Neuroradiological Institute of the University Hospitals in Homburg for their work to evaluate the screw positions with spiral CT scans.

The advantages of »virtual fluoroscopy« are [7, 8, 17]:

- presence of a fluoroscope in an operation where spine surgery is performed,
- automatic registration process without time-consuming matching procedure,
- imaging of the recent anatomical situation,
- updates of the anatomy are possible at any time.

The main problems with the use of fluoroscopic images as a base for navigation are [7,8]:

- changing of the shape of the radiation cone in different positions of the fluoroscope,
- various distorsions of the fluoroscopic image,
- geometrical errors caused by the reduction of the three-dimensional reality into a two-dimensional image.

Therefore, a genuine fluoroscopic image does not reflect the real anatomy with enough accuracy to be used for image-guided surgery.

This accuracy can only be achieved by calibrating the system, which means an exact calculation of the radiation cone in the different positions of the fluoroscope and an elimination of the distorsions.

This is achieved by a calibration target.

The exact position of the fluoroscopic image intensifier can be determined by active LED trackers and a radiation sensor allows an automatic registration of the position of the fluoroscope whenever an image is obtained (Fig. 72.1a).

With the information of the exact shape of the lead balls in the two planes of the calibration target and their defined position, the shape of the radiation cone is calculable and the image distorsions can be eliminated (Fig. 72.1b).

Although the in vitro accuracy of the used navigation system and the used software is proven and published [8], a prospective study with a larger number of screws and the aim to evaluate the in-vivo accuracy of pedicle-screw placement at the thoracic and lumbosacral spine was missing.

Therefore, a prospective study was designed using postoperative CT evaluation of the position every single pedicle screw placed with virtual fluoroscopy. An established reconstruction mode [6, 13] was used to avoid the inaccuracy of the determination of the screw position with plain radiographs [6].

Materials and Methods

After being available at the authors institution, a fluoroscopic-based navigation system (ION; Medtronic Surgical Navigation Technology; Louisville, CO) with the software FluoroNAV Ver. 3.0 (Medtronic Surgical Navigation Technology; Louisville, CO) was used to guide the insertion of pedicle screws at the thoracic and lumbar spine in patients undergoing spinal fusion procedures without limitations to certain pathologies.

Patients were positioned on a Wilson frame for surgeries from TH10 to the sacrum. In cases where the higher thoracic levels were addressed, the patients were positioned on two rigid foam cushions, one under the sternum, the second under the pelvis. This resulted in a better image quality otherwise lowered by the superposing aluminia struts of the Wilson frame.

After the surgical approach with preparation of the processi spinosi, the lamina and the capsules of the small vertebral joints, the reference arc was attached to a stable spinous process making the automatic registration of the patient possible (Fig. 72.2).

Then the fluoroscopic images were acquired, activated and used for navigation. In multilevel cases the screws were placed in up to 3 vertebral bodies with one registration process. If necessary, a second registration with a new set of images was used.

According to the results of Ebraheim et al. [4] showing that at the thoracic levels a true a.p. and a true lateral fluoroscopic image represents the real anatomical situation, these projections were used at the thoracic spine, whereas at the lumbosacral spine an additional oblique view (»owl's eye-view«) was obtained according to Robertson et al. [21] who found that only with this view the true center of the pedicle can be properly visualized radiographically.

After determination of the screw entry point with a trackable pointer (Fig. 72.3) and simulation of both screw length and diameter (Fig. 72.4), the pedicle was opened with a trackable awl/probe/tap instrument. The pedicle was then probed and the thread was cut. Then the screw was inserted with a trackable screw inserter (Fig. 72.5).

Every step (opening of the pedicle, probing, thread cutting, screw insertion) was performed with the guidance of the navigation system.

Pedicle screws of the TENOR-system (Medtronic Sofamor Danek, Memphis TN) or M8 (Medtronic Sofamor

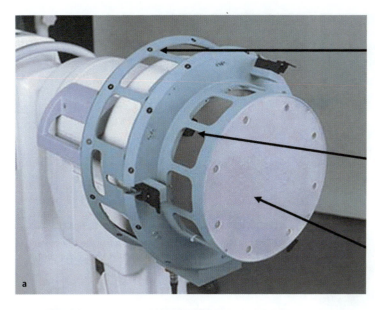

━ LED Tracking
enables exact localisation of the
fluoroscope in all positions

━ Radiation Sensor
enables automatic aquisition
of the pictures

━ Calibration Grid
markers are electronically removed in
the activation process of the image

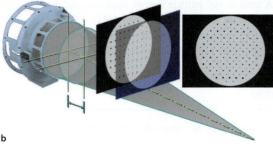

Fig. 72.1a,b. a Calibration target. **b** Using two planes with embedded lead balls of to different diameters in a defined distance the X-ray cone can be calculated and distorsions can be eliminated

Danek, Memphis TN) were used in a diameter of 5.5, 6.5 or 7.5 mm according to the simulation of the screw-diameter with the FluoroNAV software.

After introducing all screws, a final fluoroscopic view in the a.p. and lateral projection was obtained.

The evaluation of the screw position was prospectively done by 2 independent neuroradiologists in the first consecutive 30 patients with spiral CT scans (1.3 mm slice thickness) and reconstructions along the screw and perpendicular to the pedicles in accordance to Laine et al. [13] for each screw.

A screw was considered ideally placed when it was found to be complete inside the cortical borders of the pedicle. Mal-placement was graded in superior, inferior, lateral or medial and the distance between the thread of the screw and the cortical border was measured for quantification (■ Fig. 72.6).

The postoperative neurological examination was correlated with the findings of the screw-position analysis and thus a possible relation was determined.

The pathologies leading to spinal surgery of the study cohort consisted in 7 patients with failed back surgery syndrome, 8 patients with spinal stenosis often requiring multilevel decompression and stabilization, a degenerative scoliosis with a Cobb angle >40° in 2 cases, a spondylolisthesis (Grade I–III) in 4 cases, a fracture in 3 patients and metastases in 6 patients.

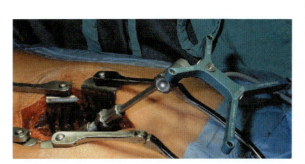

Fig. 72.2. Intraoperative view: The reference arc is attached to a spinous process

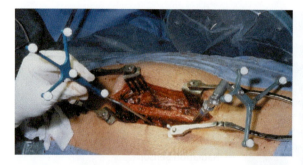

Fig. 72.3. Intraoperative view: Determination of the screw-entry point with the pointer

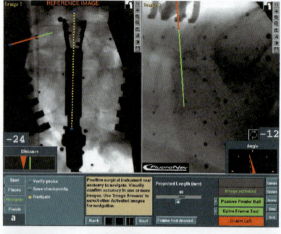

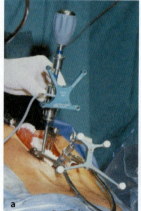 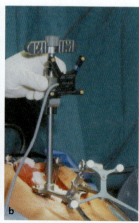

Fig. 72.5a,b. a Intraoperative view: Preparation of the pedicel with a trackable tool (Awl/Probe/Tap). **b** Intraoperative view: Placement of the screw with a trackable screwdriver

A total of 160 pedicle screws were inserted: 54 screws in 20 patients at the thoracic spine (TH4-TH12) and 106 screws in 27 patients at the lumbosacral area (■ Table 72.1).

The screws were inserted by 4 different surgeons.

Results

All screws could be inserted with guidance of »virtual fluoroscopy«.

A conversion to the conventional insertion technique due to technical problems with the guiding system was never necessary.

All screws could be left in place because the intraoperative fluoroscopic examination after placement of all screws per case did not show a gross screw mal-position.

The CT evaluation showed that 151 (94.4%) of the 160 screws were ideally positioned.

At the thoracic spine 49 of the 54 screws (91%) and at the lumbosacral area 102 of the 106 screws (96.2%) were ideally inserted (■ Fig. 72.7).

A superior or inferior mal-positioning never occurred but 1 (0.6%) medial and 8 (5%) lateral mal-positoned screws were determined.

The only medial mal-placed screw was found at the TH5 level.

4 of the 8 lateral mal-placed screws were noticed at the thoracic spine (4/54=1.8%) and 4 at the lumbar spine (4/106=3.8%; ■ Table 72.2).

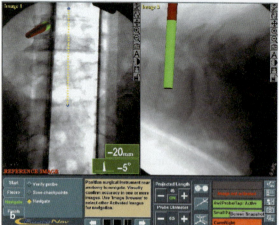

Fig. 72.4a,b. a »Virtual fluoroscopy«: Simulation of the screw lenght; *red:* actual position of the pointer; *green:* simulated screw lenght. **b** »Virtual fluoroscopy«: Simulation of the screw – diameter (6.5 mm in this case); the simulation of the screw-diameter shows that the screw will fit into the pedicle in both dimensions

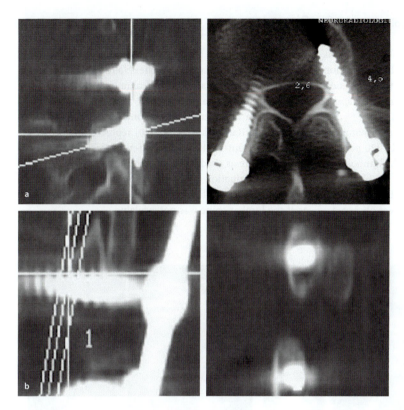

Fig. 72.6a,b. Scheme of the evaluation of the screw position with a postoperative spiral – CT scan. **a** *Left:* Definition of the reconstruction along the screw axis. *Right:* Resulting CT image. **b** *Left:* Definition of the reconstruction perpendicular to the pedicle. *Right:* Resulting CT-image.

Table 72.1. Segmental distribution of the screws placed with »Virtual Fluoroscopy«

	Number of screws
TH 4	6
TH 5	6
TH 6	4
TH 7	10
TH 8	6
TH 9	4
TH 10	4
TH 11	6
TH 12	8
L 1	8
L 2	12
L 3	14
L 4	28
L 5	32
S 1	12

Table 72.2. Direction and quantity of screw mal-placement

	Overall	Thoracic spine	Lumbosacral spine
Ideally placed [n]	150/160	49/54	101/106
Medial mal-placement [n]	1	1	0
0–2 mm [n]	0	0	0
3–4 mm [n]	1	1	0
5–6 mm [n]	0	0	0
>6 mm [n]	0	0	0
Lateral mal-placement [n]	9	4	5
0–2 mm [n]	0	0	0
3–4 mm [n]	3	1	2
5–6 mm [n]	4	1	3
>6 mm [n]	2	2	0

In the study cohort screw-related neurologic disorders were not observed.

Since the study showed excellent results and it was observed that using »virtual fluoroscopy« both radiation exposure and operating time can be saved the navigation system was used as a routine procedure in every spinal case with pedicle screws up to the level of TH2.

Since September 2000 up to now a total of approximately 1200 screws were inserted in approximately 220 patients with a distribution of about 800 screws at the lumbosacral spine and 400 screws at the thoracic spine.

Clinically since the use of »virtual fluoroscopy« a screw related neurologic deficiancy was never observed.

Discussion

Data concerning the accuracy of pedicle-screws installed with »virtual fluoroscopy« are rare. Nolte et al. [17] published 30 in vitro placements of aluminum-cylinders in pedicles using virtual fluoroscopy, one series of screw placement in 11 patients and a second series of 25 screws.

Recently Rampersaud et al. [20] reported an accuracy rate of 89% out of 40 pedicle screws inserted with the same software as used in this study from TH3 to L1.

But an evaluation of a larger number of pedicle screws inserted with »virtual fluoroscopy« at the thoracic as well as at the lumbar spine was not available.

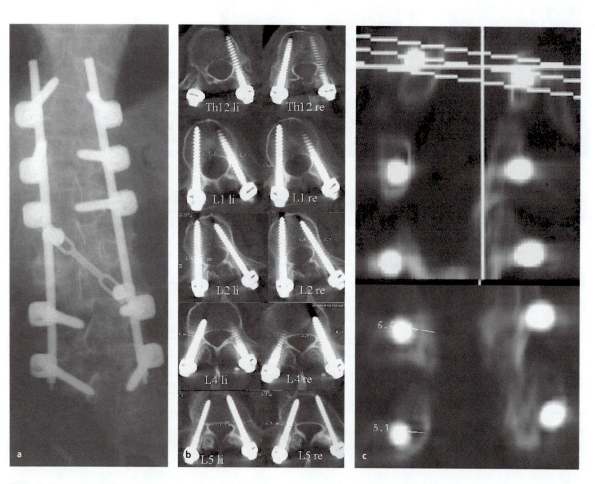

Fig. 72.7a–c. a Standard a.p. X-ray after multisegmental correction of a severe de-novo scoliosis. **b** Reconstruction of all 10 pedicle screws along the screw axis: all screws are ideally placed. **c** Reconstruction of all 10 pedicle screws perpendicular to the pedicle axis: all screws are ideally placed

Therefore the accuracy rates found in this study can only be compared to data of accuracy rates achieved with CT-based navigation.

Kalfas et al. [12] reported a rate of 91.3% ideally placed pedicle screws (n=150) at the lumbar spine utilizing CT-based navigation. Amiot et al. [1] found 95% of 292 pedicle screws between TH2 and S1 ideally placed with CT guidance and Schlenzka et al. [23] installed 95.7% of 139 screws ideally using CT-based image-guided surgery but pointed out, that in 20.1% of the planned screws the insertion could not be done with navigation due to technical problems with the system.

Recently Amiot et al. [2] and Laine et al. [14] conducted prospective randomized studies comparing the accuracy rated of pedicle screws installed with CT-based navigation vs. screws inserted without navigation.

At the thoracic spine Amiot et al. [2] found a difference of 87.1% vs. 98.3% in advantage for CT-based navigation (TH2-Th12 addressed with CT navigation; TH5-TH12 addressed conventionally). Laine et al. [14] found a difference at the thoracic spine (TH8-TH12) of 73.5% in the conventional group vs. 91% in the CT-navigated group. At the lumbar spine the difference between the two groups was 85.4% vs. 93.2% in the investigation of Amiot et al. [2]; the results of Laine et al. [14] were 88.6% vs. 95.3% ideally placed screws in advantage for the CT-guided group.

The comparison of the presented own results especially with the very differentiated findings of Amiot et al. [2] and Laine et al. [14] reveal no significant differences between the rates of ideally placed screws with »virtual fluoroscopy« and CT-based navigation.

A remarkable increase of the rates of ideally placed screws with reported results for conventional screw placement [11] is also obvious for »virtual fluoroscopy«.

With respect to the not ideally placed screws, in accordance to Schlenzka et al. [23] a shift towards the less dangerous lateral screw mal-placement could also be shown for »Virtual Fluoroscopy«.

But, reviewing literature, a rate of 100% ideally placed screws seems not to be achievable neither with CT-based navigation nor with »virtual fluoroscopy«.

One of the reasons might be seen in the findings of Rampersaud et al. [19] showing that especially at the levels TH4, TH7, TH6, TH3, TH12, L1, TH 11 (descending order) the accuracy requirements for navigation cannot be met neither by CT-based navigation nor by »virtual fluoroscopy«.

Considering the disadvantages of CT-based navigation and the irradiation dose accompanied with the planning CT scan [25], »virtual fluoroscopy« appears to be superior to CT-based navigation at the lumbar and thoracic spine because of the equal accuracy and the minimized irradiation dose.

The easy setup, the automatic registration process and the fact that a planning is not necessary makes »virtual fluoroscopy« suitable for the every day routine use in spinal fusion procedures.

But despite of the help of »virtual fluoroscopy« high surgical skills of the spine surgeon are mandatory.

Furthermore, a profound knowledge of the radiological anatomy [4, 21] which must be properly addressed at all times is essential for the successful use of virtual fluoroscopy.

References

1. Amiot L-P, Labelle H, DeGuise JA, Sati M, Brodeur P, Rivard CH (1995) Computer assisted pedicle screw fixation. Spine 20: 1208–1212
2. Amiot L-P, Lang K, Putzier M, Zippel H, Labelle H (2000) Comparative results between conventional and computer-assisted pedicle screw installation in the thoracic, lumbar and sacral spine. Spine 25: 606–614
3. Dickman CA, Yahiro MA, Lu HTC, Melkerson MN (1994) Surgical treatment alternatives for fixation of unstable fractures of the thoracic and lumbar spine. Spine 19 [Suppl]: 2266–2273
4. Ebraheim NA, Xu R, Ahmad M, Yeasting RA (1997) Projection of the thoracic pedicle and its morphometric analysis. Spine 22: 233–238
5. Esses SI, Sachs BL, Dreyzin V (1993) Complications associated with the technique of pedicle screw fixation. Spine 18: 2231–2239
6. Farber GL, Place HM, Mazur RA, Jones CDE, Damiano TR (1995) Accuracy of pedicle screw placement in lumbar fusions by plain radiographs and computed tomography. Spine 20: 1494–1499
7. Foley KT, Rampersaud YR, Simon DA (2000) Virtual fluoroscopy. Oper Tech Orthop 10: 77–81
8. Foley KT, Rampersaud YR, Simon DA (2001) Virtual Fluoroscopy: computer-assisted fluoroscopic navigation. Spine 26: 341–351
9. Gebhard F, Kinzl L, Arand M (2000) Grenzen der CT basierten Computernavigation an der Wirbelsäule. Unfallchirurg 103: 696–701
10. Gertzbein SD, Robins SE (1990) Accuracy of pedicle screw placement in vivo. Spine 15: 11–14
11. Jerosch J, Malms J, Castro WH, Wagner R, Wiesner L (1992) Lagekontrolle von Pedikelschrauben nach instrumentierter dorsaler Fusion der Lendenwirbelsäule. Z Orthop 130: 479–483
12. Kalfas ICH, Kormos DW, Murphy MA et al. (1995) Application of the frameless stereotaxy to pedicle fixation of the spine. J Neurosurg 83: 641–647
13. Laine T, Mäkilato K, Schlenzka D, Tallroth K, Poussa M, Alho A (1997) Accuracy of pedicle screw insertion: a prospective CT-study in 30 low back patients. Eur Spine J 6: 402–405

14. Laine T, Lund T, Ylikoski M, Lohikoski J, Schlenzka D (2000) Accuracy of pedicle screw insertion with and without computer assistance. A randomised controlled clinical study in 100 consecutive patients. Eur Spine J 9: 235–240

15. Nolte L-P, Steffen R, Kramer J, Jergas M (1993) Fixateur interne; Eine vergleichende biomechanische Studie mit verschiedenen Systemen. Aktuelle Traumatol 23: 20–26

16. Nolte L-P, Zamoranol, Jiang Z, Wang Q, Langlotz F, Berlemann U (1995) Image-guided insertion of transpedicular screws: A laboratory setup. Spine 20: 497–500

17. Nolte L-P, Slomoczykowski MA, Berlemann U et al. (2000) A new approach to computer-aided spine surgery: fluoroscopic based surgical navigation. Eur Spine J 9 [Suppl 1]: 78–88

18. Rampersaud YR, Foley KT, Shen AC, Williams S, Solomito M (2000) Radiation exposure to the spine surgeon during fluoroscopically assisted pedicle screw insertion. Spine 25: 2537–2645

19. Rampersaud YR, Simon DA, Foley KT (2001) Accuracy requirements for image-guided spinal pedicle screw placement. Spine 26: 352–359

20. Rampersaud YR, Montanera W, Salonen D (2001) Computer assisted cervicothoracic (3D) and thoracic (2D) pedicle screw placement: a prospective clinical study. CAOS -USA Pittsburgh, 6.–8.July; Conference Syllabus: 213–215

21. Robertson PA, Stewart NR (2000) The radiologic anatomy of the lumbar and lumbosacral pedicles. Spine 25: 709–715

22. Roy-Camille R (1970) Oseosynthese du rachis dorsal, lombaire et lombo-sacre par plaques metalliques vissees dans les pedicules vertebraux et les apophyses articulaires. Presse Med 78: 1448

23. Schlenzka D, Laine T, Lund T(2000) Computer-assisted spine surgery. Eur Spine J 9 [Suppl 1]: 57–64

24. Schulze CJ, Munzinger E, Weber U(1998) Clinical relevance of accuracy of pedicle screw placement. A computertomographic-supported analysis. Spine 23: 2215–2220

25. Slomoczykowski M, Roberto M, Schneeberger P, Ozdoba C, Vock P (1999) Radiation dose for pedicle screw insertion. Fluoroscopic method vs. computer-assisted surgery. Spine 24: 975–82

26. Vaccaro AR, Rizzolo SJ, Allardyce TJ (1995) Placement of pedicle screws in the thoracic spine: Part 2. An anatomical and radiographic assessment. J Bone Joint Surg [Am] 8: 1200–1206

27. Vahldiek MJ, Panjabi MM (1998) Stability potential of spinal instrumentations in tumor vertebral body replacement surgery. Spine 23: 543–550

28. Yuan HA, Garfin SR, Dickman CA, Mardjetko SM (1994) A historical cohort study of pedicle screw fixation in thoracic, lumbar, and sacral spinal fusions. Spine 19 [Suppl]: 2279–2296

72

Navigation on the Thoracic and Lumbar Spine

P.A. Grützner, K. Wendl, J. von Recum, A. Wentzensen, L.-P. Nolte

Introduction

Using pedicle screws for dorsal fusion of the spine is an accepted standard method for various spine diseases like instabilities through trauma, scoliosis or degenerative instabilities.

Pedicle screw placement for dorsal instrumentation of vertebral fractures makes great demands on the surgeons three-dimensional orientation ability. This applies especially to the thoracic spine with it's narrow pedicle diameters [37]. Possible complications through misplacement of pedicle screws concern spinal canal, nerve roots, and the biomechanical stability of instrumentation. For the implantation of pedicle screws a range of techniques has been developed. The intra-operative use of a conventional C-arm for visualization and position control of the pedicles is a common method. Important for the preparation of the pedicle is consolidated anatomic knowledge and the connection of optic information and the surgeons senses. Visualization of pedicles, to be instrumented, especially within this area as well as for scoliosis, spondylitis, adiposity, and osteoporosis with the C-Arm is very demanding [29, 37]. In extensive clinical studies with experienced surgeons a misplacement rate of 4% to 40% was reported for this technique in the thoracic and lumbar spine [13, 36]. Fortunately, not every misplaced screw leads to clinical consequences. On the other hand there are no reports about intra-operative misplacements that can cause complications, but can be recognized by intra-operative imaging, and hence be corrected. One must assume that there is a high number of unreported cases.

For these reasons, an increasing number of pedicle screws have been implanted with the help of a navigation system since their introduction in clinical application in 1995 [1, 26]. The navigation at the spine with the help of a CT-based navigation, or the navigation using a 2D data set, from a conventional image converter, have become established methods at centers working with navigation. Numerous publications proof that these systems can be utilized in clinical practice, and in most cases contribute to a more accurate placement of pedicle screws, compared to what can be achieved with conventional surgery techniques [2, 34]. A disadvantage of the CT-based navigation is the necessity of manual data registration [6, 11, 15].

The navigation with images from an fluoroscopic image intensifier does not have this disadvantage. Here the present situation can be depicted intra-operatively through new images. But the restriction of the image information to 2 dimensions limits the application on complex anatomic structures like the spine. Another limiting factor is the bad image quality of the upper thoracic spine and the thoracolumbar transition of adipose patients.

The mobile isocentric 3D-C-arm SIREMOBIL® ISO-C-3D (Siemens AG, Medical solutions, Erlangen, Germany) combines three-dimensional visualization as in a CT-data set with the flexibility of the intra-operative data acquisition of the C-arm.

In the following we present our experience with the ISO-C-3D in combination with an optoelectronic navigation system (SurgiGATE®, Praxim – Medivision, Grenoble, France) for the placement of pedicle screws in the thoracic and lumbar spine. The primary objective of this study was to evaluate the accuracy of pedicle screw placement with this new method, and to document the effects on the intra-operative workflow.

Material and Methods

An optoelectronic navigation system was used in the study. The instruments used (awl, probe, screwdriver, and T-grip) were tracked by active markers of an Optotrak™ 2030 camera (Northern Digital Inc. Ontario, Canada). For the dorsal instrumentation a fixed-angle screw-rod construct was applied in all cases (USS™, Synthes – Stratec, Oberdorf, Switzerland). The intra-operative imaging with the ISO-C-3D was used for the 2D fluoroscopy for the segment localization and the repositioning control as well as for the 3D imaging for navigation and control of the instrumentation. 100 2D single images from the ISO-C-3D are used to calculate a high-resolution 3D data cube with an edge length of approximately 12 cm. The data were imported through a network protocol into the navigation system. The starting point of the ISO-C-3D at the data acquisition is registered by the camera of the navigation system through markers on the C-Arm. Simultaneously, the position of the vertebral body is registered by a reference base (DRB, Dynamic Reference Base) fixed at the processus spinosus. It is important to establish a stable fixation. The reproducibility of the automatic registration and the precision of the complete system was secured in preclinical tests [30].

The adjustment and location of the data cube in relation to the starting position of the ISO-C-3D is defined. Thus the position of the data cube, analogical to the 2D C-arm navigation, can be directly transferred (automatic registration). The localization of the instruments tracked by the camera is depicted in the 3D image. During the recording of the single images it has to be guaranteed that the spatial position of the anatomic structure is not altered. A change of position, e.g. through respiratory movements during the scan causes a significant decrease of image quality, and a correct registration is not guaranteed. Those movements were measured in a study finding about 1.3 mm at the lower lumbar spine [14]. At the thoracic spine those movements are more extensive and pertain all three axis (own surveys).

Keeping these restrictions in mind, the registration and the ISO-C-3D scan were conducted in all cases with the patient in apnea. The pre-oxygenation with 100% oxygen was carried out accurately timed before the scan. Under this precondition the oxygen reserves are sufficient for an adult to stay in apnea for approximately 10 minutes. During the scan continual monitoring of the oxygen saturation was performed. In collaboration with the anes-

thetist specific stopping criteria for the apnea phase were defined [8, 23,25]. The determination of the beginning of the apnea is also very important regarding the breathing cycle. To assure that the theoretical change of the intra-thoracic volume is as small as possible, and thus no change to the position of the spine occurs, apnea is carried out in expiration in each case. The ISO-C-3D navigation was conducted only under these preconditions.

After the registration and recording of the data set the transfer of the DICOM raw data of the ISO-C-3D into the navigation system took place. There the data set is treated like a CT data set and directly used for navigation. In addition to that it is possible to schedule trajectories into the pedicles within the data set. Despite, or perhaps because of the automatic registration the surgeon has to carefully verify the accurateness prior to beginning navigation. The visualization of different positions of an instrument on screen is compared to the real position on exposed anatomic structures. All surgeons of the study have had experiences with conventional pedicle instruments as well as with CT- and fluoroscopy-based navigation at the spine.

In instable situations it is not possible to transfer the registration over several segments [4]. Therefore a repositioning of the DRB especially at the thoracic spine is necessary if there are fractures. Since these ruins registration, a re-registration has to take place through the recording of a second data set.

Thus it became necessary during long-segment fusions to record a second ISO-C-3D scan.

After the instrumentation in most cases the control of the pedicle screw position took place intra-operatively and if applicable the reposition of the fracture through a new ISO-C-3D scan. The conventional 2D pedicle imaging in the axial view was not used. If the pedicle diameter was smaller than 4 mm, the technique of the lateral parapedicular screw placement in the pre-operative CT was used. In all cases, in which a screw was not centrally visualized in the pedicle, a screenshot was taken and it was documented separately.

Surgery time, blood loss, number of ISO-C-3D scans and total fluoroscopy time of every patient was recorded. A pre- and post-operative neurologic status was ascertained. If a ventral fusion was performed in the same session, the time for the mere dorsal procedure was recorded separately to provide for a better comparability of all patients.

All post-operative complications during in-house clinical treatment were recorded, a neurologic status was ascertained, and a CT examination of the instrumented segments was conducted. The CT analysis was made according to a standardized protocol by an independent radiologist. At the spine a transgression of more than 2 mm of the pedicle wall was interpreted as misplacement. This classification is used by most of reference studies [32, 34].

Ventral screw perforations were interpreted as misplacements, too. Misplacements were classified as medial, lateral, caudal, cranial and ventral and qualified in mm. For this measuring the view in which the misplacement was best visible was chosen and the point of the most extensive perforation was measured from the cortical bone. If a screw was positioned less than 2/3 in the spine body, this was also recorded as misplacement.

The primary parapedicular inserted screws were assessed separately. Here the intra-operative screenshot was compared to the post-operative. Discrepancies over 2 mm were interpreted as misplacement.

The connection of the 3D-arm to the navigation system is used in our clinic since January 2002. Within the scope of a prospective study a total of 61 patients, in whose cases the navigation of the pedicle screws was conducted using an ISO-C^{3D} data set, were included until December 2003 (24 months). The application of the system requires a team of experts and therefore the method presented here could not be used for all emergency patients. But whenever a team was available an ISO-C-3D based navigation was carried out in all cases.

Results

A total of 302 pedicle screws were implanted using navigation in 61 patients with 73 fractures. In a further 3 patients the ISO-C-3D navigation was aborted intra-operatively. In one case the network connection between the navigation system and the ISO-C-3D could not be established due to a hardware failure. One case showed an insufficient precision during verification, attributed to a decalibration. In another case a malfunction of the DRB occurred.

61 (25 men, 36 women) patients with 73 fractures on the thoracic und lumbar spine were operated. The mean age of the patients was 48.6 years (min. 16 years, max. 82 years). The mean BMI was 26.58 (min. 19.7, max. 39.2). 9 patients (14.8%) suffered from polytrauma. Surgery was carried out at the day of accident in 10 cases (emergency indication), 8 patients showed symptoms of paraplegia. On 2 further patients with paraplegic symptoms surgery was delayed because of the transfer from

another hospital. The mean time between accident and surgery was 5.5 days (0–19). 31 patients suffered from fractures of the thoracic spine, and 42 in the lumbar spine. 7 patients had multi-segmental fractures of the thoracic spine and 5 patients had multi-segmental fractures of the lumbar spine. All fractures were categorized according to the AO classification on the basis of the preoperative images. 37 patients showed A-fractures (13 A2, 24 A3), 10 patients had B-fractures and 14 C-fractures (□ Fig. 73.1).

4 surgeons participated in this study. A total of 302 pedicle screws were placed. Dorsal stabilizing was performed with the USS System with 4 mm pedicle screws and 5 mm to 6 mm Schanz screws. On 6 of the 8 patients with paraplegic symptoms and emergency surgery, a laminectomy was carried out. On the 2 patients with paraplegic symptoms and secondary surgery curettage of the spinal canal was realized from ventral in the same session. Surgery time was 98 min +/− 31 min (47–230 min), mean blood loss was 580 ml +/− 203 (300–1200 ml). Navigation took 45 min +/− 13 (30–90 min). Mean intra-operative fluoroscopy time was 1.4 min +/− 0.6 (0.7–3.7 min). Fluoroscopy time for each implanted pedicle screw was 0.3 min +/− 0.1 min (0.2–0.9 min). The fluoroscopy time before the first ISO-C-3D was 0.2 min +/− 0.2 (0.1–1.0 min), after the last ISO-C-3D scan the time was 0.5 min +/− 0.5 (0.1–2.8 min). On average, 2.7 (2–5) scans were performed with the ISO-C-3D. 1.7 scans (1–4) were used for navigation, and 1.0 scans (0–2) for the verification of the screw position and repositioning as well as for curettage of the spinal canal. In one case 3 pedicle screws had to be exchanged, due to the intra-operative information of the ISO-C-3D.

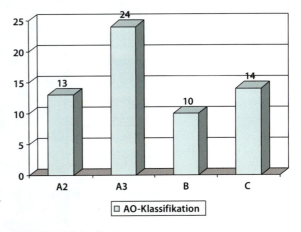

□ **Fig. 73.1.** AO classification

These screws were classified in the analysis as misplacements under navigation, although their position in the post-operative CT was correct. A flawed verification was noticed in one patient. Intra-operative analysis identified the initiation of the apnea phase during maximum inspiration as the reason. After registration, air had leaked from the thorax at the middle thoracic spine, which altered the position of the spine during the ISO-C-3D scans. The scan was repeated in exhalation, and the navigation performed without any troubles. An abort of the ISO-C-3D scans due to a drop in the oxygen saturation was never required (◘ Fig. 73.2).

No case showed a post-operative neurological worsening. Post-operative complication could not be observed. During the analysis of the post-operative CT, 3 misplaced screws were discovered. One screw was misplaced in T12 by 2–3 mm to medial. This was overlooked in the intra-operative control scan. In the same patient, two screws were misplaced in T7 and T8. One screw had a medial deviation of 2–3 mm, the other screw a lateral deviation of 3–4 mm. These screws were not included in the intra-operative control scan. In the long segment instrumentation the intra-operative control scan did not record this,

and the screws placements were judged as correct in the 2D fluoroscopy. Overall 5 of 302 pedicle screws were misplaced (1.7%). Broken down into patients, this means misplacements in 3 of 61 patients (4.9%).

Discussion

The conventional placement of pedicle screws has, according to a meta-analysis of Laine, a misplacement ratio of up to 40% [13, 32]. Even in cadaver studies this rate can be as high as 31%. This bears the risk of a worsening of the neurological symptoms and an insufficient mechanical stabilization [19]. Placing pedicel screws on the spine, especially on the thoracic spine is a demanding and technically challenging task for every surgeon. The thoracic pedicle anatomy is complex and variable [27]. The pedicle, especially in the middle area of the thoracic spine, is only marginally wider than the implant. Therefore, the parapedicular instrumentation method is recommended for extremely tight pedicle [18]. This method helps to avoid the danger of pedicle destruction, while reducing the risk of intra-spinal screw placement, and to achieve comparable

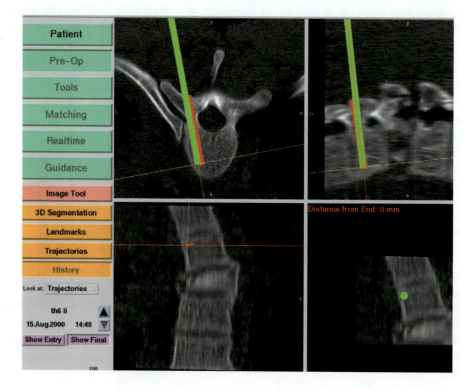

◘ **Fig. 73.2.** CT-based navigation on the spine

stability. Nevertheless this method is also very challenging.

Thus, pedicle screw placement is the perfect field of application for navigated surgery, with the aim to maximize the amount of accurately placed screws. Common navigation systems capture data with a pre-operative CT or an intra-operative 2D image with a conventional C-arm. CT-based and C-arm-based navigation systems facilitate a quality increase in screw placement in complex anatomic areas of the musculoskeletal system and a reduction of intra-operative fluoroscopy time [3, 20, 21, 32].

The only randomized prospective study showed a significant decrease of the misplacement ratio from 14.4% to 4.3% [20]. Only electively operated patients were included. Conducting such studies in trauma surgery is conceptually extremely difficulty and has so far been impossible. The main reason being, that not all surgeons are trained in the use of the navigation system in emergency situations. This deficit leads to uncertainty, expectable additional work load and thus to the refusal to use the navigation system in particular cases. Our series demonstrated that, on the other hand, trained surgeons used the navigation system even in emergency situations.

Most studies concerning this method showed a clear advantage of the navigate procedure compared to the conventional method. However, the misplacement ratios of up to 11% mentioned are relatively high [3, 34]. Problematic are the varying misplacement definitions. The analysis in clinical studies can only be performed using post-operative CT diagnosis. The informative value of conventional fluoroscopic images is simply not high enough for a precise evaluation [5, 31]. An experimental study on cadavers showed, that there is a tendency to judge the misplacement ratio in the CT higher than the actual one found in the anatomic specimen [4]. The reason for this is the forming of artifacts and the over-radiating of the screws in the CT. Because of that, the analysis can only be carried out by an experienced radiologist and should include a pedicle reconstruction.

Strictly speaking, only a precise central position of the screw should be defined as an accurate placement. This must be put into perspective for the clinical point of view. A precise central position of the screw without damage to the pedicle wall is often impossible due to the bend of the pedicles, especially at the thoracic spine, together with the small diameter [7, 9, 22, 35]. Planed parapedicular instrumentation must therefore be evaluated under these aspects, and incisions of the screw thread into the pedicle wall cannot be labeled as incorrect placement. Schulz did

an evaluation of misplacements, although a differentiation between the risk of neurological dysfunctions and the impact on biomechanics is necessary [33]. In our study, as in most clinical studies, a transgression of the pedicle wall of less than 2 mm was labeled as a correct placement.

A very important aspect of pedicle instrumentation is often not taken into account. With the conventional instrumentation method, there is the intra-operative danger, that misplacement is recognized and corrected. This can lead to a weakening of the bone structure or even lesions of the neurovascular structure through incorrect drilling and placement. Since the cases are recognized and correct during surgery, they are not included in the statistic. Our study included such cases, two screws were recognized intra-operatively by the ISO-C-3D imaging system as being 2 mm and 3 mm to far lateral and were corrected. These screws are part of the statistic, even though the post-operative CT scan showed a correct placement (Figs. 73.3–73.5).

CT-based navigation, in successful clinical use since 1995, has lead to an increase of precision. However, certain disadvantages are connected to this method, which impair widespread and everyday use. The CT must be carried out in accordance to a special protocol. Patients often have a CT scan, which is sufficient for the preoperative diagnosis, but totally useless for navigation. Pre-operative preparation of the dataset, including segmenting and planning of landmarks requires special training and is time-consuming. In general, a CT is not available for intra-operative updates or control scans of the implant position. This is the reason, why registration-free 2D C-Arms have been developed and implemented into clinical use [10, 17]. This method allows a simultaneous display of various 2D layers, providing a virtual fluoroscopy. This can enhance the screw placement precision [3, 10, 15, 16]. Yet, the 2D fluoroscopy has distinct disadvantages. Axial projection of the pedicle, possible in the 3D dataset, is not available. The technique to display the pedicle in true axial position is helpful, but is very demanding for the imagination of the surgery assistant. In the conventional technique, just like for the fluoroscopic-based, different factors, like adiposity, osteopenia, and deformities can complicate the interpretation of the 2D images.

Intra-operative 3D imaging of bone structures with an especially designed C-arm is an important step in the development of computer-based techniques for the spine. Some principles have to be considered for a useful data registration. Patients must lie on a metal-free table.

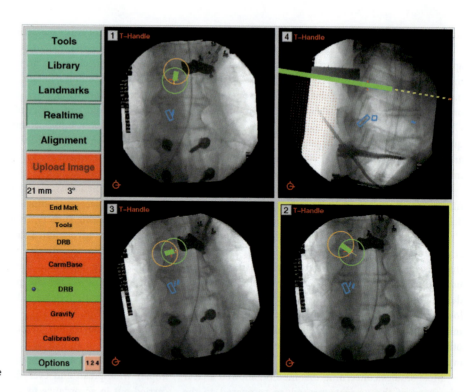

Fig. 73.3. Image amplifier-based navigation on the spine

73

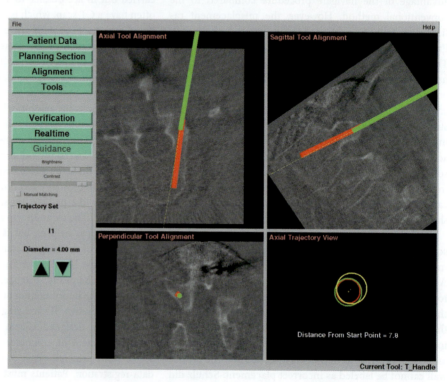

Fig. 73.4. ISO-C-3D-based navigation on the spine

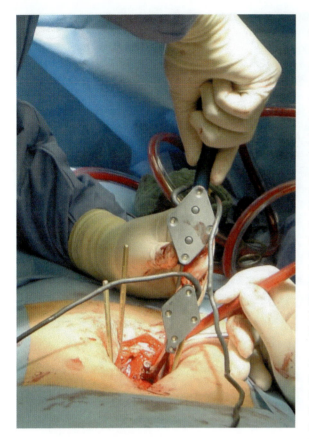

Fig. 73.5. Pedicle instrumentation with navigated instruments

The metals present in typical surgery tables can produce artifacts, which significantly impair the data evaluation. Even the fastening of the DRB can produce artifacts, to avoid this, a special alignment is necessary. The use of a DRB, which is transparent for X-rays, would be a huge improvement. The covering of the surgical area with compresses with a contrast strip should be avoided completely. Moving the object during the scan has drastic consequences on the quality of the image. The respiratory movement of the patient renders an accurate data set reconstruction impossible. The images are out of focus and full of artifacts. Naturally the most extensive respiratory movement can be found at the thorax. An extremely high image quality, which cannot be translated to intra-operative situations, can be achieved with cadavers. Based on these experiences, data acquisition in every patient is performed during respiratory arrest. A pre-oxygenation with

100% oxygen has to be carried out 5 to 10 minutes before beginning the scan. A pulsoxymeter was used to check the oxygen saturation during acquisition. According to the figures given in literature and for further safety, the criteria for aborting the scan were set to a drop of the oxygen saturation below 90% [8, 23–25]. None of the 164 scans performed in the study had to be aborted, even though 7 patients had a thoracic trauma. On the first patient with thoracic instrumentation a high imprecision was found during data verification. The initiation of the respiratory arrest during inspiration was made out as the cause immediately during surgery. Air had leaked out slowly during the scan, and the registration of the data set, done automatically at the beginning of every scan, did no longer match the position of the spine during the scan. The scan was repeated at the same patient during exhalation. The verification and the post-operative CT control scan showed excellent precision. This experience made us do all scans during exhalation since then. We think that this limiting factor of the prototype version can be overcome by further improving the hardware and software.

The intra-operative fluoroscopy time with the ISO-C-3D-based navigation was on average 1.4 min. The fluoroscopy is necessary even in CT-based navigations for the intra-operative height positioning of the vertebral body and for the documentation of the exact screw placement after completed instrumentation. During 2D fluoro-navigation significant fluoroscopy times are required for the recording of the correct positions and for documentation purposes [3, 4, 10, 28]. The intra-operative exposure to radiation for ISO-C-3D navigation can be calculated. Cause for this is the standardized fluoroscopy procedure of the ISO-C-3D, no further scans besides the focusing of the area to be registered is necessary. Especially the »search« for the best fluoroscopic angel can be left out. The latter can be extremely difficult for inexperienced personnel, particularly in the area of the thoracic spine and results in increased fluoroscopy times. No further fluoroscopies are required after data set registration. The reduction of the exposure to radiation, not only for the patient but also for the surgery personnel is an important improvement. The exposure to radiation for the personnel is further reduced, if the fact that everybody can leave the controlled area during the ISO-C-3D data acquisition is taken into account. In his clinical trial, Gebhard demonstrated a reduction by the factor of 11 with the ISO-C-3D navigation, compared to conventional instrumentation [12]. This matches our experiences.

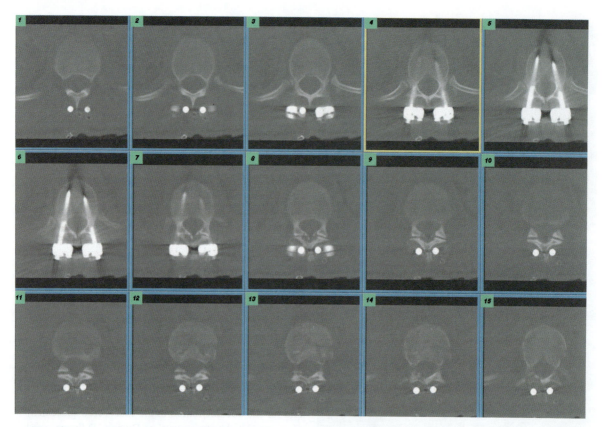

Fig. 73.6. Post-operative CT analysis. Correct screw placement

73

In our opinion, intra-operative verification of the registration is essential. The precision of the systems in influenced by a variety of factors and today's versions are prone to malfunction. A decalibration of the system was noted in one patient. The surgery had to be continued the conventional way. Since then, regular consistency tests are performed using a special calibration model. It became clear that the precision is influenced by the intrinsic calibration of the ISO-C-3D data cube and the calibration of the inherent registration.

In our study 3 screws were evaluated as misplaced by radiologists. 2 further screws were evaluated as being to far lateral in the intra-operative ISO-C-3D scans and therefore labeled as misplaced. 16 screws distributed on 3 patients were implanted in the area of the thoracic spine using the parapedicular technique. The reason was always a pedicle width of less than 4 mm. A correct trans-pedicular placement using 4 mm screws was therefore technically impos-

sible. Eminent for this method is a lateral alteration of the pedicle wall, without any biomechanical disadvantages. Without a 3D navigation, this technique is very challenging, as you move away from the anatomic and fluoroscopic landmarks. The advantage is that medial pedicle lesions or pedicle destructions can be avoided nearly completely. Kothe succeeded in proofing the biomechanical advantages and usefulness of navigation for this technique [18, 19, 27]. The apparent 2 mm alterations of the pedicle, which were identified in the post-operative CT and documented during surgery, were not labeled as misplaced screws (Fig. 73.6).

The technique of dorsal instrumentation was modified and standardized in our clinic through the combination of intra-operative 3D fluoroscopy and passive navigation with automatic registration. Conventional 2D fluoroscopy is used to define the iso-center of the image amplifier and for reposition control. Besides the already described case, no further intra-operative position changes for screws had

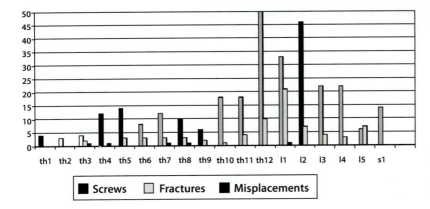

Screws ☐ **Fractures** ■ **Misplacements**

☐ **Fig. 73.7.** Fracture distribution (n=73 on 61 patients), pedicle instrumentation (n=302) and misplacements (n=5) related to spinal segments

to be performed, which not only resulted in an increase in patient safety, but also in a time reduction. The ISO-C-3D navigation did not cause a relative increase in surgery time. Complications, like for example an increased infection rate could not be found in our group (☐ Fig. 73.7).

We think that the decisive advantage of the ISO-C-3D navigation in our group was however the accuracy of the pedicle screw placement, compared to the conventional and other navigation methods. Complications connected to the misplacements could not be observed.

A practiced user can operate the system with ease. The user guidance of the combination of Siemens ISO-C-3D and navigation system in the current version still leaves room for improvements. Only after intensive introduction and training is the safe and error-free use of the system possible. Consequently, use of the system is reserved for only a small group, and thus is limited especially during the night, when trained surgeons and nurses are not present. An improved system handling could help to increase the acceptance of the system and to streamline the training process.

The substantial investment costs of the ISO-C-3D are put back into perspective by the fact, that besides the possible use as a conventional C-Arm, an ISO-C-3D navigation in other areas then the spine is possible, one example would be the implantation of IS lag screws.

Conclusion

The ISO-C-3D navigated placement of pedicle screws, performed by an experienced surgeon, is a very reliable procedure, and incorrect screw placement can be near-

ly completely avoided. The intra-operative information gained is of great important especially for fractures, as it allows for an evaluation of the bone structure of the spinal canal. The exposure to radiation can be minimized without relevant increase of the surgery time. For an increased use of the system additional software improvements, particularly concerning user-friendliness would be required.

References

1. Amiot LP, Labelle H, De Guise JA, Bellefleur C, Rivard CH (1996) Computer assisted pedicle screw installation. Our first 3 cases. Ann Chir 50: 626–630
2. Amiot LP, Lang K, Putzier M, Zippel H, Labelle H (2000) Comparative results between conventional and computer-assisted pedicle screw installation in the thoracic, lumbar, and sacral spine. Spine 25: 606–614
3. Arand M, Hartwig E, Hebold D, Kinzl L, Gebhard F (2001) Präzisionsanalyse navigationsgestützt implantierter thorakaler und lumbaler Pedikelschrauben. Unfallchirurg 104: 1076–1081
4. Austin MS, Vaccaro AR, Brislin B, Nachwalter R, Hilibrand AS, Albert TJ (2002) Image-guided spine surgery: a cadaver study comparing conventional open laminoforaminotomy and two image-guided techniques for pedicle screw placement in posterolateral fusion and nonfusion models. Spine 27: 2503–2508
5. Berlemann U, Heini P, Muller U, Stoupis C, Schwarzenbach O (1997) Reliability of pedicle screw assessment utilizing plain radiographs versus CT reconstruction. Eur Spine J 6: 406–410
6. Berlemann U, Monin D, Arm E, Nolte LP, Ozdoba C (1997) Planning and insertion of pedicle screws with computer assistance. J Spinal Disord 10: 117–124
7. Cinotti G, Gumina S, Ripani M, Postacchini F (1999) Pedicle instrumentation in the thoracic spine. A morphometric and cadaveric study for placement of screws. Spine 24: 114–119
8. Duda D, Brandt L, Rudlof B, Mertzlufft F, Dick W (1988) Effekt verschiedener Präoxygenierungsprotokolle auf den arteriellen Sauerstoffstatus. Anaesthesist 37: 408–412

9. Ebraheim NA, Jabaly G, Xu R, Yeasting RA (1997) Anatomic relations of the thoracic pedicle to the adjacent neural structures. Spine 22: 1553–1556

10. Foley KT, Smith MM (1996) Image-guided spine surgery. Neurosurg Clin N Am 7: 171–186

11. Gebhard F, Kinzl L, Arand M (2000) Grenzen der CT-basierten Computernavigation in der Wirbelsäulenchirurgie. Unfallchirurg 103: 696–701

12. Gebhard F, Kraus M, Schneider E et al. (2003) Strahlendosis im OP – ein Vergleich computerassistierter Verfahren. Unfallchirurg 106: 492–497

13. Gertzbein S, Robbins S (1990) Accuracy of pedicular screw placement in vivo. Spine 15: 11–14

14. Glossop N, Hu R (1997) Assessment of vertebral body motion during spine surgery. Spine 22: 903–909

15. Grützner PA, Köhler T, Vock B, Wentzensen A (2001) Rechnergestütztes Operieren an der Wirbelsäule. OP Journal 17: 185–190

16. Grützner PA, Vock B, Wentzensen A (2001) C-Arm Navigation an der LWS. Osteologie 10: Suppl 2

17. Hofstetter R, Slomczykowski M, Sati M, Nolte LP (1999) Fluoroscopy as an imaging means for computer-assisted surgical navigation. Comput Aided Surg 4: 65–76

18. Kothe R, Matthias SJ, Deuretzbacher G, Hemmi T, Lorenzen M, Wiesner L (2001) Computer navigation of parapedicular screw fixation in the thoracic spine: a cadaver study. Spine 26: E496–E501

19. Kothe R, Panjabi MM, Liu W (1997) Multidirectional instability of the thoracic spine due to iatrogenic pedicle injuries during transpedicular fixation. A biomechanical investigation. Spine 22: 1836–1842

20. Laine T, Lund T, Ylikoski M, Lohikoski J, Schlenzka D (2000) Accuracy of pedicle screw insertion with and without computer assistance: a randomised controlled clinical study in 100 consecutive patients. Eur Spine J 9: 235–240

21. Laine T, Schlenzka D, Makitalo K, Tallroth K, Nolte LP, Visarius H (1997) Improved accuracy of pedicle screw insertion with computer-assisted surgery. A prospective clinical trial of 30 patients. Spine 22: 1254–1258

22. Liljenqvist U, Hackenberg L, Link T, Halm H (2001) Pullout strength of pedicle screws versus pedicle and laminar hooks in the thoracic spine. Acta Orthop Belg 67: 157–163

23. Merkelbach D, Brandt L, Mertzlufft F (1993) Verhalten der arteriellen und gemischt-venösen Sauerstoff- und Kohlendioxidpartialdrücke sowie der pH-Werte während und nach einer Intubationsapnoe. Untersuchungen zum in vivo Auftreten des Christiansen-Douglas-Haldane-Effekts. Anaesthesist 42: 691–701

24. Mertzlufft F, Brandt L (1989) Hyperoxic intubation apnoea: an in vivo model for the proof of the Christiansen-Douglas-Haldane effect. Adv Exp Med Biol 248: 397–405

25. Mertzlufft F, Krier C (2001) Präoxygenierung – ein Muß. Aber wie? Anasthesiol Intensivmed Notfallmed Schmerzther 36: 451–453

26. Nolte LP, Zamorano L, Visarius H et al. (1995) Clinical evaluation of a system for precision enhancement in spine surgery. Clin Biomech (Bristol, Avon) 10: 293–303

27. Panjabi MM, Takata K, Goel V et al. (1991) Thoracic human vertebrae. Quantitative three-dimensional anatomy. Spine 16: 888–901

28. Rampersaud YR, Foley KT, Shen AC, Williams S, Solomito M (2000) Radiation exposure to the spine surgeon during fluoroscopically assisted pedicle screw insertion. Spine 25: 2637–2645

29. Rampersaud YR, Simon DA, Foley KT (2001) Accuracy requirements for image-guided spinal pedicle screw placement. Spine 26: 352–359

30. Ritter D, Mitschke M, Graumann R (2002) Markerless Navigation with the intraoperative Imaging Modality SIREMOBIL Iso C3D. electromedica 70: 31–36

31. Sapkas GS, Papadakis SA, Stathakopoulos DP, Papagelopoulos PJ, Badekas AC, Kaiser JH (1999) Evaluation of pedicle screw position in thoracic and lumbar spine fixation using plain radiographs and computed tomography. A prospective study of 35 patients. Spine 24: 1926–1929

32. Schlenzka D, Laine T, Lund T (2000) Computer-assisted spine surgery. Eur Spine J 9 (Suppl 1): S57–S64

33. Schulze CJ, Munzinger E, Weber U (1998) Clinical relevance of accuracy of pedicle screw placement. A computed tomographic-supported analysis. Spine 23: 2215–2220

34. Schwarzenbach O, Berlemann U, Jost B et al. (1997) Accuracy of computer-assisted pedicle screw placement. An in vivo computed tomography analysis. Spine 22: 452–458

35. Ugur HC, Attar A, Uz A, Tekdemir I, Egemen N, Genc Y (2001) Thoracic pedicle: surgical anatomic evaluation and relations. J Spinal Disord 14: 39–45

36. Weinstein J, Spratt K, Sprengel D, Brick C, Reid S (1988) Spinal pedicle fixation: Reliability and validity of roentgenogram, based assessment and surgical factors on successful screw placement. Spine 13: 1012–1018

37. Zindrick MR, Wiltse LL, Doornik A et al. (1987) Analysis of the morphometric characteristics of the thoracic and lumbar pedicles. Spine 12: 160–166

73

Navigation of Tumor and Metastatic Lesions in the Thoracolumbar Spine

F. Gebhard, M. Arand

Introduction

Since the description of transpedicle fixation of posterior spinal implants by Roy-Camille et al. [22], this procedure has gained general acceptance for rigid segmental fixation. Correct implantation of the screws without perforation of the pedicle is difficult and requires detailed anatomic knowledge and good surgical skills. The identification of the correct entry point for the pedicle screw and the angle of inclination in the sagittal and transverse planes are crucial. A standard technique for pedicle screw insertion is done with an image intensifier in the lateral and antero-posterior (AP) views. In osteolytic tumors identification of anatomical landmarks is difficult and intra-operative imaging can be impossible due to increased radio trans-lucent vertebrae.

Computed tomography (CT)-controlled studies have had significant rates of incorrect placement of lumbar tran-spedicle screws [6, 10, 29]; implant-related and neurologic complications have also been reported [7, 30]. The central implant placement in the thoracic pedicle is a more diffi-cult procedure [32], and an increasing rate of misplace-ment can be expected in this region.

Within the past years, computer-aided systems for CT-based freehand navigation have been introduced [19, 28]. With this technique, a pre-operative CT scan (CT dataset) is superimposed onto the intra-operative rigid body (the spinal vertebra). As long as the navigated vertebra is non-deformable, online visualization of the instruments within the preoperative data set is possible. In addition, it is important to have intact posterior structures for stable fixation of the minimal invasive reference array (MIRA)

Using these new techniques, experimental [1, 5, 20] and initial clinical [16, 18] results have shown significantly reduced misplacement rates in the lumbar spine pedicle and a decrease in neurologic complications [2].

Additionally, very recently an imaging intensifier provi-ding modality-based 3D-navigable datasets has been in-troduced [9]. As a very useful alternative, intra-operative fluoroscopy based 3D imaging (see Fig. 74.1) has replaced CT-based navigation in our department for thoracic and lumbar spine applications.

First results showed a high accuracy with misplacements rates of > or = 2 mm in 1.7% [12, 13].

Depending on the extent of the disease, the main goals of tumor surgery of the spine are tumor reduction, decom-pression of the neural structures, and stable fixation of a malignancy-induced destabilized spine. As tumor localiza-tion in the spine is predominantly in the anterior column, posterior treatment is palliative only or is done as a first step in a double intervention approach. In corpectomies of tumors of the cervical [21, 27] and thoracic spine [27], initial clinical studies have shown possible applications of image-guided surgery using an anterior approach. Only one clinical study has been published regarding posterior treatment of the thoracic spine so far [3].

Another disadvantage in standard spine tumor surgery is that the extension of the tumor cannot be accurately de-termined intra-operatively, and therefore, the surgeon can-not do procedures such as neural decompression, hemila-minectomy, or laminectomy in complete safety. However, accurate visualization of the tumor can be obtained preoperatively using CT or magnetic resonance imaging (MRI) scans, which can provide safer surgery for the patient.

The aim of this clinical feasibility study was to investigate the efficacy of a computer-aided visualization technique during neural decompression and transpedicle stabilization in patients who require tumor-related surgery of the spine.

Materials and Methods

From 1999 to 2004, an optoelectronic navigation system (SurgiGATE©, Medivision, Oberdorf, Switzerland) has been used by the authors. Starting in 2004, another navigation system (Vectorvision©, BrainLAB, München, Germany) has replaced the optoelectronic system. The navigable data sets have been generated on a four-gantry spiral CT (MX 8000©, Marconi, Hofheim-Wallau, Germany) or in a 40 row scanner (Philips Brilliance) in our radiology department and intra-operatively using a isometric motor driven fluoroscope (Siremobil Iso-C-3D©, Siemens, Germany, ◘ Fig. 74.1). 12 patients with tumors of the spine and acute instability or myelopathy underwent posterior decompression and stabilization using the non modality based CT process and 8 patients using the modality based Iso-C-3D fluoroscopic image related navigation system. In 8 patients two or more vertebrae were involved and in 8 patients the tumor was located in one vertebra only. Twelve tumors were in the thoracic level, 4 in the lumbar area (◘ Fig. 74.2). In all patients advanced metastatic disease was diagnosed, therefore, surgical intervention was palliative and no anterior procedure followed the posterior intervention.

In all non-modality-based navigated posterior decompression and computer-guided pedicle screw implantations were planned (◘ Fig. 74.3).

After footside installation of the navigation camera and the navigation computer with the screen, correct fluoroscopic identification of the involved spinal region in the lateral and AP views was ensured in all patients.

Positioning, covering and the surgical approach corresponded to the standard technique in each patient. To achieve computer guidance, matching of the CT dataset and the patient was done in case of pre-operative non-modality-based imaging, a matching was not necessary in the patients obtaining an intra-operative Iso-C-3D scan (only one scan per patient). Having fixed the MIRA, the point matching procedure was done using four points and a surface matching was added. After achieving an acceptable matching result, verification was done to recheck the accuracy of registration of the CT dataset and the vertebra on the posterior laminar surfaces of the registered vertebra.

Transpedicle instrumentation of the matched vertebra was done with a tracked pedicle awl to have access to the pedicle followed by a tracked pedicle probe to generate the screw hole, in which the 5-mm Schanz screws were implanted with a tracked T handle. After instrumentation of one vertebra, the same procedure was done for the next vertebra.

The second step of the operation consisted of decompression. Therefore, in the non modality based procedure, a third matching was done for metastatic vertebrae after fixation of the dynamic reference base to its spinal process, if the latter was intact (n=8). In 4 cases the MIRA was fixed at the cranial or caudal neighbor vertebra. In the modality based navigated patients, dynamic reference base was placed on the spinal process placed caudal to the tumor, then a small piece of the medio-cranial edge of the left or right lamina was resected by an Hayek dissector with intermittent application of the pedicle awl in the guidance or real-time mode of the navigation system. On the screen of the navigation system, the real-time position of the tracked pedicle awl was observed in relation to the tumor on the pre-operative CT dataset or the fluoroscopical 3D dataset. This mode was used to get biopsies of the tumor (◘ Fig. 74.4).

Complete posterior decompression can be controlled and ensured by the surgeon as well.

The following data were recorded for each patient:

1. the time required for data transfer and planning the intervention (only non-modality-based navigation);
2. the time required for intra-operative installation of the computer system;
3. the time required for vertebral matching and instrumentation (only non-modality-based navigation); and
4. the subjective (surgeon) and objective (history mode) performance of the navigation system.

Post-operatively CT-based analysis of localization of the pedicle screws and the status of decompression in each patient was confirmed by two independent observers (radiologist and trauma surgeon). Correct pedicle screw insertion was reported in all cases where the patient had a successful intraosseous implant, or where patients experienced perforation less than a screw thread in the case of a pedicle breadth that was smaller than the implant diameter.

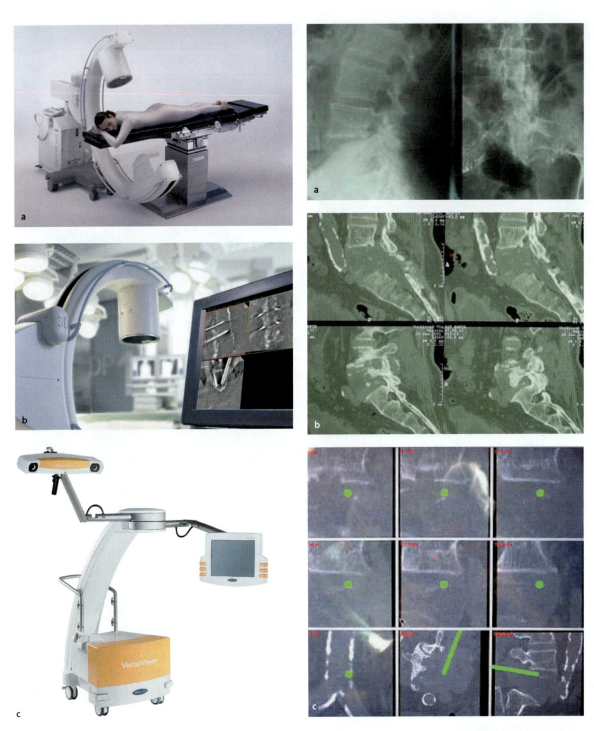

▣ **Fig 74.1a–c.** Intra-operative 3D imaging using a fluoroscope (Siemens ISO C-3D) with the patient placed on a carbon fiber table (**a**) and transferring the dataset via NaviLink (**b**) to the BrainLab VV² system (**c**)

▣ **Fig 74.2a–c.** Metastasis of a spino-cellular tumor in the lumbar spine in standard X-rays (**a**) and CT (**b**). Intra-operative position of the biopsy forceps (**c**)

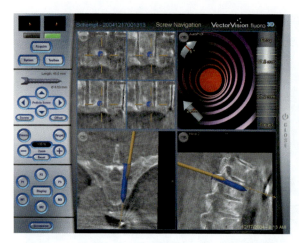

Fig 74.3. Intra-operative pedicle screw planning in the 3D dataset of the cranial vertebra next to the tumor (metastasis of lung carcinoma)

To evaluate the quality of decompression, in the transverse scans the original vertebral tumor extension was identified in the spinal canal. The rim of the tumor, intruding into the canal was marked and translated posteriorly by graphics software (volume matching, MX-view, Marconi, Hofheim-Wallau, Germany). This was implemented into sagittal and frontal reconstructions and consecutive observation showed if the posterior laminar structures were resected completely, referring to the anterior tumor extension.

Results

Inclusion criteria in this study was palliative posterior tumor treatment of the spine and intra-operative CT-based navigation.

One patient with extensive disease that extended to the posterior spinal structures (not listed above) was excluded from the study before surgery, because a rigid connection between the affected vertebra and the data reference base was not possible due to instability of the spinous process. Six thoracic screws had to be placed in standard technique, because no successful matching procedure could be achieved in the non modality based navigation technique. All 16 screws of the 8 patients receiving an intra-operative Iso-C-3D scan were navigated.

The aim of computer-aided decompression and hemilaminectomy was realized in all patients. The average

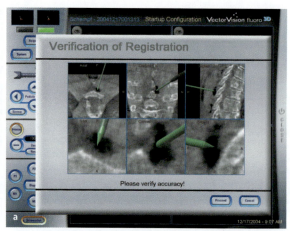

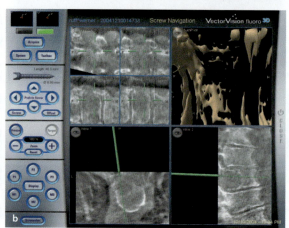

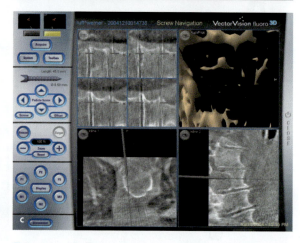

Fig 74.4. a Verification and accuracy check of the 3D fluoroscopy image after transfer to the navigation system in the area of the tumor bearing spine segment. Transpedicular aiming to the tumor (**b**) and guided insertion of the biopsy probe into the tumor (**c**)

time of data transfer in the non modality based technique was 11 min (range 8–15 min), and the average planning time for the operation was 35 min (range 13–90 min). In the modality-based technique, performance and transmission of the ISO-C-3D scan into the navigation system took 3 min. Intra-operative installation of both systems took approximately 5 min and the final matching time per vertebra was 7 min in the non modality based navigation (range 5–10 min); an average re-matching frequency of one procedure with paired point and surface matching was seen in the pre-operative acquired datasets, no second Iso-C-3D scan was necessary in a patient using the modality based technique. Using computer-guided implantation in the non-modality-based navigation, 86% of pedicle screws were positioned centrally as seen on the post-operative CT scan. However, three pedicle screws were placed eccentrically, although in all three patients the history mode showed correct matching results and no faults in the intra-operative application of the navigation system could be found. It is possible that in these initial two patients, operated on with computer guidance, the MIRA loosened during surgery. However, a radicular neurologic disorder of the focal nerve root was not observed in any of the patients with eccentric pedicle screw placement. Based on the modality based Isc-C-3D navigation, two (12%) of the transpedicle screws showed a moderate breach.

In all patients the post-operative CT scan showed accurate decompression of the neural structures (◻ Fig. 74.5). Regarding the pre-operative neurologic findings [8], three patients were classified as having Frankel-B lesions, three had Frankel-C lesions and one patient had a Frankel-D lesion. Five patients had no neurologic disorders pre-operatively. Post-operatively, two patients with a Frankel-B lesion had improvement of the lesion to Frankel-C, and two of the three patients with Frankel-C lesions and the patient with the Frankel-D lesion had no neurologic signs. No neurologic deterioration occurred.

The illustration of the tumor in relation to the implant allowed exact and stable positioning of the transpedicle screws in both navigated techniques, based on different modalities on image acquisition.

Intra-operatively, biopsies could be taken in the center of tumor lesion in all cases.

The main intra-operative pitfalls were the difficulties in thoracic paired-point matching attributable to missing landmarks on the posterior vertebral structures.

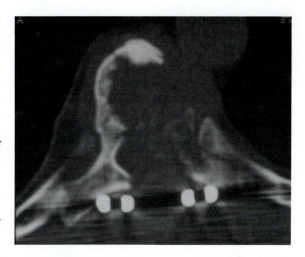

◻ **Fig 74.5.** Post-operative control of CAS guided complete decompression of the posterior structure at the most significant extension of the tumor at Th9 level

Discussion

In this clinical feasibility study, non-modality and modality CT-based verification of the efficacy of navigated decompression and pedicle screw placement in patients who had tumor-related posterior surgery has been demonstrated. Eighty-six percent of the non modality pre-operative CT data set based navigated pedicle screws were positioned centrally in the bone without perforation, 88 percent of the implants were placed intra-osseously using the modality based Iso-C-3D technique. In all patients accurate decompression was seen.

The accuracy of transpedicle screw implantation post-operatively has been investigated in vitro and in vivo with CT-scans [11, 16, 18, 24], plain radiographs [15, 29], MRI [2, 33], and via dissection [20]. In several studies a significant percentage (21% [29], 23% [23], 40% [14], 41% [26,] and 42% [17], respectively) of conventional implanted transpedicle screws were inserted incorrectly. However, other reports have indicated that perforation rates of the lumbar pedicle were as low as 10% [25] to 15% [2]. In vitro and in vivo computer-aided navigation studies, have shown an increased accuracy of transpedicle implant fixation with perforation rates from 2.7% to 11.3% [2, 15, 16, 24]. In addition, Zippel et al. [33] achieved in a MRI-controlled study a better reduction of thoracic misplacement rates (11.4%) than for lumbar misplacement rates (16%).

Authors with comparable studies [2, 16, 33] have observed higher rates of misplacement in their conventionally treated cohorts (range, 14.3%-42%) as in the navigated groups. In very recently published modality based cohorts, the rate of »misplacement« (perforation of 2 mm maximum) was reported as low as 1.7% [12].

However, the accuracy of the computer-guided insertion of transpedicle screws in this series was higher than in some published reports of studies which used conventional fluoroscopic positioning [14, 23, 26, 29]. Moreover, and unlike other published studies [4, 5, 31], no post-operative neurologic deterioration and no implant loosening were seen in the patients as a result of using computer-aided surgical procedures. At the same time we were able to achieve complete decompression of the neural structures.

Because of inaccurate registration, it was not possible to use computer-aided implantation surgery for 15% of the pedicles and, therefore, a conventional fluoroscopic approach was used. These data compare favorably with the findings of other investigators who observed rates of non-navigable pedicles as high as 32% [16, 24]. An advantage of the modality based navigation with intra-operative acquisition of the dataset was the accurate navigation in all patients without re-imaging the spine in one patient. The average intra-operative time for navigated instrumentation of the spine was 7 minutes for the matching per vertebra in the non modality based technique, which is slightly higher than that reported in the literature (5.5 min) [16].

Our initial results indicate that non modality and modality-based computer-aided frameless navigation of tumor surgery of the spine is a safe technique which improves surgical performance during posterior decompression and transpedicle stabilization. In addition, CAS surgery improved the intra-operative information about the tumor and the current surgical intervention during decompression. In contrast to other authors [11, 24], a learning curve was observed for processing and interpretation of the intra-operative matching, the crucial part of non modality based spinal navigation. Imaging quality on the other side is essential in the modality-based Iso-C-3D technique; a carbon table without metal interference with regard to the scan field is required as well as the exclusion of local motions during scanning (rest of respiration during scanning in the thoracic spine) [9].

In general the described techniques should be used only by experienced surgeons who can, if required, continue the operation using conventional techniques. Furthermore, the surgeon should have a complete theoretical understanding of the navigation system to minimize possible misinterpretation of computer guidance information.

In future we think that the fluoroscopy-based 3D imaging is the most preferable technique in the above described cases.

References

1. Amiot LP, Bellefleur C, Labelle H (1997) In vitro evaluation of computer-assisted pedicle screw system. Ann Chir 51: 854–860
2. Amiot LP, Lang K, Putzier M, Zippel H, Labelle H (2000) Comparative results between conventional and computer-assisted pedicle screw installation in the thoracic, lumbar, and sacral spine. Spine 25: 606–614
3. Arand M, Hartwig E, Kinzl L, Gebhard F (2002) Spinal navigation in tumor surgery of the thoracic spine: first clinical results. Clin Orthop Rel Res: 399: 211–218
4. Bauer HC (1997) Posterior decompression and stabilization for spinal metastases: Analysis of sixty-seven consecutive patients. J Bone Joint Surg 79A: 514–522
5. Carl AL, Khanuja HS, Sachs BL et al. (1997) In vitro simulation: Early results of stereotaxy for pedicle screw placement. Spine 22: 1160–1164
6. Castro WH, Halm H, Jerosch J et al. (1996) Accuracy of pedicle screw placement in lumbar vertebrae. Spine 21: 1320–1324
7. Esses SI, Sachs BL, Dreyzin V (1993) Complications associated with the technique of pedicle screw fixation: A selected survey of ABS members. Spine 18: 2231–2238
8. Frankel HL, Hancock DO, Hyslop G et al. (1969) The value of postural reduction in the initial management of closed injuries of the spine with paraplegia and tetraplegia. Paraplegia 7: 179–192
9. Gebhard F, Weidner A, Liener UC, Stockle U, Arand M (2004) Navigation at the spine. Injury: 35S: 35–45
10. Gertzbein SD, Robbins SE (1990) Accuracy of pedicular screw placement in vivo. Spine 15: 11–14
11. Girardi FP, Cammisa FP, Sandhu HS, Alvarez L (1999) The placement of lumbar pedicle screws using computerised stereotactic guidance. J Bone Joint Surg 81B: 825–829
12. Gruetzner PA, Beutler T, Wendl K, von Recum J, Wentzensen A, Nolte LP (2004) Intraoperative three-dimensional navigation for pedicle screw placement. Chirurg 75: 967–975
13. Hott JS, Papadopoulos SM, Theodore N, Dickman CA, Sonntag VK (2004) Intraoperative Iso-C C-arm navigation in cervical spinal surgery: review of the first 52 cases. Spine 29: 2856–2860
14. Jerosch J, Malms J, Castro WH, Wagner R, Wiesner L (1992) Lagekontrolle von Pedikelschrauben nach instrumentierter dorsaler Fusion der Lendenwirbelsäule. Z Orthop 130: 479–483
15. Kamimura M, Ebara S, Itoh H et al. (1999) Accurate pedicle screw insertion under the control of a computer- assisted image guiding system: Laboratory test and clinical study. J Orthop Sci 4: 197–206
16. Laine T, Schlenzka D, Makitalo K et al. (1997) Improved accuracy of pedicle screw insertion with computer-assisted surgery: A prospective clinical trial of 30 patients. Spine 22: 1254–1258

74

17. Merloz P, Tonetti J, Pittet L et al. (1998) Pedicle screw placement using image guided techniques. Clin Orthop 354: 39–48
18. Merloz P, Tonetti J, Pittet L et al. (1998) Computer-assisted spine surgery. Comput Aided Surg 3: 297–305
19. Nolte LP, Visarius H, Arm E et al. (1995) Computer-aided fixation of spinal implants. J Image Guid Surg 1: 88–93
20. Nolte LP, Zamorano LJ, Jiang Z et al. (1995) Image-guided insertion of transpedicular screws: A laboratory set-up. Spine 20: 497–500
21. Roessler K, Ungersboeck K, Dietrich W et al. (1997) Frameless stereotactic guided neurosurgery: Clinical experience with an infrared based pointer device navigation system. Acta Neurochir 139: 551–559
22. Roy-Camille R, Roy-Camille M, Demeulenaere C (1970) Osteosynthesis of dorsal, lumbar, and lumbosacral spine with metallic plates screwed into vertebral pedicles and articular apophyses. Presse Med 78: 1447–1448
23. Saillant G (1995) Complications de la visee pediculaire, echecs et complications de la chirurgie du rachis. Montpellier Sauramps
24. Schwarzenbach O, Berlemann U, Jost B et al. (1997) Accuracy of computer-assisted pedicle screw placement: An in vivo computed tomography analysis. Spine 22: 452–458
25. Sim E (1993) Location of transpedicular screws fixation of the lower thoracic and lumbar spine. Acta Orthop Scand 64: 28–32
26. Vaccaro AR, Rizzolo SJ, Balderston RA et al. (1995) Placement of pedicle screws in the thoracic spine. Part II: An anatomical and radiographic assessment. J Bone Joint Surg 77A: 1200–1206
27. Vinas FC, Holdener H, Zamorano L et al. (1998) Use of interactive-intraoperative guidance during vertebrectomy and anterior spinal fusion with instrumental fixation: Technical note. Minim Invasive Neurosurg 41: 166–171
28. Visarius H, Gong J, Scheer C, Haralamb S, Nolte LP (1997) Man-machine interfaces in computer assisted surgery. Comput Aided Surg 2: 102–107
29. Weinstein JN, Spratt KF, Spengler D, Brick C, Reid S (1988) Spinal pedicle fixation: Reliability and validity of roentgenogram- based assessment and surgical factors on successful screw placement. Spine 13: 1012–1018
30. West JL, Bradford DS, Ogilvie JW (1991) Results of spinal arthrodesis with pedicle screw-plate fixation. J Bone Joint Surg 73A: 1179–1184
31. Wise JJ, Fischgrund JS, Herkowitz HN, Montgomery D, Kurz LT (1999) Complication, survival rates, and risk factors of surgery for metastatic disease of the spine. Spine 24: 1943–1951
32. Zindrick MR, Wiltse LL, Doornik A et al (1987) Analysis of the morphometric characteristics of the thoracic and lumbar pedicles. Spine 12: 160–166
33. Zippel H, Putzier M, Lang K (2000) Computerassistierte Wirbelsäulenchirurgie. In: Reichel H, Zwipp H, Hein W (eds) Wirbelsäulenchirurgie. Standortbestimmung und Trends. Steinkopff, Darmstadt, 174–201

Part VII   Future Perspectives in CAOS

Alternatives to Navigation

M.A. Hafez, B. Jaramaz, A.M. DiGioia III

Introduction

Computer-assisted orthopaedic surgery (CAOS) has become a reality and its tools, especially surgical navigation, have become a part of the toolbox of many orthopaedic surgeons. However, CAOS technologies encompass a wide spectrum of devices that are still unknown to most orthopaedic surgeons. These devices have been designed to assist at different stages of surgical management of orthopaedic conditions such as preoperative planning, operative performance, postoperative measurement, training, telesurgery, etc. Some of them are in clinical use but many are still under laboratory testing. With the broad spectrum and continuous expansion of CAOS technologies and applications it is difficult for researchers to have a precise definition or a standard classification of CAOS. We envisage that CAOS may be defined as the use of computer-enabled technology at pre, intra and/or postoperative stages in the management of surgical conditions using active or passive systems, and performed for various applications such as planning, simulation, guidance, robotic, telesurgery and/or training [9].

There are many technical classifications for CAOS tools but surgeons generally prefer simple and clinically based classifications such as that of Picard et al. [18] who classified CAOS devices based on their actions (active, semi-active and passive) and then sub-grouped them based on their need for imaging (image free or image based). Using this classification, surgeons in many surgical disciplines can easily differentiate between main categories, such as active robotics and passive navigation systems.

However, CAOS is an emerging and expanding field and it is expected that hybrid devices and new systems may appear in future. In our institute, several CAOS devices (other than navigation) have been developed. Based on our experience and on the literature review, we grouped CAOS devices on the basis of their functionality and clinical use into 6 categories, which are then sub-grouped on technical basis (■ Table 75.1). In future, new devices can be added under new categories or subcategories. This grouping scheme is meant to provide a simple guide on orthopaedic systems rather than a comprehensive classification for all computer assisted systems in surgical practice. For example, the number and diversity of tasks of surgical robots is enormous, as shown by Pott et al. [20] who identified 159 surgical robots with different mechanisms and functions. These can be classified according to their tasks, mechanism of actions, degree of freedom and level of activity but for the purpose of simplicity we sub-categorized the orthopaedic robots to only industrial, hand-held and bone-mounted.

Robotics

Robotic technology was introduced to orthopaedics in early 1990s (before navigation), when Robodoc (Integrated Surgical Systems, Sacramento, California) was used for milling of femoral canals during total hip arthroplasty [17]. Few other robotic systems have been developed for orthopaedic use and tested clinically [13, 25]. Although both navigation and robotic technologies have been successfully applied to several procedures world-

▫ Table 75.1. Categories of different CAOS systems

#	Categories Clinically based	Subcategories Technically based	Examples	Mechanism
1	Robotics	Industrial Hand-held Bone-mounted	ROBODOC [17] PFS [2] MINARO2 [4] MBARS [28]	Actively perform surgical actions, sub-classified based on ergonomics
2	Navigation	Image free Image-based (preop) Image-based (intraop)	Most navigation systems can be adapted to be image- based or im-age free [5, 7, 26]	Passively acts as Position tracking devices and information systems, sub-classified based on imaging needs
3	Hybrid techniques	Image free Image based	ROBONAV [27] PRAXITELES [19] PI GALILEO [22] PFS [2]	Combine features of robotic and navigation, sub-classified based on imaging needs
4	Templating	Guide Tool	Individual templating [21] Patient-specific templating (TKA) [8]	Provide guidance and/or tooling, sub-classified based on the mechanism of action of the templates
5	Simulation	Planning simulators Virtual reality Augmented reality	ROM simulators [23] Knee arthroscopy simulators [15] Image overlay [1]	Improve visualization through intuitive user interfaces ± interactive animation, sub-classified based on the way data are manipulated
6	Telesurgery	Telepresence Telementoring	Under development [29]	Allows the surgeon to remotely operate or mentor other surgeons

Preop pre-operative, *Intraop* intra-operative, *TKA* total knee arthroplasty.

wide, universal acceptance has not been forthcoming. Inherent complexity, cost, set up time and learning curves dissuade many potential users. Current navigation techniques require the insertion of tracking targets into bone and robotics require rigid fixation of the limb, thus adding invasiveness and risk, and extending OR time. Image-based systems may require preoperative CT or MRI scans, or intra-operative X-rays, which are not a part of the normal routine. All of these considerations contribute to the cautious environment in adopting new CAOS technologies. Comprehensive cost effectiveness analysis may be required before these emerging technologies are widely accepted.

New Generation of Robotic Devices

The robots initially introduced into orthopaedic surgery were large industrial robots adapted for surgical use. Despite their high bone shaping accuracy they were surpassed by navigation systems that are less expensive and more acceptable to ordinary surgeons on safety and ease-of-use basis. However, a new generation of smaller robots designed specifically for surgical use is currently under development and testing. Because orthopaedic surgery deals with the hardest structure (bone) that requires cutting and machining, unique robotic devices have been developed in the form of bone mounted and hand held robots. MINARO2 [4] is an example of a bone mounted orthopaedic robot that is based on a parallel robotic structure. Initially, it was designed to be mounted to the OR table before it was developed further to be bone mounted and smaller in size. The device was tested for cement removal during revision total hip arthroplasty (THA) (▫ Fig. 75.1). Another miniature bone attached robotic system (MBARS) [28], was developed for preparation of the femoral bed in patello-femoral arthroplasty (see Fig. 75.1). The robot is attached to the femur using 3 pins and directly palpates the bone surfaces with no need for imaging or tracking in the operating room. The robot directs a conventional cutting burr based on the planning procedure. Laboratory experiments supported the feasibility of this approach.

Brisson et al. [2] described a handheld robot called »Precision Freehand Sculptor« (PFS). It is closer to the size of a micro-drill that is frequently used in hand and feet surgery. The surgeon can hold the robot in one hand while the working end (rotating burr) performs the surgical action. The burr can be inserted through arthroscopic incisions allowing the performance of minimally invasive surgery. The device was tested under laboratory condition for bone preparation of unicompartmental arthroplasty (UKA). Haider et al. [10] reported the use of freehand navigation cutting for TKA without using surgical jigs. The project aimed at developing a bone cutting simulation presented on a regular PC to provide the surgeon with a real-time feedback and corrections for instrument alignment and bone cutting accuracy.

Alternative Technologies

Hybrid Techniques

Ongoing research is now directed towards combining different features of CAOS tools, particularly robotics and navigation. This development may broaden the range of applications of these systems and allow procedures to be performed less invasively. Currently, there are few examples of hybrid techniques in orthopaedic surgery that are in clinical testing or awaiting clinical development.

PRAXITELES [19] is a hybrid manual/motorized device for knee arthroplasty that is positioned in the frontal and axial planes with the aid of a navigation system. The authors justified this approach on the basis of minimizing the size, weight, and number of motorized degrees of freedom of the robot. The project was developed for knee surgery using an image-free navigation system while a bone-mounted robot is allowed to orient cutting blocks (◨ Fig. 75.2). The position of the implant can either be adjusted manually following the planning performed by the navigation system or automatically adjusted by the robot to follow the anatomical axis. The system was tested on plastic and cadaveric specimens for TKA and UKA and authors reported satisfactory results.

Precision Freehand Sculptor (PFS) [2] combines active features of robotics with navigation. It helps the surgeon to perform bone cutting according to pre-operative planning. Although it actively performs the surgical action, the surgeon has full control of the tool's position while holding the device. The rotating burr removes only the

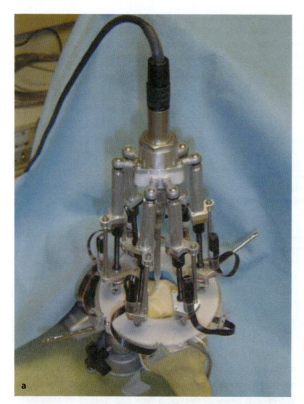

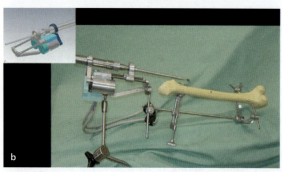

◨ **Fig. 75.1a,b.** Example of bone mounted robots. **a** »MBARS« robot positioned for patello-femoral arthroplasty (with permission from Elsevier [9]). **b** »MINARO« robot positioned for cement removal in revision THA (with permission from Prof K. Radermacher)

bone that was planned to be removed as it retracts inside a guard when placed beyond the planned cutting zone. Similar to navigation systems, the freehand placement of the tool is tracked and displayed on a computer screen in real time providing the surgeon with a feedback and

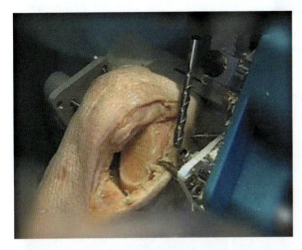

◨ **Fig. 75.2.** An example of a hybrid device (PRAXITELES), while tested for a cadaveric knee experiment (with permission from PRAXIM medivision, France)

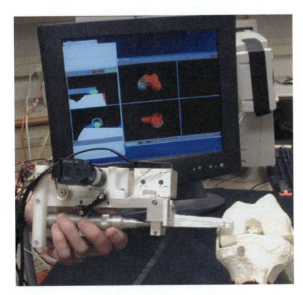

◨ **Fig. 75.3.** A prototype of the Precision Free Hand Sculptor (a handheld robot) (with permission from Elsevier [9])

allowing the surgeon to stop or continue bone cutting as needed. The PFS was experimentally tested for UKA (◨ Fig 75.3) but authors believe that it can potentially be used for TKA and patello-femoral arthroplasty.

PI GALILEO NAV [22] uses a 2 perpendicular linear axis robot with a navigation system to automatically orient the cutting block for knee replacement. *ROBONAV* [27] is a combination of the orthopaedic robot (ROBODOC) and a navigation system allowing an optical tracking of bone and patient's alignment during surgery.

Templating Techniques

The term »templating« is not unfamiliar to orthopaedic surgeons who use radiographic templates to preoperatively select types and sizes of implants and also use templates intra-operatively for sizing fixation plates. Computer-assisted templating techniques are different as they rely on CT-based pre-operative planning to provide patient-specific templates (guides or tools) that can be used during surgery. These templates are typically manufactured using rapid prototyping (RP) machines that act as a 3D printer to transform the computer-aided design (CAD) of the templates to physical and identical models. This technique is more user-friendly than robotics and navigation since it requires no additional equipments in the operating room and no tracking or registration. Radermacher et al. [21] reported the first use of this technology in spine, hip and knee surgery. The templates were used as guides for pedicle screw fixation, pelvic osteotomy (◨ Fig. 75.4) and to align traditional cutting blocks in knee surgery. The use of CT scan and the time involved for preoperative planning and production of the templates have to be weighed against the benefit of using these extra guides.

Hafez et al. [8] reported a new generation of templating techniques where a complete pre-operative planning for TKA was performed, including sizing of the implant, bone cutting and alignment. Simulation of surgery and virtual evaluation of the results can be demonstrated on the computer screen allowing the surgeon to identify and correct errors before real surgery. Based on the final planning, patient-specific templates (cutting blocks) were designed and then produced by RP machines. Then, the surgery can be performed using only femoral and tibial patient specific cutting blocks eliminating the use of conventional jigs or medullary guides (◨ Fig 75.5). Authors justified the drawbacks of using CT scan on the basis of

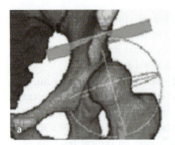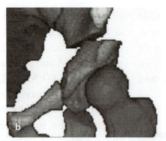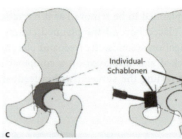

Fig. 75.4a–c. Templating technique for peri-acetabular osteotomy. **a** CT-based pre-operative planning. **b** Pre-operative 3-D simulation of osteotomy. **c** Using the template as a guide during surgery (with permission from Prof K. Radermacher)

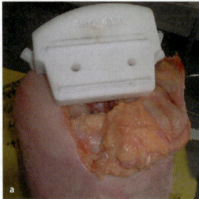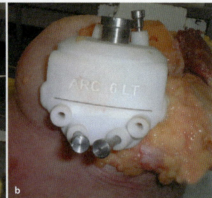

Fig. 75.5a,b. Patient-specific templates for TKA while positioned on a cadaveric knee. **a** Femoral template, **b** tibial template (with permission from Elsevier [9])

the reduction of operative (bone cutting) time to half, the complete elimination of jigs and subsequently the cost reduction.

Simulation

With the introduction of computers and subsequently CT scans, several attempts have been made to simulate the anatomy of the human body and to add animations and interactive programs. Real anatomical images from radiographs, CT scans and MRI scans were used in addition to computer-generated data. Virtual reality has also been introduced to medicine following its successful use in aviation, in which flight simulators have been used for decades as an essential part of training junior pilots before flying. There are obvious advantages of using simulators before practicing on real patients, first is improving patients' safety and second is reducing cost

and time. However, the main challenge for the currently available simulators is to be realistic and offer relevant and accurate information.

Preoperative Planning Simulators

The range of motion simulator described by Jaramaz et al. [14] is an example of a planner component of an image-base navigation system (HipNav) [5]. The planner component allows surgeons to virtually plan a procedure such as THA using the desired implants (Fig. 75.6). The pre-operative planning can be used per se to help the surgeon in selecting the proper type and size of implants, accurately aligning the implants and then testing the ROM, impingements and stability of the hip joint [23]. Moreover, the planning can be transferred to the operating room and used as a road map to help the surgeon in achieving a more accurate performance.

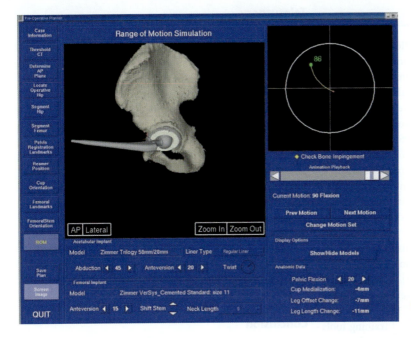

■ **Fig. 75.6.** ROM Simulator while testing impingement and stability for THR

Virtual Reality Simulators

Virtual reality simulators became popular after the successful introduction of laparoscopic surgery. They are superior to cadaveric and plastic bone workshops, as they offer a cost-effective alternative to these traditional training methods. They are typically used in training junior orthopaedic surgeons on arthroscopic knee procedures. They may eliminate the need for the classic intra-operative training on real patients. However, virtual reality simulators are still under development and require further improvement of the visual and tactile properties. According to Satava [6], one of the pioneers in virtual reality in surgery »there are two generic requirements for any surgical simulator; it must have accurate detail and must be highly interactive. Specifically, the image must be anatomically precise and the organs must have natural properties such as the ability to change shape with pressure and to behave appropriately in gravity. All the body parts that are represented must be able to be manipulated by grasping, clamping, or cutting, and they must be able to bleed or leak fluids«. Several systems have been reported in literature [3, 12, 15, 16, 24] but many are still at the experimental phase (■ Fig 75.7).

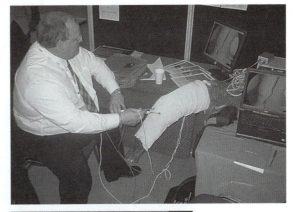

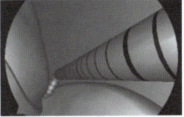

■ **Fig. 75.7.** An example of a virtual reality knee arthroscopy system (*left*) and a probe locating a loose body (*right*) (with permission from Lippincott Williams & Wilkins [16])

Augmented Reality

Augmented reality (AR) is the combination of real world and computer-generated data. In orthopaedic surgery, this computer display technique can superimpose computer images over the surgeons' direct view of the real anatomy. Since images are transformed in real-time, the user interface appears to be an integral part of the surrounding environment. There are few examples in CAOS with alternative terminology being used such as image overlay or image fusion. Heining et al. [11] explained the need for AR in a specialized field such as thoracoscopic spine surgery where, AR could provide a more intuitive user interface by fusing pre- and intra-operative 3-D images, endoscopic camera view, visualization of instrument position and planning of procedures. Using AR, these different imaging modalities can be visualized in their actual location overlaid into a stereoscopic video view. Blackwell et al. [1] described a prototype AR system »Image Overlay« that was experimentally tested for hip and knee surgery (◘ Fig. 75.8) and showed the potential to be used as educational and training tools by clearly visualizing the anatomical and technical aspects of THA. By using »Image Overlay« with three-dimensional medical images such as CT reconstructions, a surgeon could visualize the data »in vivo«, exactly positioned within the patient's anatomy, and potentially enhance the surgeon's ability in performing complex procedures.

Telesurgery

Using robotics and/or other computer-assisted devices experienced surgeons can supervise, assist or perform surgical procedures at remote locations. The first telesurgical procedure across the Atlantic was reported in 2001 when surgeons from New York operated on 68-year-old lady in Strasbourg, France to remove her gall bladder by remotely manipulating robotic tools. Telesurgery has been used in several other surgical procedures such as Nissen fundoplication, hernia repair and bowel resection in addition to other specialties such as urology and neurosurgery. In orthopaedics, telesurgery is not well developed and peer reviewed publications are lacking. Yang et al. [29] introduced an image-based simulated system for telesurgery in kyphoplasty, giving special attention to security problems. Their system allows remote experts in turn to work in a secured surgery room.

Conclusion

While the surgical navigation has become a mainstream CAOS technology, there are other technologies that encompass a wide spectrum of applications and devices. Many of these are technically capable and potentially useful tools that can revolutionize the surgical management

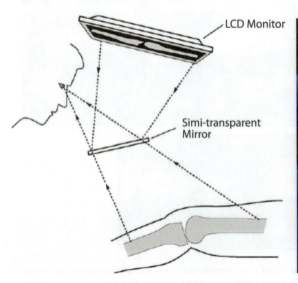

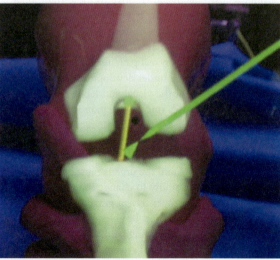

◘ **Fig. 75.8.** An example of augmented reality system (Image Overlay) (with permission from Elsevier [9])

of orthopaedic conditions. However, the challenges that remain for the clinicians and developers of these systems are not only to understand what these new technologies and tools can accomplish, but also to understand their limitations. It is expected that these systems will gradually evolve in future to become more user friendly, less invasive and less expensive. Eventually these assisting technologies will permit the development of new generation of surgical procedures that surgeons are not capable of performing today because of surgical limitations.

References

1. Blackwell M, Nikou C, DiGioia AM III, Kanade T (2000) An Image Overlay system for medical data visualization. Med Image Anal 4: 67–72

2. Brisson G, Kanade T, DiGioia AM (2003) Precision handheld sculpting of bone. CAOS, Marbella, Spain, pp 36-37

3. Cannon WD, Eckhoff DG, Garrett WE Jr, Hunter RE, Sweeney HJ (2006) Report of a group developing a virtual reality simulator for arthroscopic surgery of the knee joint. Clin Orthop Relat Res 442: 21–29

4. de-la-Fuente M, Ohnsorge J, Bast P, Wirtz DC, Radermacher K (2002) Minaro – new approaches for minimally invasive roentgen image based hip prosthesis revision. Biomed Tech (Berl) 47 (Suppl 1): 44–46

5. DiGioia AM, III et al. (1998) Image guided navigation system to measure intraoperatively acetabular implant alignment - The Otto Aufranc Award. Clin Orthop Relat Res 355: 8–22

6. Green PE, Piantanida T, Hill JW, Simon IB, Satava RM (1991) Telepresence: Dexterous procedures in a virtual operating field. Am Surg 57: 192

7. Grutzner PA, Zheng G, Langlotz U (2004) C-arm based navigation in total hip arthroplasty – background and clinical experience. Injury 35 (Suppl 1): S-A90–95

8. Hafez MA, Chelule KL, Seedhom BB, Sherman KP (2006) Computer-assisted total knee arthroplasty using patient-specific templating. Clin Orthop Relat Res 444: 184–192

9. Hafez MA, Jaramaz B, Di Gioia AM III (2006) Computer Assisted Surgery of the Knee: An overview. In: Insall JN, Scott N (eds) Surgery of the Knee, 4th edn. Churchill Livingston, Philadelphia, pp 1655–1674

10. Haider H et al. (2004) Freehand navigation cutting for TKA surgery without jigs: Simulation of bone saw cutting. CAOS International, Chicago, pp 69–70

11. Heining SM et al. (2004) Augmented reality and in-situ-visualization in thoracoscopic spine surgery. CAOS International, Chicago, pp 335–357

12. Heng P, Cheng C, Wong TT, Wu W, Xu Y, Xie Y, Chui YP, Chan KM, Leung KS (2006) Virtual reality techniques. Application to anatomic visualization and orthopaedics training. Clin Orthop Relat Res 442: 5–12

13. Jakopec M, Harris SJ et al. (2001) The first clinical application of a «hands-on» robotic knee surgery system. Comput Aided Surg 6: 329–339

14. Jaramaz B, Nikou C, DiGioia AM III (1997) A pre-operative computerized range of motion simulator for total hip replacement. 43rd Annual Meeting, Orthopaedic Research Society, San Francisco, CA

15. Mabrey J, Gillogly SD, Kasser JR et al. (2002) Virtual reality simulation of arthroscopy of the knee. Arthroscopy 18: E28

16. McCarthy AD, Moody L, Waterworth AR, Bickerstaff DR (2006) Passive haptics in a knee arthroscopy simulator: is it valid for core skills training? Clin Orthop Relat Res 442: 13–20

17. Paul HA, Bargar WL, Mettelstadt BD, Musits B (1992) Development of a surgical robot for cementless total hip arthroplasty. Clin Orthop Relat Res 285: 57–66

18. Picard F, Moody JE, DiGioia AM I, Jaramaz BJ (2004) Clinical classification of CAOS systems. In: DiGioia AM I, Jaramaz BJ, Picard F, Nolte L (2004) Computer and robotic assisted knee and hip surgery ed. Oxford University Press, Oxford, pp 43–48

19. Plaskos C et al. (2004) PRAXITELES: A universal bone mounted robot for image free knee surgery – Report on First cadaver trials. CAOS International, Chicago, pp 67–68

20. Pott PP, Scharf HP, Schwarz ML (2005) Today's state of the art in surgical robotics. Comput Aided Surg 10(2): 101–132

21. Radermacher K, Portheine F, Anton M, Zimolong A, Kaspers G, Rau G, Staudte H-W (1998) Computer assisted orthopaedic surgery with image-based individual templates. Clin Orthop 354: 28–38

22. Ritschl P Jr, Fuiko R, Zettl R, Kotten B (2004) The Galileo system for implantation of total knee arthroplasty. In: Stiehl JB, Konermann WH, Haaker RG (eds) Navigation and robotics in total joint and spine surgery. Springer, Berlin Heidelberg New York Tokyo, pp 282–286

23. Seel MJ, Hafez MA, Eckman K, Jaramaz B, Davidson D, DiGioia AM (2006) 3-D planning and virtual X-ray in revision hip arthroplasty for instability. Clin Orthop Relat Res 442: 35–38

24. Sherman KP, Ward JW, Wills DP (2001) Surgical trainee assessment using a VE knee arthroscopy training system (VE-KATS): experimental results. Stud Health Technol Inform 81: 465–470

25. Siebert W, Mai S, Kober R, Heeckt PF (2002) Technique and first clinical results of robot-assisted total knee replacement. Knee 9(3): 173–180

26. Stulberg SD, Loan P, Sarin V (2002) Computer-assisted navigation in total knee replacement: results of an initial experience in thirty-five patients. J Bone Joint Surg Incorporated 84-A (Suppl 2): 90–98

27. Witherspoon L (2004) ROBONAV-Robotic system for minimally invasive surgery. Robotic and navigation. International symposium. Nuremberg, Germany

28. Wolf A, Jaramaz B, DiGioia AM III (2005) MBARS: mini bone-attached robotic system for joint arthroplasty. Int J Med Robot Comput Ass Surg 1(2): 101–121

29. Yang Y et al. (2003) Secure an image-based simulated telesurgery system. Institute of Infocomm Research, Singapore. Available at: http://icsd.i2r.org.sg/publications/BaoFeng_2003_telesurgery.pdf

Advanced Technologies in Navigation

F. Langlotz, G. Zheng, L.-P. Nolte

Introduction

Since the first presentation of intra-operative navigation systems for supporting orthopaedic surgery in the 1990's these devices follow the same conceptual design [13] that is defined by the need to visualize surgical action with respect to the operated anatomy respecting the constraints of the orthopaedic operating room and the available technology. So far, technological advancements of CAOS systems have usually been driven by improvements of the underlying technology, i.e., radiographic imaging devices or infrared light based tracking systems. Examples were the introduction of three-dimensional fluoroscopy that allowed navigation with intra-operative images to be performed in three dimensions [9], as well as the development of passive optical tracking – the Polaris System (Northern Digital Inc., Waterloo, Canada), the core optical technology inside the majority of today's computer assisted therapy systems, was designed to track not only wired but also wireless instruments for the surgical navigation market.

In contrast to this technology driven improvement of CAOS systems, research groups constantly explored and evaluated possibilities to integrate new devices, methods, algorithms, or philosophies into surgical navigation in order to overcome existing deficiencies, to enhance workflow or precision, to reduce invasiveness, or to expand the range of applicability of existing systems.

It is the aim of this chapter to review some of the successful and less successful of those approaches of the past and to present current research that may potentially become the state-of-the-art of surgical navigation in the future.

Imaging

The optimal choice of the image modality for a computer assisted orthopaedic navigation system depends on a number of aspects. The image must be able to act as a useful virtual object [13], i.e., it must provide a clear and exact representation of the anatomical structures that are operated. Computed tomography (CT) was therefore the method of choice for the CAOS pioneers. CT scans were either available from the diagnosis of a given case or needed to be acquired specifically to enable surgical navigation for this patient. As for each preoperative image acquisition, intra-operative registration using interactively digitized features of the exposed bone was required and presented one of the most critical and error-prone steps in each navigated surgery.

Magnetic Resonance Imaging (MRI) although being much less invasive due to the absence of ionizing radiation has been proposed for orthopaedic navigation by some authors [14, 19], but did not become widely available. Standard MRI tomographies lack detailed information about bony structures and high-contrast representation of soft tissues makes 3D segmentation of the bony surface a very challenging undertaking. Moreover, they are geometrically less accurate when compared to CTs.

At the end of the 1990's intra-operative imaging means were proposed for a number of orthopaedic and traumatological applications. Ultrasonography was suggested to be used for intra-operative registration. However, the algorithm for calibration of the device and for segmenting the low-quality images resulted in a rather cumbersome usage with considerable user interaction involved. Therefore, this technique was not successful at that time.

Using intra-operatively acquired images as virtual objects initiated a first revolution in orthopaedic navigation. X-ray fluoroscopy was widely available and was an established imaging device during many types of surgery. The principle of fluoroscopy-based navigation can be summarized by three key steps: (1) track the fluoroscope during image acquisition, (2) calibrate the fluoroscope to account for distortions and mechanical effects and to determine the projection parameters of the acquisition, and (3) transfer the corrected image and projection parameters to a surgical navigation system. The major advantage of this technique is that steps 1 and 2 make a subsequent, manual registration of the image with the patient obsolete. Not only does this let the surgeon skip the error prone procedure of feature based registration, but it also permits easy re-acquisition of images of the patient throughout the course of the surgery. This is of significant importance in procedures that alter the surgical scene considerably (e.g., the reduction of fractures) because the updated images are available for navigation immediately after acquisition. With the introduction of three-dimensional fluoroscopy as provided, e.g., by Siemens's Iso-C-3D system, these advantages became available for 3D navigation, too.

Recent developments suggest tracked and calibrated 2-D or 3-D ultrasound to serve as virtual objects. Although this technology is still in its infancy, it can be expected that it will find appropriate fields of application within the domain of CAOS.

Tracking

The tracking device is the component in each navigation system that relates surgical instruments to the operated anatomy. Mathematically spoken it enables transferring the instrument's shape in the coordinate space of the patient, from where an interactive or inherent registration allows projecting it into the right position within the virtual object. Accuracy and usability in the operating room pose some restrictions on the tracker, but a considerable number of measuring principles are potential candidates for successful tracking systems.

Early navigation systems for orthopaedics used active optical tracking. Light emitting diodes (LEDs) were attached to the objects of interest and registered by a camera. In order to power and control the LEDs all instruments were equipped with cables making them less flexible to be used in a free-hand manner. One company is still using LED based instrument tracking. However, their tools are equipped with batteries allowing the emission of infrared light without external power supply.

Similarly, passive tracking permits cable-less instruments. Reflective markers are used instead of LEDs and allow for the construction of very light-weight navigated instruments. This technique is nowadays implemented by most of the navigation products.

There are a number of alternative approaches for remote tracking that can potentially by employed as part of a navigation system, but have up to now not been used in any products in a wide-spread manner. Video-based tracking is very common in applications such as gait analysis [3] or virtual reality. The principle is comparable to optoelectronic tracking using infrared LEDs or reflective markers: calibrated cameras detect special objects that can be identified in a video scene unambiguously yielding the 3-D location of the tracked object. Although experimental setups have proven that such an approach is practical [7, 21] no video-based tracking system is currently available that could meet the accuracy and performance requirements of orthopaedic navigation.

Electromagnetic tracking has been proposed in the early years of CAOS [1], but was soon discontinued due to the uncontrollable influence of metallic objects on tracking accuracy. Recently, new concepts for electromagnetic tracking have been presented both by manufacturers of stand-alone trackers as well as producers of navigation technology using proprietary tracking technology. Special calibration algorithms have been implemented and the electromagnetic field generators are suggested to be placed in close proximity to the tracked objects. Both efforts are meant to decrease the adverse effects of surrounding ferromagnetic items and enable reliable and precise tracking. Up to date, there is no published information that would allow proving if the claims of this new breed of electromagnetic trackers are valid and they can be advocated for navigation in orthopaedics without restrictions. The possibility to trace tiny coils without the need for a direct line-of-sight to the field generator is alluring: it could revolutionize computer assisted traumatology in particular allowing, e.g., tracking of deep-seated bone fragments during fracture reduction.

Shape Modeling

Statistical shape modeling (SSM, also referred to as »shape prediction« [20] or »bone morphing« [18]) describes a method to reconstruct the geometrical shape of an object from sparse input data using a previously generated statistical shape atlas. In the context of orthopaedic navigation, the shape of the operated bone is predicted based on a collection of sample bones that reflect the morphological variance found in a given population. In order to create a good estimation of the individual patient's bone, a rather small number of morphological features (surface points, rotation centers, anatomical axes, etc.) are acquired by the surgeon intra-operatively and enable the underlying algorithms to select parameters that guarantee precise shape prediction. This method therefore differs from the previously proposed »surgeon-defined anatomy« method [8], in which abstract bone models were constructed from the acquired data following simple instructions. In contrast, the input data to an SSM algorithm is used to extract the individual deviations of a particular patient from the statistical mean and to deform that mean accordingly. So far, this method is heavily employed in so-called »image-free« navigation systems for knee surgery. However, with the availability of statistical shape atlases of other anatomical regions, the technique could by applied to any part of the skeleton. Such approaches bear a huge potential for future developments of CAOS technology since they are not at all bound to the classical pointer-based acquisition of bony features. In principle, the reconstruction algorithms can be tuned to any type of patient-specific input such as, e.g., preoperative calibrated images or intra-operative tracked ultrasound thereby potentially enabling new minimally invasive procedures. Moreover, prediction from statistical atlases is possible not only for the geometric shape of an object. Given a three-dimensional radiological atlas, »synthetic CT scans« could be predicted from intra-operatively recorded data [24].

Intelligent Sensors and Instruments

Classical orthopaedic navigation systems provide a means to receive intra-operative positional feedback in real-time and to relate this information to a preoperatively made surgical plan, thus acting as a guidance device. However, all involved information is of a purely geometrical nature

and the navigation system aims at guaranteeing precise spatial realization of the surgery.

Recent developments suggest integrating other entities such as forces, moments, loads, pressures, or tensions to be controlled and optimized by means of computer assistances. Spine surgery and total knee replacement (TKR) have so far been identified as possible fields of application for this new group of computer assisted surgery devices. Force sensors can be used to facilitate ligament balancing in TKR surgery [5] or to enable further study of the loading characteristics of the knee [11] or the spine [2]. This field is certainly still in its infancy and the possible applications for combining electronic data acquisition with existing surgical navigation can hardly be foreseen at this point in time.

Introducing computer assisted metrology into orthopaedics will also lead to new surgical instruments that can support the surgeon's tactile capabilities. They can help applying intra-operative forces in a controlled manner [6, 12] when excessive manipulation has been identified as a possible source of complication.

Combining such sensing capabilities with robotic actuation yields so-called »active constraint« devices, a sub-specialty of surgical robots. Load sensors detect small forces applied by the surgeon's hand and activate the robot's actuators letting the machine follow the motion of the human's hand. Such robotic devices can be used, e.g., for precise milling tasks the advantage being that the robot can actively interfere when the surgeon is about the mill outside predefined safety margins [4, 22].

A last group of devices combines the worlds of surgical navigation and surgical robotics. The robotic component is that small that it can be mounted directly onto the operated bone. Optional surgical navigation techniques can be employed to position the robot coarsely onto the bone and the apparatus then carries out a drilling, milling, or positioning task autonomously and in accordance with a computer assisted planning. Such devices are currently available for TKR [16, 17] and prototypes have been presented for hip surgery [10, 23] and spinal application [15].

Conclusions

Surgical navigation combines and is driven by technological developments in the areas of imaging, tracking, image processing, sensor technology, and robotics. Corresponding prototype systems and commercial products have been presented, and some of them are currently in clinical evaluation to prove or disprove their clinical value. It can be foreseen already now that the integration of new algorithms, measurement systems, mechatronic devices, and smart instruments will push CAOS beyond the capabilities of today's navigation systems. It will remain the surgeons' responsibility to evaluate these new developments clinically and to separate the wheat from the chaff.

References

1. Amiot LP, Labelle H, DeGuise JA, Sati M, Brodeur P, Rivard CH (1995) Computer-assisted pedicle screw fixation. A feasibility study. Spine 20(10): 1208–1212
2. Brown MD, Holmes DC (2002) Intraoperative measurement of lumbar spine motion segment stiffness. Spine 27(9): 954–958
3. Castro JL, Medina-Carnicer R, Galisteo AM (2006) Design and evaluation of a new three-dimensional motion capture system based on video. Gait Posture 24(1): 126–129
4. Cobb J, Henckel J, Gomes P, Harris S, Jakopec M, Rodriguez F, Barrett A, Davies B (2006) Hands-on robotic unicompartmental knee replacement: a prospective, randomized controlled study of the Acrobot system. J Bone Joint Surg Br 88(2): 188–197
5. Crottet D, Maeder T, Fritschy D, Bleuler H, Nolte LP, Pappas IP (2005) Development of a force amplitude- and location-sensing device designed to improve the ligament balancing procedure in TKA. IEEE Trans Biomed Eng 52(9): 1609–1611
6. Demetropoulos CK, Truumees E, Herkowitz HN, Yang KH (2005) Development and calibration of a load sensing cervical distractor capable of withstanding autoclave sterilization. Med Eng Phys 27(4): 343–346
7. de Siebenthal J, Grützner PA, Zimolong A, Rohrer U, Langlotz F (2004) Assessment of video tracking usability for training simulators. Comput Aided Surg 9: 59–60
8. Dessenne V, Lavallée S, Julliard R, Orti R, Martelli S, Cinquin P (1995) Computer-assisted knee anteriore cruciate ligament reconstruction: first clinical tests. J Imag Guid Surg 1: 59–64
9. Euler E, Heining S, Riquarts C, Mutschler W (2003) C-arm-based three-dimensional navigation: a preliminary feasibility study. Comput Aided Surg 8(1): 35–41
10. Hahndorff M, de la Fuente M, Wirtz DC, Radermacher K (2005) Development of a new miniaturized robotic device for the removal of femoral bone cement. In: Langlotz, Davies, Schlenzka (eds) Computer Assisted Orthopaedic Surgery – 5th Annual Meeting of CAOS-International (Proceedings). Pro Business, Berlin, pp 138–139
11. Kirking B, Krevolin J, Townsend C, Colwell CW Jr, D'Lima DD (2006) A multiaxial force-sensing implantable tibial prosthesis. J Biomech 39(9): 1744–1751
12. Klockner C, Rohlmann A, Bergmann G (2003) Instrumented forceps for measuring tensile forces in the rod of the VDS implant during correction of scoliosis. Biomed Tech (Berl) 48(12): 362–364
13. Langlotz F, Nolte LP (2004) Technical approaches to computer assisted orthopedic surgery. Eur J Trauma 30: 1–11
14. Martel AL, Heid O, Slomczykowski M, Kerslake R, Nolte LP (1998) Assessment of 3-dimensional magnetic resonance imaging fast low angle shot images for computer assisted spinal surgery. Comput Aided Surg 3: 40–44
15. Natanzon A, Vitchevsky A, Silberstein B, Batkilin E, Burman M, Shoham M (2005) Validation of robotically assisted system for spinal procedures. In: Langlotz, Davies, Schlenzka (eds) Computer Assisted Orthopaedic Surgery – 5th Annual Meeting of CAOS-International (Proceedings). Pro Business, Berlin, pp 371–375
16. Plaskos C, Cinquin P, Lavallée S, Hodgson AJ (2005) Minimal access total knee arthroplasty using a miniature robot and a new side milling technique. In: Langlotz, Davies, Schlenzka (eds) Computer Assisted Orthopaedic Surgery – 5th Annual Meeting of CAOS-International (Proceedings). Pro Business, Berlin, pp 368–371
17. Ritschl P, Machacek F et al. (2004) The Galileo system for implantation of total knee arthroplasty – an integrated solution comprising navigation, robotics and robot-assisted ligament balancing. In: Stiehl, Konermann, Haaker (eds) Navigation and robotics in total joint and spine surgery. Springer, Berlin Heidelberg New York Tokyo, pp 281–361
18. Stindel E, Briard JL, Merloz P, Plaweski S, Dubrana F, Lefevre C, Troccaz J (2002) Bone morphing: 3D morphological data for total knee arthroplasty. Comput Aided Surg. 7(3): 156–68
19. Suhm N, Simeria A, Hügli R, Messmer P, Bongartz G, Regazzoni P (2003) MR-imaging of bone cements as a first step towards MR-guided vertebroplasty. In: Langlotz F, Davies BL, Bauer A (eds) Computer Assisted Orthopaedic Surgery – 3rd Annual Meeting of CAOS-International (Proceedings). Steinkopff, Darmstadt, pp 146–147
20. Talib H, Rajamani K, Kowal J, Nolte LP, Styner M, Ballester MA (2005) A comparison study assessing the feasibility of ultrasound-initialized deformable bone models. Comput Aided Surg 10: 293–299
21. Tonet O, Ramesh TU, Megali G, Dario P (2006) Tracking endoscopic instruments without localizer: image analysis-based approach. Stud Health Technol Inform 119: 544–549
22. Van Ham G, Denis K, Vander Sloten J, Van Audekercke R, Van der Perre G, De Schutter J, Simon JP, Fabry G (2005) A semi-active milling procedure in view of preparing implantation beds in robot-assisted orthopaedic surgery. Proc Inst Mech Eng 219(3): 163–174
23. Wolf A, Jaramaz B (2005) Mini bone-attached robot for joint arthroplasty. In: Langlotz, Davies, Schlenzka (eds) Computer Assisted Orthopaedic Surgery – 5th Annual Meeting of CAOS-International (Proceedings). Pro Business, Berlin, pp 513–515
24. Yao J, Taylor R (2003) Assessing accuracy factors in deformable 2D/3D medical image registration using a statistical pelvic model. Proceedings of the 9th IEEE International Conference on Computer Vision (ICCV 2003), 14–17 October 2003, Nice, France, S 1329–1334

Measuring Cup Alignment from Radiographs after THR

B. Jaramaz, K. Eckman

Introduction

After total hip replacement, standard AP radiographs are typically used to evaluate implant alignment, particularly the alignment of the acetabular cup. While cup version can only be assessed qualitatively, the abduction (inclination) of the cup can be measured directly on a given radiograph with a high degree of repeatability, even with simple tools. For this reason, radiographic measurements of cup orientation are a part of standard THR follow-up procedure. In most cases, the X-ray measurements are sufficiently accurate to either confirm that the implants are placed within a desired range or to detect serious misalignment. Unfortunately, measurements from standard radiographs can suffer from inaccuracies due to different reasons. While the order of these errors does not typically affect the qualitative assessment, they become apparent when the radiographic measurements are expected to yield accurate quantitative measurements. One such example is when a cup alignment achieved using surgical navigation is inconsistent with the postoperative radiographic measurements. Surgical navigation systems claim an angular accuracy on the order of one to two degrees, and the radiographic measurements of cup abduction can be performed manually with the repeatability of the same order. It may therefore be difficult for surgeons to understand the much larger discrepancies that can be observed between the two measurements. Several different sources may contribute to this outcome – most notably using a different anatomic reference, different definitions of cup orientation, and ignoring the effects of X-ray source position and variations in pelvic flexion. In the following, we will try to explain some methodological differences in the two measurement approaches and the sources of inaccuracy in radiographic measurements.

Pelvic Reference System

All currently used surgical navigation systems for THR have adopted the same reference system to measure the cup orientation. The reference system is based on the anterior pelvic plane (APP) defined by the anterior superior iliac spines (ASIS) and the pubis symphysis points. The transverse axis is defined as a line connecting the two ASIS points. The reference transverse axis used in the radiographic measurements is often defined by the teardrop image artifacts (◘ Fig. 77.1). While these two axes are close to being parallel in most cases, some variation may occur. Additionally, errors in localization of the ASIS points, to which image-free navigation may be prone, may contribute to these discrepancies. The angular difference between the two transverse references directly affects the cup abduction measurements.

X-ray Source Position and Perspective Distortion

Radiographs are inherently two-dimensional perspective projection images, and the parameters of the projection need to be considered when the measurements are made on the radiograph. Consider the following example: Assume the central X-ray beam is placed in the mid sagittal plane, the patient is of average size and the source-to-film distance is 1 m. As a result, the hip is imaged at an angle of approximately 10°. Consequently, a cup anteverted 10 degrees will appear as having zero anteversion (◘ Fig. 77.2). Changing the location of the source position will change the geometry of the features in the resultant X-ray.

This effect is further illustrated in ◘ Fig. 77.3. An X-ray image of a cup oriented at 45° abduction and 25° version was synthesized. This image was produced with the pelvic plane parallel to the film plane (i.e. zero pelvic flexion and zero degrees of pelvic superior-inferior rotation). The actual source position was marked on the image with a white circle. Next, a 3D CAD model was matched to this

image to measure the cup's orientation. This measurement was repeated while varying the source position used by the measuring program. The source position was changed in 50 mm increments. Both the x and y coordinates (the in plane coordinates) of the source position were changed. The figure shows how the measurements of cup orientation would be affected if the X-ray source was assumed to be at different positions within the 50 mm interval grid. It can be seen that 100 mm movement of the X-ray source along the mid-sagittal plane would produce 1.8° in difference in abduction measurements and 4.2° in version measurements. Similarly, placing the X-ray source centered at the pelvis vs. centered on the hip would result in 1.1° of abduction and 8.3° of version difference. Clearly, the variation of the X-ray source position within a typical range affects the version measurements significantly more than the abduction.

Definition of Cup Orientation

Three definitions of cup orientation are commonly used in clinical practice, each derived from a related application in THR: radiographic, operative and anatomical [3]. These definitions can be easily visualized as two sequential rotations that will take the cup from the initial position to its final position. Assuming the cup is initially in the face down position, with the axis of symmetry aligned with the long body axis, the first rotation is abduction (inclination) of the cup, i.e., rotation around the sagittal axis (◘ Fig. 77.4, 1). The three definitions differ in the second rotation after initial abduction of the cup, as they use different axes for that rotation.

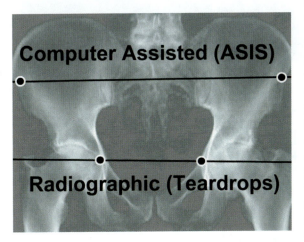

◘ **Fig. 77.1.** The CAOS (ASIS) and radiographic (teardrop) transverse axes

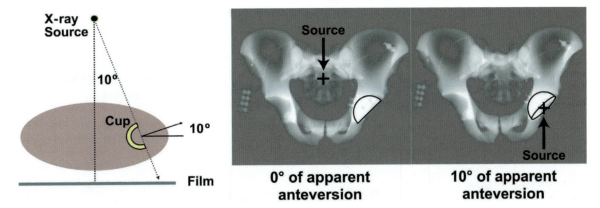

◘ **Fig. 77.2.** Effect of the X-ray source the perceived cup anteversion

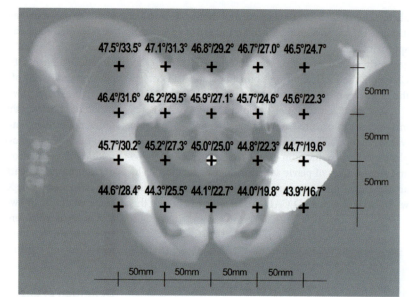

Fig. 77.3. Cup abduction/version measurements versus source position. The actual orientation of the cup is 45°/25°. The implant was imaged with the X-ray source located above the white-circled plus sign. The values above each cross mark indicate what the measured cup orientation would be if the source position was assumed at that location

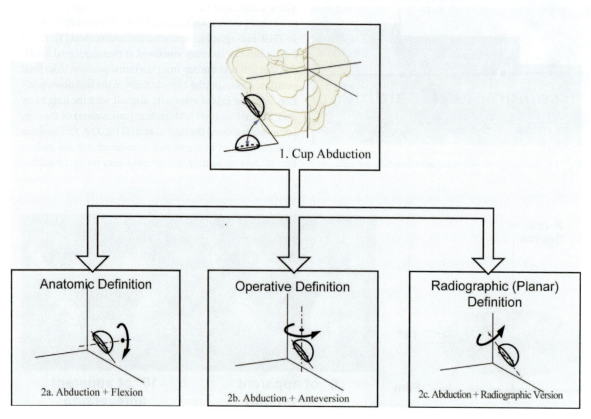

Fig. 77.4. Definitions of cup orientation

In the anatomic definition the cup is anteverted by rotating around the long body axis (■ Fig. 77.4, 2a). The operative orientation is associated with the majority of mechanical guides used to align the cup in the operating room. After initial abduction, the cup is rotated around the transverse axis, in the hip extension direction (■ Fig. 77.4, 2b). In the radiographic definition this rotation is performed around the abducted transverse axis (■ Fig. 77.4, 2c). The radiographic definition is used for interpretation of X-rays, since the radiographic version can be reconstructed from the ratio of the short and long axis of the elliptic projection of the cup opening. Although references and conversion tables exist [3], these definitions are often mixed, assuming they represent the same orientation of the cup. If different definitions of cup orientation are used, this may be one of the reasons why the reported surgical navigation values of cup orientation disagree with the radiographic measurements, especially if the cup is more anteverted.

Pelvic Orientation

It is commonly assumed that the anterior pelvic plane is parallel to the X-ray film plane. Unfortunately, this is not guaranteed by the standard radiographic protocol, and the variation in pelvic pose, especially the flexion/extension, can have a significant effect on the radiographic measurements. In fact, in one study of 101 patients, the standing AP radiographs showed a mean pelvic flexion angle of 3° with a standard deviation of +/−11.9° [3]. These pelvic flexion measurements ranged from −46° to 33°. This study also compared the change in pelvic flexion angle between preoperative and postoperative radiographs of the same patient taken in the same posture. The mean change in standing pelvic flexion was found to be −2° +/− 7.5°. The changes in standing pelvic flexion ranged from −26° to +15°. Thus, pelvic flexion can vary considerably even for the same patient. These pelvic pose variations will negatively impact implant measurement accuracy.

Using custom software, it was possible to determine the effect of pelvic flexion on cup measurement errors. An X-ray of a cup implant with an actual orientation of 45° abduction and 25° version was synthesized with the pelvis in a state of 0° flexion. The cup orientation was measured by matching a 3D CAD model of the implant to the synthesized image using an automatic method based on mutual information (MI) [5]. Multiple measurements were acquired while varying the amount of pelvic flexion in the measurement software. A pelvic flexion range of -25° to 25° was used. This range corresponds to approximately 2 standard deviations of standing AP pelvic flexion. The effects of pelvic flexion on implant orientation measurements can be seen in Figures 5 and 6. The effects are significant for both abduction and version measurements. With a cup oriented at 45° of abduction and 25° of anatomic version, the radiographic version measurements will be more sensitive to source position errors.

For example, if an implant appears to be oriented at 45°/25° on an X-ray film and the pelvis was in 10° of flexion with respect to the film plane, from ■ Fig. 77.5, we find that abduction has to be adjusted by +5°. Likewise, using ■ Fig. 77.6 we determine that version should be adjusted by +8°.

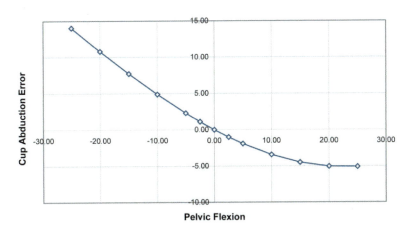

■ **Fig. 77.5.** Effect of pelvic flexion on cup abduction measurements (cup is oriented to 45.0°/25.0° abduction/version)

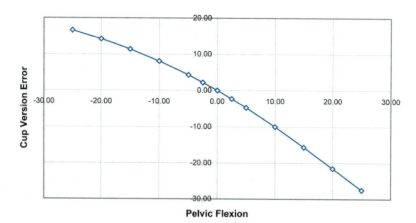

■ **Fig. 77.6.** Effect of pelvic flexion on cup version measurements (cup is oriented to 45.0°/25.0° abduction/version)

Better Measurements

A custom software program, Xalign, has been developed for measuring implant orientation from conventional radiographs with improved accuracy. By co-registering a radiograph with both a synthetic X-ray, which is generated from a CT scan of the patient, and a projection of the implant CAD model, Xalign recovers the true pose of the implant with respect to the patient's anatomy using the following protocol (■ Figs. 77.7, 77.8):

1. An anatomic reference system for the pelvis is defined in the CT scan using the CT-based THR planning software.
2. A real pelvic AP radiograph is digitized. The source-to-film distance is recorded and the X-ray source location is marked on the film using small metallic washer.
3. A synthetic pelvic AP radiograph is generated from the CT scan, with known projection parameters.
4. Image similarity is evaluated using a mutual information method [5]. The two images (real and synthetic radiograph) are registered by maximizing mutual information.
   The pose of the CT scan in the projection space is manipulated until the best match between the real and the synthetic X-ray is found.
5. A virtual projection of the CAD graphic cup model was generated for a given position and spatial orientation of the cup.
6. The cup position and orientation relative to the X-ray film is iteratively modified using an automatic method

until the virtual projection best matches the projection of the cup in the real radiograph.

7. Cup orientation relative to the anatomic reference system of the pelvis is calculated. In addition, pelvic flexion (inclination of the APP plane relative to the radiographic plane) is calculated.

True anatomic measurements of cup orientation are obtained, and inaccuracies due to a different reference system, X-ray source effects, and pelvic orientation are eliminated. A single CT scan, preoperative or postoperative, can be used to analyze an entire series of radiographs.

Xalign produces good results with a variety of source positions and pelvic orientations. In an experimental validation study, the average error between the 2D/3D registration measurements and the CT Planner measurements was -0.05° in abduction and -0.37° in version with a standard deviation of 0.16° and 0.94° respectively. The range of values for abduction was -0.49° to 0.21° and -3.10° to 1.68° for version. In the clinical experiment, using direct postoperative CT scan measurements as a reference, the accuracy of Xalign was similar. Here, the mean (± standard deviation) acetabular cup abduction was 52.9° ± 4.8°, ranging from 46.0° to 60.1°. The cup version ranged from 3.1° to 29.7°, with a mean (± standard deviation) of 18.7° ± 6.6°. The measurement differences, compared to CT measurements, were 0.4° ± 0.8° (mean ± standard deviation) for cup abduction and 0.6° ± 0.79° for cup version. The maximum absolute errors were 2.15° for abduction and 2.03° for version.

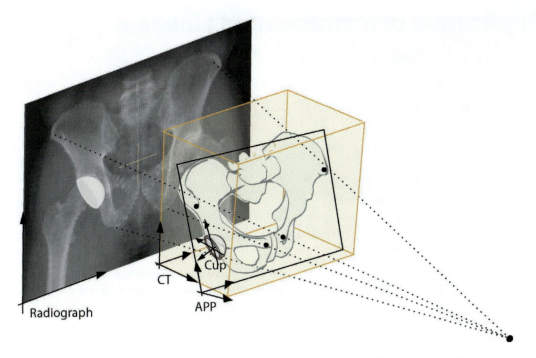

■ **Fig. 77.7.** Reference systems in the synthetic x-ray projection environment. The CT scan (CT) and the cup model (Cup) are placed relative to the X-ray film (Radiograph) in order to create a synthetic projection. The anatomic reference plane of the pelvis (APP) is specified in the CT scan

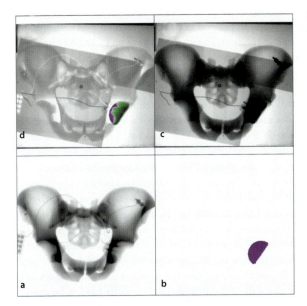

■ **Fig. 77.8a–d.** Color-inverted and labeled view of the Xalign program. The four main windows are for the synthetic X-ray (**a**), the implant (**b**), the real X-ray (**c**), and the combined view (**d**)

References

1. Eckman K, Mor A, Jaramaz B (2004) Xalign validation: accurately recovering implant pose from a single anteroposterior radiograph. Submitted for CAOS, Chicago, Illinois
2. Kennedy JG, Rogers WB, Soffe KE et al. (1998) Effects of acetabular component orientation on recurrent dislocation, pelvic osteolysis, polyethylene wear, and component migration. J Arthoplasty 13: 530–534
3. Murray DW (1993) The definition and measurement of acetabular orientation. J Bone Joint Surg. 75-B: 228–232
4. Nishihara S, Sugano N, Nishii T, Ohzono K, Yoshikawa H (2003) Measurements of pelvic flexion angle using three-dimensional computed tomography. Clin Orthop 411: 140–151
5. Viola PA, Wells WM (1995) Alignment by Maximization of Mutual Information. Fifth International Conference on Computer Vision, 16–23, IEEE, Cambridge, MA

Application of Instrumented Linkage for TKR Surgery

R.E Forman, M.A. Balicki, P.S Walker, C.-S. Wei, G.R. Klein

Introduction

Coordinate-measuring machines (CMMs) are mechanical systems that use a measuring probe to determine the coordinates of points on the surface of a workpiece. They are used for dimensional measurement, profile measurement, angularity or orientation measurement, depth mapping, digitizing or imaging, and surface definition. An instrumented linkage is a portable CMM with a number of revolute joints, each with encoders to monitor its angular position, thus the orientation as well as the position of the measuring probe can be determined in 3D space. Usually, one end of the linkage is fixed rigidly to a reference table or in some cases to the object being measured. A typical application is the measurement of accuracy of machined parts or surfaces in situ. Since these instruments provide continuous real time feedback and measurement accuracy even down to 0.01 mm they are good candidates for tracking applications.

We are currently developing an instrumented linkage that can be used as a navigation tool in total knee replacement (TKR) surgery. This linkage is not unlike a commercial CMM arm such as the Microscsribe (Immersion Corp), with six joints (six degrees-of-freedom) required to fully track the position (x, y, z) and orientation of the end of the arm (roll, pitch, and yaw). Rigid links are joined by revolute joints (◘ Fig. 78.1) to allow for the manipulation of a digitizing and navigation tool attached to the last link. The design specifications call for a lightweight arm that has the empirically determined range of motion required for the surgical environment, and generates real-time tool position

and orientation within 1 mm and half a degree. The tools that are attached to the last link of the arm should be interchanged quickly and the base mount should allow for rigid connection with the bone.

Design and Calibration of the Linkage

The linkage incorporates sensors consisting of optical incremental rotary encoders that use light to determine the speed, angle and direction of a rotary shaft. Six of these devices are implanted to track the angular position of the 6 axes of rotation. The encoders have up to 32,000 discrete positions per revolution which yields an angular resolution of 0.01 degrees. Each incremental encoder has a zero index which allows the encoder to provide an absolute position. A hardware module counts the signals produced by the encoders, these counts are then acquired by the PC via a USB connection and used by the linkage software model as input for joint angles. To simplify fabrication the joints are grouped into a two-axis modular unit. The joint module was designed around two encoders with minimal housing size without compromising rigidity. High strength and precision ball bearing assemblies were used as the mating rotary mechanism. The joint housing is machined from titanium while the links are carbon fiber tubing, making the linkage rigid but lightweight.

In order to compute the position and orientation of the tool end of the linkage relative to its base, a forward kinematics model was developed [7]. Each link was represented by a matrix transform, or a frame, that mathematically describes the location and orientation of the

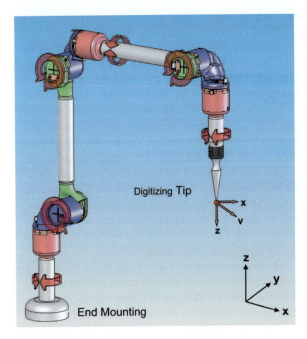

Digitizing Tip

x
v
z

z

y

x

End Mounting

Fig. 78.1. A diagram of the instrumented linkage designed for TKR surgery. The link at the end mounting block is fixed to plates on the medial sides of the femur and tibia. The digitizing tip can be exchanged with a drill guide or other tools

software. During regular usage, a homing procedure is required after each power-up to reset all the angular encoders, which involves the rotation of each joint through its full range of motion.

Each attachment requires a calibration procedure which includes registering the location of a custom block relative to the linkage. The block accepts the active end of the tool and its location relative to the linkage is recorded. This is then included in the forward kinematics model of the linkage. The standard attachment to the last link of the arm is a digitizing probe. Other instruments such as a drill guide, oscillating saw or burr can be attached to the end of linkage as long as their connection is rigid and their active areas are calibrated with respect to the linkage. A method of quickly releasing these tools from the arm is preferred, especially for surgical applications. A very rigid base mount is required for maximum accuracy as the misalignment and flexion errors are compounded when the errors are nearer to the base. Device accuracy is calculated by using the arm to digitize a precision machined block. The orientation measurements are inherently built into the procedure since they affect the resulting point measurements.

Calibration and Accuracy

Full linkage calibration involves the process of first measuring the geometry of the linkage using a precise CMM device. This data is then fed into a commercial robot calibration system which uses sophisticated mathematical routines and a displacement measurement system to further correct for any discrepancies due to manufacturing tolerances. Finally, the resulting geometrical parameters are used in the kinematic model in our custom link relative to the previous link. The model incorporates the physical parameters of the arm such as link lengths, link-link orientations and offsets, as well as joint angles which are updated continuously via feedback from the six angular encoders. By multiplying all the transforms, a relationship between the base frame and the tool frame was calculated. Software was written in C++ to compute the kinematics of the linkage and OpenGL was applied to display this data via a 3-D Graphical User Interface.

Evaluation of the System

In order to provide an easy transition from a technique using standard jigs and fixtures, we decided to use the linkage initially to navigate a drill guide for the placement of pins onto which slotted cutting guides would be placed [4]. Hence the concept was to digitize key points on each bone, to compute the cutting planes, and then to compute the locations of the pins. A single tool was used on the end of the linkage which incorporated a digitizing pointer and a dual drill guide, the spacing of the two holes the same as the slotted cutting guide. This methodology was evaluated for resecting the upper tibia by performing cuts and measuring the accuracy of the depth of the cut and the frontal and sagittal plane angles.

A six degree-of-freedom MicroScribe G2LX instrumented linkage (Immersion Corporation) with a point accuracy of 0.23 mm RMS was rigidly anchored next to a foam plastic tibia (Sawbone) (▪ Fig. 78.2). Points on the tibia holder and on the upper tibia were used to define the target resection plane 10 mm below the tibial surface. A dual drill guide with holes corresponding to those of the slotted saw guide was attached on the end of the linkage. Software was written to determine the location of the tibia, to track the drill guide and to navigate the placement of the drill guide against the anterior tibia. The task of the surgeon was to position the guide in order to align a set of circles on the computer screen, one representing target hole position on the bone and another representing target orientation (■ Fig. 78.3). First, the drill guide was moved

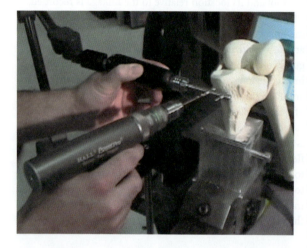

■ **Fig. 78.2.** Experimental set-up showing the dual drill guide attached to the linkage. The pins were later tapped into the holes. As an alternative the pins can be drilled directly into the bone

over the bone surface until the position was correct. The castellated end of the guide was then pressed into the bone surface to hold it in position, and then the drill guide was tilted until the orientation was correct. The surgeon then drilled a hole through the guide into the anterior tibia. A pin was tapped into the hole. While the first guide was located over the first pin, the second hole was then drilled. This constrained the motion of the guide to one degree of freedom about pin one, making the second pilot hole easier to align and drill. The slotted saw guide was placed over the pins and the upper tibial resection made. The MicroScribe was then used to digitize a plate placed on the cut surface to measure the accuracy of the cut. Both the depth and the angle in frontal and sagittal planes were analyzed. The system was tested by three surgeons of varying experience, each cutting 10 tibias.

All three operators were able to complete the drilling procedure with minimal learning curve and obtained similar overall results. ■ Figure 78.4 shows the errors in the final resection cuts for the 30 cases. The errors in the depth of cut were mostly less than 1 mm. For the sagittal plane angles there was a bias towards a posterior tilt of around 1 degree, and for the frontal plane angles, a bias towards a varus tilt of around 1 degree. Although these results are of acceptable accuracy, methods for further improvements have been investigated as described in the next section.

■ **Fig. 78.3.** The graphical user interface which guides the placement of the drill guide. Aligning the upper yellow and black circles gives position on the anterior tibia; aligning the bottom circles gives rotational orientation

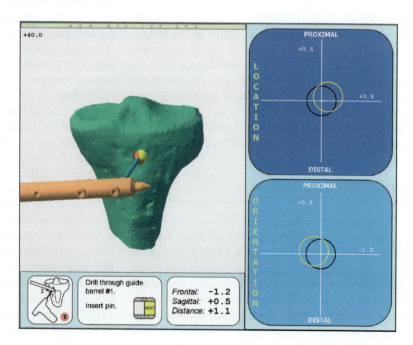

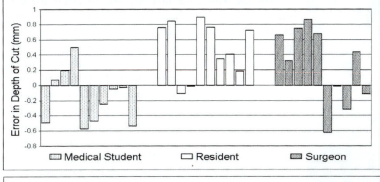

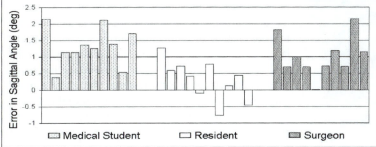

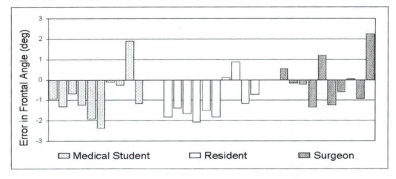

Fig. 78.4. The errors in depth of cut, sagittal angle, and frontal angle for each of the 10 sawbones cut by the three surgeons. Positive values represent an excessive cut, a posterior tilt, or a varus tilt. The absence of a »learning curve« is notable

Application to TKR Surgery

There are different methods that can be used to reference the location of the bone with respect to the tool. One possibility is to clamp the linkage to the operating table and then clamp the femur and tibia to the table until the drilling procedure has been completed. However, subsequent checking of the cuts and making other measurement would be impractical since these techniques require tracking of the relative motion of the bones. An alternative that provides continuous tracking of the femur and tibia is the attachment of the linkage directly to the bone. Hence it was necessary to design small mounting plates that fit

the medial sides of the femur and tibia onto which the linkage could be rigidly fixed using a quick release mechanism. For the tibia, the linkage was used to digitize the lateral and medial malleoli (**□** Fig. 78.5) and the center of the anterior cruciate attachment, which defined the mechanical axis. Other points included the center of the PCL attachment and the medial border of the patella ligament to define the AP direction [1], the lowest points on the condyles for depth of cut, and points on the periphery. The pins were then inserted for a medially placed upper tibial cutting guide and the resection made. A flat on the side of the drill guide was then used to check the depth and orientation of the cut.

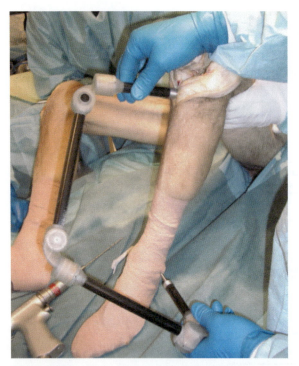

Fig. 78.5. The base of the linkage is attached to a plate fixed to the proximal medial tibia, while the tip is extended to digitize the malleoli

For the femur, the first step was to determine the center of the femoral head using the kinematic method [8, 10]. This was accomplished by placing the digitizing pointer into a small puck fixed to the operating table, and rotating the leg (■ Fig. 78.6). The mathematical routines were modified from the previous methods [8]. The pointer was then used to digitize the center of the distal femur for the mechanical axis, points on Whitesides line [2], the distal and posterior condyles, and the medial and lateral extreme points (■ Fig. 78.7). Pins were placed for the distal femoral cutting guide and the orientation checked with the linkage. After distal resection, the drill guide was then used to place the pins into the distal resected surface for the four-in-one cutting guide. In order to subsequently measure varus-valgus rotations during the ligament balancing procedure, or alignment and flexion angles at the trial and final component stages, the linkage has to be affixed to the sideplate of the femur or tibia and the digitizing pointer docked into the sideplate of the other bone.

The system can be adapted for carrying out the bone cuts in any required order, or carrying out cuts based on ligament tensions [3, 13] with anterior or posterior femoral referencing. In terms of improving accuracy of pin placement, several schemes were tested. A single drill guide was more convenient to use than a dual for ease of

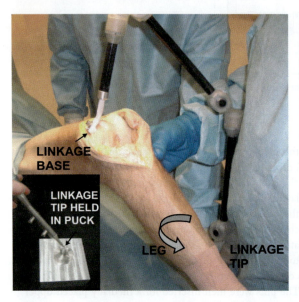

Fig. 78.6. The base of the linkage is attached to the medial side of the femur, while the tip is held into a puck fixed to the operating table. The leg is then rotated to locate the center of the femoral head

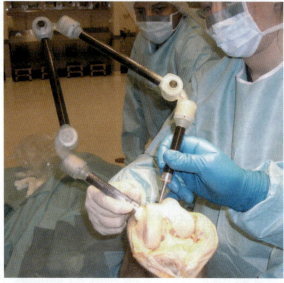

Fig. 78.7. The tip of the linkage is used to digitize the reference points on the femur

access to the required locations on the femur or tibia. The method of drilling the hole and then tapping in the pin led to some error. One promising method was to grind a cutting tip on to a solid 3.2 mm pin and to drill this directly through the drill guide into the bone.

Discussion

An instrumental linkage, clamped to the operating table, has already been used in surface hip surgery [5]. There are a number of options to applying an instrumented linkage to total knee surgery. Initially, we envisaged navigating an oscillating saw directly, so that after determining the cutting planes on the bones from a sequence of digitized points, the cuts would be made directly without the use of slotted cutting guides [11]. One of the disadvantages at present is the necessity to watch the computer screen for saw direction data, whereas full attention should ideally be given to the saw itself. Another option is to navigate a burring tool [6, 12]. The difficulty is the large volume of bone material to be removed with present-day square cut total knees. This takes too much time and results in excessive particulate debris. The linkage could be attached to the operating table but the requirement to clamp the bone prevents intra-procedural measurements from being taken, hence the preference for fixing the linkage to the femur or tibia by use of side plates which remain in place until the end of the procedure.

An advantage of a linkage over an optical system is the lack of the line of sight problem, while metallic components do not affect the linkage as they do for electromagnetic systems [9]. A linkage is likely to be more accurate than both optical and electromagnetic techniques. The particular configuration of the linkage, where the points being digitized are close to the fixation point on the bone, is a definite advantage for accuracy. Also the linkage may be less expensive, simpler, and quicker to operate than the other systems. There is a slight disadvantage however in the procedure necessary to monitor the relative motion between the femur and the tibia at any time during the procedure.

It is concluded that the use of a purpose-built instrumented linkage is a useful and convenient tool for performing navigated total knee surgery. Such a linkage can be readily adapted to other knee procedures, and to many other bone and joint problems. Options such as freehand navigation of saws, burrs, or other cutting tools, expand the versatility.

References

1. Akagi M, Mori S, Nishimura S, Nishimura A, Asano T, Hamanishi C (2005) Variability of extraarticular tibial rotation references for total knee arthroplasty. Clin Ortho Relat Res 436: 172–176
2. Arima J, Whiteside LA, McCarthy DS, White SE (1995) Femoral rotational alignment, based on the anteroposterior axis, in total knee arthroplasty in a valgus knee. J Bone Joint Surg (A) 77-A (9): 1331–1334
3. Asano H, Hoshino A, Wilton TJ (2004) Soft-tissue tension total knee arthroplasty. J Arthroplasty, 19(5): 558–561
4. Balicki MA, Forman RE, Walker PS, Wei CS, White B, Roth J, Klein GR (2006) A navigated drill guide using an instrumented linkage for the placement of cutting jigs during total knee arthroplasty, vol. 31. Trans Orthopaedic Research Society, Chicago, IL, USA
5. Barrett ARW, Cobb JP, Baena FMR, Jakopec M, Harris SJ, Davies BL (2005) The Tubes™ System for Minimally Invasive Computer-Assisted Hip Resurfacing Surgery. 5th Annual Meeting of the International Society for Computer Assisted Orthopaedic Surgery (CAOS), Helsinki, Finland
6. Brisson G, Kanade T, DiGioia A, Jaramaz B (2004) Precision freehand sculpting of bone. In: Barillot C, Haynor DR, Hellier P (eds) MICCAI 2004, LNCS 3217. Springer, Berlin Heidelberg New York Tokyo, pp 105–122
7. Craig JJ (2005) Introduction to robotics – mechanics and control. 3rd edn, Pearsons Prentice Hall, Upper Saddle River, NJ
8. Krackow KA, Bayers-Thering M, Phillips MJ (1999) A new technique for determining proper mechanical axis alignment during total knee arthroplasty: progress toward computer-assisted TKA. Orthopedics 22(7): 698–702
9. Poulin F, Amiot L-P (2002) Interference during the use of an electromagnetic tracking system under OR conditions. J Biomech 35: 733–737
10. Siston RA, Delp SL (2006) Evaluation of a new algorithm to determine the hip joint center. J Biomech 39: 125–130
11. Walker PS, Wei CS, Forman RE (2005) Freehand navigation for bone shaping. In: Hozack WJ, Krismer M, Nogler M, Bonutti PM, Rachbauer F, Schaffer JL, Donnelly WJ (eds) Minimally invasive total joint arthroplasty. Springer, Berlin Heidelberg New York Tokyo, pp 232–234
12. Wolf A, Mor B, Jaramaz B, DiGioia AM III (2005) How can CAOS support MIS TKR and THR? – Background and significance. In: Hozack WJ, Krismer M, Nogler M, Bonutti PM, Rachbauer F, Schaffer JL, Donnelly WJ (eds) Minimally invasive total joint arthroplasty. Springer, Berlin Heidelberg New York Tokyo, pp 182–185
13. Zalzal P, Papini M, Petruccelli D, deBeer J, Winemaker MJ (2004) An in vivo biomechanical analysis of the soft-tissue envelope of osteoarthritic knees. J Arthroplasty 19(2): 217–223

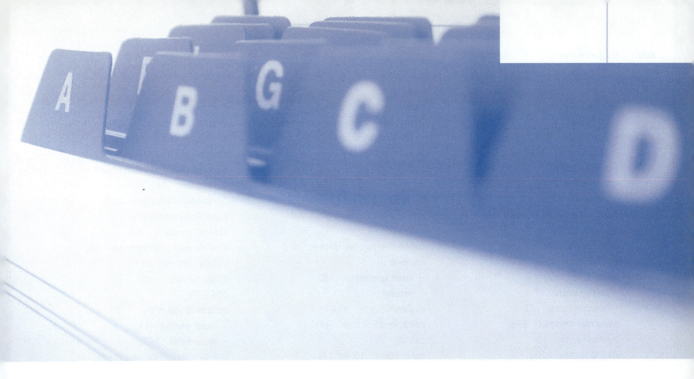

A

Q

R

U

V

W

X

Y

Z

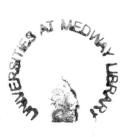